SARA

*Health Psychology*

# CHARLES K. PROKOP
TRINITY UNIVERSITY, SAN ANTONIO

# LAURENCE A. BRADLEY
UNIVERSITY OF ALABAMA, BIRMINGHAM

# THOMAS G. BURISH
VANDERBILT UNIVERSITY

# KAREN O. ANDERSON
UNIVERSITY OF MASSACHUSETTS MEDICAL CENTER

# JUDITH E. FOX
UNIVERSITY OF COLORADO HEALTH SCIENCES CENTER, DENVER

# *Health Psychology*

## *Clinical Methods and Research*

MACMILLAN PUBLISHING COMPANY
NEW YORK
COLLIER MACMILLAN CANADA
TORONTO

Editor: Christine Cardone
Production Supervisor: Charlotte Hyland
Production Manager: Nicholas Sklitsis
Cover Designer: Jane Edelstein
Cover photograph: Marjory Dressler
Illustrations: FineLine Inc.

This book was set in Baskerville by V&M Graphics, and was
printed and bound by R.R. Donnelley & Sons Company.
The cover was printed by New England Book Components.

Macmillan Publishing Company
866 Third Avenue, New York, New York 10022

Collier Macmillan Canada, Inc.
1200 Eglinton Avenue East, Suite 200
Don Mills, Ontario M3C 3N1

LIBRARY OF CONGRESS CATALOGING-IN-PUBLICATION DATA

Health psychology: clinical methods and research / Charles K. Prokop
. . . [et al.].
        p.      cm.
    Includes bibliographical references.
    Includes index.
    ISBN 0-02-313480-1 (case)
    1. Clinical health psychology.      I. Prokop, Charles K.
    [DNLM: 1. Behavioral Medicine.   2. Disease — psychology.   3. Health
    Behavior   4. Psychology, Medical.     WM 90 H4338]
R726.7.H4336   1991
616′.0019 — dc20
DNLM/DLC
for Library of Congress             90-6429
                                    CIP

Printing:  1 2 3 4 5 6 7     Year:  1 2 3 4 5 6 7

# *Preface*

*Health Psychology: Clinical Methods and Research* examines the contributions of psychology to the treatment, prevention, and assessment of physical distress and disease. The relationship between psychological and physical functioning has occupied the minds of scientists and philosophers as have few other questions, and health care providers have recognized the existence of important links between personality, behavior, and health since the time of Hippocrates. However, recent years have been witness to an exponential growth in explicit knowledge about these links. The research and clinical activities of psychologists in health care have made significant contributions to this knowledge base, and this book summarizes these contributions.

This text is appropriate for courses in Health Psychology or Behavioral Medicine. These courses are often taken by students with a wide range of interests and backgrounds. Some take the courses as part of the psychology major. Students majoring in fields such as biology, sociology, and health care management enroll to broaden their perspective. Still other students register because of personal interest or curiosity; the material discussed in these courses makes up a major part of today's health news, and it is the rare student who has not had a close friend or family member experience at least one of the diagnostic procedures, disorders, or therapies discussed in this text.

In recognition of the variety of backgrounds and interest areas of the students reading this text, we have minimized the level of psychological and biological prerequisites for the reader. The first section of the book puts the field of health psychology into historical context and introduces basic principles of psychological research. The coverage of research methods in Chapter 2 has a dual purpose. Students with little background in research methods are exposed to the research techniques referred to later in the text, and students with more research training may review basic research concepts and see how they are applied to problems in health psychology. Practical and ethical problems in health psychology research are discussed in detail in this chapter, and a sense of the relationship between clinical practice and research is communicated.

The second section of the text introduces psychological and biological concepts basic to health psychology. Chapter 3 presents basic biological and anatomical information, and Chapter 4 reviews learning theory and behavioral and cognitive-behavioral therapy techniques. Once again, illustrations of these basic processes are drawn from health psychology practice and research. Chapter 5 discusses and illustrates the interrelationships of psychological and biological factors in health and illness.

The major section of the text examines the contributions of health psychology to the understanding, prevention, and treatment of health problems. Chapters 6 through 16 review specific areas of application, ranging from health-enhancing and health-endangering behaviors to major disease entities such as cancer. Relatively common health problems such as heart disease and headache receive extensive coverage, but less well-known disorders, such as Raynaud's disease and gastroesophageal reflux, are also discussed. Chapters 15 and 16 present the contributions of health psychology in pediatric and geriatric populations. Finally, Chapter 17 discusses health psychology training and career opportunities.

Each chapter includes a chapter outline and a summary. The summaries review the most important concepts and conclusions of the chapter, and may be used as a study guide. Important key words and concepts are highlighted throughout the text. Clinical case examples and samples of research projects breathe life into the presentation and stress the continuity between theory, research, and practice.

We are all clinical psychologists with experience in health care settings, and this text reflects our clinical perspective. The promotion of health-enhancing behaviors and prevention of health-endangering behaviors receive attention, but psychological contributions to the causes, assessment, and treatment of disorder also receive extensive coverage. Topics such as stress and its management, the effects of smoking and alcohol on health, and relationships between diet, exercise, and health are receiving increasing attention in courses in health promotion, introductory psychology, and adjustment. Information on these topics also permeates the popular media. However, information that helps students become knowledgeable evaluators and critical consumers of psychological health care services is less available. We hope that this book helps to fill this gap.

Any project of this type would be impossible without extensive help from many sources, and this book is no exception. We would particularly like to thank the following reviewers, whose suggestions contributed immeasurably to the accuracy and completeness of the material:

· Felipe G. Castro, University of California, Los Angeles
· Frank L. Collins, West Virginia University
· Leonard Doerfler, University of Massachusetts–Medical School
· Robert Hoff, Mercyhurst College

· David I. Mostofsky, Boston University
· Michael Strube, Washington University

The editorial and production staff at Macmillan, especially Christine Cardone, Charlotte Hyland, and Tony English, showed patience above and beyond the call of duty. Without their forbearance and continued interest, the project would never have come to fruition. We also acknowledge the support of our home institutions, noted on the title page. The senior author wishes to especially recognize the support of the University of North Carolina, Asheville. Although now at Trinity University, he completed most of the text while at UNCA. Finally, each of us owes a personal debt of gratitude to our professional mentors and family members. Without their support and encouragement, we would never have involved ourselves in health psychology or felt free to commit our time to its pursuit.

# Contents

CHAPTER 7

# Psychological Preparation for Stressful Medical and Dental Procedures                                                              *159*

CHAPTER 8

# Cardiovascular Disease                                                              *197*

CHAPTER 9
# *Cancer*                                                                                          *238*

# PART I

# Introduction

# CHAPTER 1

# Health Psychology and the Health Care Delivery System

Imagine yourself lying in a hospital bed. It is late afternoon, and you just have been brought to your room in a wheelchair even though you are capable of walking by yourself. You feel embarrassed about being forced to ride in the chair because you had only gone to see the doctor at the student health service that morning to have your headache treated. An apparently simple problem is beginning to look very complicated, and by now you're wondering if you made a big mistake by going at all. After all, you tell yourself, a headache is just a headache, not really something serious.

Although the headaches have persisted, intermittently, for several months, you are not particularly concerned about them because you are in the middle of your toughest year at college and you assumed the headaches were just ordinary "tension headaches." You have been under a lot of stress trying to keep your grade point average up and participate in all your other activities;

on top of that, you have just broken up with the person you had been dating for the last two semesters. The stress from that relationship was pretty intense for a while. You had visited the student health service several times before, and they suggested that you needed to relax. They also gave you some medication for the pain, but the headaches still bothered you at times.

This morning the pain seemed different. The pain was so bad that you were nauseous, and you couldn't stand to open the blinds because the light made the pain worse. You remember that your mother used to complain about headaches; could this be what she was experiencing? After you describe your symptoms to the family practice resident at the student health service, she suggests that you check in to the university hospital for some tests because what had been tried so far had not solved the problem. You spend the evening in bed, reviewing the last few days and trying to rest.

The next morning a bewildering array of people come through your room. They all appear to be doctors, and they all ask similar questions, but each has a few slightly different questions, too. It's hard to tell which parts of your history you should tell the different doctors, and some of them don't seem too interested in what you think is important and are very interested in what seem like unimportant details. By the time the student health doctor comes by to check on you in the afternoon, you're exhausted. She tells you that today you saw an internist, a neurologist, and one of her associates in family practice, and tomorrow you'll have some lab tests. Later in the afternoon, she expects that a clinical psychologist will be by to see you. You begin to wonder if they think you are imagining the pain.

The psychologist comes by and talks to you for a while. As he leaves he gives you a few questionnaires to fill out, and it's hard for you to see what some of the questions have to do with your headaches. By the time the second day is over, you've also seen an anesthesiologist; you know that anesthesiologists are the people who administer the anesthetic in surgery, and you are beginning to get pretty worried about how serious they think your headaches might be. Do they think you might have a brain tumor that's causing the pain?

You leave the hospital after three days and are presented with a bill on your way out. You know that your insurance will pay some of this, but it's up to you to file the forms, and in the interim the hospital wants you to set up a payment plan for the portion not covered by your insurance. The doctors have told you that you have migraine headaches and that you can take some medicine to relieve them. However, a lot of the treatment will involve learning some ways you can relax and practicing different ways to handle the stress that you're under. They've set up a few appointments for you over the next few weeks so you can get started on this part of the treatment. They have also stated that there's a chance you will have the headaches on and off all your life, particularly considering that your mother had them. Thus, learning different coping strategies may be very important for your long-term health. The headache you feel beginning as you look over the bill suggests they may be right.

What you have just experienced is an imaginary, but not entirely atypical, hospital evaluation for headaches. Of course, not all of these experiences happen to everyone, but the case presented illustrates many of the topics that will be discussed later in this chapter and discussed in more detail in the following chapters of this text. Not only has attention to the interplay of psychological, social, and medical factors become an increasingly important aspect of the health care process, but also the practice of medicine itself has become more specialized and complex. The following sections provide a history of how medicine and psychology have been drawn closer together, and they describe the assets and liabilities of the current health care delivery system.

# Toward a Science of Health Psychology

Two major trends are apparent in the history of the struggle to understand the relationship between the physical and the psychological aspects of human functioning. First, the question of the relationship between mind and body, between psychological and somatic processes, has occupied the energies of a great many thinkers and health practitioners. Second, there has been debate as to whether health and illness are concerns of science or whether they are in the province of religion. Although medicine and psychology are today considered to be scientific pursuits, this is a relatively new development when viewed in a historical perspective. At many times in the past, physical and psychological disorders were treated in religious rites rather than by scientifically-based procedures. The following section provides a brief overview of the major events in the history of civilizations's attempts to understand and deal with health, illness, and behavior.

## From the Ancient Greeks to the Enlightenment

It has long been recognized that health, behavioral, and psychological processes are related, even though the underlying mechanisms of the relationship among these processes are only now becoming apparent. Even the earliest conceptions of disease, in which injury or illness was often attributed to the actions of gods or demons, suggested a link between health and psychology in that thoughts and behaviors displeasing to the gods might be punished with illness. However, the application of the scientific method to problems of health and illness may be said to have begun at the time of the ancient Greek physician Hippocrates, who was born in 459 or 460 B.C. and lived for about 100 years.

Before Hippocrates' lifetime, the dominant force in Western medicine was the cult of Aesculapius. Aesculapius was said by some to be mortal and by others to be the son of the god of medicine Apollo. In the temples of this cult, healing was accomplished through ceremonies and fasting and was often guided by the patient's dreams. History suggests that Hippocrates was a major figure in the development of an alternative approach to the practice of medicine and the understanding of human behavior. Hippocrates acknow-ledged Aesculapius in his recommendations concerning the ethical practice of medicine; the well-known Hippocratic Oath begins "I swear by Apollo the physician, and Aesculapius, and Hygeia, and Panacea." However, the views of the causes of health and illness Hippocrates developed were a major step away from priestly medicine and toward scientific medicine.

Hippocrates emphasized the role of observation and experience in under-standing and treating health problems. He believed health to be the result of a balance between four bodily humors: blood, phlegm, black bile, and yellow bile. He asserted that imbalances affected not only physical health but also behavior and personality. Hippocrates stated that disease is a natural process; that is, it is the result of natural causes rather than of divine intervention. He further stated that symptoms are the reaction of the body to illness, and the role of the physician is to aid the natural healing forces of the body. To aid these natural forces, Hippocrates prescribed medicines and surgery, changes in diet and exercise, and such activities as gymnastics and sea bathing (Castig-lioni, 1958).

Although Hippocrates' methods are indeed primitive forms of treatment, they were clearly precursors of more modern emphases on behavior as a means of promoting and restoring health. Recommendations for dietary changes and exercise for health maintenance are common today, and many people who experience health problems are given such recommendations as a part of their treatment program. How frequently have we heard of someone who, after suffering a heart attack or receiving a diagnosis of high blood pressure, is told to begin a regular exercise program, lose weight, and avoid foods high in salt and saturated fats? The details of this treatment program may be different from what Hippocrates would have prescribed, but the areas of change in the person's life-style are strikingly similar.

The relative influences of religion and empiricism continued to vary after Hippocrates' time, and knowledge regarding anatomy and physiology in-creased gradually. By the Renaissance period, the fourteenth to seventeenth centuries, medical treatment was primarily in the hands of the laity rather than the clergy. Perhaps the most significant shift in medical thought came at the end of the Renaissance, with the philosophy of René Descartes (1596–1650). Descartes argued that mind and body were separate entities. *Psyche* and *soma* were the two basic constituents of the universe, and the realms of each were entirely different. What little interaction that could occur between mind and body took place in the pineal gland. Descartes's influence moved the study of medicine in the direction of the physical sciences, such as chemistry and physics, and thus encouraged the accumulation of knowledge regarding the physiological bases of health and illness. However, his philosophy also served to drive a wedge between psychological and somatic functioning, thus complicating the scientific study of psychological and behavioral influences on health.

During the Renaissance, individuals suffering from psychological disorders were frequently treated as if they were possessed by demons or persecuted for being in league with the devil. Even if they were not treated as if their disorder was due to demonic factors, they seldom received humane care. Asylums for psychologically disturbed persons were oriented toward restraint rather than treatment, and sometimes patients were exhibited to the public as a form of entertainment.

A landmark in the care of the mentally ill came in the late eighteenth century. Philippe Pinel (1745–1826), a French physician who was serving as the director of Bicêtre, a hospital in Paris, removed the shackles from patients and provided sanitary, humane conditions. Pinel argued that psychologically disturbed people were ill and deserved to be treated humanely rather than as if they were possessed by demons or subhuman. The patients released from their chains improved dramatically, and there began a gradual change toward seeing psychological disturbance as a condition deserving and requiring treatment rather than punishment and isolation.

## Psychosomatic Medicine and Clinical Psychology

With psychological and medical dysfunction entering the realm of science, and thus open to empirical study, the way was cleared for investigations into the relationships between psychological and physical health and illness. In 1852 the physician Henry Holland stated, in his book *Mental Physiology*, that

> Human physiology comprises the reciprocal actions and relations of mental and bodily phenomena, as they make up the totality of life.—Scarcely can we have a morbid affection of the body in which some feeling or function of mind is not concurrently engaged-directly or indirectly-as cause or as effect. (Grinker, 1953, p. 12)

Perhaps the major stimulus to the modern study of mind-body interactions came with the influence of Sigmund Freud. Freud was quite interested in cases in which physical symptoms exist despite the absence of a biological cause. Freud believed such symptoms to be a reflection of the presence of unconscious conflicts, commonly associated with sexual feelings. He hypothesized that unacceptable and disturbing thoughts and emotions were kept unconscious in order to reduce anxiety, but the pressure of these conflicts led to the appearance of the physical disorder. For example, a shy and isolated person might feel anxious and guilty about expressing his feelings of love for others because he learned from his parents that sexual desire was unacceptable. If this person developed a paralyzed arm with no physical reason for the paralysis and became Freud's patient, Freud might have concluded that the paralyzed arm was a symbol for the anxiety the person feels about making contact with others. If the patient's arm is paralyzed, he cannot reach out, hug, or touch anyone, so he is protected from the anxiety and guilt he would feel if he became involved in an intimate relationship. In such a case, Freud argued, psychological conflicts were converted into physical symptoms. He therefore labeled the psychological defense mechanism under-lying the development of this type of symptom *conversion*. As Freud's psychoanalytic theory became increasingly prominent, the field of psychosomatic medicine was born.

Early psychosomatic medicine was particularly interested in the study of "vegetative" responses to emotions, the physical changes that occur as a natural part of emotional experience. Individuals suffering from neurotic conflicts were hypothesized to be unable to express emotions normally. The inhibition or blockage of emotional expression caused continuing vegetative responses, which could lead to physical disturbance. Thus, prolonged and unexpressed anger in an adult could eventually lead to irreversible high blood pressure, or a child experiencing fears of rejection and abandonment by his or her mother might express this fear indirectly through an asthma attack. Psychological conflicts were proposed as important factors in disorders as diverse as peptic ulcer, asthma, diabetes, and glaucoma (Alexander & French, 1948).

The range of topics encompassed by modern psychosomatic medicine has expanded far beyond its psychoanalytic heritage. As Wittkower and Warnes (1977) noted, the current psychosomatic approach focuses on psychological and psychosocial factors evident in any patient suffering from any disorder, and therapies other than psychoanalysis are also frequently employed.

Coincident with the development of psychosomatic medicine, psychologists were becoming increasingly involved in the assessment and treatment of individuals suffering from psychological and physical disorders. This is particularly true of clinical psychology, in which the application of psychological knowledge to the adjustment problems of individuals is investigated and practiced (Sundberg & Tyler, 1962). Clinical psychology may be said to have had its beginnings in the 1890s when Lightner Witmer studied children with learning and school problems. Clinical psychology has shown steady growth since that time, particularly stimulated by the influence of World Wars I and II. At the beginning of the First World War, there was a need for the development of an instrument to screen potential soldiers for the presence of psychological problems that might interfere with their ability to function in the military. This led to the development of tests of intelligence known as the Army Alpha and Army Beta and a test of emotional functioning conceived by Robert Woodworth that was known as the Psychoneurotic Inventory.

Between the two World Wars, clinical psychologists became increasingly involved in the assessment of psychological disorders, and they were also heavily influenced by the same psychoanalytic tradition as their medical colleagues. Psychologists frequently served as the experts on diagnosis in treatment teams in hospitals and clinics but were involved in treatment to a relatively limited degree. However, with the coming of the Second World War and the consequent increase in the need for psychological treatment of returning veterans, training programs in clinical psychology became more clearly defined (Schofield, 1979), and clinical psychologists became increasingly involved in treatment as well. (Readers interested in more detail concerning the history of clinical psychology will find an interesting and personal report in Korchin, 1983.)

Psychologists have also been highly involved in the study of the more normal aspects of human behavior, especially learning. Classical conditioning—initially demonstrated by the Russian physiologist and psychologist Ivan Pavlov and discussed in detail in Chapter 4—provided a scientific basis for psychosomatic medicine by illustrating how behavior and physiological responses may be correlated (Grinker, 1953). In addition, B. F. Skinner's demonstrations of operant conditioning, also discussed in Chapter 4, provided a powerful tool for the study of human behavior, as behavior change and maintenance were potentially reducible to the selection and presentation of the appropriate stimuli.

In the 1960s evidence accumulated indicating that humans and animals could learn to control autonomic nervous system responses. Such responses had previously been thought to be impossible to control voluntarily. For example, Shapiro, Crider, and Tursky (1964) demonstrated that humans could learn to control changes in skin potential, or fluctuations in the electrical conductivity of the surface of the skin of their palm, when provided with monetary rewards for successfully doing so. The electrical conductivity of the skin is related to sweat gland activity, a function controlled by the autonomic nervous system. Neal Miller and his associates conducted a series of experiments that suggested animals could learn to control responses such as heart rate even when they were paralyzed by the drug curare if the animals were rewarded with direct stimulation of pleasure centers in the brain (Miller, 1969). Although it has been difficult to successfully replicate the results of the studies with curarized animals, the human and animal studies stimulated interest in the application of operant conditioning procedures to medical problems (Shapiro & Surwit, 1979). Biofeedback—a technique in which individuals are provided with information regarding physiological reponses so they may begin to alter them—grew out of this early research. Recommendations for changes in behavior had been a standard part of medical treatment throughout history, and psychology began to provide a technology that might help transform these recommendations into actual behavioral changes.

## The Emergence of Health Psychology

The realization of the potential implications of psychological knowledge for medical practice led to the employment of psychologists in medical schools. In 1953 there were 255 psychologists identified who worked in medical schools in the United States (Mensh, 1953). However, by 1976 there were 2,336 psychologists employed in American schools of medicine (Lubin, Nathan, & Matarazzo, 1978).

The field of behavioral medicine evolved in response to this growing interaction between psychology and medicine. The term *behavioral medicine* was initially used by Birk (1973) in reference to biofeedback, but its meaning today is significantly broader. Behavioral medicine has been defined as

> the interdisciplinary field concerned with the development and integration of behavioral and biomedical science knowledge and techniques relevant to health and illness and the application of this knowledge to prevention, diagnosis, treatment, and rehabilitation. (Schwartz & Weiss, 1978, p. 250)

Behavioral medicine, then, is a field that serves as a point of integration for knowledge from many different disciplines, including medicine and psychology as well as sociology, education, nutrition, and all other scientific fields that may provide information relevant to health and illness.

In order to more clearly delineate preventive and treatment efforts, Matarazzo (1980) suggested that the term *behavioral health* be used to refer to a parallel field emphasizing prevention of illness and health maintenance. Matarazzo has defined behavioral health as the

> interdisciplinary field dedicated to promoting a philosophy of health that stresses *individual responsibility* in the application of behavioral science knowledge and techniques to the *maintenance* of health and the *prevention* of illness and dysfunction by a variety of self-initiated individual or shared activities. (Matarazzo, 1980, p. 813)

There has been some debate as to the most appropriate label for the field encompassing the contributions of psychology to behavioral medicine and behavioral health (Bradley & Prokop, 1981). The term *health psychology* has been selected by the American Psychological Association, and this text will use that term. Health psychology is defined as

> the aggregate of the specific educational, scientific, and professional contributions of the discipline of psychology to the promotion and maintenance of health, the prevention and treatment of illness, the identification of etiologic and diagnostic correlates of health, illness, and related dysfunction, and to the analysis and improvement of the health care system and health policy formation. (1981, p. 6)

The field of health psychology therefore provides a focus for the contributions of psychologists to behavioral medicine.

As is apparent from the foregoing, the field of health psychology represents the current state of an extended evolutionary process and may be expected to continue to change with the passage of time. In noting this historical progression, Gentry and Matarazzo (1981) referred to the current emphasis on the integration of psychology and medicine as the reemergence of a persistent human interest rather than the emergence of a new idea. This text will present an overview of the primary methods used by today's health psychologists in their practice and research and the promise of these procedures for the future.

# The Health Care Delivery System

When an individual is in need of health care, whether it is preventive care, such as a regular physical or dental examination, or acute care for an illness or accident, he or she typically turns to some socially sanctioned healer for help. Earlier, we presented a hypothetical case of a student with headaches. This case illustrates that the process of finding and receiving care can be quite complex. The array of practitioners and services involved in this process constitutes the health care delivery system. Steven Jonas (1981) listed eleven significant problems confronting the health care delivery system in the United States. These are summarized in Table 1.1 and include factors related to economics and psychology as well as medicine itself. Although not all of the problems are directly relevant to health psychology, many do involve psychological and behavioral components and will be discussed in more detail.

Perhaps the most notable current difficulty involves the increasing cost of health care. As of 1986, it was estimated that 8,129,000 people were employed in health care in the United States, and $458.2 billion, or 10.9% of the gross national product, was spent on health care. This compares to expenditures of about $12.7 billion in 1950, or 4.4% of the gross national product (National Center for Health Statistics [NCHS], 1989).

Several factors are related to this increase in health care costs, ranging from advances in medical technology to increasing malpractice suits brought against doctors (Kurtz & Chalfant, 1984). Technological advances have led to significant improvements in medicine's ability to treat disease and accidental injury. However, these advances have also increased the cost of medical care by making treatment possible for people with diseases that were formerly untreatable

TABLE 1.1  Problems Confronting the Health Care System

1. The rising cost of health care
2. Geographic maldistribution of manpower and facilities
3. Overspecialization of providers
4. Overutilization of hospitals
5. Deficiencies in quality and quality control
6. The tendency, especially among physicians, to stress the unusual at the expense of the commonplace
7. The presence of barriers to effective provider-to-patient communication
8. An emphasis on treatment rather than prevention
9. An orientation toward patients with acute physical problems at the expense of patients who are chronically ill or who have mental problems
10. Training, education, and research programs that are not directly relevant to patient needs
11. Financial and other barriers to care

SOURCE: Jonas, S. (1981). *Health care delivery in the United States* (2nd ed.). New York: Springer.

and by extending the life span of those requiring chronic care. For example, before the development of renal dialysis and transplant procedures, individuals suffering from kidney failure had few treatment options available. With the advent of these lifesaving procedures, Medicare payments in 1978 to individuals in the final stages of kidney disease were $947 million. Medicare expenditures for the same disease in 1990 are expected to exceed $3.4 billion (Orr, 1984). The actual national expenditure should be higher, as this estimate only includes government-sponsored payments through Medicare.

As these data suggest, one of the major reasons for the increase in medical care expenditures is the growing proportion of patients who are suffering from chronic illnesses. Medicine has become increasingly successful in the treatment of infectious diseases and injuries, but a common element in both these conditions is that they tend to be time limited. A patient recovers from strep throat in a relatively short time and a broken arm mends. However, an individual suffering from chronic kidney dysfunction must make many difficult life-style changes, and the continuing nature of the disease increases the chances for adjustment problems as well (Ford & Castelnuovo-Tedesco, 1977). There is also relatively little, if any, implication of patient responsibility in the cause or treatment of injuries or infections. All people are subject to infections at some time, and accidents often are unavoidable; all the patient must do to recover is take antibiotics or submit to treatment for the injury.

However, the leading causes of death today are not related to infectious illneses or accidents. Instead, heart disease, cancer, and stroke are the three leading killers in the United States. Not only do these disorders have a chronic course, but they also appear to be related to life-style and behavior, such as alcohol abuse, smoking, and obesity. Similarly, Acquired Immune Deficiency Syndrome (AIDS) is associated with sexual behavior and drug use. Reported AIDS cases have increased from 664 in 1982 to 21,123 in 1987 (NCHS, 1989). A health care delivery system oriented toward treatment of acute disorders has difficulty dealing with chronic disorders related to behavioral factors. Thus, the system is prone to the delivery care directed toward the results rather than the causes of chronic disorders. The health care system is admirably equipped to remove a cancerous lung but less well equipped to prevent cigarette smoking or to help smokers to break the habit.

The health care delivery system in the United States is much more focused on treatment rather than prevention of disease. As Albino (1983) has noted, most physicians and other health care professionals have come to define successful treatment as the elimination of symptoms, and prevention of disease does not fit this model. If a physician is presented with a full appointment calendar and two new patients call, one requesting an appointment to discuss an exercise program and the other an appointment to have an examination for an irregular heartbeat, the physician will understandably give precedence to the patient with the already existing symptoms. Not only is it harder to justify time spent with healthy people, it is also difficult to measure success when success is the maintenance of health rather than the relief of suffering.

A further complicating factor is that insurance often does not reimburse subscribers for health maintenance visits, such as regular physicals, but instead reimburses only for the treatment of definable, already existing illness. Thus, people are often reluctant to seek preventive health care when the expense will not be reimbursed as their other medical expenses commonly are.

Even if an individual waits until the appearance of symptoms to seek medical care, they will be unable to benefit from the contact with the health care system unless they are able to effectively communicate their symptoms and concerns to the provider. The health care system has been criticized for the existence of barriers to effective patient–provider communication (Jonas, 1981). Indeed, it has been suggested that the rapid advances in medical technology have not been accompanied by similar advances in the human aspects of patient care. The degree to which patients experience a satisfying interpersonal relationship with their physician might seem to be a rather trivial matter in comparison to the technical quality of the medical care itself. The evidence suggests, however, that the personal aspects of care are as important, if not more so, than the technical aspects. For example, Doyle and Ware (1977) found that the physician's conduct toward the patient was the strongest determinant of patient satisfaction. Patient satisfaction may have a significant impact on the health care process, as it has been suggested that unsatisfied patients are more likely to file malpractice suits and to seek care from quacks or charlatans (DiMatteo, 1979).

Effective communication with the physician may also have a measurable effect on the process of recovery. Egbert, Battit, Welch, and Bartlett (1964) found that patients who met with their anesthesiologist prior to surgery and received explanations of what to expect during recovery requested less pain medication after surgery and were discharged from the hospital sooner than those who did not receive such explanations. Rapport between the provider and patient is also important if the patient is to have the best chance of understanding his or her condition and following the provider's recommendations (Francis, Korsch, & Morris, 1969). Poor adherence to medical instructions has been found to be a major problem. Davis (1966) found that estimates of patient nonadherence range from 15% to 94%, dependent upon the study at issue. In a review of the literature regarding adherence, Masur (1981) noted improved adherence to health care suggestions would be likely to substantially reduce health care costs. (These issues are discussed in more detail in Chapter 6.)

Patients may also have difficulty in selecting the type of health care provider they should see without regard to the quality of the interpersonal relationship they may have with the provider. Although there was a time when the general practitioner provided almost all necessary health care for a person or a family, and often came to know that person or family well, there has been a tremendous increase in specialization in the medical field in the last several decades. Table 1.2 presents a partial listing of the health care specialties existing today.

TABLE 1.2  A Noncomprehensive Listing of Health Care Provider Specialities

| | | |
|---|---|---|
| Anesthesiology | Naturopathy | Pediatrics |
| Biomedical Engineering | Neurology | Physical Therapy |
| Cardiology | Nurse Practitioner | Preventive Medicine |
| Clinical Psychology | Nutrition | Psychiatry |
| Dentistry | Obstetrics and Gynecology | Radiology |
| Dermatology | Occupational Therapy | Radiologic Technician |
| Endocrinology | Oncology | Registered Nursing |
| Family Practice | Opthalmology | Rheumatology |
| Gastroenterology | Optometry | Sports Medicine |
| Health Psychology | Orthopedics | Surgery |
| Hematology | Osteopathy | Social work |
| Internal Medicine | Otorhinolaryngology | Urology |
| Licensed Practical Nursing | Pathology | |

Imagine that you are a patient suffering from back pain and muscle spasms. Which type of provider would you initially contact for help? A family practitioner, considering you may have already established a relationship with one? An orthopedist, because you know of a friend with a back problem who saw an orthopedist and recovered? A clinical psychologist, because you believe the spasms are caused by stress and you might benefit from biofeedback or some other technique to help you better handle stress? As health care providers have become increasingly specialized, it has become more difficult for the consumer to make an informed decision about the choice of providers and treatments. Additionally, increasing specialization has made it difficult for patients to feel that their provider is aware of all their health needs, because the provider may be associated with only a portion of their health care. Linn (1977) has suggested that physicians experience similar difficulties, as increasing specialization complicates their ability to view the patient in his or her entirety and in the context of the social environment.

In summary, although the health care delivery system of today is very effective in the treatment of acute illnesses and accidents and scientific and technical advances have greatly increased the range of disorders that may be successfully treated, the system has also been criticized for a variety of other reasons. Particularly relevant to psychology are problems relating to rising cost, an emphasis on treatment rather than prevention, the problems of the chronically ill, and barriers to effective patient–provider communication. These and other concerns are discussed in more detail in the chapters to follow.

# Summary

The ancient Greek physician Hippocrates is recognized as the first to understand that health and illness are determined by natural, rather than supernatural, forces. He believed that imbalances in the bodily humors (blood, phlegm, yellow bile, and black bile) caused illness. Hippocrates' treatment procedures included medicine, surgery, and changes in diet and exercise.

Near the end of the Renaissance, René Descartes proposed that the mind and body were separate entities. Descartes argued that *psyche* and *soma* were the two basic constituents of the universe, interacting to a limited degree in the pineal gland. Although Descartes' viewpoint stimulated scientific study in medicine, it retarded the study of the interaction of psychological events and physical health. The examination of psychological disorders became a more legitimate area of scientific study after Pinel provided humane treatment for psychologically disturbed patients. Pinel believed that psychological disturbance was a form of illness, and patients should not be treated as if they are subhuman or possessed by demons.

Studies of the relationship between psychological and physical functioning became more common in the nineteenth century. Henry Holland's book *Mental Physiology* and Sigmund Freud's investigations into the fact that physical symptoms apparently are caused by psychological conflicts were particularly influential. Psychosomatic medicine focused on the study of vegetative responses, or the physical changes accompanying emotional arousal.

Modern clinical psychology began with Lightner Witmer's studies of children with learning and school problems. Psychological assessment and treatment needs increased during and following World War I and World War II, and clinical psychologists played a large role in meeting these needs. Advances in learning theory also contributed to the development of new applications of psychological principles to health problems. Ivan Pavlov's studies of the classical conditioning of physiological processes provided an empirical demonstration of how physical responses may by influenced by environmental events. Skinner's operant conditioning paradigm was applied in treatment procedures such as biofeedback, in which subjects learn to control physiological responses.

The increasing recognition of the applications of psychological principles to medicine was reflected in an expansion of the number of psychologists working in medical settings. Behavioral medicine evolved as an interdisciplinary field integrating behavioral and biomedical science. In 1981, health psychology was defined as a specialty area in psychology. Health psychology encompasses the contributions of psychology to health maintenance, the treatment of illness, and the causes and diagnostic correlates of health and illness. Health psychology also studies the applications of psychological principles to the health care system.

The United States health care system has been criticized on several levels. Health care costs have increased rapidly as a result of medical technology becoming more complex and a greater proportion of patients suffering from long-term, chronic diseases. The health care system has been largely successful in treating accidents and infectious illnesses, but the leading causes of death today are chronic diseases related to life-style and behavior. Changes in behavior could reduce the health-care burden by preventing illness, but the system is better equipped for treatment than it is for prevention.

The health care system has also been criticized for overemphasizing technical procedures and underemphasizing the human aspects of health care. Patients may find it difficult to communicate with health care providers. A good provider–patient relationship plays a large role in patient satisfaction, recovery time, and adherence to medical instructions. Increasing provider specialization has complicated communication because more providers may be involved in the care of a single patient. Increasing specialization has made it more difficult for one provider to be aware of all of a patients's health care needs. Specialization has also made it more difficult for patients to make informed choices about which provider they should see.

# References

ALBINO, J. E. (1983). Health psychology and primary prevention: Natural allies. In Felner, R. D., Jason, L. A., Moritsugu, J. N., & Farber, S. S. (Eds.), *Preventive psychology: Theory, research, and practice* (pp. 221–233). New York: Pergamon.

ALEXANDER, F., & FRENCH, T. M. (1948). *Studies in psychosomatic medicine.* New York: Ronald Press.

AMERICAN PSYCHOLOGICAL ASSOCIATION, DIVISION 38. (1981). *The Health Psychologist, 3*(2), 6.

BIRK, L. (Ed.). (1973) *Biofeedback: Behavioral medicine.* New York: Grune and Stratton.

BRADLEY, L. A., & PROKOP, C. K. (1981). The relationship between medical psychology and behavioral medicine. In C. K. Prokop & L. A. Bradley (Eds.), *Medical psychology: Contributions to behavioral medicine* (pp. 1–4). New York: Academic Press.

CASTIGLIONI, A. (1958). *A history of medicine* (2nd ed.) (E. B. Krumbhaat, Trans.). New York: Knopf.

DAVIS, M. S. (1966). Variations in patient's compliance with doctors' orders: Analysis of congruence between survey responses and results of empirical investigations. *Journal of Medical Education, 41,* 1037–1048.

DiMATTEO, M. R. (1979). A social-psychological analysis of physician-patient rapport: Toward a science of the art of medicine. *Journal of Social Issues, 35,* 12–33.

DOYLE, B. J., & WARE, J. E. (1977). Physician conduct and other factors that affect consumer satisfaction with medical care. *Journal of Medical Education, 52,* 793–801.

EGBERT, L. D., BATTIT, G. E., WELCH, C. E., & BARTLETT, M. K. (1964). Reduction of postoperative pain by encouragement and instruction of patients: A study of doctor-patient rapport. *New England Journal of Medicine, 270,* 825–827

FORD, C. V., & CASTELNUOVO-TEDESCO, P. (1977). Hemodialysis and renal transplantation: Psychopathological reactions and their management. In E. D. Wittkower & H. Warnes (Eds.), *Psychosomatic medicine: Its clinical applications* (pp. 74–83). Hagerstown, MD: Harper & Row.

FRANCIS, V., KORSCH, B. M., & MORRIS, M. J. (1969). Gaps in doctor-patient communications. *New England Journal of Medicine, 280,* 535–540.

GENTRY, W. D., & MATARAZZO, J. D. (1981). Medical psychology: Three decades of growth and development. In C. K. Prokop & L. A. Bradley (Eds.), *Medical psychology: Contributions to behavioral medicine* (pp. 6–14.) New York: Academic Press.

GRINKER, R.R. (1953). *Psychosomatic research.* New York: Norton.

JONAS, S. (1981) *Health care delivery in the United States* (2nd. ed.). New York: Springer.

KORCHIN, S. (1983). The history of clinical psychology: A personal view. In M. Hersen, A. E. Kazdin, & A. S. Bellack (Eds.), *The clinical psychology handbook.* New York: Pergamon.

KURTZ, R. A., & CHALFANT, H. P. (1984). *The sociology of medicine and illness.* Boston: Allyn and Bacon.

LINN, L. (1977). Basic principles of management in psychosomatic medicine. In E. D. Wittkower & H. Warnes (Eds.) *Psychosomatic medicine: Its clinical applications* (pp. 2–14). Hagerstown, MD: Harper & Row.

LUBIN, B., NATHAN, R. G., & MATARAZZO, J. D. (1978). Psychologists in medical education: 1976. *American Psychologist, 33,* 339–343.

MASUR, F. T. (1981). Adherence to health care regimens. In C. K. Prokop & L. A. Bradley (Eds.), *Medical psychology: Contributions to behavioral medicine* (pp. 441–470). New York: Academic Press.

MATARAZZO, J. D. (1980). Behavioral health and behavioral medicine: Frontiers for a new health psychology. *American Psychologist, 35,* 807–817.

MENSH, I. N. (1953). Psychology in medical education. *American Psychologist, 8,* 83–85.

MILLER, N. E. (1969). Learning of visceral and glandular responses. *Science, 163,* 434–445.

NATIONAL CENTER FOR HEALTH STATISTICS (1989). *Health, United States, 1988.* (DHHS Publication No. PHS 89–1232). Washington, DC: U.S. Government Printing Office.

ORR, M. L. (1984). Public policy issues in ESRD care. In L. E. Lancaster (Ed.), *The patient with end stage renal disease* (2nd ed.) (pp. 335–348). New York: Wiley.

SCHOFIELD, W. (1979). Clinical psychologists as health professionals. In G. C. Stone., F. Cohen, & N. E. Adler, *Health psychology: A handbook* (pp. 447–464). San Francisco: Jossey-Bass.

SCHWARTZ, G. E., & WEISS, S. M. (1978). Behavioral medicine revisited: An amended definition. *Journal of Behavioral Medicine, 1,* 249–251.

SHAPIRO, D., CRIDER, A. B., & TURSKY, B. (1964). Differentiation of an autonomic response through operant reinforcement. *Psychonomic Science, 1,* 147–148.

SHAPIRO, D., & SURWIT, R. S. (1979). Biofeedback. In O. V. Pomerleau & J. P. Brady (Eds.), *Behavioral medicine: Theory and practice* (pp. 45–74). Baltimore: Williams and Wilkins.

SUNDBERG, N. D., & TYLER, L. E. (1962). *Clinical psychology: An introduction to theory and practice.* New York: Appleton, Century, Crofts.

WITTKOWER, E. D., & WARNES, H. (Eds.) (1977). *Psychosomatic medicine: Its clinical applications.* Hagerstown, MD: Harper & Row.

# Research Methods in Health Psychology

The preceding chapter has reviewed the growth of health psychology. From its beginnings in Hippocrates' hypotheses integrating personality and physiology, health psychology has advanced to its present position as a scientific and clinical specialty within modern psychology. This progression has been fueled by knowledge arising from varied sources. Many important advances had their beginnings in the day-to-day activities of health care providers; regular contact with patients often led to insights into the causes and treatment of health problems. The psychoanalytic movement and much of psychosomatic medicine had its roots in such speculations. Other diagnostic and treatment innovations developed from data collected in tightly controlled scientific experiments. This research often followed ideas generated in clinical practice, as experiments were designed to test and refine the hypotheses developed during daily contact with patients. An initial association between life-style and heart disease may have been noted by a physician treating patients who suffered heart attacks, but an understanding of the components of the Type A behavior pattern and the physiological mechanisms through which life-style and health are related must come from controlled scientific research examining both healthy people and heart disease patients.

All research strategies, from case studies to tightly controlled laboratory experiments, have their own assets and liabilities. An acquaintance with the relative merits of these varying procedures is thus crucial for the effective evaluation and application of the knowledge gained from research efforts. This chapter provides an overview of the research methods used by health psychologists.

# Research Designs in Health Psychology

## Case Studies

The experiences of a single physician or psychologist with a single patient have often provided the first hints leading to an understanding of previously baffling disorders. In the *case study*, observations made in the course of the diagnosis or treatment of one patient are reported in detail. If the techniques used with the patient presented in the case study prove useful for other patients with similar problems, then advances in treatment or diagnosis may result. The case study approach possesses a variety of distinct advantages. It is especially useful in the early phases of research, when little is known about a problem area. Hypotheses may be generated from the detailed study of one case, and these leads may then be followed up with more carefully controlled research (Kazdin, 1980). The following example illustrates the use of case studies in early psychosomatic medicine.

Franz Alexander, one of the pioneers of psychosomatic medicine, reported the treatment of a 47-year-old male suffering from essential hypertension, or high blood pressure, with no known cause (Alexander, 1948). The patient was seen for psychoanalysis on a daily or nearly daily basis, and his blood pressure was measured at the beginning and end of each therapy session. The emotional state of the patient during the session was also rated by Alexander. From a comparison of the emotional and physiological data, Alexander concluded that emotional disturbance was related to the patient's hypertension; blood pressure readings were highest on days when he was rated as "very disturbed" and lowest on days when he was rated as "calm." In addition, Alexander reported that the material discussed in the analytic sessions revealed that the patient's emotional tension was a reflection of inhibited aggressive impulses that could be traced to intimidating childhood experiences. As these experiences were discussed in therapy, the patient's emotional tension was relieved, and his blood pressure declined.

The Alexander study is a good example of the case study in its classic form. Detailed observations from the treatment of a single patient were reported, and hypotheses concerning the causes and treatment of hypertension were generated from these observations. From this and other cases, it was concluded that hypertension may be related to inhibited aggressive feelings, and psychoanalytic treatment of the inhibited aggressive urges was suggested as a method to reduce blood pressure in patients suffering from essential hypertension. The case thus shed some light on a previously confusing medical condition.

Case studies also demonstrate unique applications of already existing therapies or provide early trials for innovative therapies (Kazdin, 1980). An example of this use of a case study is presented in Boxed Highlight 2.1. As you can see, the authors of this study (Bird & Colborne, 1980) used thermal, or temperature, biofeedback and relaxation in the treatment of a patient who had experienced a serious electrical burn to the left hand. Thermal biofeedback is a procedure in which a subject learns to increase the temperature of some area of the body, usually the finger, and was initially developed as a treatment for migraine headaches (Sargent, Green, & Walters, 1972). (A more complete discussion of this use of thermal biofeedback is provided in Chapter 14.)

Skin temperature is an indirect measure of blood flow. If an individual learns to increase finger temperature, he or she has learned to increase blood flow to that finger. Adequate blood flow to a wound is extremely important in the healing process because blood carries oxygen and nutrients to the healing tissue. Bird and Colborne (1980) reasoned that finger temperature biofeedback might be helpful in wound healing by increasing the flow of blood to the wound site. The progress of the patient reported in the case study does suggest that temperature biofeedback was useful in reducing pain and as an aid to the healing process. It therefore might be useful to study the utility of this treatment with other wound patients, even though finger-temperature biofeedback was developed as a treatment for migraine headache.

Although case studies often provide insights into the causes and treatment of disorders, they suffer from several disadvantages. In particular, it may be questionable to assume that the subject of the case study is representative of all other patients experiencing similar problems. Thus, the conclusions drawn from a case study may not easily be applied to other cases. That is, the results may have *limited generalizability*. It may be that high blood pressure and repressed anger were related in the case of the patient reported by Alexander (1948), but this relationship may be unusual. If the connection between blood pressure and inhibited anger is unusual, it would be incorrect to generalize from this single patient and assume that other patients suffering from high blood pressure are also characterized by the presence of repressed anger and resentment.

A second disadvantage of the case study is the possibility of *alternative explanations*. The explanation developed in the case study may be only one of several possible interpretations of the events reported. This risk is especially noteworthy in cases in which retrospective accounts, or memories of past events, are relied on to reconstruct the past in an effort to explain the present. Memory may not be entirely accurate, and events other than those reported may be responsible for the condition being investigated. For example, that a patient "remembers" a consistent feeling of anger at his or her parents and an inability to express this anger is not a guarantee that this anger was as constant in childhood as it is now remembered to be, nor is it a certainty that the anger in childhood is the cause of the patient's difficulty with emotional expression in adulthood. Alternative explanations may be easily generated: The patient may have been warned against impulsive behavior at school or been rejected when he expressed his feelings for several girlfriends during adolescence. Any, all, or none of these factors could be related to later difficulties with emotional expression.

That parallels are drawn between the past and the present does not constitute incontrovertible evidence that the past events caused the present problems. This weakness of the case study is counteracted somewhat when it can be shown that improvement was closely associated with treatment of the proposed causes of the symptoms. That the patient's blood pressure decreased as he became more calm strengthens the suggestion that emotional tension was related to his increased blood pressure. However, it is more questionable to assume that childhood anger at his parents was the major cause of this emotional tension, and it is even more indefensible to argue that repressed anger toward parents is a common cause of high blood pressure.

A related limitation of the case study is found in the *difficulty in specifying essential elements* in a treatment program. That is, it is often impossible to specify which part or parts of a treatment are responsible for the changes that are observed. In the wound-healing study discussed previously, both relaxation and temperature biofeedback were used. Could the same results have been obtained if only relaxation had been used? What if only biofeedback had been used? As we will see later, there is considerable debate as to which parts of the frequently used biofeedback treatment programs are the most critical and which parts may be expendable. Answers to these and similar questions may lead to the development of more effective therapies and may also help to hold down health care costs as unnecessary treatments may be eliminated. Indeed, in some cases the passage of time alone may have led to the changes observed. Because case studies have no other patient or group of patients to use for comparison purposes, it is often not possible to answer these questions.

*Placebo effects* refer to changes that appear to be due to the treatment but are instead due to factors such as the patient's expectations for change or faith in the health care provider. For example, in the burn study just described it is impossible to know whether or not the same improvement would have occurred with another treatment, such as biofeedback for muscle tension rather than skin temperature. If the patient believed that muscle tension feedback might lead to relaxation and thus an increased chance of healing, might that belief have been translated into physical changes and improved recovery? Placebo effects are more effectively dealt with in controlled experimental studies.

BOXED HIGHLIGHT 2.1

# A Case Study of Biofeedback and Wound Healing

A twenty-two-year-old male suffered high voltage electrical burns to his left wrist in an accident. Seven months after the injury he continued to experience pain, reduced movement, and limited sensation in his fingers. Blood flow to his left hand was restricted, he had been scheduled for a skin graft. At this point he began a treatment program in which he was trained to increase the temperature, and thus the blood flow, in his left hand by using thermal biofeedback and relaxation techniques.

The patient practiced with biofeedback and relaxation on fourteen days, and on three other days practiced relaxation without the aid of the biofeedback equipment. At the beginning of treatment the temperature of his left hand was between 77 and 80 degrees Fahrenheit, whereas the temperature of his undamaged right hand was between 93 and 95 degrees. By the ninth day of treatment he was able to raise the temperature of his left hand above that of his right hand, and after the full seventeen days of treatment he was able to raise the temperature of his damaged hand by 21 degrees Fahrenheit. Pain decreased noticeably when the temperature of his left hand reached the 90 to 93 degree range. Figure 2.1 illustrates the progress and results of the treatment program.

Six weeks after the conclusion of the treatment, the patient went to his physician for the scheduled skin graft. After an examination, the physician noted a "rare regrowth of nerves," and the skin graft was canceled because it was now unnecessary. Recovery of motion and sensation was reported in the patient's middle, ring, and little fingers, although no recovery was reported in the index finger.

Case studies are also limited by the *possibility for bias*. When a new treatment is tried, it is often the case that both the patient and the provider are quite hopeful that the treatment will be a success, and this hope may lead one or both of them to be less than objective in their evaluation of the results. This problem is magnified when the symptoms being treated are difficult to observe or fluctuating. For example, very few patients experiencing chronic headaches are always in pain or always have equally severe headaches. It is easy in such a case for both the patient and the provider to rate the headache problem as improving, even though what may actually be occurring represents a normal fluctuation in the headaches' severity and frequency. Before a new treatment was attempted, the change might have been interpreted as a welcome, but relatively insignificant, event. However, after a new treatment begins, it can easily be viewed as a response to the treatment.

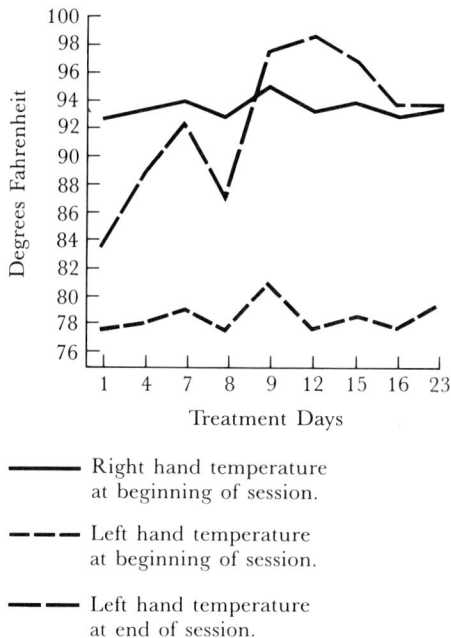

FIGURE 2.1   Progress of thermal biofeedback and relaxation treatment on patient with electrical burns. Data from "Rehabilitation of an Electrical Burn Patient Through Thermal Biofeedback" by E. I. Bird and G. R. Colborne, 1980. *Biofeedback and Self Regulation, 5*, pp. 283–288.

## Descriptive Group Studies

It is apparent from the foregoing discussion that case studies are limited in that only one subject or patient is involved. The generalizability of conclusions derived from these approaches is thus limited by the possibility that what is true of the subject under study may not be true of all, or even most, other individuals. It is therefore desirable to examine more than one person for more confident generalizability to other persons. The *descriptive group study* offers such an opportunity.

A descriptive group study allows an investigator to construct a portrait of a sample of subjects who all share some similar attribute or attributes. A group of individuals sharing one or more characteristics is sometimes referred to as a *cohort*. For example, if an investigator is interested in studying the possibility that interpersonal factors may be related to the risk of developing cancer, a group of cancer patients may be interviewed regarding their family life, friendships, and social activities for the two years immediately preceding their diagnosis. A summary description of this cohort of cancer patients is developed. It might be reported that 50% of the cancer patients experienced the loss of a family member or close friend within these two years. The investigators may then suggest that a significant interpersonal loss contributes to the development of cancer.

As with case studies, descriptive group studies are most useful in the early stages of a research program. Although they can provide an excellent over-

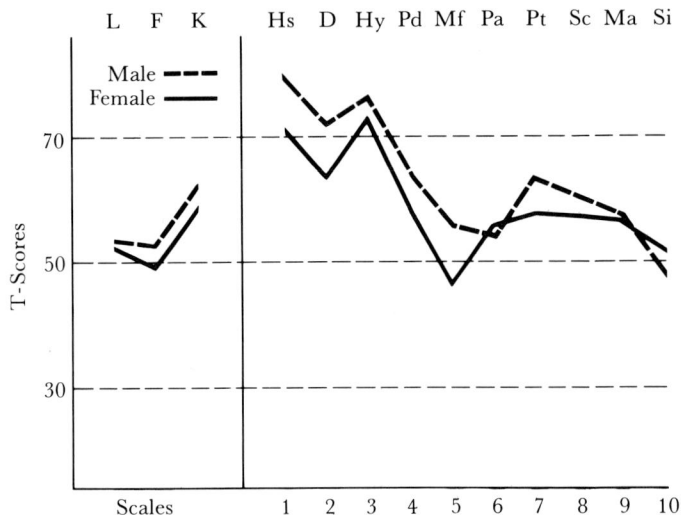

FIGURE 2.2   Minnesota Multiphasic Personality Inventory (MMPI) profiles of male and female low back pain patients. From "Chronic Low Back Pain: A Psychological Profile" by W. D. Gentry, W. D. Shows, and M. Thomas, 1974. *Psychosomatics, 15*, 174–177. Reprinted with permission of *Psychosomatics*.

view of the average subject or patient, they suffer from one major drawback. Without the presence of a second group for comparison purposes it may be quite difficult to say whether or not the characteristics found in the study are specific to the group under study. It may be that 50% of *all* people about the same age as the patients in the hypothetical cancer study experience interpersonal losses in a two-year period, without regard to health status. If this is the case, it is unlikely that interpersonal losses are an important risk factor for cancer because they occur equally in cancer patients and persons without cancer. It is therefore important to compare the results of descriptive group studies to averages for the general population whenever possible.

*Standardized tests* are sometimes used in place of population averages in descriptive group studies. A standardized test has been administered to a cross section of the general population or some other large group. The results of these administrations, called normative data, are therefore available so the score of a single subject or a group of subjects may be compared to the scores of the population as a whole. It is thus possible to say with more confidence that the characteristics of the experimental group are or are not different from the average for the general population and to say to what degree they are different if variations are apparent.

As an example of this use of standardized testing, consider the following study of low back pain patients by Gentry, Shows, and Thomas (1974). As we will see later in Chapter 14, patients suffering from chronic low back pain often pose serious treatment problems. Pain may continue in the absence of clearly diagnosable or treatable physical problems, and this pain may be severe enough to disable the patient and seriously compromise his or her family and social life. In an effort to determine the psychological characteristics of such patients, Gentry, Shows, and Thomas administered a standardized psychological test, the Minnesota Multiphasic Personality Inventory (MMPI), to a group of fifty-six chronic low back pain patients. The average length of time the patients had suffered from back pain was 7.5 years. They had undergone an average of 2.4 surgical operations without significant relief.

The MMPI profiles found to be characteristic of male and female low back pain patients are presented in Figure 2.1. As is clear from the figure, a V-shaped profile in which the Hypochondriasis (*Hs*) and Hysteria (*Hy*) scales are elevated whereas the Depression (*D*) scale remains lower is present in both the male and female patients. The conclusion that this profile differs from what would be obtained from a sample of fifty-six individuals without low back pain is strengthened by the fact that the MMPI is standardized such that a score of fifty on any scale is average for the general population, and a score of seventy is two standard deviations above the mean of the general population. That is, scores above seventy on any particular scale would be expected to be seen in only about 2.2% of the population. This MMPI profile suggests that the individual is preoccupied by physical problems and prone to deny the presence of any other difficulties, such as family, work, or psychological problems. Based on this evidence, Gentry, Shows, and Thomas hypothesized that the presence of these psychological characteristics might be contributing factors in the chronic pain syndrome and should be studied as potential predictors of treatment outcome. This suggestion has resulted in a significant body of research, some of the conclusions of which will be discussed in more detail in Chapter 14.

The descriptive group study thus offers several advantages, as it may be relatively easily conducted by studying an already existing group of subjects and it may have greater generalizability than case studies or single-subject designs. Its major weaknesses are related to its lack of a control group for comparison purposes, although this weakness may be at least partially counteracted by the use of standardized testing or comparison to population norms. However, one more serious drawback exists. Even with the use of standardized testing, the descriptive group study does not allow for inferences regarding causality to be confidently drawn. That cancer patients are found to be depressed on a standardized measure of depression does not necessarily mean that depression is a risk factor for the development of cancer. Instead, depression may be a common result of cancer. Descriptive group studies may provide useful information about the problems likely to need attention in a group of patients but provide less information about the causes of these problems.

# Correlational Studies

Many questions in health psychology may be framed in the form: "Is the magnitude of variable $X$ related to the magnitude of variable $Y$?" Is the number of days per week a person exercises (variable $X$) related to their risk of heart disease (variable $Y$)? Is the number of cigarettes a person smokes per day related to the risk of lung cancer? However, many of these questions are quite difficult to investigate by changing a behavior and observing changes in the variable of interest. It may be quite difficult to intervene with many people in such a way that their level of exercise is reliably changed, and it may take many years for lung cancer to appear as a result of cigarette smoking. It would also be unethical to ask people to smoke more to see if lung cancer rates increase. Instead, information on excercise habits and heart condition, or smoking history and lung cancer, are more easily collected simultaneously, without making any effort to change behavior. In cases such as these, a *correlational study* is often appropriate.

In a correlational study, data relating to two or more variables are collected. These variables are then compared to one another, and relationships between them are noted. The degree of relationship present between the variables is usually presented in the form of a *correlation coefficient*. Correlation coefficients range from $-1.00$ to $+1.00$; the sign indicates the direction of the relationship between variables, and the absolute magnitude of the coefficient indicates the strength of the relationship. A perfect positive relationship between variables is represented by a correlation of $+1.00$. Thus, if an increase in caloric intake of 3,500 calories always resulted in a weight gain of 1 pound and a decrease in caloric intake of 3,500 calories always resulted in a weight loss of 1 pound, the correlation between weight change and caloric intake would be $+1.00$. Conversely, if each cigarette smoked decreased life span by 10 minutes, so that a person who smoked 30 cigarettes would be expected to live 5 hours less than a person who never smoked, the correlation between cigarette consumption and reduction in life span would be $-1.00$. This type of relationship, in which an increase in one variable is associated with a decrease in another variable, is also referred to as an *inverse* relationship. If there is no relationship between two variables, the correlation coefficient is 0.

Very few events are perfectly related to one another, so it is exceptionally rare to see a correlation coefficient as high as $+1.00$ or as low as $-1.00$. Instead, important relationships in health psychology research are much more likely to be represented by correlation coefficients with absolute values in the range of .20 to .50. It is usually the case that more than one factor is an important determiner of most events. For example, it is not just caloric intake that determines weight change. Many other factors, such as exercise and metabolic rate, are also important. For this reason, the correlation between weight change and caloric intake will not be $+1.00$. Similarly, life span is related to many factors in addition to cigarette smoking, including dietary habits and occupation. Thus, the correlation between number of cigarettes smoked and life span will not be $-1.00$.

Correlational studies may be *univariate* or *multivariate*. In a univariate study, only two variables are investigated. Thus the relationship between anxiety and tension headache frequency may be studied by having subjects complete an anxiety scale and estimate the number of tension headaches they experience each week. No other variables are studied. In a multivariate correlational study, more than two variables are measured. Multivariate studies allow an investigator to examine the possibility that more than one variable is important in the understanding of a phenomenon. For example, it may be that anxiety is not the only important variable in headache frequency but that a family history of headaches is also quite important. The overall correlation between anxiety and headache frequency may be quite low, but when family history is taken into account, it may be found that persons with a family history of headaches are much more likely to report an increase in headache frequency as anxiety increases than are people who do not have a family history of headaches. Multivariate correlational studies allow an investigator to discover such relationships.

Research investigating the relationship between Type A behavior and heart disease provides an excellent example of the use of univariate and multivariate correlational studies. The Type A behavior pattern, discussed in more detail in Chapter 8, has been suggested to be associated with the development of coronary heart disease. However, evidence for this association has not been uniformly positive. MacDougall, Dembroski, Dimsdale, and Hackett (1985) were interested in investigating the possibility that one of the reasons for this inconsistency in the research may be related to the existence of many different behavioral styles, including impatience, irritability, ambition, hostility, and an unwillingness to express anger, are all involved in Type A behavior. Therefore, it is possible that a univariate correlational approach, in which an overall measure of Type A behavior is correlated with signs of heart disease, may fail to reliably uncover a relationship if only some aspects of Type A behavior are related to heart disease. A multivariate correlational approach, which examines the components of Type A behavior separately and in combination, may reveal relationships that a univariate approach obscures.

The authors examined a group of 125 patients who had been admitted to Massachusetts General Hospital for diagnostic testing. All patients underwent cardiac catheterization, a test that reveals the degree to which the major blood vessels in the heart are blocked by fatty deposits. Before undergoing catheterization, the patients were assessed for the presence of Type A behavior. Finally, correlations between the number of blocked blood vessels, overall Type A rating, and the separate components of Type A behavior were computed.

A summary of the results of this study is presented in Table 2.1. When a univariate strategy was used, no significant correlation was found between overall Type A behavior and heart disease. In fact, the correlation coefficient

TABLE 2.1   A Correlational Study of Type A Behavior and Heart Disease

| Type A component | Correlation with number of diseased vessels |
|---|---|
| Global Type A rating | − .02 |
| Potential for hostility | .18* |
| Anger-in | .28** |
| Time pressure | − .18* |
| Loudness | − .03 |
| Competitiveness | − .14 |
| Multivariate correlation (includes potential for hostility, anger-in, time pressure) | .51** |

\*   $p < .05$
\*\*  $p < .01$

SOURCE:   J. M. MacDougall, T. M. Dembroski, J. E. Dimsdale, & T. P. Hackett (1985). Components of Type A, hostility, and anger-in: Further relationships to angiographic findings. *Health Psychology, 4*, 137–152.

was − .02; remember that a correlation coefficient of zero indicates that variables are not related. However, when a multivariate strategy was used, and Type A behavior was broken down into its components, it was found that difficulty in expressing anger (anger-in), a tendency to become angry in daily activities (potential for hostility), and a consistent sense of time pressure taken together significantly predicted the presence of heart disease; the multivariate correlation coefficient was .51. This type of strategy, in which several variables are used to predict one target variable, is referred to as *multiple correlation.*

A surprising finding in this study was that one of the components of Type A behavior, time pressure, was related inversely to heart disease. Note that the correlation between time pressure and the number of diseased arteries was − .18. This indicates that as time pressure increased the number of blocked blood vessels decreased. It is in this type of situation that a multivariate correlational study may be particularly useful. If one of the components being combined to yield the total Type A score actually predicts heart disease in the direction opposite than expected, use of the total score will act to obscure the relationships that are present. A multivariate strategy allows such unexpected findings to be uncovered.

Table 2.1 also illustrates another important concept in health psychology research, that of *statistical significance.* It is possible in any research project that the results obtained are not reliable. If the results are unreliable and the study is conducted again with a different group of subjects, the results will not be similar. The likelihood that a finding in an experiment is unreliable, or due to chance factors, is expressed by probability values. These values are noted in Table 2.1 by the footnotes "$p < .05$" and "$p < .01$." This indicates that there is less than a 5% probability that the relationships between time pressure and potential for hostility with heart disease reported in this study were due to chance and less than a 1% probability that the relationship between anger-in and heart disease was due to chance. The correlation coefficients not noted with asterisks have a greater than 5% probability of being due to chance. For a finding to be considered to be significant in most psychological research, it generally has to have less than a 5% probability ($p < .05$ or smaller) of being due to chance. When a finding is referred to as "significant," this usually means that it is statistically significant: unlikely to be due to chance. Statistical significance is generally reported in correlational studies and controlled experimental studies, discussed later in this chapter.

Correlational studies are typically conducted as was the MacDougall et al. (1985) study just discussed. Two or more variables are measured at the same or nearly the same time, and associations between the two variables are investigated. This type of strategy may be very useful for prediction. For example, the MacDougall et al. study suggests that individuals with symptoms of heart disease who score high on anger-in and hostility and low on time pressure are more likely to suffer from blocked coronary arteries than patients whose scores do not fit this pattern. However, a correlational study of this type does not allow statements regarding causality to be made. It is not possible to say with certainty that these psychological differences increase the risk for the development of heart disease. Instead, blocked coronary arteries may affect a person's outlook on life such that hostility increases and his or her sense of time pressure decreases. Thus, the physical dysfunction might be the cause of the psychological and behavioral characteristics rather than the other way around. Indeed, MacDougall et al. (1985) suggested that "severe artery disease or its concomitants may dampen enthusiasm for time pressured activity" (p. 150). A third possibility also remains, as it may be that both the blocked arteries and these behavioral styles are caused by some other, unmeasured variable, such as a physiological predisposition.

When two or more variables are said to be causally related, it is usually meant that change in one variable is followed by change in another variable. For example, a causal interpretation of the MacDougall et al. (1985) data is that an increase in hostility is followed by an increase in the risk of heart disease. However, most correlational studies provide little information about the temporal sequence of the development of a relationship because all the data are usually collected simultaneously, or nearly so. In order to make more confident inferences regarding causality, an experimental strategy in which variables are actually manipulated or controlled and changes are observed over time is often employed.

## Controlled Experimental Studies

In a controlled experimental study, an investigator controls or manipulates one or more variables and observes changes in another variable or group of variables. For example, if an exercise instructor wished to determine the relationship between physical condition and self-esteem, he or she might assess the self-esteem of two groups of people. One group would then participate in a three-month physical conditioning program, such as jogging or aerobics, whereas the other group continued their normal life-style. At the conclusion of the three-month conditioning program, the self-esteem of both groups would again be assessed. If the group in the physical conditioning program showed an increase in self-esteem during this period whereas the group that did not participate showed little or no change, this would be evidence suggesting that improved physical condition leads to increased self-esteem.

The strength of the experimental study is in its control. Because the physical conditioning program was under the control of the experimenter and measurements were taken immediately prior to and following the program, it is difficult to argue that the differences between the groups in self-esteem change were due to factors other than participation or nonparticipation in the conditioning program. If a correlational design had been applied to the same problem, group members might have been surveyed regarding participation in some form of physical conditioning program and measured for self-esteem. However, if a positive correlation between conditioning and self-esteem were found, this would not justify the conclusion that exercise leading to better physical condition increases self-esteem. Instead, it may be that those with high self-esteem are more likely to exercise and take better care of themselves.

It is very important to understand the difference in these two approaches. In the experimental study the investigator manipulated one variable, participation in an exercise program, and measured a second variable, self-esteem. The variable that was manipulated is the *independent variable*, and the variable that was measured but not directly controlled by the experimenter is the *dependent variable*. An easy way of remembering this distinction is to note that the level of the dependent variable *depends on* the independent variable: self-esteem depends on participation in the physical conditioning program.

This dependence becomes clear by comparing the two groups, the group participating in the conditioning program and the group not participating. In all experiments, the group that is exposed to an experimental manipulation, such as the exercise program in the above example, is called the *experimental group*. The group that is not exposed to a manipulation and serves as a comparison group is referred to as the *control group*. In most controlled experiments, experimental and control groups are compared on one or more dependent variables. If a difference not present at the beginning of the study is present at the end of the study, it is concluded that the differences in the independent variable caused the change in the dependent variable.

In the correlational study there is no manipulation and control of an independent variable. Thus, there are no clear experimental and control groups and no clear dependent and independent variables. Variables are measured but not manipulated. Relationships may be uncovered, but it is difficult to draw conclusions regarding how these relationships developed. Correlational studies provide information that may be very useful in prediction, but this information is often less useful in understanding the factors causing the relationships.

Controlled experiments are particularly useful in health psychology because they provide an excellent model for investigating the effects of a treatment program or searching for the factors responsible for the change produced by a treatment, sometimes referred to as the active elements in a treatment program. An excellent example of using this design in the search for the active elements in a treatment is provided by Andrasik and Holroyd (1980).

Electromyographic (EMG) biofeedback provides an individual with information, or feedback, concerning the level of tension that exists in specific muscles of the body. It would therefore seem to be an ideal treatment for tension headache; if a subject can learn to control and reduce his or her level of muscle tension, then this should result in a decrease in the frequency and intensity of tension headaches. As we will see later in Chapter 14, the use of EMG biofeedback in tension headache is not as universally accepted as this would imply. Frank Andrasik and Kenneth Holroyd have been among the most active invetigators in the attempt to understand the mechanisms underlying tension headache and its treatment.

In their 1980 study, Andrasik and Holroyd exposed twenty-nine tension headache sufferers to one of three EMG biofeedback programs. One group received the standard treatment, in which they used the biofeedback signal to learn to reduce the tension in the muscles in their forehead. In EMG biofeedback, the pitch of a tone typically lowers or the rate of a tone's pulses becomes slower as muscles become more relaxed. Thus, the subjects could listen to the tone, learn what they needed to do to alter the tone in the appropriate manner, and thereby learn to reduce their levels of muscle tension. Two other groups also received biofeedback, but with a difference. One group was led to believe that the biofeedback equipment was indicating a decrease in muscle tension when it was actually indicating an increase. This second group of subjects was actually learning to increase the tension in their muscles while they believed they were learning to decrease tension. The third group also believed that they were learning to decrease the tension in the forehead, or frontal, muscles. However, in their case the feedback was actually related to the level of tension in the muscles of their forearm, so they were not learning to control the level of tension in their frontal muscles. All three groups received seven treatment sessions, scheduled at the rate of two sessions per week, and made daily recordings of the frequency and intensity of their headaches.

You will note that this design is structured to provide information about the importance of actually learning to decrease muscle tension in biofeedback treatment. If learning to decrease muscle tension in the biofeedback session is the active element in treatment, then the first group described above should show more improvement in headache activity than the other two groups. In fact, it might be expected that the second group, the one learning to increase muscle tension, should experience an increase in headache activity. Andrasik and Holroyd (1980) were aware of this possibility, and they regularly evaluated the subjects' headaches so treatment could be stopped if discomfort was increasing.

One final group is needed to complete this design if the investigators wish to be able to confidently attribute to the biofeedback programs whatever changes may be seen. This is the control group, which you will remember from the previous discussion is a group that receives no treatment yet is measured on the dependent variable. Holroyd and Andrasik used a common form of the control group, in which ten tension headache sufferers did not participate in biofeedback sessions but met weekly with the experimenters and turned in records of their headache activity for the previous week. If participation in biofeedback without regard for the nature of the learning that occurs is the important factor in treatment, then it would be expected that all three experimental groups would improve while the control group remains the same.

The results of the treatments were evaluated immediately after the end of the biofeedback sessions and six weeks after the end of the treatment. No significant differences were found to be present between the three experimental groups on any indicators of headache activity immediately after treatment. All three groups improved in comparison to the control group. However, the group that learned to decrease muscle tension improved on more measures of headache activity than the other two experimental groups. The similarities between the three experimental groups increased with the passage of time, so that by the six-week follow-up all three experimental groups were equivalent and improved in headache activity in comparison to the control group.

Based on the similarities in the responses of the three experimental groups and their differences from the control group, Andrasik and Holroyd (1980) were able to conclude that there is something involved in the biofeedback treatment process that facilitates a reduction in headache symptoms, but this important element is not simply learning to reduce levels of muscle tension. The careful reader may have thought, But couldn't the subjects in the increase and in the no-change experimental groups have really been using the biofeedback signal to lower muscle tension even if the signal was inaccurate? If the increase group, for example, had sensed that muscle tension increased as the tone decreased in pitch, might they not have learned to make the tone increase in pitch, thereby lowering their muscle tension? And mightn't learning to relax forearm muscles, like the no-change group did, transfer to an ability to relax forehead muscles?

That such questions may be asked illustrates another important feature of many experiments, namely, the need for a *manipulation check*. In a manipulation check, an investigator determines whether or not the independent variable had the effect on the subjects that the experimenters intended. Andrasik and Holroyd employed a manipulation check to deal with these problems. They checked to see if the subjects actually learned muscle tension control as they were intended to. Indeed, the increase group demonstrated the highest level of muscle tension and the decrease group the lowest level. It thus appears that the changes in headache symptoms were in fact unrelated to learned decreases in frontal muscle tension. Holroyd and Andrasik suggested that all three biofeedback programs provided the subjects with an experience of success at monitoring and controlling their physiological responses. The successes encouraged the subjects to apply active coping strategies when they experienced signs of a headache. These conclusions were supported by the comments of the subjects. All three groups reported learning to use similar coping strategies during the biofeedback sessions, which they later applied to headaches. These strategies included such activities as using fantasy and imagery and focusing attention on bodily sensations. Thus, their success during treatment encouraged them to engage in active coping strategies to deal with their headaches rather than passively accepting the headaches as inevitable.

However, there is an alternative interpretation of the data. Because all subjects learned control of muscle tension, perhaps the important factor in headache improvement was not the perception of success in controlling physiological responses but was instead learned control over muscle tension. Might any type of muscle tension control lead to headache improvement? The Andrasik and Holroyd (1980) study is unable to shed light on which of these interpretations is correct. Instead, an additional study in which the type of learned control of muscle tension _and_ perceived success at muscle tension control are both manipulated as independent variables is required. This type of experiment, in which more than one independent variable is used, is referred to as a _factorial design_. In health psychology, factorial designs are often used to determine the relative contributions of several factors to the results of a treatment program or the causes of a disorder.

Holroyd et al. (1984) used a factorial design to investigate the relative contributions of perceived success and learned control of muscle tension to reductions in headache symptoms. The design was somewhat similar to the previously discussed experiment by Andrasik and Holroyd (1980). Two groups of headache sufferers believed they were receiving biofeedback indicating reductions in frontal muscle tension, but one of these groups actually received feedback for increasing muscle tension. Additionally, half of each group was lead to believe that they were very successful in learning to decrease muscle tension, and half of each group was lead to believe that they were moderately successful. Four groups were thus created: (1) decrease tension/high success, (2) decrease tension/moderate success, (3) increase tension/high success, and (4) increase tension/moderate success. This design is illustrated in Table 2.2. The numbers inside the boxes refer to the average number of headaches per week the subjects in each group reported at the conclusion of treatment.

A look at the number of headaches per week suggests that the most important factor in headache improvement was not whether the subjects learned to increase or decrease muscle tension but instead whether they believed they were successful at reducing muscle tension. This conclusion was supported by other data concerning headache activity, such as headache intensity and hours of headache activity per week. Additionally, subjects who received high-

TABLE 2.2   A Factorial Design: The Effects of Perceived Success and
Biofeedback Strategy on Tension Headaches Per Week

|  |  | *Biofeedback* | |
| --- | --- | --- | --- |
|  |  | *Increase Muscle Tension* | *Decrease Muscle Tension* |
| Perceived Success | High | 5.2 | 3.4 |
|  | Moderate | 6.3 | 7.6 |

SOURCE:   Holroyd et al. (1984). Change mechanisms in EMG biofeedback training: Cognitive changes underlying improvements in tension headache. *Journal of Consulting and Clinical Psychology, 52,* 1039–1053

success feedback felt more confident in their ability to control their headaches, and increases in confidence were positively correlated with improvements in headache symptoms. That is, the greater the increase in confidence, the greater the improvement in headache symptoms. Improvements in headache symptoms were not significantly correlated with changes in muscle tension. Holroyd et al. (1984) were thus able to conclude that an increased sense of competence regarding the ability to control headaches is a more important factor in biofeedback treatment than is the ability to control muscle tension.

Note that this final conclusion illustrates the use of a correlational strategy within a controlled experiment. Reporting a correlation coefficient does not automatically mean that the experimental design precludes an understanding of causality. The important factor is what the experimenter actually did in the experiment. In the case of Holroyd et al. (1984), the independent variables (direction of EMG change and perceived success) were controlled by the experimenters. They could measure perceptions of confidence, muscle tension changes, and headache activity and confidently conclude that their manipulation of the independent variables caused the changes in the dependent variables. The use of the correlation coefficient provided a means of confirming that the degree of change in one dependent variable (headache symptoms) was associated with change in a second dependent variable (confidence in controlling headaches) but not with changes in a third (muscle tension).

The most serious disadvantage to any experiment concerns the generalizability of the results of the study. In the act of exerting control over the experimental setting, the investigator must be careful to keep the experiment as similar as possible to the setting to which he or she wishes to generalize. For example, it is very important that Andrasik and Holroyd's (1980) subjects were all college students who had a problem with headaches. If they had used college students without headache problems similar to those of most patients who seek treatment voluntarily, the applicability of their results to actual headache patients would have been questionable. The degree of resemblance between the experimental setting and the setting to which the results are to be applied is often referred to as the *external validity* of the experiment.

# Practical and Ethical Considerations in Health Psychology Research

No matter which research design is used, research in health psychology is complicated by a variety of factors that all investigators must consider before and during any study. Problem areas studied in health psychology often involve health maintenance or treatment of illness and may require that the investigator collect information regarding or exert control over relatively private aspects of an individual's life. Issues demanding consideration in health psychology research may be generally classified as practical or ethical in nature.

## Practical Issues in Health Psychology Research

NEED FOR FOLLOW-UP   One of the most difficult issues in any health psychology research project concerned with the causes, prevention, or treatment of an illness is related to the need to collect data over a long time-span, frequently during a time after the conclusion of the experiment itself. Collecting data after the conclusion of the formal study is commonly referred to as *follow-up*. Consider the question of the importance of Type A behavior in the development of heart disease. The ideal design for studying this issue would involve measuring a large number of individuals for the presence of Type A behavior, then observing them for the development of heart disease. However, heart disease develops gradually, and the effects of Type A behavior on coronary functioning may appear only after many years have passed. It will therefore be quite difficult for the investigator to follow the original subjects for a long enough period of time to clearly conclude that Type A behavior is a major factor in heart disease.

In a similar vein, imagine the difficulties of a psychologist who has developed a children's behavioral and educational program designed to promote healthy dietary habits in adulthood. Although it may be true that the first and second graders who participate in the program show more knowledge about nutrition and are more likely to choose healthy foods in the school cafeteria, this provides little evidence relevant to the dietary habits these children may possess five, ten, or twenty years later. A follow-up period of many years may be required to fully assess the success of the program. In addition, the reason that dietary changes are considered to be important enough to target in such a program is the expectation that better diet leads to enhanced health in adulthood. Enhanced health should be reflected in fewer illnesses, lower medical bills, and a longer life span. Although many intermediate studies may shed light on the health status and dietary habits of the participants, the ultimate success of the program may best be judged over the entire life-span of the participants. Such problems are not insurmountable, but a Herculean effort may be required to maintain contact with subjects, keep records, and pass the administration of the study along to subsequent investigators.

Although such a project may appear impossible on the surface, long-term follow-up studies have been conducted and are still in operation. These studies, in which subjects are followed over several or many years, are referred to as *longitudinal studies*. They contrast to the more common *cross-sectional studies*, in which subjects are observed for a relatively brief period. Much of our current knowledge concerning the long-term relationships between diet, behavior, and heart disease has come from one longitudinal project: the Framingham study. A group of 2,282 male and 2,845 female citizens of Framingham, a city in Massachusetts, volunteered for this study. Data concerning their psychological adjustment, life-style, health habits, and medical condition have been regularly collected since 1949, and a multitude of research has been generated from the information collected in the course of this project (e.g., Haynes, Levine, Scotch, Feinleib, & Kannel, 1978).

Follow-up is also a very important issue in treatment research, even though the length of time at issue may not be of the same magnitude as in preventive research or a longitudinal project like the Framingham study. Anyone who has tried to make a change in their own behavior is aware that short-term success does not guarantee long-term success. As the joke goes, "It's easy to stop smoking. I've done it a hundred times myself." A similar problem exists in many health psychology treatment studies. It is much more convincing to demonstrate that a treatment has resulted in long-term changes in health or behavior than merely to report that changes were present at the conclusion of a treatment program. Many treatments may be temporarily effective as a result of the presence of a placebo effect. You will remember that the placebo effect refers to the phenomenon by which patients often improve simply because they believe they are receiving effective treatment or because they have faith in the provider. Placebo responses typically fade with time, so the presence of a treatment effect in a follow-up assessment strengthens the conclusion that the treatment's success was more than a placebo effect. For example, the argument presented by Andrasik and Holroyd (1980) for the equal effectiveness of biofeedback designed to increase, decrease, or maintain muscle tension is made even more convincing because they conducted a three-year follow-up study (Andrasik & Holroyd, 1983). All three experimental groups maintained their improvement in headache symptoms over a three-year period, and subjects with similar symptoms who had received no treatment had not improved. It is thus highly unlikely that the improvements seen were placebo effects.

DIFFICULTIES RELATED TO DEPENDENT VARIABLES    Other practical difficulties in health psychology research are related to the nature of the dependent variables commonly seen in the research projects. Studies of an intervention program, be it a preventive or a treatment program, need to specify at some point what a successful outcome is considered to be. In some cases this may be a very complex issue, and the answer may vary dependent upon the person being asked the question. For example, consider the case of an individual being treated for pain following a back injury on the job. If the patient is asked to define a successful treatment, he or she is likely to say that the absence of pain is the major factor determining the success or failure of the treatment. A return to work is likely to be mentioned but not seen as the most important factor. However, if the insurance company and employer are asked the same question, the answer given is more likely to stress coping with pain so that the person may return to work and stop drawing disability payments. The elimination of pain is likely to be secondary in their eyes. In addition, the family may see a reduction in the patient's depression and irritability as very important. Which, if any, of these factors is the most important indicator of treatment success?

Problems such as these are most effectively dealt with by the use of *multiple dependent variables* in a research project. Data concerning several areas of functioning are collected, and the success or failure of a treatment or prevention program is evaluated on several dimensions. The apparently simple question, "Does this program work?" thus becomes "What behaviors, psychological factors, and/or physical measures does this program alter, and to what degree?"

Dependent variables in health psychology research projects may also be difficult to measure. Pain is an obvious example, as pain is an experience that may be directly observed by only one person, the sufferer. Many innovative approaches to measuring pain have been developed and are discussed further in Chapter 14. No single technique is universally accepted as the best, and more than one measurement approach is often used. Another dependent variable that is often of interest in health psychology research concerns "quality of life." It is often important to know to what degree the overall life situation of a person has improved or deteriorated, yet this is a very difficult concept to measure. This issue becomes particularly important in rehabilitation, as with improving medical technology patients are much more likely to survive serious illness and trauma, yet their survival may be plagued by a variety of disabling conditions that reduce the quality of their life.

Procedures have been developed to measure such global concepts as quality of life, but some controversy exists regarding their utility. The Karnofsky Performance Status (in Grieco & Long, 1984) is a frequently used indicator of quality of life. Points are assigned on a 0–100 point scale based on the presence of disease symptoms and the degree to which a person is able to carry on daily activities without assistance. For example, "dead" earns 0 points, "requires occasional assistance but is able to care for most of own needs" earns 60 points, and "normal, no complaints, no evidence of disease" earns 100 points. However, the scale provides little information regarding the internal state of the person rated, and problems such as pain may be missed by the rating. Grieco and Long (1984) pointed out that two persons with ratings of 60 might actually have quite different qualities of life if one suffered moderate pain and the other was pain free. They suggested collecting multiple indicators of quality of life, with some measures drawn from observers and some from self-ratings by the person being observed. Once again, multiple measures of a dependent variable provide a more accurate assessment.

# Ethical Issues in Health Psychology Research

Ethical considerations must play a prominent part in the design and conduct of many health psychology investigations due to the nature of the subject matter under study. Relatively sensitive information concerning the life-style and psychological adjustment of individuals may need to be collected in studies attempting to document important factors contributing to health or illness. Confidentiality may thus be a major concern, as it is important that the information collected about the subjects in a study not be used for any purposes other than what were originally intended. An additional problem may arise in treatment studies, as treatment may need to be withheld or modified in research projects investigating the effectiveness of or the active elements in therapeutic strategies. In these studies, the health of an individual must take precedence over ideal research design considerations, and subjects must be informed as to the possibility that treatment may temporarily be withheld. The importance given to ethical considerations in psychological research is reflected in that the Ethical Principles of Psychologists (APA, 1981) refer directly to standards that must be adhered to in the conduct of research with human subjects. Relevant portions of these principles are presented in Boxed Highlight 2.2. Membership in the American Psychological Association commits a psychologist to these principles.

CONFIDENTIALITY    Maintaining the *confidentiality* of participants' data is one of the most important concerns in many research projects. It will become clear in later chapters that very personal information is sometimes collected in the course of a health psychology research program. For example, we will see in Chapter 9 that the collection of data concerning sexual habits has been useful in research regarding certain forms of cancer. The psychological adjustment of family members has also been studied, as illustrated by the discussion of asthma in Chapter 11. A variety of procedures are commonly used to protect the confidentiality of such personal information.

Case studies present some of the most difficult problems for the maintenance of confidentiality. Detailed presentation of the important information concerning a case may carry the risk that the subject will be identified by some of the readers. In order to reduce this risk, details not directly relevant to the case being described may be altered so as to disguise the subject. Thus, a 40-year-old twice-married male head of an insurance firm in New York may become a 38-year-old divorced vice president of a bank in Des Moines when the case study is published. Another strategy that is sometimes used involves

# Ethical Principles of Psychologists: Research with Human Participants

*Principle 9*
*Research with Human Participants*
The decision to undertake research rests upon a considered judgment by the individual psychologist about how best to contribute to psychological science and human welfare. Having made the decision to conduct research, the psychologist considers alternative directions in which research energies and resources might be invested. On the basis of this consideration, the psychologist carries out the investigation with respect and concern for the dignity and welfare of the people who participate and with cognizance of federal and state regulations and professional standards governing the conduct of research with human participants.

a. In planning a study, the investigator has the responsibility to make a careful evaluation of its ethical acceptability. To the extent that the weighing of scientific and human values suggests a compromise of any principle, the investigator incurs a correspondingly serious obligation to seek ethical advice and to observe stringent safeguards to protect the rights of human participants.

b. Considering whether a participant in a planned study will be a "subject at risk" or a "subject at minimal risk," acccording to recognized standards, is of primary ethical concern to the investigator.

c. The investigator always retains the responsibility for ensuring ethical practice in research. The investigator is also responsible for the ethical treatment of research participants by collaborators, assistants, students, and employees, all of whom, however, incur similar obligations.

d. Except in minimal-risk research, the investigator establishes a clear and fair agreement with research participants, prior to their participation, that clarifies the obligations and responsibilities of each. The investigator has the obligation to honor all promises and commitments included in that agreement. The investigator informs the participants of all aspects of the research that might reasonably be expected to influence willingness to participate and explains all other aspects of the research about which the participants inquire. Failure to make full disclosure prior to obtaining informed consent requires additional safeguards to protect the welfare and dignity of the research participants. Research with children or with participants who have impairments that would limit understanding and/or communication requires special safeguarding procedures.

e. Methodological requirements of a study may make the use of concealment or deception necessary. Before conducting such a study, the investigator has a special responsibility to (i) determine whether the use of such techniques is jusified by the study's prospective scientific, educational, or

*continued*

*BOXED HIGHLIGHT 2.2 continued*

applied value; (ii) determine whether alternative procedures are available that do not use concealment or deception; and (iii) ensure that the participants are provided with sufficient explanation as soon as possible.

f. The investigator respects the individual's freedom to decline to participate in or to withdraw from the research at any time. The obligation to protect this freedom requires careful thought and consideration when the investigator is in a position of authority or influence over the participant. Such positions of authority include, but are not limited to, situations in which research participation is required as part of employment or in which the participant is a student, client, or employee of the investigator.

g. The investigator protects the participant from physical and mental discomfort, harm, and danger that may arise from research procedures. If risks of such consequences exist, the investigator informs the participant of that fact. Research procedures likely to cause serious or lasting harm to a participant are not used unless the failure to use these procedures might expose the participant to risk of greater harm, or unless the research has great potential benefit and fully informed and voluntary consent is obtained from each participant. The participant should be informed

of procedures for contacting the investigator within a reasonable time period following participation should stress, potential harm, or related questions or concerns arise.

h. After the data are collected, the investigator provides the participant with information about the nature of the study and attempts to remove any misconceptions that may have arisen. Where scientific or humane values justify delaying or witholding this information, the investigator incurs a special responsibility to monitor the research and to ensure that there are no damaging consequences for the participant.

i. Where research procedures result in undesirable consequences for the individual participant, the investigator has the responsibility to detect and remove or correct these consequences, including long-term effects.

j. Information obtained about a research participant during the course of an investigation is confidential unless otherwise agreed upon in advance. When the possibility exists that others may obtain access to such information, this possibility, together with the plans for protecting confidentiality, is explained to the participant as part of the procedure for obtaining informed consent.

SOURCE: American Psychological Association, Council of Representatives (1981). *Ethical principals of psychologists.* Washington, D.C.: Author. Copyright (1981) by the American Psychological Association. Reprinted by permission.

merging two similar cases in such a way that identifying details are obscured while data relevant to the purpose of the case history are maintained. Thus, if a psychoanalyst treated two persons suffering from high blood pressure in which the analyst believed repressed hostility was involved, the historical data illustrating this hypothesis might be drawn from both cases yet presented as a single case. In general, the simplest solution is to avoid the presentation of any information not considered necessary to an understanding of the principles illustrated in the case.

Because most research in modern health psychology involves more than one subject, confidentiality is not likely to be breached by the reader identifying the subject. Instead, the major concerns relate to minimizing or eliminating the risk that data collected solely for research are used for other purposes. In a study of psychological adjustment and gastrointestinal disorders such as peptic ulcer it would be very important that information concerning psychological problems not go beyond the researcher's files, considering the difficulties such information might cause for the subjects. In order to avoid such difficulties, records are maintained anonymously, usually by code number rather than by name. In some cases, it may be necessary that a name be at least temporarily retained. For example, in the preceding study the medical records of a subject may need to be examined for indicators of gastric disease in order to relate the information to psychological status. In these studies, confidentiality is maintained by using a system in which very few people (or no one individual) have access to all the information associating the name of an individual with the data. Questionnaires may be identified only by code number and the medical record reviewer may know the record only by code number. The person assigning code numbers to names may never see the data itself. Thus, the only person with the ability to identify the subjects is not privy to the data. After all data are collected and collated, the records connecting the code numbers and names are destroyed, and data analysis proceeds with only code numbers identifying the subjects. In any research project, confidentiality is routinely maintained by entering only identifying numbers into research records. The more sensitive the nature of the information collected and stored, the more elaborate the safeguards employed. A study of quality of life after heart attack (Follick et al., 1988; discussed in more detail in Chapter 8) illustrates how confidentiality can be maintained. In this study, names were never attached to questionnaire response sheets, and the data were stored in a locked file at a hospital that did not have patients participating in the study.

ALTERATIONS OF BEHAVIOR AND HEALTH CARE DELIVERY Many health psychology research projects require changes in the normal course of the subjects' life-style or health care. The intrusions may be quite minor, as in cases in which a subject may be required to complete one or more questionnaires regarding behavior, health status, and /or psychological adjustment. Other studies may require alterations of a much larger magnitude. For example, in studies of the effectiveness of a new therapy, patients seeking treatment may be administered a presumably inactive placebo treatment in order to accurately assess the effectiveness of the new treatment. Studies requiring significant alterations in the health care or health-related behavior of subjects raise particularly difficult ethical considerations.

A variety of issues must be considered by any investigator embarking on a research project requiring subjects to make potentially health-altering life changes. Before any such program is begun, a *risk-benefit analysis* must be performed. A risk-benefit analysis delineates the potential risks the project may pose to the experimental subjects, including factors such as delayed treatment of a disease and temporary discomfort during the experiment itself. Benefits to the subject and to society as a whole are also noted, such as the development of a more effective therapy for a disorder that has resisted treatment or education of the subjects in a relaxation strategy they may find useful outside the confines of the experiment. Risks are weighed against benefits, and the study proceeds only if there appears to be good reason to expect that the long-term benefits of the study outweigh the risks. As the Ethical Principles of Psychologists indicate, the investigator has the responsibility of detecting and removing or correcting any undesirable consequences of the experiment.

The principle of *informed consent* is also of great importance in any study carrying potential risks. Investigators are required to inform the subjects of the presence of significant risks and allow the potential subject to make an informed decision concerning willingness to participate. For example, if a project is investigating the effectiveness of relaxation for treating high blood pressure and the study requires a control group, the investigator is required to inform the prospective subject that he or she may receive an inactive treatment, thus delaying effective treatment of his or her high blood pressure. If a subject declines to participate or requests to withdraw from the study at any time during the experimental procedure, the investigator respects these wishes and allows the subject to withdraw. As the requirement to remove undesirable consequences suggests, active treatment is typically offered to any subject who may have received an inactive treatment during the course of the experiment.

The decision to expose some subjects who might benefit from treatment to a procedure expected to be a placebo or inactive treatment requires special care on the part of the investigator. It is clearly unethical to withhold treatment from a patient desperately in need of treatment and correspondingly unethical to expose that same patient to an experimental treatment when an effective treatment already exists. Some potential subjects may therefore be lost to an experiment as a result of the seriousness of their illness. In contrast, if research results are to be generalizable, it is important that subjects being experimentally treated approximate as nearly as possible the patients expected to be treated in the clinical environment. This need to balance ethical concerns with the need for external validity may lead to screening procedures that rule out many more subjects than are accepted; the aforementioned headache treatment study of Andrasik and Holroyd (1980) began with 1,221 potential subjects and ended with 39 subjects completing the experiment.

In the case of many innovative treatment programs, the question at issue is not simply "Does this treatment work?" but rather "Is this treatment more effective than the existing therapies?" A modified form of a control group may be used in studies comparing the effectiveness of a new treatment to that of an existing therapy, so no subject is denied treatment. Instead, the already existing therapy with known effectiveness is used as the control against which the new treatment is evaluated.

Another alternative that demands consideration, particularly in the early stages of a research program, is the possibility that an *analogue study* may be conducted. In an analogue study a treatment is evaluated under conditions that are similar, but not identical, to those existing in the clinical setting. For example, experimental subjects may be solicited by means of an advertisement announcing an experimental treatment to help people stop smoking. It is hoped that the results will generalize to the clinical setting, in which a physician may order a patient to stop smoking. By beginning the investigation of an experimental therapy in a population with little risk, such as healthy individuals, and gradually increasing the similarity of the experimental and clinical settings, a research program may minimize risks to ill patients and effectively evaluate the utility of an innovative therapy.

Consider the case of an investigator interested in teaching relaxation techniques to people suffering from high blood pressure. Some individuals suffering from high blood pressure are unable to tolerate treatment using medication because of the possibility of serious side effects; the investigator is hopeful that relaxation will provide an effective treatment for these individuals. As a first step, the investigator might assemble a group of volunteer subjects with normal blood pressure, then determine whether or not relaxation training lowers blood pressure in normals. If this experiment is a success, the technique might then be tried in a group of individuals suffering from borderline high blood pressure who do not require medication, because they control their blood pressure through diet and exercise. If both of these studies indicate that relaxation training does lead to a reduction in blood pressure, then the investigator is on firmer ground in making the decision to attempt to use the treatment in a group of high blood pressure patients who would normally be prescribed medication but experience side effects of sufficient intensity to make medication an undesirable alternative. In fact, there is evidence based on such a research tradition that relaxation and stress management training can lead to a reduction in the need for medication in patients with high blood pressure (Crowther, 1983; and see also Chapter 8).

There are some important problems in health psychology in which there are no ethically justifiable methods for using humans as research subjects. Determining the causes of disease and the physiological consequences of health-endangering behaviors under controlled conditions are primary illustrations of these areas. Animal analogue studies, in which nonhuman species are used as research subjects, are frequently conducted in such cases. However, the use of animals as research subjects does not eliminate the need for consideration of ethical principles, and the elimination or minimization of pain and discomfort in animal subjects is of major importance. Ethical princi-

*BOXED HIGHLIGHT 2.3*

# Ethical Principles of Psychologists: Care and Use of Animals

*Principle 10*
*Care and Use of Animals*

An investigator of animal behavior strives to advance understanding of basic behavioral principles and/or to contribute to the improvement of human health and welfare. In seeking these ends, the investigator ensures the welfare of animals and treats them humanely. Laws and regulations notwithstanding, an animal's immediate protection depends upon the scientist's conscience.

a. The acquisition, care, use, and disposal of all animals are in compliance with current federal, state or provincial, and local laws and regulations.

b. A psychologist trained in research methods and experienced in the care of laboratory animals closely supervises all procedures involving animals and is responsible for ensuring appropriate consideration of their comfort, health, and humane treatment.

c. Psychologists ensure that all individuals using animals under their supervision have received explicit instruction in experimental methods and in the care, maintenance, and handling of the species being used. Responsibilities and activities of individuals participating in a research project are consistent with their respective competencies.

d. Psychologists make every effort to minimize discomfort, illness, and pain of animals. A procedure subjecting animals to pain, stress, or privation is used only when an alternative procedure is unavailable and the goal is justified by its prospective scientific, educational, or applied value. Surgical procedures are performed under appropriate anesthesia; techniques to avoid infection and minimize pain are followed during and after surgery.

e. When it is appropriate that the animal's life be terminated, it is done rapidly and painlessly.

SOURCE: American Psychological Association, Council of Representatives (1981). *Ethical principles of psychologists*. Washington, D.C.: Author. Copyright (1981) by the American Psychological Association. Reprinted by permission.

ples concerning the care and use of animals in research are presented in Boxed Highlight 2.3 (APA, 1981).

One of the newer and more innovative uses of animal analogue studies has been proposed by Straub, Singer, & Grunberg (1986). These investigators have reported the development of strains of Type A and Type B Mongolian gerbils; Type A gerbils were bred to be more dominant and prone to more rapid responses than Type B gerbils. Questions not easily studied in humans may be studied in these animals. For example, is a significant component of Type A behavior inherited, or is it largely determined by learning processes? It would obviously be unethical to force Type A humans to marry other Type A humans and reproduce, and correspondingly unethical to control an individual's environment in order to force the learning of Type A behavior. However, such control may be obtained with gerbils, and thus important information regarding Type A behavior and heart disease may be obtained. Important uses of animal analogue studies in cancer research are discussed in Chapter 9.

Of course, the ultimate usefulness of any animal analogue research is determined by the degree to which the animal data collected are generalizable to humans. It must be determined that the Type A gerbils of Straub, Singer, and Grunberg show cardiovascular responses to stress that are similar to those of humans before research using the gerbils as subjects may be seen as applicable to humans. However, the development of potential animal models of Type A behavior and other human behavior patterns could provide previously unavailable methods for studying important health issues.

# Summary

A variety of research designs are used in health psychology. All have specific advantages and disadvantages. The *case study* is most useful during the early stages of research. Case studies often provide insights into previously confusing conditions, allow for the development of new therapeutic approaches, and demonstrate innovative uses of already existing therapies. However, case studies are limited in that the findings may not be generalizable to other cases, alternative explanations for the results may be developed, it is often difficult to specify the essential elements in the treatment program reported, and a possibility for bias exists. The interpretation of case studies is also complicated by the possibility that *placebo effects* may have been responsible for the improvement seen.

*Descriptive group studies* increase the likelihood that generalizable results will be obtained, since more than one subject is studied. In these studies, a group of individuals sharing a common attribute, such as a health-enhancing behavior or an illness, are described on several dimensions, such as personality or family history. The major drawback of the descriptive group study is the lack of a comparison or control group. This disadvantage may be minimized by comparing the results to population averages or by using standardized tests. Descriptive group studies also do not allow for inferences regarding causality to be confidently drawn.

*Correlational studies* allow an investigator to search for relationships between two or more variables. Such information allows for prediction of the values of a target variable when the values of another variable or group of variables are known. Studies with only one predictor variable and one target variable are *univariate* studies. *Multivariate* studies use more than one predictor or target variable. Correlational studies are very useful for exploring the relationships between variables; however, inferences regarding the causes of these relationships must be drawn cautiously, if at all.

The *statistical significance* of a finding is the probability that the finding is due to chance factors and thus not reliable. Statistical significance is commonly reported in correlational studies and controlled experiments.

*Controlled experimental studies* allow for a more confident attribution of causality. In these studies, one or more *independent variables* are manipulated or controlled and the effect of the independent variable(s) on one or more *dependent variables* is observed. Studies with more than one independent variable are referred to as *factorial designs*. A control group that is not exposed to the experimental manipulation is usually compared to one or more experimental groups. Controlled experiments are often used in health psychology to demonstrate the effectiveness of a treatment or to search for the elements in a treatment most responsible for the observed effects. The major risk in a controlled experiment is that the results will not be generalizable if the experimental control applied reduces the *external validity* of the findings. This may be true if the experimental setting bears little or no relationship to the clinical setting.

Health psychology investigators must also consider a variety of practical and ethical issues as they conduct their research. *Follow-up* is often necessary in order to uncover the long-term effects of health-promoting or health-endangering behaviors. *Longitudinal studies* follow groups of individuals over long time-spans. Follow-up may also demonstrate that the benefits derived from a treatment program are not transient. This is important because placebo effects commonly fade with time.

Many of the dependent variables seen in health psychology complicate the conduct of the research itself. It may be difficult to specify exactly what a successful treatment outcome is, and it is difficult to objectively measure dependent variables such as pain and quality of life. *Multiple dependent variables* are often used to alleviate measurement problems.

One of the major ethical issues in health psychology research concerns the need to protect the *confidentiality* of the subjects' data. Information collected in health psychology research projects may be personal or sensitive, involving the life-style and psychological adjustment of the subjects. A variety of procedures are routinely followed to assure the confidentiality of research files.

Alterations in life-style and health care delivery may be required in some health psychology research. A *risk-benefit analysis* compares the potential risks to the subjects to the potential benefits to subjects and society. The potential benefits must outweigh the risks for a research project to be considered ethical. If subjects experience any undesirable consequences, it is the investigators' responsibility to correct these.

Subjects must also give *informed consent* when they participate in a research project. This is especially important in projects requiring the potential withholding or delaying of effective treatment. The health status of the individual subject takes precedence over the need for controlled research. In some cases, people in good health or only slightly ill may serve in *analogue studies* before the techniques are applied to higher-risk groups. When ethical considerations rule out the use of human subjects, animal analogue studies may be conducted.

# *References*

ALEXANDER, F. (1948). Psychoanalytic study of a case of essential hypertension. In F. Alexander & T. M. French, *Studies in psychosomatic medicine: An approach to the cause and treatment of vegetative disturbance* (pp. 298–315). New York: Ronald.

AMERICAN PSYCHOLOGICAL ASSOCIATION, COUNCIL OF REPRESENTATIVES. (1981). *Ethical principles of psychologists.*Washington DC: Author.

ANDRASIK, F., & HOLROYD, K. A. (1980). A test of specific and nonspecific effects in the biofeedback treatment of tension headache. *Journal of Consulting and Clinical Psychology, 48*, 575–586.

ANDRASIK, F., & HOLROYD, K. A. (1983). Specific and nonspecific effects in the biofeedback treatment of tension headache: 3-year follow-up. *Journal of Consulting and Clinical Psychology, 51*, 634–636.

BIRD, E. I., & COLBORNE, G. R. (1980). Rehabilitation of an electrical burn patient through thermal biofeedback. *Biofeedback and Self Regulation, 5*, 283–288.

CROWTHER, J. H. (1983). Stress management training and relaxation imagery in the treatment of essential hypertension. *Journal of Behavioral Medicine, 6*, 169–187.

FOLLICK, M. J., GORKIN, L., SMITH, T. W., CAPONE, R. J., VISCO, J., & STABLEIN, D. (1988). Quality of life post-myocardial infarction: Effects of a transtelephonic coronary intervention system. *Health Psychology, 7*, 169–182.

GENTRY, W. D., SHOWS, W. D., & THOMAS, M. (1974). Chronic low back pain: A psychological profile. *Psychosomatics, 15*, 174–177.

GRIECO, A., & LONG, C. J. (1984). Investigation of the Karnofsky Performance Status as a measure of quality of life. *Health Psychology, 3*, 129–142.

HAYNES, S. G., LEVINE, S., SCOTCH, N., FEINLEIB, M., & KANNEL, W. B. (1978). The relationship of psychosocial factors to coronary heart disease in the Framingham study: I. Methods and risk factors. *American Journal of Epidemiology, 107*, 362–383

HOLROYD, K. A., PENZIEN, D. B., HURSEY, K. G., TOBIN, D. L., ROGERS, L., HOLM, J. E., MARCILLE, P. J., HALL, J. R., & CHILA, A. G. (1984). Change mechanisms in EMG biofeedback training: Cognitive changes underlying improvements in tension headache. *Journal of Consulting and Clinical Psychology, 52*, 1039–1053.

KAZDIN, A. E. (1980). *Research design in clinical psychology.* New York: Harper & Row.

MACDOUGALL, J. M., DEMBROSKI, T. M., DIMSDALE, J. E., & HACKETT, T. P. (1985). Components of Type A, hostility, and anger-in: Further relationships to angiographic findings.*Health Psychology, 4*, 137–152.

SARGENT, J. D., GREEN, E. E., & WALTERS, E. D. (1972). The use of autogenic feedback training in a pilot study of migraine and tension headaches. *Headache, 12*, 120–125.

STRAUB, R. O., SINGER, J. E., & GRUNBERG, N. E. (1986). Toward an animal model of Type A behavior. *Health Psychology, 5*, 71–85.

# PART II

# Models in Health Psychology

# Physiological Bases of Health and Illness

This chapter will examine the major physiological bases of health and illness behavior. First, the genetic bases for behavior will be examined. This will be followed by brief discussions of the central and peripheral nervous systems, the endocrine system, the cardiovascular system, the respiratory system, and the gastrointestinal tract. Finally, the immune system will be discussed and important interactions between the brain and immune processes will be discussed.

## Genetic Bases of Behavior

Psychology is often described as the study of human behavior. Thus, health psychologists tend to emphasize the importance of behavioral factors in the promotion and maintenance of health as well as in the prevention and treatment of illness (cf. Matarazzo, 1980). These behavioral factors, such as the role of environmental events in learning, are reviewed in Chapter 4. It is important to remember, however, that human behavior is influenced by both genetic and environmental factors. Indeed, genetic and environmental factors interact in a very complex fashion in the development and behavior of human beings. The current view among psychologists is that genetic factors, or heredity, set the limits for what an individual's potential behavior can be. However, favorable or unfavorable environmental conditions influence the expression of behavior within those limits.

An example of the interaction between heredity and environment may be found in the development of peptic ulcers. There is consistent evidence that high levels of *pepsinogen*, the precursor of a gastric enzyme (pepsin) that aids in digestion, are associated with the development of peptic ulcers and that pepsinogen level is an inherited characteristic (Mirsky, 1958; Mirsky et al., 1952; Pilot et al., 1957). However, not all people with high levels of pesinogen develop ulcers. The eventual development of peptic ulcers, then, is determined by both heredity and other factors, such as environmental conditions (see Chapter 13 for further discussion of environmental conditions related to peptic ulcer development). Moreover, once a person has developed a peptic ulcer, his or her health care behavior, which is shaped by environmental factors such as previous experience with physicians, will influence the degree to which the ulcer improves or worsens. The individual's health care behavior includes actions such as following carefully the medication and diet regimens prescribed by the physician and altering environmental conditions or one's responses to those conditions that are associated with increased ulcer activity.

## Chromosomes and Genes

The hereditary units that we receive from our parents and transmit to our children are carried by structures, known as *chromosomes*, that are found within the nucleus of each body cell. Among human beings, each cell contains twenty-two pairs of somatic chromosomes and one pair of sex chromosomes (XY in males and XX in females) for a total of forty-six chromosomes.

Each chromosome is composed of several thousand hereditary units known as *genes*. These genes are actually large molecules of *deoxyribonucleic acid*, or *DNA*. Each molecule resembles a twisted ladder, or double helix (see Figure 3.1). The sides of the ladder are composed of chains of alternating sugar and phosphate and the rungs that attach the sugars consist of matched pairs of adenine and thymine or guanine and cytosine. The specific sequence in which the rungs of the double helix are arranged within the molecule determines the instructions for the development of cells into the different structures of our bodies. Given the large number of genes within each chromosome, it is very unlikely that any two individuals, even among brothers or sisters, will have exactly the same hereditary features. Only identical twins, who develop from the same fertilized ovum, carry exactly the same genes and hereditary traits.

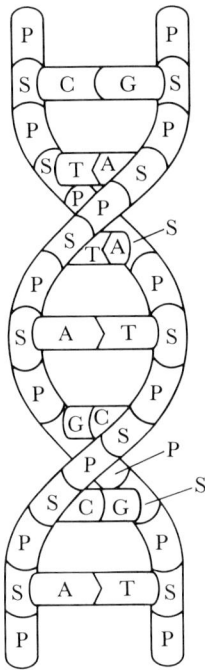

FIGURE 3.1 The Structure of the DNA Molecule. The strands of the molecule are composed on an alternating sequence of sugar (S) and phosphate (P). The rungs that attach the strands are composed of adenine (A) and thymine (T) or guanine (G) and cytosine (C). Adapted from R. L. Atkinson, R. C. Atkinson, and E. Hilgard, 1983, *Introduction to Psychology* (8th ed.) (p. 54), New York: Harcourt, Brace Jovanovich.

## Hereditary Transmission

Similar to chromosomes, genes are also found in pairs. One gene is contributed by the father and one is contributed by the mother. The specific genetic constitution of an individual is known as the person's *genotype*. The physiological state or physical appearance of the individual is known as the *phenotype*.

Genes may be either *dominant* (e.g., brown eye color) or *recessive* (e.g., blue eye color). When the genes of any given gene pair are both alike, regardless of whether they are dominant or recessive, the individual will display the trait that is determined by the gene pair. The phenotype, then, will be consistent with the genotype. However, when the gene pair consists of one dominant and one recessive gene, the phenotype will be determined by the dominant gene although the recessive gene may be transmitted to the individual's children. The trait associated with the recessive gene may be displayed by one or more of the children if both the mother and father carry the same recessive gene.

SEX-LINKED GENES   It was noted earlier in this chapter that the twenty-third pair of chromosomes in each cell determines the individual's sex. Thus, the genes found in the pair 23 position are said to be sex-linked. A normal female carries two similar chromosomes in pair 23 called X chromosomes (XX). Normal males, however, have one X chromosome and a different chromosome, Y, in pair 23 (XY).

The X chromosome may carry either dominant or recessive genes whereas the Y chromosome carries primarily recessive genes. There are several disorders associated with defective, recessive genes on the X chromosome that appear primarily in males because the Y genes found on the other chromosome cannot block the expression of the disorders. These are termed *recessive X-linked disorders* and include color blindness, Duchenne muscular dystrophy, and classical hemophilia. Sons of mothers who carry the defective gene have a 50% chance of receiving the X chromosome with the defective gene and thus displaying the disorder. One-half of the daughters of these mothers also carry the defective gene and also have a 50% probability of producing abnormal sons. In addition, there is an X-linked dominant inheritance pattern in which the mothers display the abnormal phenotype associated with a defective dominant gene; the sons who carry the defective gene on their X chromosome are also affected by this gene.

## Chromosomal Imbalance Syndromes

There are several disorders that are caused by various forms of *aneuploidy*, or deviations from the normal number of forty-six chromosomes. These disorders are usually associated with varying degrees of mental retardation as well as abnormal physical appearance.

The most common aneuploidy involves the presence of three chromosomes in what ordinarily would be the pair 21 position. The result is *Down's syndrome*, or Trisomy 21. There are three forms of this disorder, all of which are associated with slanting eyes, thickened eyelids, folded ears, and a high risk for congenital heart disease. Most of these children are moderately to severely retarded (i.e., IQ scores ranging between three and five standard deviations below the normative mean and significant deficits in social functioning).

Another aneuploidy involves a missing X chromosome in what would normally be pair 23. The resulting condition, *Turner's syndrome*, occurs only among females. The affected individuals tend to be short, sexually underdeveloped, with broad chests and low posterior hairlines. Mental retardation is present in about 10% of these people, and approximately one-third of those with Turner's syndrome have congenital heart defects, neurosensory hearing loss, or disorders involving the urinary tract.

There are also several disorders that arise from the presence of an extra chromosome in the pair 23 position. *Klinefelter's syndrome* is characterized by the presence of two X chromosomes and one Y. People with this disorder are generally phenotypically male, but they also have feminine sexual features, including enlarged breasts and small testicles that do not produce sperm. Mental retardation is found in about 50% of persons with Klinefelter's syndrome. There are also a few females with the XXY gene configuration, however, who do not experience the physical or mental problems encountered by XXY males.

A small number of males are born with an extra Y chromosome (type XYY). These men tend to be taller and to have stronger sexual drives than normal XY males. Several early studies found that the prevalence of XYY males within the prison population, especially among violent offenders, was several times that expected by chance alone (Jacobs et al., 1965, 1968; Jarvik et al., 1973). Although these early findings have not been replicated consistently, there has been a great deal of speculation that the extra Y chromosome may lead to excessive productions of testosterone and highly aggressive antisocial behavior. It must be remembered, however, that the aggressiveness that has been observed among XYY males may be due, in part, to environmental factors. For example, the unusual height of XYY males, coupled with the mental retardation that is sometimes associated with this disorder, may provoke negative reactions from persons in the environment that can lead to aggressive reponses and possibly to arrest and imprisonment (Wiggins et al., 1976). Moreover, not all XYY males have been found to be highly aggressive or violent, indicating that the presence of an extra Y chromosome alone does not reliably predict antisocial behavior.

Finally, there are many disorders that are caused by mutations of single genes or interactions among multiple genes. Mutations are caused by changes in the DNA sequence of a gene that, in turn, alter the structure and function of the protein whose production is governed by that gene. If the affected protein is an enzyme, abnormalities in body metabolism may reult. This process is exemplified by *phenylketonuria* (PKU). This is a metabolic disorder characterized by a deficiency in the liver enzyme phenylalanine hydroxylase. The enzyme deficiency leads to the production of excessive amounts of phenylalanine in the blood stream, which causes damage to the brain. The end result is mental retardation, irritability, seizures, or autistic behavior.

Gene mutations that alter structural proteins can also produce harmful effects such as sickle-cell anemia. In this disorder, Hemoglobin S molecules take on a curved, sicklelike shape that entraps red blood cells in the small blood vessels. This process inhibits the flow of oxygenated blood to certain body areas, causing the patient to suffer from recurrent painful episodes involving the back, chest, limbs, or abdomen. Severe cases of sickle-cell anemia may lead to life-threatening health problems such as kidney failure, strokes, or liver and bone damage (Cozzi et al., 1987). It should be noted, however, that not all gene mutations produce negative results. Some produce no harmful effects, or others may be beneficial to the individual.

Unlike single-gene mutations, interactions among multiple genes may directly and negatively affect entire organ systems and adjacent organ structures. Disorders produced by multiple-gene interactions include cleft palate, clubfoot, congenital hip dislocation, some forms of congenital heart disease, and various types of neural tube defects such as hydrocephalus and anencephaly. As in the case of single-gene mutations, it should be emphasized that there are many neutral and positive human traits that result from multiple-gene interactions. Intelligence, height, body frame, and emotional reactivity are determined by a large number of genes. The effects of these genetic interactions, in turn, are modified by the individual's interactions with his or her environment.

# Genetic Studies of Human Behavior

Three major methods have been used to study the extent to which genetic factors account for certain behavioral traits among humans. This area of study is called *behavioral genetics*. The three study methods are family studies, twin studies, and adoption studies. The behaviors that have been investigated include intelligence, aggression, psychiatric disorders, and criminality.

FAMILY STUDIES    Family studies evaluate the genetic basis of a behavioral trait by examining the incidence of the trait among the biological relatives of an affected individual during a designated period of time. The incidence rate within the family members is then compared with the incidence rate in the general population. For example, it has been found that children's IQ scores are more highly correlated with those of their parents than with those of randomly selected nonrelatives (Mussen et al., 1979). Similarly, early studies of schizophrenia revealed that the risk of developing this condition was substantially higher among the biological relatives of affected individuals than the risk in the general population (Kallman, 1938).

TWIN STUDIES    Identical twins are said to be *monozygotic* because they develop from a single fertilized ovum and share the same genetic material. Fraternal twins are said to be *dizygotic* because they develop from different ova and are no more alike genetically than ordinary siblings. Thus, twin studies compare the incidence of a behavioral trait among both members of monozygotic and dizygotic twin pairs. If there is a significant genetic component to the behavioral trait, that trait will be shared much more frequently among the monozygotic twin pairs. For example, it has been found that the IQ scores of monozygotic twins reared together are more highly correlated than those of both dizygotic twins and nontwin siblings who also are reared together (Crampton et al., 1981).

   Another approach to twin studies involves studying the incidence of behavioral traits between twins raised together and twins raised apart. Bouchard and McGue (1981), for example, summarized the results of 111 studies of genetic influences on intelligence. They found that the correlations in intelligence scores between monozygotic twins raised together (.86) and between those raised apart (.72) were substantially higher than those of dizygotic twins raised together (.60) and non-twin siblings raised together (.47).

ADOPTION STUDIES    Adoption studies examine the incidence of a trait among adopted children as well as among their biological and adoptive parents. If genetic factors play a large role in the development of a behavioral trait, then the incidence of a trait among adopted children of the affected biological parents will be higher than that among adopted children whose biological parents do not show the trait. It is also possible to study the incidence of the trait among biological parents of adopted children who show the trait. The influence of genetic factors may be established if the incidence of the trait among the biological parents exceeds that in (a) the biological parents of adopted children without the trait and (b) the nonbiological relatives of adopted children, regardless of whether or not the children display the trait.

Adoption studies have been used successfully in establishing a genetic basis for schizophrenia. Heston (1966), for example, examined the incidence of schizophrenia among children who were given up for adoption soon after birth by schizophrenic or nonschizophrenic mothers. It was found that adopted children of the schizophrenic biological mothers later showed a much higher incidence of schizophrenia and other forms of psychiatric disturbance than the adopted children of the normal biological mothers. Another series of studies, performed in Denmark (Kety, 1975; Tsuang, 1976), found that the incidence of schizophrenia in the biological relatives of adopted children with this disorder (8%) was significantly greater than that in the biological relatives of adopted children without schizophrenia (2%). The incidence of schizophrenia in the adoptive relatives of the schizophrenic and nonschizophrenic children was 1.5% and 3%, respectively.

These adoption studies clearly reveal, then, that genetic factors play an important role in the development of schizophrenia. However, it is also clear that many biological relatives of schizophrenic children are not affected by the disorder and that children of schizophrenic mothers do not necessarily develop the disorder themselves. Thus, environmental factors must moderate the relationship between heredity and schizophrenia. Indeed, Zubin and Spring (1977) have proposed a *diathesis-stress* model of schizophrenia in which it is assumed that some persons inherit a predisposition (diathesis) for the development of schizophrenia. However, it is also proposed that only those vulnerable individuals who are also exposed to stressful environmental conditions with which they cannot adequately cope actually develop the disorder. A similar diathesis-stress model for the development of medical disorders is described in Chapter 5.

## The Nervous System and Organ Systems of the Body

We have learned that behavior is influenced by both genetic factors and environmental events. However, we must also examine how various organ systems within the body operate to produce human behavior. An understanding of these systems is essential to fully comprehend the diseases that affect these systems and the role of psychological factors in the development, course, and treatment of these diseases, as well as in the maintenance of health.

# The Nervous System

The primary determinant of human behavior is the nervous system, which comprises the *central nervous system* (CNS) and the *peripheral nervous system*. Unless the nervous system is structurally intact and functions properly, an individual cannot interact successfully within his or her environment.

CENTRAL NERVOUS SYSTEM   The CNS comprises the brain and the spinal cord. It may be thought of as the center for integrating and coordinating all bodily functions and behavior. The peripheral nervous system, then, is primarily responsible for transmitting information into and away from the CNS.

During the prenatal development period among mammals, the CNS begins to form as a tubular structure called the *neural tube.* The anterior portion of the neural tube develops into the brain while the remainder becomes the spinal cord. As the prenatal development period continues, the brain becomes subdivided into several regions with specialized functions. The outer portion of the brain forms the *cerebral hemispheres,* or *cerebrum,* which form the largest portion of the brain in human beings. Figure 3.2 shows that they are con-

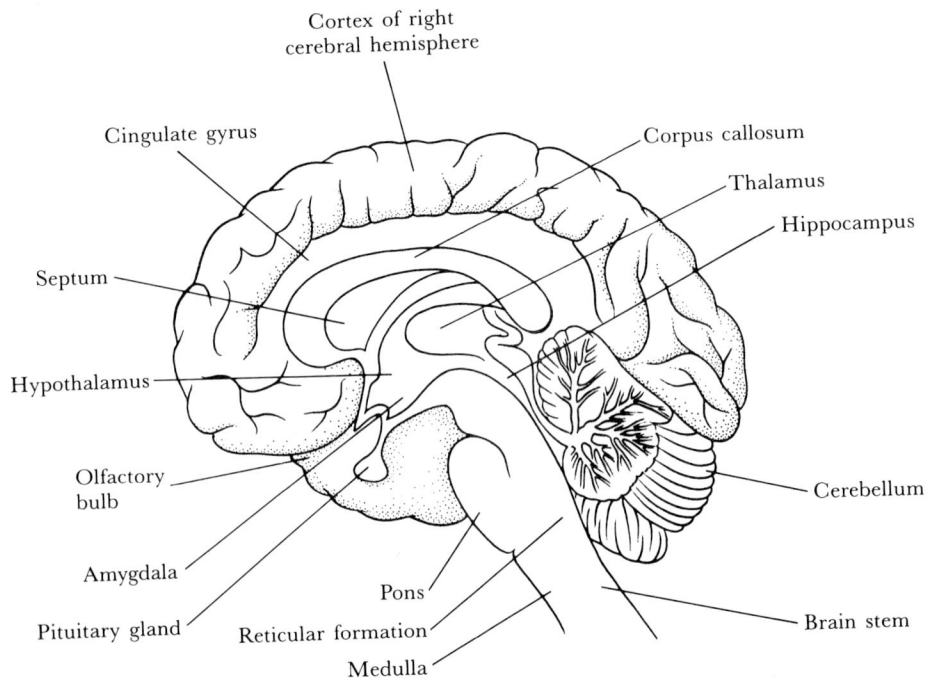

FIGURE 3.2   Midline view of the brain depicting the cerebrum and deeper brain structures. Adapted from *Psychology and Medicine* (p.58) by D. A. Bakal, 1979, New York: Springer.

nected by a band of fibers termed the *corpus callosum*. The cerebral hemispheres are responsible for controlling many bodily functions. These include voluntary motor movements, sense perception involving temperature, touch, body movement, pain, vision, hearing, taste, and smell, and learning, memory, thinking, and consciousness.

The deeper portions of the brain below the cerebrum are responsible for the basic bodily processes and survival. The *limbic system* is composed of several structures that lie along the innermost edge of the cerebral hemispheres. The major limbic structures include the hippocampus, cingulate gyrus, olfactory bulb, septum, and amygdala. The functioning of the limbic system structures is not well understood. However, it is known that the hippocampus plays a special role in memory. People who sustain damage to the hippocampus are unable to store new information in memory although they retain skills and information learned prior to the brain injury. The limbic system also appears to be involved in regulating emotional reactions and instinctive behaviors such as eating, exhibiting aggression, and fleeing from danger. Lesions of the amygdala have been found to inhibit predatory behaviors in many animal species (Gay, Cole, & Leaf, 1976) and surgical lesions of the cingulate gyrus have been used in a small number of humans to reduce or eliminate chronic, severe pain that has been unresponsive to other treatments (Foltz, 1976).

Below the limbic system are the deepest and oldest portions of the brain. Figure 3.2 shows that these portions include the *brain stem, hypothalamus, thalamus, medulla, reticular activating system*, and the *cerebellum*. The brain stem is the oldest part of the brain and is located at the point at which the spinal cord enters the skull. Most of the activities controlled by the brain stem are reflexive in nature rather than voluntary. In addition, the brain stem is responsible for relaying incoming or afferent sensory messages from the spinal cord to the upper portions of the brain.

The medulla appears as a swelling on the lower portion of the brain stem. It is involved in the control of breathing, heart rate, and blood pressure. The cerebellum is located slightly above the medulla and is dedicated primarily to the coordination of movement. Although voluntary movements are initiated in the cerebral hemispheres, the cerebellum regulates muscle tone and coordinates the various muscle activities that allow us to perform complex voluntary movements as well as to maintain our balance and stand erect. The two lobes of the cerebellum are connected by a set of nerve fibers called the *pons*.

The thalamus and hypothalamus are located just above the brain stem. One region of the thalamus receives sensory information from the eyes and projects this information to the portions of the cerebrum responsible for vision. Other areas of the thalamus project information from the ears and the spinal cord to the portions of the cerebrum responsible for hearing, touch, and body position. In addition, the thalamus is involved in the regulation of sleep and wakefulness in conjunction with the reticular activating system.

The hypothalamus is located between the thalamus and the pituitary gland. It is a vital structure in the regulation of sexual, drinking, and feeding activity. It is also involved in the regulation of body temperature and metabolism. Moreover, it regulates the endocrine system by means of its influence on the nearby pituitary gland.

The reticular activating system (RAS) is a tangled mass of nerve fibers that extends from the lower brain stem up to the thalamus and projects to the cerebrum. The primary function of the RAS is to regulate arousal levels, ranging for sleep to states of high alertness. The RAS may also play a role in our ability to focus attention on some aspects of sensory information and to ignore others. That is, the RAS appears to serve as a filter for incoming sensory information, allowing some of the sensory messages to reach the cerebral hemispheres and blocking the transmission of other messages.

PERIPHERAL NERVOUS SYSTEM    As noted earlier, the peripheral nervous system brings information (afferents) into the central nervous system and transmits commands (efferents) back to the muscles. The portion of the peripheral nervous system that connects the CNS with voluntary msucles is known as the *somatic system*, and the portion that connects the CNS with involuntary muscles, such as the heart and lungs, is called the *autonomic* system. The term *autonomic* is used because it usually appears to operate independently, without conscious awareness or control. Thus, we do not usually need to think about regulating the activities of our hearts, lungs, or glands, which are controlled by the autonomic nervous system. However, it is necessary for us to learn to control such autonomic functions as urination and defecation. Furthermore, it is possible for us to learn to exert some control over other autonomic functions using techniques such as biofeedback and deep muscle relaxation. These autonomic functions include blood pressure, muscle tension levels, and peripheral blood flow. Learning to control these functions are important components of behavioral treatments for essential hypertension and headaches. This topic is discussed in detail in Chapters 8 and 14.

The autonomic nervous system is further divided into two parts, the *sympathetic* and *parasympathetic* systems. Many organs receive efferents from both the sympathetic and parasympathetic systems but the two systems have entirely different functions. The sympathetic system is responsible for increasing organ activity in order to prepare the individual for responding to states of excitement such as sexual situations and to stressors such as threats to life. For example, the sympathetic system increases heart rate and blood pressure as well as the secretion of epinephrine and norepinephrine, which further increase arousal levels.

The sympathetic system tends to influence several different organ systems at one time. However, its counterpart, the parasympathetic system, tends to affect organs in a more piecemeal fashion. Its function is to reduce the activity of organs and to allow the body to restore energy that has been depleted by the actions of the sympathetic system. It is also involved in regulating digestion, directing tissue repair, and enabling wastes to be eliminated from the body.

It should be noted that the sympathetic and parasympathetic systems do not always act in an entirely antagonistic fashion. For example, coordination of the two systems is necessary for successful sexual functioning among males. The parasympathetic system is involved in the erection of the penis whereas the sympathetic system controls the ejaculatory response. Interaction of the two systems is also seen in the digestive process, which will be discussed in greater detail later in this chapter.

## The Endocrine System

It was noted earlier that the autonomic nervous system regulates the activities of some glands as well as voluntary muscles. Indeed, many of the bodily responses that are initiated by autonomic nervous system activity are mediated by the effects of the nervous system on the endocrine glands. These endocrine glands, which are shown in Figure 3.3, secrete *hormones* that are carried throughout the body by the bloodstream. These hormones, then, influence a wide variety of bodily reponses, but they act more slowly than does the autonomic nervous system.

The *pituitary gland* is located near the hypothalamus and is controlled by this brain structure. This has been termed the *master gland* because it produces at least eight hormones and controls the activity of several other endocrine glands, including the thyroid gland, sex glands, and the outer portions, or *cortex*, of the adrenal glands.

The *adrenal glands* lie on top of the kidneys and, together with the hypothalamus and pituitary gland, play an important role in determining an individual's response to stress. The integrated activity of these structures has been termed the *hypothalamic-pituitary-adrenal axis*. Each adrenal gland contains an inner core, the *medulla*, and an outer layer, the cortex. Stimulation of the sympathetic nervous system causes the adrenal medullae to secrete two hormones, *epinephrine* (adrenaline) and *norepinephrine* (noradrenaline). These two hormones are called *catecholamines* and circulate throughout the body's blood vessels. Epinephrine often works in conjunction with the sympathetic portion of the autonomic nervous system in preparing the individual for emergency action. Epinephrine increases the heart rate and the activity of the sweat glands. In addition, it stimulates the RAS, which, in turn, further excites the sympathetic system; the end result is that the adrenal glands secrete even more epinephrine, and emotional arousal is maintained for a sustained period of time.

Norepinephrine, similar to epinephrine, increases heart rate and generally causes the same effects as does stimulation of the sympathetic nervous system. In addition, it stimulates the pituitary gland to release *adrenocorticotrophic hormone* (ACTH). This hormone acts on the adrenal cortex, which releases a group of hormones called the *corticosteroids*. One subgroup of the cortico-

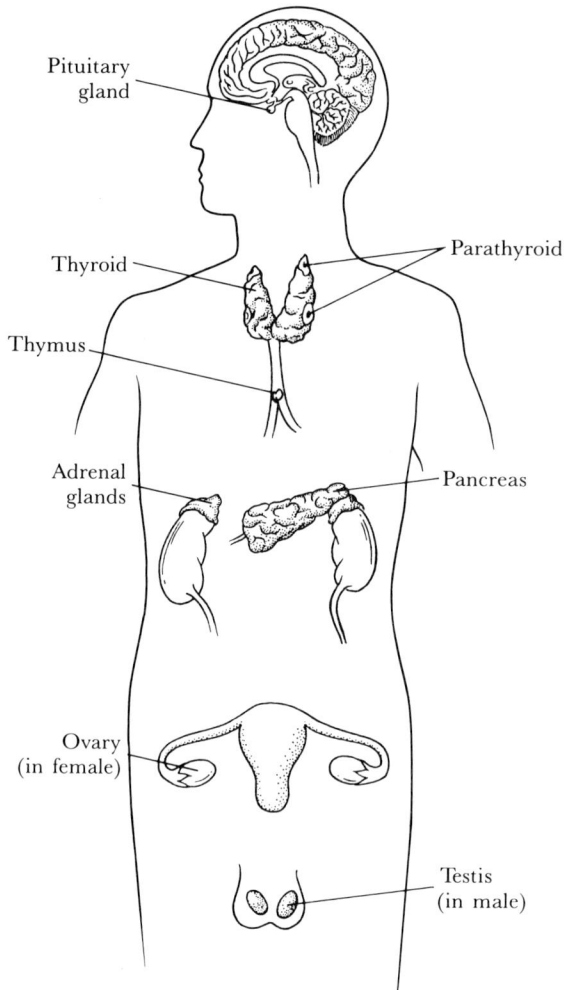

FIGURE 3.3   The major endocrine glands that interact with the nervous system in the regulation of bodily activity. Adapted from *Introduction to Psychology* (8th ed.) (p. 52) by R. L. Atkinson, R. C. Atkinson, and E. Hilgard, 1983, New York: Harcourt, Brace Jovanovich.

steroids is known as the *glucocorticoids*. The major glucocorticoid is *cortisol*, which produces a rapid release of glucose from the liver and inhibits inflammatory processes in damaged tissue.

In summary, then, there are an important series of interactions that take place between the central and peripheral nervous systems and the endocrine system. Stimulation of the sympathetic nervous system by stressful or other arousing environmental events directly causes the adrenal medullae to release

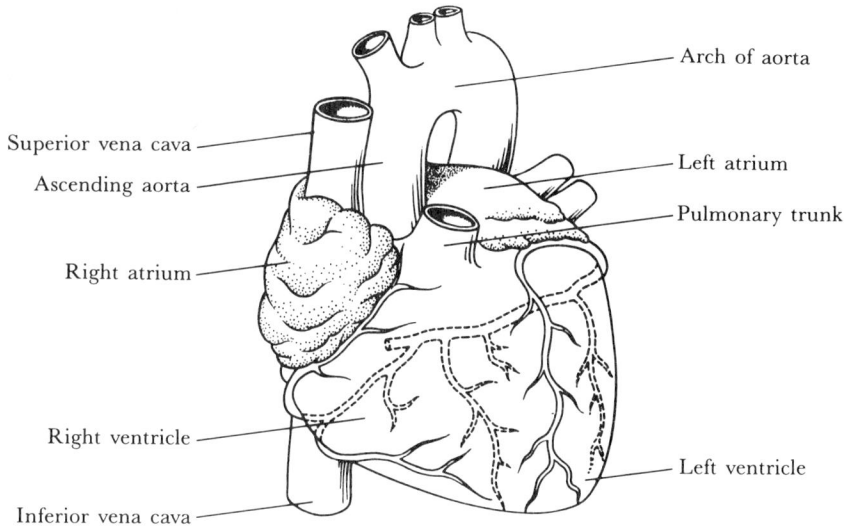

FIGURE 3.4   Illustration of the heart and coronary circulation system. Adapted from *Laboratory Exercises in Human Anatomy with Cat Dissections* (p. 315) by J. G. Tortora, 1984, New York: Macmillan.

catecholamines into the bloodstream. Moreover, norepinephrine release indirectly affects the adrenal cortex. It stimulates the pituitary gland to release ACTH, which, in turn, causes the adrenal cortex to secrete the corticosteroids. The hypothalamus also causes the pituitary gland to release ACTH and activates corticosteroid production in the adrenal cortex. Hence, the hypothalamic-pituitary-adrenal cortex axis forms a self-sustaining system that maintains emotional arousal. This system accounts in large part for the power of stressful or excitatory stimuli to produce prolonged periods of emotional arousal even after the stimuli have been removed from the environment (e.g., the sustained arousal that is felt after viewing a frightening movie or witnessing an exciting athletic contest).

## The Cardiovascular System

The cardiovascular system consists of the heart, the blood, the arteries that transport oxygenated blood throughout the body, the smaller capillaries, and the veins that carry blood back to the heart. The heart is the most important muscle in the body and the most important organ in the cardiovascular system. It functions as a pump that circulates blood throughout the body. Figure 3.4 shows a diagram of the heart. Newly oxygenated blood in the lungs enters the left atrium and is then pumped from the left ventricle through the aorta and then throughout the arterial system. The circulation of the blood carries oxygen and nutrients to all portions of the body. The oxygen and nutrients are exchanged for the waste materials of the cells and the blood returns by means of the venous system to the right side of the heart. The blood then enters the right atrium and is pumped to the lungs via the pulmonary artery by the right ventricle. Once the blood is again oxygenated, it returns to the left atrium through the pulmonary veins.

The flow of blood to and from the heart is regulated by the opening and closing of valves that connect the ventricles with the atria and with the aorta in the pulmonary artery. The blood flow is also controlled by the regular phases of contraction and relaxation of the heart itself. These phases, which consist of the *systole* and *diastole*, are known as the *cardiac cycle*. The heart contracts during the systolic phase and pumps blood through the arterial system; pressure in the blood vessels increases during this phase. The relaxation of the heart muscle, or diastolic phase, allows blood to return to the heart and blood pressure decreases.

Blood pressure is the force that the blood exerts against the arterial and venous walls. The blood pressure measurement obtained during a physical examination is a ratio, measured in millimeters of mercury, of maximum blood pressure during the systolic phase to minimum blood pressure during the diastolic phase. Blood pressure measures are recorded by inflating an air-filled cuff around the arm in order to constrict an artery. The cuff then is slowly deflated until the sound of the blood flow through the artery is heard through a stethoscope. Systolic blood pressure is the pressure displayed in the *sphygmomanometer* at which the sound of the blood flow (Korotkoff sounds) is first detected. Diastolic blood pressure is that at which the Korotkoff sounds disappear. For most individuals, systolic blood pressure may range from 100 mm Hg to 145 mm Hg; diastolic blood pressure will vary from 60 mm Hg to 95 mm Hg.

Blood pressure can be affected by several factors. One factor is the volume of blood, or cardiac output. An increased rate of pumping or increased strength of the heart contractions will increase cardiac output. Thus, stressful situations that produce excitation of the sympathetic nervous system will increase the release of catecholamines, which, in turn, will increase heart rate, cardiac output, and blood pressure. Another factor is the thickness, or viscosity, of the blood. This thickness is determined by the amount of red blood cells, or *erythrocytes*, within the liquid plasma. As blood viscosity increases, blood pressure tends to increase. A third important factor that influences blood pressure is the structure of the arterial walls. Again, stressful situations that heighten activity of the sympathetic nervous system will result in the release of catecholamines that constrict most blood vessels and contribute to an increase in blood pressure. Narrowing of the arteries, or *atherosclerosis*, is produced by thick deposits of cholesterol and other substances on the arterial walls. These deposits become hard *plaques* that reduce arterial blood flow and contribute to increases in blood pressure. The formation of plaque, which can begin late in childhood or during early adolescence, may also lead to permanent damage to the arterial walls because the plaque interferes with the passage of oxygen and nutrients from the capillaries to cells of the arterial wall.

# The Respiratory System

The respiratory system is described in Chapter 11. It is sufficient, at this point, to note that the primary functions of the respiratory system are to provide oxygen to and eliminate carbon dioxide from the blood. Air is inhaled through the nose and mouth and passes through the pharynx, larynx, and trachea to the bronchi that lead to the lungs. Oxygen enters the small blood vessels within the lungs and circulates through the body. At the same time, carbon dioxide passes from these small vessels to the lungs for removal from the body in exhaled air.

# The Gastrointestinal System

The gastrointestinal (GI) tract is composed of two overlapping layers of muscle. The inner layer consists of circular muscle that contracts in order to mix the contents of the bowel, propel the contents down the GI tract, or prevent passage of additional bowel contents. The outer layer is composed of longitudinal muscle. Contractions of this muscle layer also contribute to the downward movement of bowel contents and increase the tone of the gut. The inner surface of the circular muscle is covered with mucosa that contain secretory cells and numerous nerve endings (Whitehead & Schuster, 1985).

Figure 3.5 shows a diagram of the anatomy of the GI tract. There are four major portions of the GI tract, each of which is bounded by two sphincters. These major portions are the esophagus, stomach, small intestine (duodenum, jejunum, and ileum), and colon.

ESOPHAGUS   The esophagus is a simple tubelike structure that functions to transport food to the stomach and prevent the contents of the stomach from backing up or refluxing into the esophagus. It is bounded by an upper and a lower esophageal sphincter. The esophagus accomplishes food transport by a series of peristaltic contractions that push the food downward toward the stomach. It should be noted that the peristaltic contractions are initiated by parasympathetic nerve fibers and inhibited by sympathetic nerve activity. Sympathetic nerve fibers are also responsible for contracting the upper and lower esophageal sphincters. The relationship between autonomic nervous system activity and muscle contractions found in the esophagus generally hold true throughout the GI tract.

STOMACH   The stomach is a stretchable sack that is bounded by the lower esophageal sphincter and by the pyloric sphincter. The pyloric sphincter regulates the rate at which the stomach contents are released into the small intestine and prevents reflux from the intestine into the stomach. The stomach's functions are the mixing and digesting of food as well as the breakdown of protein. These functions are accomplished by the secretion of hydrochloric

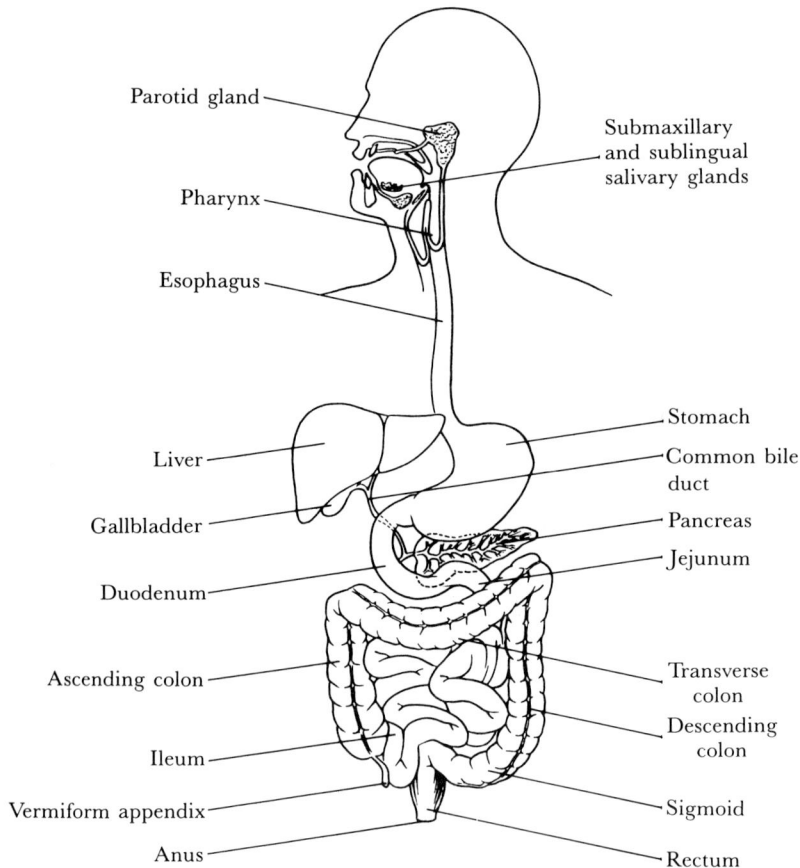

FIGURE 3.5 The organs of the digestive system. Adapted from *Functional Gastrointestinal Disorders* (p. 5) by P. R. Latimer. 1983, New York: Springer.

acid and the enzyme pepsin from the mucosal lining of the stomach as well as by the contractions of the stomach.

SMALL INTESTINE    The small intestine, which is bounded by the pyloric sphincter and the ileocecal sphincter, is responsible for digestion and absorption of food nutrients. It is considered to be subdivided into the duodenum, jejunum, and the ileum. There are no structures that mark these divisions; rather, they are categorized by function. The duodenum is the area in which the bowel duct and pancreatic ducts join the intestine. It, along with the jejunum, regulates contractions and enzyme production in the stomach and small intestine. The ileum is primarily responsible for nutrient absorption.

COLON    The colon, or large intestine, is bounded by the ileocecal sphincter and by both an internal and external anal sphincter. The functions of the colon are to absorb water, store fecal material prior to defecation, and to control defecation. It is divided into four sections based on the positions of these sections: ascending, transverse, descending, and sigmoid. Little contractile activity occurs in the ascending and transverse colon. However, there do occur brief periods of propulsive activity once or twice each day that push the colon contents into the descending colon. There is a greater amount of contractile activity in the descending and sigmoid colon, but these contractions serve to retard the passage of the colon's contents toward the rectum.

# The Immune System

The immune system is somewhat different from the organ systems just described. That is, it is composed of specialized cells that are produced in the bone marrow and are stored in specific organs—such as the thymus, lymph nodes, and spleen—before they are released into the blood. The function of the immune system is to recognize and eliminate foreign microorganisms and their toxins that enter the body. The immune system is divided into two subsystems that are responsible for *cell-mediated* and *humoral immunity*. Cell-mediated immunity refers to the direct action of a type of white blood cell, the *T cell lymphocytes* on foreign cells. Humoral immunity is mediated by the *B cell lymphocytes* that release into the bloodstream antibodies, or substances called *immunoglobulins*, that attack specific foreign cells called *antigens*. Other immunologic functions are performed by another type of white blood cell, the *phagocytes*, that ingest foreign cells. However, cell-mediated and humoral-immune functions as well as phagocytosis must work together in order to protect us from infection and illness.

The lymphocytes involved in cell-mediated immunity are called *T cells* because they mature in the thymus gland. These T cells are further divided into three categories. First, there are *cytotoxic* cells that directly destroy invading cells. Second, there are helper T cells that come into contact with antigens and release several chemicals called *lymphokines*. Several of these lymphokines kill foreign cells directly whereas others attract and activate phagocytes that engulf and ingest the invading cells. There are also additional forms of lymphokines that aid in the development of cytotoxic cells and the B cell lymphocytes that are involved in humoral immunity. The third type of T cell consists of suppressor T cells, which inhibit the development of the B cells and the activity of the helper T cells. These suppressor T cells, then, turn off the immune response once the organism has defended itself successfully against the invading foreign cells. Together, all three forms of the T cells are particularly effective in defending the body against viral and fungal infections, parasites, foreign tissue (such as transplanted organs), and cancerous tumor cells.

It was noted above that the lymphocytes involved in humoral immunity are known as *B cells*. These lymphocytes are produced in the bone marrow and carried to the lymph nodes, spleen, and tonsils. When B cells recognize the presence of foreign cells, they release antibodies (immunoglobulins) from their surfaces. These antibodies combine with the target antigens, and the antigens are destroyed by one of several different means. For example, the immunoglobulin IgG combines with antigens in such a manner as to allow the phagocytes to recognize and destroy the antibody-antigen complex. IgM, however, is capable of directly destroying bacterial cells. The immunoglobulin IgA is found primarily in bodily fluids such as tears, saliva, and the secretions of the respiratory and gastrointestinal tracts. It is believed that IgA does not directly kill invading cells; rather, it denies these cells access to the mucosal linings of the body. IgE is involved in allergic reactions. It attaches to antigens and then to the surface of tissue cells known as basophils and mast cells. These tissue cells, in turn, release histamine and prostaglandins. However, little is known about the actions of the fifth class of immunoglobulins, IgD. Humoral immunity mediated by B cells is particularly effective in defending the body against bacterial infections and viruses that have not yet invaded cells, as well as carrying out immediate allergic reactions.

Recently, a form of non-B, non-T lymphocytes has been identified. These have been termed *natural killer cells*. They have been found to directly kill virus-infected cells and cancerous tumor cells by secretion of the lymphokine *interferon*. Therefore, interferon has been administered in experimental clinical trials to patients with various types of malignancies (Calabrese, Kling, & Gold, 1987).

STRESS, THE ENDOCRINE SYSTEM, AND IMMUNE FUNCTION    We learned earlier in this chapter that stressful situations activate interactions between (a) the sympathetic nervous system and the adrenal medullae and (b) the hypothalamic-pituitary-adrenal cortex axis. It is now known that activation of these two systems and the subsequent release of catecholamines and corticosteroids exert direct effects on the functioning of the immune system. It has been found, for example, that injection of epinephrine increases the release of suppressor T cells and reduces the number of mature helper T cells (Crary, Borysenko, Sutherland, et al., 1983). Corticosteroids inhibit the functioning of certain types of phagocytes, T cells, and natural killer cells (Cupps & Fauci, 1982; Meuleman & Katz, 1985). The study of the relationships between the central nervous system, the endocrine system, and the immune system is termed *psychoneuroimmunology* (Ader, 1981).

A growing number of correlational investigations have also demonstrated relationships between several clinical stressors and depressed immune responses. For example, Locke and his colleagues (1984) reported that psychological distress, such as anxiety and depression, was associated with decreased levels of natural killer cell activity among college students. Similarly, Kiecolt-Glaser, Garner, and their colleagues (1984) reported that medical students showed significant reductions in natural killer cell activity during their final examinations. The reductions in natural killer cell activity were also correlated positively with students' scores on the UCLA Loneliness Scale. These investigators found in an independent study that psychiatric patients' scores on the Loneliness Scale were associated with high levels of urinary cortisol, reduced natural killer cell activity, and reduced lymphocyte responsiveness (Kiecolt-Glaser et al., 1984).

Two studies have produced evidence that clinical interventions can enhance immune functioning among college students. Peavey, Lawlis, and Goven (1985) reported that biofeedback-assisted relaxation training produced significant increases in phagocyte immune functioning among college students with high levels of recent life stress and depressed phagocytic activity. More recently, Pennebaker and his colleagues (1988) asked college students to write essays on four consecutive days regarding either their most traumatic personal experiences or on neutral topics. Those students who wrote about their traumatic experiences showed greater responsiveness on an immunologic measure of helper T cell proliferation than did students who wrote about neutral experiences. The former students also made fewer visits to the University Health Center during the six weeks following the essay-writing task. It was suggested that the immunoenhancing effects of self-disclosure might help mediate the documented relationship between psychotherapy and decreased usage of medical services (e.g., Mumford et al., 1981).

Effects of stress and clinical interventions on immune system functioning have also been found in older adult populations. Several studies, for example, have found that disruptions of marital relationships due to divorce or separation (Kiecolt-Glaser et al., 1987) or bereavement (Irwin et al., 1987) produced decreases in helper T cells and natural killer cell activity, respectively. For several years, Andrew Baum and his colleagues have been studying the stressful long-term effects of the Three Mile Island (TMI) nuclear accident on residents of the area surrounding the power plant. Relative to control individuals, the TMI residents have shown a lower level of B cells and T cells (Baum, 1985). It should be noted, however, that the number of subjects studied thus far has been small. Finally, it has been found consistently that major affective disorder (i.e., a psychiatric diagnosis of depression) is associated with decreases in T cells (Schleifer et al., 1984, 1985).

With regard to clinical interventions, Kiecolt-Glaser and her colleagues (1985) have demonstrated that, relative to attention-placebo and no-treatment control conditions, relaxation training enhanced natural killer cell activity among geriatric residents of independent living facilities. It has also been found consistently that psychological interventions that include a strong emphasis on relaxation training produce significant decreases in measures of joint inflammation among patients with rheumatoid arthritis (Achterberg et al., 1981; Bradley et al., 1987; O'Leary et al., 1988). However, only one of these studies with rheumatoid arthritis patients has examined immune functioning at the cellular level (O'Leary et al., 1988); unfortunately, this investigation did not show any evidence of changes in T cell activity.

ACQUIRED IMMUNE DEFICIENCY SYNDROME    The acquired immune deficiency syndrome (AIDS) was first described in 1981. It was identified originally among gay men and intravenous drug users, and these persons remain at greatest risk for acquiring AIDS (McKusick, Horstman, & Coates, 1985). However, AIDS is now recognized as a worldwide epidemic that may also be transmitted to male and female heterosexuals by sexual contact or sharing a needle with infected individuals. To illustrate the scope of the AIDS epidemic, it should be noted that the number of new cases in the United States alone doubles every 12 to 14 months and at least 270,000 cases are expected by 1991 (Kelly et al., 1989).

The current evidence indicates that the causative agent in AIDS is a single virus or a family of viruses that is termed the *human immune deficiency virus*, or HIV. The most striking abnormality of the immune system associated with AIDS is a deficiency in helper T cells. However, alterations of natural killer cell cytotoxicity as well as impaired production of interferon have also been reported (Seligmann et al., 1984).

It was not until 1983 that techniques were available to determine the presence of antibodies to HIV in human blood. It has been recognized for several years, however, that the course of AIDS is profoundly negative. Most persons with HIV infection remain asymptomatic for various lengths of time. However, the early stages of AIDS are characterized by weakness, frequent infections, anorexia, weight loss, swollen lymph glands, and pain. As the disease progresses, more frequent infections, especially pneumonia and herpes simplex virus, and nutritional depletion occur. An otherwise rare form of cancer, Kaposi's sarcoma, is also frequently found in people with AIDS (Holland & Tross, 1985). At the present time, no one has been found to recover from AIDS or the diseases that accompany it, even with massive antiinfectious chemotherapy. In San Francisco, 45% of all reported patients have died; more than 76% of all patients diagnosed before July 1982 are now dead (McKusick et al., 1985).

In addition to patients with AIDS, there are also individuals with milder forms of the syndrome, known collectively as AIDS-related complex (ARC). ARC is characterized by swollen lymph glands, fever, fatigue, weight loss, anorexia, and diarrhea (Seligmann et al., 1984). A high percentage of these persons also carry antibodies to HIV. However, it is unknown at present how many persons with ARC will go on to develop the full-blown AIDS syndrome.

The detection of antibodies to HIV, or the detection of ARC or full-blown AIDS, is a highly traumatic event. Each new symptom, infection, or alteration in weight tends to be viewed by individuals as evidence of potential disease progression (Holland & Tross, 1985). Among those who are HIV positive but without symptoms, common psychological reactions include depression, anger, denial, and perceptions of hopelessness (Catalan, 1988). Evidence of cognitive impairment has been found in 44% of HIV-positive gay men compared to 9% of HIV-negative males. Abnormalities in the cerebral spinal fluid of HIV-positive males have also been reported (Goudsmit et al., 1986), and it has been assumed that these abnormalities and cognitive impairments reflect the effects of HIV on the central nervous system.

As one might expect, the psychological and neuropsychological difficulties of persons with ARC are greater than those of asymptomatic HIV-positive individuals. The major psychological disturbances are depression and anxiety; common neuropsychological impairments include slowness in carrying out tasks and abnormalities in abstract thinking, learning, and memory (Catalan, 1988). Finally, among those with full-blown AIDS, depression, suicidal thoughts, guilt, social isolation, perceptions of the illness as retribution, and concern about the effects of the illness on loved ones are common (Catalan, 1988). The most common neurological problem associated with AIDS is a diffuse encephalopathy (i.e., inflammation or degeneration of the brain). As time passes, the neuropsychological symptoms change in most patients from psychomotor retardation and apathy to disorientation, seizures, and profound mental confusion (Holland et al., 1985).

Most of the psychological investigations performed with AIDS patients thus far have been cross-sectional studies that have identified the psychosocial problems that confront these individuals. However, a few longitudinal investigations recently have been completed. For example, McKusick, Wiley, and their colleagues (1985) examined the effects of an intensive media education campaign in San Francisco upon the self-reports of sexual behavior of 454 men at risk for the development of AIDS. Over a six-month period, there were substantial changes in reported sexual behavior. There were significant decreases in the average number of male partners and in high-risk sexual behaviors such as receptive anal intercourse with someone other than the primary partner. However, although there was also a significant decrease in sex with primary partners, there was no change in high-risk sex behaviors with these partners. Reductions in the number of male partners accompanied by relatively small decreases in high-risk sexual behaviors also have been found among homosexual men in New York City (Siegal et al., 1988), Vancouver, Canada (Schechter et al., 1988), and Amsterdam, The Netherlands (van Griensven et al., 1988).

A more promising investigation recently was described by Kelly and his colleagues (1989). This study examined the effects of a twelve-session group intervention for homosexual men that included AIDS risk education, behavioral self-management and assertiveness training for reducing high risk sexual behavior, and development of social support and relationship skills. It was found that compared to a waiting-list control condition, the intervention produced a significant reduction in the frequency of unprotected anal intercourse and a significant increase in the use of condoms during intercourse. These effects were maintained at an eight-month follow-up assessment. However, the intervention failed to influence other high risk sexual behaviors such as oral/anal and oral/genital practices, as well as contact with multiple sexual partners.

# Summary

It is necessary for health psychologists to understand the physiological bases of health and illness in order to help people engage in actions that will help them maintain their health or to recover or cope with illnesses. We have reviewed genetic bases for behavior as well as several organ systems and the immune system.

Human behavior is influenced both by genetic and environmental factors. The study of behavioral genetics suggests that heredity sets the limits for what an individual's potential may be but environmental conditions influence the expression of behavior within those limits. The basic units of heredity are genes that are carried on twenty-three pairs of chromosomes within each cell nucleus of the body. The three major methods of studying the extent to which genetic factors account for behavioral traits among humans are family studies, twin studies, and adoption studies.

All human behavior is controlled primarily by the nervous system, which comprises both the central nervous system and the peripheral nervous system. The central nervous system consists of the brain and spinal cord. The peripheral nervous system includes the somatic and autonomic systems; the latter is also divided into two parts—the sympathetic and parasympathetic systems. The sympathetic system generally increases organ activity, whereas the parasympathetic system tends to reduce the activity of organs. The nervous system and the endocrine system act together to maintain normal functioning and to respond quickly during periods of danger, stress, or excitement. These two systems also interact with the immune system to influence the body's ability to defend itself against invading microorganisms.

The cardiovascular system is responsible for carrying oxygen and nutrients to cell tissues and for removing carbon dioxide and other wastes from these tissues and expelling them from the body. The respiratory system is also involved in this process, as it is responsible for providing oxygen to and eliminating carbon dioxide from the blood. Finally, the gastrointestinal system allows us to break down food so that the nutrients may be absorbed by the body for the production of energy and the growth and repair of cells.

One of the greatest challenges facing health psychologsists is the development of interventions that will influence the sexual behaviors of people who are at high risk for contracting AIDS. It is clear that current attempts to change these behaviors through the provision of information are not sufficient. In the absence of an effective vaccine against HIV, health psychologists may play a key role in slowing the spread of the AIDS epidemic by devising effective preventive interventions.

# References

ACHTERBERG, J., MCGRAW, P., & LAWLIS, G. F. (1981). Rheumatoid arthritis: A study of relaxation and temperature biofeedback training as an adjunctive therapy. *Biofeedback and Self-Regulation, 6*, 207–223.

ADER, R. (Ed.). *Psychoneuroimmunology.* New York: Academic Press, 1981.

BAUM, A., SCHAEFFER, M. A., LAKE, C. R., FLEMING, R., & COLLINS, D. L. (1985). Psychological and endocrinological correlates of chronic stress at Three Mile

Island. In R. Williams (Ed.), *Perspectives on behavioral medicine* (Vol. 2.). New York, Academic Press.

BOUCHARD, T. J., & McGUE, M. (1981). Familial studies of intelligence: A review. *Science, 212,* 1055–1059.

BRADLEY, L. A., YOUNG L. D., ANDERSON, K.O., TURNER, R. A., AGUDELO, C. A., McDANIEL, L. K., PISKO, E. J., SEMBLE, E., & MORGAN, T. M. (1987). Effects of psychological therapy on pain behavior of rheumatoid arthritis patients: Treatment outcome and six-month follow-up. *Arthritis and Rheumatism, 30,* 1105–1114.

CALABRESE, J. R., KLING, M. A., & GOLD, P. W. (1987). Alterations in immunocompetence during stress, bereavement, and depression: Focus on neuroendocrine regulation. *American Journal of Psychiatry, 144,* 1123–1134.

CATALAN, J. (1988). Psychosocial and neuropsychiatric aspects of HIV infection: Review of their extent and implications for psychiatry. *Journal of Psychosomatic Research, 32,* 237–248.

COZZI, L., TRYON, W. W., & SEDLACEK, K. (1987). The effectiveness of biofeedback-assisted relaxation in modifying sickle cell crises. *Biofeedback and Self-Regulation, 12,* 51–61.

CRAMPTON, D. R., BENKE, P. J., & BRAUNSTEIN, J. J. (1981). Genetics, development, and behavior. In J. J. Braunstein & R. P. Toister (Eds.), *Medical applications of the behavioral sciences.* Chicago: Yearbook Medical Publishers.

CRARY, B., BORYSENKO, M., SUTHERLAND, D. C., KUTZ, I., BORYSENKO, J. Z., & BENSON, H. (1983). Decrease in mitogen responsiveness of mononuclear cells from peripheral blood after epinephrine administration in humans. *Journal of Immunology, 130,* 694–697.

CUPPS, T. R., & FAUCI, A. S. (1982). Corticosteroid-mediated immunoregulation in man. *Immunological Review, 65,* 133–155.

FOLTZ, E. L. (1976). Psychosurgical approach to chronic pain (cingulumotomy). In J. F. Lee (Ed.), *Pain management: Symposium on the neurosurgical treatment of pain.* Baltimore: Williams & Wilkins.

GAY, P., COLE, S. O., & LEAF, R. C. (1976). Interactions of amygdala lesions with effects of pilocarpine and d-amphetamine on mouse killing, feeding, and drinking in rats. *Journal of Comparative and Physiological Psychology, 90,* 630–642.

GOUDSMIT, J., WOLTERS, E., BAKKER, M., SMIT, L., NOORDA, J., HISCHE, E., TUTUARIMA, J., & HELM, H. VAN DER. (1986). Intrathecal synthesis of antibodies to HILV-III in patients without AIDS or ARC. *British Medical Journal, 292,* 1231–1234.

HESTON, L. L. (1966). Psychiatric disorders in foster home reared children of schizophrenic mothers. *British Journal of Psychiatry, 112,* 819–825.

HOLLAND, J. C., & TROSS, S. (1985). The psychosocial and neuropsychiatric sequelae of the acquired immunodeficiency syndrome and related disorders. *Annals of Internal Medicine, 103,* 760–764.

IRWIN, M., DANIELS, M., SMITH, T. L., BLOOM, E., & WEINER, H. (1987). Impaired natural killer cell activity during bereavement. *Brain, Behavior, and Immunity, 1,* 98–104.

JACOBS, P. A., BRUNTON, M., & MELVILLE, M. M. (1965). Aggressive behavior, mental subnormality, and the XYY male. *Nature, 208,* 1351–1352.

JACOBS, P. A., PRICE, W. H., COURT A., BROWN, W. M., BRITTAIN, R. P., & WHATMORE, P. B. (1968). Chromosome studies of men in a maximum security hospital. *Annals of Human Genetics, 31*, 339–358.

JARVIK, L. F., KLODIN, V., & MATSUYAMA, S. S. (1973). Human aggression and the extra Y chromosome: Factor or fiction? *American Psychologist, 28*, 674–676.

KALLMANN, F. J. (1938). *The genetics of schizophrenia.* Locust Valley: J. J. Augustin.

KELLY, J.A., ST. LAWRENCE, J. S., HOOD, H. V., & BRASFIELD, T. L. (1989). Behavioral intervention to reduce AIDS risk activities. *Journal of Consulting and Clinical Psychology, 57*, 60–67.

KETY, S. S. (1976). Mental illness in the biological and adoptive families of adopted individuals who have become schizophrenic: A preliminary report. In R. Fieve, D. Rosenthal, & H. Brill (Eds.), *Genetic research in psychiatry.* Baltimore: Johns Hopkins University Press.

KIECOLT-GLASER, J. K., FISHER, L. D., OGROCKI, P., STOUT, J. C., SPEICHER, C. E., & GLASER, R. (1987). Marital quality, marital disruption, and immune function. *Psychosomatic Medicine, 49*, 13–34.

KIECOLT-GLASER, J. K., GARNER, W., SPEICHER, C. E., PENN, G., & GLASER, R. (1984). Psychosocial modifiers of immunocompetence in medical students. *Psychosomatic Medicine, 46*, 7–14.

KIECOLT-GLASER, J. K., GLASER, R., WILLIGER, D., STOUT, J. C., MESSICK, G., SHEPPARD, S., RICKER, D., ROMISHER, J. C., BRINER, W., BONNELL, G., & DONNERBERG, R. (1985). Psychosocial enhancement of immunocompetence in a geriatric population. *Health Psychology, 4*, 25–41.

KIECOLT-GLASER, J. K., RICKER, D., GEORGE, J., MESSICK, G., SPEICHER, C. E., GARNER, W., & GLASER, R. (1984). Urinary cortisol levels, cellular immunocompetency, and loneliness in psychiatric inpatients. *Psychosomatic Medicine, 46*, 15–23.

LOCKE, S. E., KRAUS, L., LESERMAN, J., HURST, M. W., HEISEL, S., & WILLIAMS, R. M. (1984). Life change stress, psychiatric symptoms, and natural killer cell activity. *Psychosomatic Medicine, 46*, 441–453.

MCKUSICK, L., HORSTMAN, W., & COATES, T. J. (1985). AIDS and sexual behavior reported by gay men in San Francisco. *American Journal of Public Health, 75*, 493–496.

MCKUSICK, L., WILEY, J. A., COATES, T. J., STALL, R., SAIKA, G., MORIN, S., CHARLES, K., HORSTMAN, W., & CONANT, M. A. (1985). Reported changes in the sexual behavior of men at risk for AIDS, San Francisco, 1982–1984: The AIDS behavioral research project. *Public Health Reports, 100*, 622–629.

MATARAZZO, J. D. (1980). Behavioral health and behavioral medicine: Frontiers for a new health psychology. *American Psychologist, 35*, 807–817.

MEULEMAN, J., & KATZ, P. (1985). The immunologic effects, kinetics, and use of glucocorticosteroids. *Medical Clinics of North America, 69*, 805–816.

MIRSKY, I. A. (1958). Physiologic, psychologic, and social determinants in the etiology of duodenal ulcer. *American Journal of Digestive Diseases, 3*, 285–314.

MIRSKY, I. A., FRITTERMAN, P., & KAPLAN, S. (1952). Blood plasma pepsinogen. II. The activity of the plasma from "normal" subjects, patients with duodenal ulcer, and patients with pernicious anemia. *Journal of Laboratory and Clinical Medicine, 40*, 188–195.

MUMFORD, E., SCHLESINGER, H. J., & GLASS, G. V. (1981). Reducing medical costs through mental health treatment: Research problems and recommendations. In

A. Broskowski, E. Marks, & S. H. Budman (Eds.), *Linking health and mental health*. Beverly Hills, CA: Sage.

MUSSEN, P. H., CONGER, J. J., & KAGEN, J. (1979). *Child development and personality*. New York: Harper & Row.

O'LEARY, A., SHOOR, S., LORIG, K., & HOLMAN, H. (1988). A cognitive-behavioral treatment for rheumatoid arthritis. *Health Psychology, 7*, 527–544.

PEAVEY, B. S., LAWLIS, G. F., & GOVEN, A. (1985). Biofeedback-assisted relaxation: Effects on phagocytic capacity. *Biofeedback and Self-Regulation, 10*, 33-47.

PENNEBAKER, J. W., KIECOLT-GLASER, J. K., & GLASER, R. (1988). Disclosures of traumas and immune function: Health implications for psychotherapy. *Journal of Consulting and Clinical Psychology, 56*, 239–245.

PILOT, M. L., LENKOSKI, L. D., SPIRO, H. M., & SCHAEFFER, R. (1957). Duodenal ulcer in one of identical twins. *Psychosomatic Medicine, 19*, 221–229.

SCHECHTER, M. T., CRAIB, K. J. P., WILLOUGHBY, B., DOUGLAS, B., MCLEOD, W. A., MAYNARD, M., CONSTANCE, P, & O'SHAUGHNESSY, M. (1988). Patterns of sexual behavior and condom use in a cohort of homosexual men. *American Journal of Public Health, 78*, 1535–1538

SCHLEIFER, S. J., KELLER, S. E., MEYERSON, A. T., RASKIN, M. J., DAVIS, K., L. & STEIN, M. (1984). Lymphocyte function in major depressive disorder. *Archives of General Psychiatry, 41*, 484–486.

SCHLEIFER, S. J., KELLER, S. E., SIRIS, S. G., DAVIS, K. L., & STEIN, M. (1985). Depression and immunity: Lymphocyte function in ambulatory depressed, hospitalized schizophrenic, and herniorrhaphy patients *Archives of General Psychiatry, 42*, 129–133.

SELIGMANN, M., CHESS, L., FAHEY, J. L., FAUCI, A. S., LACHMANN, P. J., L'AGE-STEHR, J., NGU, J., PINCHING, A. J., ROSEN, F. S., SPIRA, T. J., & WYBRAN, J. (1984). AIDS—An immunologic reevaluation. *New England Journal of Medicine, 311*, 1286–1297.

SIEGEL, K., BAUMAN, L. J., CHRIST, G. H., & KROWN, S. (1988). Patterns of change in sexual behavior among gay men in New York City. *Archives of Sexual Behavior, 17*, 481–497.

TSUANG, M. T. (1976). Genetic factors in schizophrenia. In R. G. Grennell & S. Gabay (Eds.), *Biological foundations of psychiatry* (Vol. 2). New York: Raven Press.

VAN GRIENSVENN, G. J. P., DEVROOME, E. M. M., TIELMAN, R. A. P., GOUDSMIT, J., VAN DER NOORDAA, J., DEWOLF, F,. & COUTINHO, R. A. (1988). Impact of HIV antibody testing on changes in sexual behavior among homosexual men in the Netherlands. *American Journal of Public Health, 18*, 1575–1577.

WHITEHEAD, W. E., & SCHUSTER, M. M. (1985). *Gastrointestinal disorders: Behavioral and physiological basis for treatment*. New York: Academic Press.

WIGGINS, J. S., RENNER, I. E., CLARE, G. L., & ROSE, R. J. (1976). *Principles of personality*. Reading, MA: Addison-Wesley.

ZUBIN, J., & SPRING, B. (1977). Vulnerability: A new view of schizophrenia. *Journal of Abnormal Psychology, 86*, 103–126.

# CHAPTER 4

# Behavioral and Social Learning Principles

Chapter 1 traced the evolution of health psychology from ancient times to the present. It is apparent that health psychology has been influenced by developments in many fields, ranging from psychoanalysis to laboratory psychology. During the last four decades, health psychology has been influenced particularly by developments in two fields of psychology: behavior therapy and social learning theory. This chapter traces the historical foundations of behavioral and social learning approaches, describes major mechanisms important in the development of adaptive and maladaptive behavior, and discusses therapeutic techniques in use today.

## Behavioral Models

Behavioral models of psychological disorders and their treatment stem from studies of two major forms of learning: (1) classical, or respondent, conditioning, and (2) operant, or instrumental, conditioning. These two types of learning represent very different processes, and different scientists played key roles in their historical development. However, all behavioral approaches share one common element: a focus on the environmental circumstances controlling the learning and continued emission of behavior. Behavioral theory avoids any reliance on concepts such as unconscious motivation and instead looks for observable events in the past or present that explain why a behavior first occurred and persists today. For example, a psychoanalyst might say that a man is prone to feeling ill despite the lack of any diagnosable physical disorder because he is anxious about his ability to be a competent and successful businessman. A behaviorist would be more likely to point out that when that same man stays home sick, he is paid his salary just as if he had worked that day and his family also treats him very sympathetically. The psychoanalytic explanation emphasizes unobservable causes of the man's hypochondriasis, but the behavioral explanation emphasizes the observable consequences of his behavior.

# Classical Conditioning

Ivan M. Sechenov (1829–1905) and his student Ivan P. Pavlov (1849–1936) were Russian physiologists with interests in the study of physiological reflexes and learning processes. Sechenov proposed that behavior could be accounted for by physiological reflexes of the brain and that behavior could be understood only through the examination of these reflexes. Brain reflexes were thought to develop through mechanisms of learning, such as the experience of reinforcement for the emission of specific behavioral acts. In this way, a brain reflex would develop if a human or any other organism was rewarded for the demonstration of a particular behavior. Sechenov advocated the need to apply the objective research methods of physiology to the study of psychology in order to understand how the learning of these brain reflexes occurred.

Pavlov was one of the first to apply learning principles to the experimental study of behavior. He launched a series of studies circa 1884 that investigated the role of learning in animal behavior. He was specifically interested in how the automatic reflexes, such as the salivation of a dog, could be conditioned to occur in response to stimuli that had not previously produced the reflexive response. Pavlov developed a number of surgical procedures that made it possible to observe canine digestive processes, including salivation and the secretion of gastric juices in the stomach. He was thus able to place food in a dog's mouth and measure various glandular secretions, which led to a better understanding of reflexive digestive processes.

Pavlov's interest in the psychology of learning was probably stimulated by some frustrating experiences in his laboratory as he prepared to measure the dogs' digestive secretions. Many of his animals would already be salivating before he placed food in their mouths. Pavlov thought that the animals perhaps had learned to anticipate food when they heard the sound of his footsteps approaching the laboratory. At first, he referred to the reflexes as "psychical secretions": secretions evoked by psychical as opposed to physical stimulation. Later the term *psychical secretion* was replaced with *conditioned reflex* because it was thought that the dogs were not experiencing subjective states of anticipation. Instead, they were thought to have simply learned an automatic association between one stimulus (footsteps) and another stimulus (food).

Pavlov performed several experiments to explore conditioned reflexes in dogs. He always investigated the salivary reflex because it is unlearned or innate; in other words, it occurs automatically, without the need for learning, in response to a stimulus such as food. He labeled the reflexes he studied *unconditioned reflexes,* or *unconditioned responses,* and the stimuli that naturally led to the reflexive behavior were *unconditioned stimuli.*

To study the learning process Pavlov selected a *neutral stimulus,* a stimulus that did not originally lead to any response other than an "orienting reflex" in which a dog becomes alert and attentive. For example, lights, tones, and bells are neutral stimuli. Pavlov found that if a neutral stimulus was presented simultaneously with the unconditioned stimulus, the neutral stimulus alone would eventually elicit the same response as did the unconditioned stimulus. Thus, if a bell was rung at the same time that a dog was given food, eventually the sound of the bell alone would lead the dog to salivate. In this way, the unconditioned response had become a *conditioned response.* Figure 4.1 illustrates this process.

Pavlov's discovery of conditioned reflexes revolutionized psychological thinking. It not only provided an account of how animals learned but it also provided a new way to understand and investigate complex human behaviors. If a dog could be conditioned to salivate at the sound of a bell, might it also be true that a child might be conditioned to experience an asthma attack upon entering his or her classroom at school? Figure 4.1 also includes an illustration of how this process might occur.

## Operant Conditioning

Although classical conditioning is automatic and reflexive, operant conditioning is a much more active learning process. The dogs in Pavlov's experiments learned to salivate at the sound of a bell simply because the bell and food were presented simultaneously. The dogs engaged in no active behavior in the process of learning but simply learned an association between a previously neutral stimulus and a reflexive response. In operant conditioning an organism operates actively on the environment. If a behavior results in reinforcing consequences, the behavior is more likely to occur again. If a child is praised for "being brave" at the dentist, the child is more likely to show less fear during her next dentist appointment.

B. F. Skinner (1904–     ) is the psychologist most associated with operant conditioning. Skinner's basic research paradigm involved teaching animals new behaviors by allowing them to work for rewards. To study this process, he developed an apparatus now referred to as the Skinner box. The Skinner box is simply a small, controlled environment in which the relationship be-

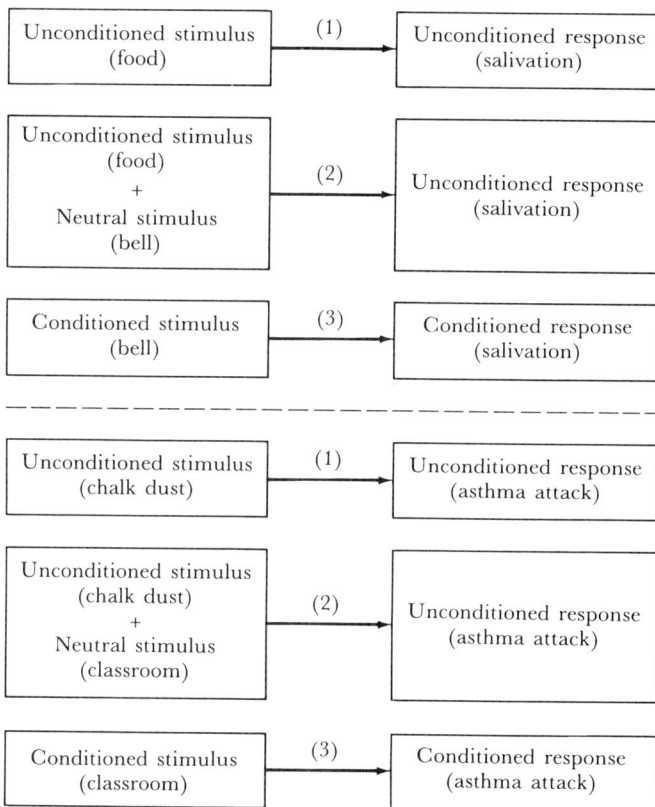

FIGURE 4.1 The classical conditioning process. The top sequence illustrates Pavlov's conditioning of salivation in dogs; the bottom sequence illustrates the conditioning of a child's asthma attacks so that the attacks are likely to occur whenever the child enters a classroom at school. Note that the conditioning process is the same.

tween an animal's behavior and environmental consequences can be studied. For example, a pigeon in a Skinner box may peck a key and receive a pellet of food, or a rat may press a bar to turn off an electric shock. Key pecking or bar pressing thus become more likely the next time the animal is placed in the Skinner box. *Reinforcement* occurs if the consequences of a behavior make that behavior more probable.

*Positive reinforcers* increase the probability of a behavior when the reinforcers are added to the environment. For example, a pellet of food delivered to a pigeon and praise for a child for brave behavior at the dentist are both positive reinforcers because when added to the environment they increase the probability of future key pecking or good behavior at the dentist. *Negative reinforcers* increase the probability of a behavior when the reinforcers are removed from the environment. The removal of electric shock from the floor of a Skinner box and the reduction of headache pain are both negative reinforcers because they make future bar pressing or aspirin taking more likely.

As we will see when behavior therapies are discussed, the emphasis of operant conditioning principles upon the consequences of behavior rather than upon the unobservable internal state of the organism has important effects on how psychological and health problems are understood and treated. If a patient does not take high blood pressure medication despite repeated instructions from his physician, it is not because he does not "want" to take the medication or is an "uncooperative patient"; it is because the consequences of taking the medication are not sufficiently reinforcing. A behavioral treatment program would thus try to find a way to increase the reinforcement value of taking the medication. Perhaps the patient's family can reward medication taking with attention and social support and thus positively reinforce healthy behavior. Alternatively, perhaps taking a medication with fewer side effects will negatively reinforce healthy behavior. In either case, the consequences of the behavior, not the patient's presumed attitude or personality, are altered.

Operant conditioning and classical conditioning processes may both be important in the learning and maintenance of a single behavior. As we will see in Chapter 11, asthma attacks similar to the one described in Figure 4.1 may develop by classical conditioning but be maintained through operant conditioning. If the child is reinforced for an asthma attack by receiving extra attention and a day off from school, then the attacks may be more likely to occur again. The symptom of a biological disorder (asthma) thus becomes a classically conditioned response (asthma attacks when the child approaches school) and the response is maintained in an operant manner by the reinforcement (attention and a holiday) the child receives.

## Social Learning Theory

Classical and operant conditioning models of learning dominated theories of behavior development and change for a significant period of time. Both models emphasized the importance of observable events and processes and avoided reliance on unobservable phenomena such as thoughts. Social learning theory developed out of a recognition that "private events," such as a person's thoughts, may influence the acquisition of behavior.

Albert Bandura was one of the first psychologists to describe learning mechanisms involving thoughts or cognitions (Bandura, 1969, 1971, 1977). He noted that learning may occur even if a person never actually engages in a behavior but instead only watches another person engaged in that same behavior. Since the observer does not emit the behavior, he or she is not directly reinforced. However, learning still occurs. Bandura labeled this type of learning *modeling*, or *observational learning*. He suggested that learning occurs through observation because the observer receives *vicarious reinforcement*. The observer is reinforced vicariously, or through the experience of another person, as he or she watches the other person engage in a behavior and receive reinforcement. Thus, children who observe a parent getting attention from others only when complaining about physical symptoms may be vicariously reinforced and learn to complain about physical symptoms themselves.

Learning may also occur even if the model is not reinforced. One of Bandura's early experiments investigated how the modeling process affects the learning of aggressive behavior (Bandura, 1965). Children watched a film of a child behaving aggressively toward an adult-sized Bobo doll. Following the aggressive behavior, the model on the film was rewarded, punished, or experienced no consequences for his behavior. Children who watched the film were then escorted to a room containing toys, including a Bobo doll, and allowed to play as they chose. Children who had seen the model rewarded or experience no consequences behaved more aggressively than did children who had seen the model punished. All children, however, had learned the model's behavior; when they were offered prizes for imitating that behavior, all differences among the reward, punishment, and no consequences groups disappeared. The reinforcement a model receives affects whether a behavior is likely to be performed, but the behavior may be acquired even if the model is punished.

The distinction between behavior acquisition and behavior performance has important implications for the prevention of undesirable or unhealthy behaviors. It suggests that educational efforts demonstrating the negative consequences of undesirable behavior may be less effective than intended because the behavior may still be learned despite the observation of negative consequences. Attempting to discourage adolescents from smoking by having them watch another person smoke and begin to cough may encourage the acquisition, if not the immediate performance, of smoking behavior. When the adolescent encounters a situation in which smoking might be rewarded, the acquired behavior may be performed.

THE MODELING PROCESS  Four features must be present for observational learning to occur (Bandura, 1977).

1. *Attention.* The observer must be attentive to the modeled behaviors in order to observe their operation and the consequences they elicit.

2. *Retention.* The observer must be able to remember what is observed. Information may be retained over long periods through either verbal means ("I heard my older brother say he felt good when he smoked"), or visual, by maintaining an image of the observed events (retaining a visual image of the brother's pleasurable expression as he smoked).

3. *Reproduction.* The observer must be able to emulate the observed behaviors and thus must have the ability to perform the observed acts. Reproduction is influenced by a number of ability factors such as physical size and skill, age, and prior experience.

4. *Motivation.* Without motivation to learn the observed behavior, minimal learning will occur. Motivation is influenced by the observed consequences of the act and the availability of those consequences to the viewer. If positive reinforcement is observed, the viewer will be most apt to display the behavior if the reinforcement is personally attainable. Observing a model receive reinforcement that is unobtainable by the viewer will decrease motivation to perform the observed act.

Bandura (1977) also emphasized the role of cognition in motivation. He particularly stressed the importance of *self-efficacy,* the degree to which an individual expects that he or she will be able to successfully perform a desired behavior. Self-efficacy is an important mediating factor in the modeling process. It includes the person's expectations for successful performance as well as the degree to which an individual anticipates that performing the behavior will result in rewarding consequences. Self-efficacy thereby influences motivation, and thus the likelihood that a person will learn and perform a modeled behavior.

Motivation also includes a self-evaluative process that in and of itself may act as a reinforcer. Learning to reproduce modeled behaviors that provide one with a positive self-evaluation can be a strong motivating factor. Behaviors that provide pride or a sense of competence will be more motivating than those that do not, and experiences that lead to a sense of mastery over new behaviors will also lead to increased self-efficacy. The importance of self-evaluation and self-efficacy has influenced the kinds of therapeutic interventions that Bandura has suggested are most effective in teaching patients to engage in more adaptable behaviors. These interventions will be described later in this chapter.

## Behavior Therapy

Behavior therapy refers to a large number of specific behavior change techniques derived from the learning principles described earlier in this chapter. Some of these techniques focus on the acquisition of skills, such as training socially inhibited individuals to be more assertive. Other techniques are used to eliminate problem behaviors, such as smoking or alcoholism, or to reduce uncomfortable affective states, such as anxiety or depression. Some behavior therapy techniques rely heavily on more traditional models of learning (classical and operant conditioning) while others emphasize the role of cognitions in learning and in behavior change.

Although the term *behavior therapy* was not introduced until the late 1950s, early experimental studies of classical and operant conditioning influenced behavior therapy development. Watson and his associates (Watson & Rayner, 1920) were among the first to actually apply learning principles to human behavior change. In a classic case report, they classically conditioned a child to fear white furry objects by pairing the presentation of a white rat with the noise made by a hammer striking a steel bar. B. F. Skinner's influential book *Science and Human Behavior* (1953) described the importance of operant conditioning in the development of learned behaviors. *Psychotherapy and Reciprocal Inhibition* (Wolpe, 1958) discussed the role of classical conditioning in the development of neurotic behavior. Perhaps more important, Wolpe also developed specific behavioral techniques aimed at eliminating neurotic behavior.

The following section reviews the contributions of behavior therapy to the treatment of psychological and psychophysiological disorders. After the assumptions of behavior therapy approaches are presented, specific behavior therapy techniques that have developed from classical conditioning, operant conditioning, and cognitive models of learning are described.

## Assumptions of Behavior Therapy

Behavior therapy differs from more traditional psychotherapeutic approaches, such as psychodynamic psychotherapy, in a number of ways. In particular, behavior therapy stresses the primary importance of the behavior itself rather than a hypothesized underlying cause for the behavior. Consider the example of the asthmatic child mentioned earlier. Although a psychodynamic therapist might emphasize the child's fear of separation from his or her mother and work to help the child feel less dependent, a behavior therapist would concentrate on the child's asthma attacks and work directly on finding ways to reduce the frequency and intensity of them. Behavior therapy assumes that maladaptive behaviors are learned in the same way that other behaviors are learned. By setting clearly defined goals and concentrating treatment efforts on observable behavior, a behavior therapist develops an individualized plan of treatment relying upon learning theory principles to help the client unlearn maladaptive behaviors and learn new, adaptive behaviors (Masters, Burish, Hollon, & Rimm, 1987, 1989). Some basic principles of behavior therapy are summarized in Table 4.1.

TABLE 4.1  Some Basic Principles of Behavior Therapy

1. Behavior itself is the main focus, rather than a presumed underlying cause.
2. Learning processes underlying the acquisition of maladaptive behaviors are largely the same as those underlying any behavior.
3. Maladaptive behaviors may be modified effectively through the application of psychological principles, especially learning principles.
4. Clearly defined and specific treatment goals are of major importance.
5. Treatment procedures are adapted to the specific client's problem and concentrate on the present rather than the past.

SOURCE:  Adapted from J. C. Masters, T. G. Burish, S. D. Hollon, and D. C. Rimm, 1987, 1989. *Behavior therapy: Techniques and empirical findings* (3rd ed.). New York: Harcourt, Brace, Jovanovich.

## Techniques for Behavior Change

Numerous behavior therapy techniques have been developed; those with particular relevance to health psychology are described here. Relaxation training and systematic desensitization are used to help patients control or eliminate an undesirable, usually anxiety-based, response. Aversive counterconditioning and covert sensitization may be useful if the goal is to eliminate an undesirable, yet temporarily pleasant behavior by associating it with an unpleasant outcome. For example, smoking or excessive drinking might come to be associated with nausea. Self-control techniques, modeling, and therapies attempting to change thought patterns may be used to encourage the acquisition of new behaviors and/or cognitive patterns.

### RELAXATION TRAINING AND SYSTEMATIC DESENSITIZATION

Relaxation training is one technique used by behavior therapists as a means of reducing arousal or anxiety. One of the first approaches to relaxation training, *progressive muscle relaxation,* was developed by Edmund Jacobson (1938). Jacobson's technique was designed to reduce central and autonomic nervous system arousal by producing a state of deep muscle relaxation; he reported significant therapeutic benefits as a result of having anxious patients practice relaxation procedures.

In Jacobson's (1938) progressive muscle relaxation procedure the subject alternately tenses and relaxes muscle groups, often pairing the relaxation of the muscles with the word *relax.* The subject is seated in a comfortable chair and the therapist explains the rationale for the use of the technique. Then, the first tension-relaxation cycle is presented: "I want you to make a fist and tense the muscles in your hand really hard. Notice how uncomfortable the tension in your hands feels." After ten seconds the therapist then says, "Now, when I say relax, I want you to let the tension go from your hands, let them feel very relaxed and heavy ... now, relax." This same procedure is performed with several muscle groups, including those of the arms, shoulders, neck, mouth, tongue, eyes and forehead, back, midsection, thighs, stomach, calves, feet, and toes. On occasion the subject is instructed to inhale deeply and then to exhale and relax.

Although other relaxation training procedures exist, progressive muscle relaxation is still the most commonly used. The popularity of progressive muscle relaxation may be attributable, at least in part, to Joseph Wolpe's (1958) development of systematic desensitization (Masters, Burish, Hollon, & Rimm, 1987, 1989). Systematic desensitization was developed as a means of reducing anxiety by replacing the anxiety with an incompatible alternative response, such as assertion or relaxation. Wolpe suggested that systematic desensitization worked through reciprocal inhibition, a term originally posed by the physiologist Sherrington in 1906. Reciprocal inhibition is a process by which an excessive level of anxiety is inhibited by a competing activity that is the opposite, or reciprocal, of anxiety. For Wolpe, excessive levels of anxiety were indicators of sympathetic nervous system activity. Other activities such as relaxation, assertion, and sexual behavior were considered competing activities in that they decrease sympathetic activity in the nervous system and increase parasympathetic activity. The process of reciprocal inhibition was also described by Wolpe as *counterconditioning*, in which adaptive or appropriate associations are learned as replacements for old, maladaptive associations.

Wolpe developed procedures designed to provide antagonistic responses to anxiety as a means of extinguishing the anxiety response. For example, he trained anxious patients to use techniques of relaxation or self-assertion whenever the maladaptive response of anxiety arose. It was thought that if a response antagonistic to anxiety could be produced in the presence of the anxiety-evoking stimuli, the strength of the bond between these stimuli and the anxiety response would be decreased. After some experimentation, Wolpe settled on an abbreviated version of Jacobson's progressive muscle relaxation as a way to induce a response incompatible with anxiety (Wolpe, 1982).

In the systematic desensitization procedure, the relaxation response is paired with imagined scenes that the patient has indicated cause him distress. Initially, the patient is taught deep muscle relaxation as a competing response to anxiety. Then, with the therapist's assistance, the patient constructs a hierarchy of scenes of anxiety-provoking situations. The scenes are ordered from least anxiety provoking to most anxiety provoking.

After learning the relaxation technique and constructing an anxiety hierarchy, desensitization proper begins. First, the patient relaxes, then the therapist describes the least anxiety-provoking situation while the patient uses imagery to visualize himself or herself in the scene. If the patient experiences any anxiety, he or she signals to the therapist, scene presentation stops, and the patient goes back to relaxing. This cycle is repeated until the patient is able to visualize the scene for about twenty-five to thirty seconds without becoming anxious, at which point treatment progresses to the next most anxiety-provoking scene in the hierarchy. This procedure continues until all scenes in the hierarchy have been visualized without an anxiety response.

Although there is some debate about exactly why or how systematic desensitization works, it is widely recognized to be an effective method of treating many anxiety-based problems (Masters et al., 1987, 1989). As we will see in later chapters, systematic desensitization has been applied to a variety of health psychology problems. It has been used in the treatment of asthma (see Chapter 11) and has been particularly useful in the treatment of the anticipatory nausea suffered by some cancer patients undergoing chemotherapy (see Chapter 9).

AVERSIVE COUNTERCONDITIONING Aversive counterconditioning is another technique developed from the classical conditioning model. It involves the elimination of a problem behavior by pairing that behavior with a stimulus that is distasteful and therefore aversive. The behavior becomes less rewarding through this process. Several kinds of aversive stimuli have been used, including electric shock, drug-induced aversive states, and imagined aversive cognitive stimuli. This procedure is in many ways the opposite of desensitization. Both follow the same model, but aversive counterconditioning has the goal of making a response unpleasant rather than pleasant and relaxing. Indeed, aversive counterconditioning is sometimes referred to as *sensitization*.

Alcoholism is one of the most common problem behaviors for which aversive counterconditioning procedures are used. A nausea-inducing drug, or *emetic*, is given to the alcoholic patient. When the drug begins to take effect and the patient feels nauseated, he or she is given several ounces of alcohol, particularly favorite types and brands. For each drink presented, the alcoholic patient is instructed to savor the alcohol, to smell, taste, and sometimes swallow the liquor. Vomiting usually occurs after the alcohol is swallowed.

Most alcoholism treatments using aversive counterconditioning methods have total abstinence as their goal. However, Masters et al. (1987, 1989) found great variability in the abstinence rates reported in studies examining the aversive treatment of alcohol. Only four of the twenty studies they reviewed between 1928 and 1977 showed abstinence rates lower than 50%. In general, abstinence is quite high immediately following treatment but declines sharply six to twelve months after treatment.

*Covert sensitization* is a cognitive aversive counterconditioning technique (Cautela, 1966). This technique involves the use of imagery of aversive stimuli together with the imagined performance of the problem behavior. The pairing of the aversive image with the maladaptive behavior reduces the attractiveness of the behavior. Relaxation is usually used to help the patient develop vivid imagery.

Janda and Rimm (1972) investigated the usefulness of covert sensitization in the treatment of obesity. The effectiveness of covert sensitization was compared to that of an attention-control group and no-contact controls. (An attention-control group receives the same amount of attention from the therapist as does a group receiving treatment; however, an attention-control group does not receive treatment. In this way, the effects of the treatment itself and attention from the therapist may be separated.) Subjects in the covert sensitization group were weighed at the beginning of each treatment session. They were given relaxation training during the first treatment session. Following this, the subjects were required to vividly imagine approaching a food to be eliminated from their diet, feeling increasingly ill, and finally vomiting just before putting the forbidden food in their mouth. Subjects then imagined resisting the food and, subsequently, feeling much better while eating a meal consistent with their diet plan, enjoying it thoroughly, and feeling proud for staying on their diet.

One week later, subjects in all three groups were weighed and various other subjective measures taken. Six weeks later a similar follow-up weight check was conducted. Results of the study indicated that following treatment the no-contact controls showed a mean weight loss of 4.5 pounds, the attention-control subjects showed one of 0.7 pounds, and the covert sensitization subjects showed one of 9.5 pounds. At the six-week follow-up, no-contact control subjects showed a mean weight loss of 0.9 pounds, attention-control subjects showed a mean gain of 2.3 pounds, and the covert sensitization group showed a mean loss of 11.7 pounds. The superiority of the covert sensitization group at follow-up was clearly significant.

Unfortunately, other studies of the effectiveness of covert sensitization in reducing problem behaviors have not consistently shown it to be more efficacious than attention-control procedures. Sipich, Russel, and Tobias (1974), for example, compared covert sensitization to a placebo, or nonspecific, treatment designed to reduce smoking. Although covert sensitization was found to be effective in reducing smoking behavior, its effects were not significantly different from those of the nonspecific treatment. Nevertheless, case studies have suggested that covert sensitization may be useful in the treatment of obesity (Cautela, 1966; Stuart, 1967), alcoholism (Anant, 1968), and cigarette smoking (Tooley & Pratt, 1967). Because of a lack of adequate controls in many studies, the efficacy of this technique awaits further empirical substantiation.

CONTINGENCY MANAGEMENT    Operant methods have been used to assist clients in developing adaptive behavioral patterns. The use of these methods is based on the assumption that a lack of adequate reinforcements and learning experiences has blocked the development of adaptive behaviors. Typical examples of these behavioral deficits include a failure to be involved in social contacts, an inability to study, problems in being appropriately assertive, and difficulties exercising effective parenting skills.

Contingency management involves the presentation and withdrawal of rewards and punishments to promote the desired behavior(s). To successfully use such a procedure to aid individuals in acquiring new behaviors, one must make a detailed analysis of the reinforcement conditions involved. When a behavioral analysis is made the following kinds of measurements are usually obtained:

1. A baseline measurement indicating the frequency or infrequency of the behaviors in question is made. This occurs before any therapeutic intervention begins.

2. An assessment is made of the antecedents (preceding events) and consequences that occur in the situation in which the behavior is performed.

3. If the contingency management procedure involves a child, any significant others, usually the parents, are trained in the use of rewards and punishments.

4. A system is implemented to monitor the effectiveness of the program to produce the desired behavior.

If a contingency management program to reduce tantrums were devised, for example, the initial frequency of the behavior would be determined and an assessment of the antecedents and consequences (e.g., the child sees some candy, has a tantrum, and the parents buy the candy) would be made. The parent would then be taught to use rewards and punishments more effectively so as to decrease the problem behavior and to monitor the frequency with which tantrums occur after the behavioral program is implemented. As we will see later in Chapter 14, contingency management procedures have been extensively applied in the treatment of chronic pain. Chronic pain often leads to social withdrawal and isolation as a person reduces activity levels. Treatment of these problems involves providing reinforcement for increased levels of activity and for decreased levels of pain-related behaviors such as complaining, resting, and taking medication.

TIME-OUT AND RESPONSE-COST PROCEDURES    *Time-out* and *response-cost* procedures use contingency management to reduce the frequency of inappropriate behaviors. In the time-out procedure, the individual is socially isolated when he or she displays the undesired behavior. Thus, an interval of time-out, wherein other reinforcers are unavailable, is scheduled as an immediate consequence of an undesired behavior. Various kinds of time-out situations have been used to reduce problematic behavior, including time-out from social interaction and time-out from desirable activities. Such undesirable behaviors as tantrums, aggressive behaviors, and alcoholism have been suppressed using this technique.

Griffiths, Bigelow, and Liebson (1977) studied the impact of the loss of socialization opportunities or restriction of physical activity on the drinking behavior of chronic alcoholics. The alcoholic subjects in the experiment had access to alcoholic drinks during the day. However, four different consequences were imposed if the alcoholic took a drink when it was available: (1) a baseline period, during which no adverse consequences followed taking a drink; (2) a social time-out, in which the alcoholic was not allowed to interact with other patients or the staff; (3) an activity time-out, during which the patient was required to sit in a chair and engage in no activities except talking to staff and/or patients; and (4) an activity and social time-out.

Results showed an average reduction in alcohol consumption to 71% of baseline for the social time-out procedure, a greater decrease to 36% of baseline for the activity time-out procedure, and an even greater decrease to 24% of baseline for the social and activity time-out combined. These results suggest that both the social and activity restriction components of contingent time-out contribute to the suppression of drinking. Although each component alone markedly reduced drinking, the combination of activity and social time-out was most effective in reducing alcohol consumption.

Response-cost, another operant technique used to eliminate problem behaviors, is a punishment procedure wherein positive reinforcements are withdrawn to suppress a problematic behavior. The majority of response-cost procedures have emphasized the removal of conditioned reinforcers, like tokens, points, or money, contingent upon an undesirable response, as opposed to physical cost or effort (Kazdin, 1972). In a discussion of the usefulness of this procedure, Kazdin has noted that it can be used in a variety of settings where it is possible to control the removal of reinforcers.

This does not mean that a patient need be in a controlled environment. If a response-cost procedure were applied to the problem of smoking, for example, control of conditioned reinforcers might occur by asking patients to pay in advance of therapy a sum of money that may be lost if the target response (smoking) is performed. The notion behind this approach is that the threat of a fine is a powerful enough punishment to inhibit performance of the undesirable response. In one study (Elliot & Tighe, 1968) 84% of smokers were abstaining from smoking after sixteen weeks of a treatment program using response-cost as a part of the treatment package.

MODELING   Modeling procedures also have been used to teach new behavior patterns. Generally they can be categorized into one of three types: (1) procedures involving simply the observation of a model enacting the desired behavior (simple modeling); (2) procedures involving the patient's enacting the modeled behaviors during the modeling treatment (participant modeling); or (3) procedures primarily involving the patient's imagining the desired behavior (covert modeling). Such techniques are often combined with modeled approximations of the desired behavior so that the patient learns in a step-by-step fashion how to perform the target behavior. Direct reinforcement also may be a component of the modeling process if the patient is reinforced for performing a desired behavior. The experience of self-mastery also has been considered as a reinforcing aspect of some modeling procedures; simply feeling confident and proud of the ability to perform a task is rewarding in and of itself.

As we will see in Chapter 6, modeling processes have been viewed as important in the development of behaviors that have an impact on health. For example, when children see adults relying on smoking as a means of tension reduction, they are vicariously reinforced for smoking. Children thus may anticipate pleasurable consequences for themselves if they smoke, and the acquired behavior (smoking) may be performed later when the circumstances are right (Evans, 1984).

Modeling is also used to prepare patients for stressful medical events such as surgery, dental treatment, and diagnostic procedures. As we will see in Chapter 7, children who view videotapes of a model going through the same experiences that they will later encounter in the hospital have been found to show less anxiety than children who do not view the same videotapes. Similar effects have been found in adults about to undergo stressful medical diagnostic procedures.

COGNITIVE AND SELF-CONTROL THERAPIES   Many of the behavior therapies used to treat psychological problems today differ in emphasis from traditional behavioral approaches. Mahoney and Arnkoff (1978) noted that two lines of thought have emerged to produce a shift in emphasis from a stimulus–response (i.e., behavioral) perspective to a more cognitive perspective. First, an emphasis on *reciprocal determinism* as opposed to environmental determinism was ushered in by an interest in the phenomenon of self-control. Reciprocal determinism refers to a complex interaction between the organism and its environment that results in learned behavior. *Environmental determinism*, the more traditional view, emphasizes a causal link between environmental stimuli and resulting behavior, with the organism being relatively passive in the learning process. An interest in self-control has focused attention on the organism as an active force in shaping its behavioral destiny. In an applied sense, such an interest has been exemplified by the development of psychotherapeutic treatments that emphasized self-control of health problems such as weight (Stuart, 1967).

Second, in the 1960s the field of psychology renewed its interest in the role of thought, or cognition, in behavior. Thoughts, or "private events," were considered to be accessible to analysis and modification. Lloyd Homme (1965), one of Skinner's students, described a technique of analyzing and modifying thoughts known as *coverant control*. Covert sensitization, described earlier in this chapter, is an example of the impact of this renewed emphasis on cognition.

Mahoney and Arnkoff (1978) drew a useful distinction among three types of current therapies that stress the importance of thought, or cognition. They suggested that therapies be classified as: (1) self-control therapies; (2) covert conditioning therapies; or (3) cognitive learning therapies. Self-control therapies generally emphasize the use of techniques that promote self-observation and regulation abilities. Covert conditioning therapies emphasize the use of imagery-based techniques to alter maladaptive behaviors. Cognitive learning therapies emphasize the role of cognitive processes in the development of behavior and emotions and may be further classified into three subcategories: cognitive restructuring therapies, coping skills therapies, or problem solving therapies.

*Self-control Therapies.*  Early research in self-control techniques examined several different approaches, including stimulus control and self-monitoring (Mahoney & Arnkoff, 1978). *Stimulus control* techniques focus on the cueing function of specific environmental events. Specific stimuli in the environment cue particular behaviors. For example, the green light at a traffic signal produces the "accelerate" response, but the red light does not. The color of the light thereby acquires a *discriminative function*. Interest in stimulus control techniques has spawned a number of investigations of the use of stimulus control in weight control programs (Stuart, 1967; Ferster, Nurnberger, & Levitt, 1962). These weight control programs attempt to alter maladaptive eating patterns by restricting the obese person to eating in very limited settings, thereby limiting the cues associated with eating. Although such self-control approaches have had some success, further investigation of their utility is warranted (Mahoney & Arnkoff, 1978).

*Self-monitoring* is another self-control method often used as a part of behavioral treatment packages. This technique involves training patients to self-observe and record behaviors under study with the hope that such self-monitoring will promote the desired behavior change. It is hoped that the use of self-monitoring will lead to an increase in patients' self-awareness. This increased self-awareness may then lead to improved self-regulation, allowing for the successful alteration of maladaptive habits such as smoking or overeating. The success of this technique, however, is thought to be limited and variable (Mahoney & Arnkoff, 1978).

Stuart (1967) described a program for weight loss exemplifying the use of both *stimulus control* and *self-monitoring* in a self-control treatment. The treatment program extended over a four to five week period with maintenance sessions afterwards, as needed. The treatment involved daily recordings of information about food intake, circumstances under which food was consumed, emotional state at the time of eating, and weight. Patients were encouraged to use numerous behaviors to help in the self-control of eating. They were encouraged (1) to put down eating utensils and sit at the table without eating for a period of time during a meal; (2) to avoid eating while doing someting else, such as reading; (3) to eat only in a particular room and thus reduce the stimuli associated with eating; (4) to take small bites; and (5) to put down eating utensils while chewing. A few patients in this study also were taught covert sensitization to aid in reducing their desire to eat. This procedure involved imagining the food paired with an image of an aversive stimulus. The success of this and similar self-control techniques for treating obesity is discussed in more detail in Chapter 6.

COGNITIVE BEHAVIORAL THERAPIES    Cognitive behavioral therapies emphasize the role that cognitive processes play in the development of behavior and emotions. These therapies work to change a person's evaluations of self, others, and life events, and thus alter emotions and behavior. Cognitive behavioral therapies work directly on thought processes by challenging and changing maladaptive cognitions. They also stress behavior change. Behavioral exercises may be suggested as a means of illustrating to patients that their cognitions may be in error, or as a way of providing experiences that allow patients to examine their thought processes more closely.

*Cognitive restructuring* therapies are based on the premise that maladaptive behaviors and emotions partially stem from errors in a person's thinking. These errors in thinking lead to the misperceptions, distortions, or overgeneralizations of everyday events. The actual event, such as failing an examination, is not what determines how we react, feel, or behave. It is, rather, our "automatic thoughts" or "self-statements" about those events that determine these results (Beck, 1976).

Aaron Beck, one of the founders of the cognitive learning therapy movement in psychology, developed a well-known cognitive theory of and therapy
for depression (Beck, 1976). His underlying assumption is that the individual's affect and behavior are largely determined by the way in which he or
she structures the world. According to Beck, the depressed person has developed a negative view of himself, the world, and the future. These negative
cognitions form the basis of schema by which the individual then perceives
external stimuli. The symptoms of depression result from the depressed person's negative views. Because the individual's cognitive system is composed of
negative views of himself or herself, new information is incorrectly processed
to confirm this view.

Beck's theory of psychotherapy stresses the need for identifying maladaptive modes of thinking and then teaching the client more realistic ways to
evaluate experiences. The treatment of depression is based on the assumption
that when a patient's negative cognitions are reversed and realigned with reality, depression will dissipate.

Beck (1976) has described several aspects of cognitive therapy as it is
applied to alleviate psychological distress through correcting faulty cognitions.
These aspects include the following:

1. Identifying misconceptions and challenging them and the maladaptive
assumptions on which they are based. Patients are encouraged to monitor
their cognitions and to recognize the connections among cognition, affect, and
behavior. They are taught to examine the evidence for and against their
distorted cognitions and to substitute more reality-based cognitions. Patients
are, in essence, taught to identify, challenge, and alter their dysfunctional
belief system.

2. Exposing the patients to experiences that demonstrate the inadequacy of
their cognitive belief. Patients are encouraged to engage in goal-directed
behaviors and they are given particular assignments to do so. Not only do
the results of these behaviors challenge negative self-cognitions, the behaviors
in and of themselves are antithetical to a depressive position. These behavioral changes, however, must be accompanied by cognitive changes in order
to endure.

*Rational-emotive therapy* (Ellis, 1970) is also based on a theory that assumes
that psychological problems arise from faulty or "irrational" patterns of thinking. Ellis suggests that individuals inherently have two types of processes that
often conflict: the predisposition to actualize their potential and the predisposition to engage in some irrationally based thinking. Irrationally based
thinking develops early in life when the individual overly values others' evaluations of him or her. The individual eventually may deny any internally felt
needs or ideas that contradict the evaluations of other people. Denial of internal needs, ideas, or perceptions of events leads to a distortion of reality that,

in turn, may create maladaptive behaviors. The irrational beliefs that underlie such denial are thought to be the cause of negative affective experiences such as anxiety and depression.

The process by which irrational beliefs influence emotion and behavior is described by Ellis (1970) in his *ABC model*. *A* refers to some event to which the individual is exposed, such as failing an exam. The event activates the thoughts, behaviors, and emotions that follow at B and C. *B* refers to the beliefs the individual holds regarding the events that occurred. *C* symbolizes the consequences of these beliefs, the emotions and behaviors that the person experiences. Much like Beck's model of intervention for depression, the therapist's interventions involve direct efforts at having the patient examine in a critical manner the validity or rationality of the self-statements at point B. Specifically, the therapist helps the patient make the very critical discrimination between those statements at B that are objectively true and those that may be irrational. For example, reactions at B to failing an exam at A might be "I'll have to work harder next time," or "I'm a worthless person for having failed that exam." The therapist would help the patient examine the rationality of each of these statements, making a distinction between them in terms of their basis in reality. In this case, the first belief would be rational, whereas the second would be irrational.

Ellis argues that some irrational beliefs are quite common. For example, many persons believe that "it is a dire necessity for an adult human being to be loved or approved by virtually every significant person in his life," or "it is awful and catastrophic when things are not the way one would like them to be" (Ellis, 1974, p. 37). Irrational beliefs are characterized by their self-defeating nature in that holding such beliefs is usually frustrating and disappointing.

*Coping skills therapies* emphasize the importance of teaching a repertoire of skills that will allow for successful coping in a variety of stressful situations (Mahoney & Arnkoff, 1978). Goldfried (1971), for example, has described a modified version of the typical systematic desensitization procedure in which patients are encouraged first to experience the anxiety associated with specific thoughts and then to try to cope with the anxiety with relaxation. Unlike systematic desensitization, the focus here is on active coping rather than passively pairing the relaxation response with an anxiety-provoking image. Similarly, Suinn and Richardson (1971) have described a procedure that emphasizes the development of skills to deal with anxiety in many situations. This procedure is called *anxiety management training*. The therapist attempts to induce stress, through imagery, and then to train patients to use a variety of effective coping strategies.

Meichenbaum (1977) has developed a treatment program designed to teach patients to cope with "small, manageable units of stress." His program, called *stress-inoculation training*, is an attempt to teach specific strategies for dealing with a variety of stressful situations. This technique has also been applied to populations with specific psychological problems, such as phobias or problems with anger control. As we will see later it has been used in health psychology to treat patients suffering from rheumatoid arthritis (see Chapter 12) and to prepare patients for stressful medical procedures (see Chapter 7).

Stress-inoculation training has three phases. In the first phase, patients are provided with a framework for understanding their stress reactions. For example, patients who experience intense anxiety related to an academic test situation might be taught that their anxious reaction involves two elements: (1) heightened physiological arousal or anxiety occurs and is experienced as increased heart rate, muscle tension, or other physiological functions; and (2) anxiety-evoking thoughts, such as thoughts of failure, precede the heightened physiological arousal and subsequent difficulty in concentrating and performing well on tests. The therapist then would explain that treatment will help the patient control his physiological arousal and anxiety by changing the thoughts or self-statements that evoke anxiety in the situation.

In the second, or rehearsal, phase, patients are taught a number of behavioral and cognitive coping skills to use at each of four stages of the coping process. It is necessary (1) to prepare for the onset of the stressor, (2) to confront and handle the stressor, (3) to cope with the feeling of being overwhelmed, and (4) to use reinforcing self-statements after completion of the coping behavior (Meichenbaum, 1977). The specific negative self-statements that might evoke anxiety during each of these stages are modified by teaching patients to employ more adaptive coping self-statements.

Meichenbaum (1977) notes that the package of self-statements (1) encourages patients to assess the reality of the situation, (2) controls negative thoughts and images, (3) helps patients acknowledge, use, and relabel the arousal they experience, (4) prepares patients to confront the stressful situation, (5) copes with the intense fear patients might experience, and (6) helps patients reflect on their performance and reinforce themselves for having tried.

In the third, or practice, phase, patients practice their coping skills during exposure to either the specific stressor or a variety of stressors. This may be done by imagining the situation(s) or by in vivo confrontation. Thus, the patients test their skills under actual stressful conditions.

*Problem-solving therapies* emphasize the need to view many psychological difficulties as deficits in problem-solving ability, with the hope that if problem-solving techniques are taught the difficulties will be eliminated. This approach was largely initiated by Spivack and his colleagues (1976) in a series of studies involving "normal" and "psychiatric" child and adolescent populations. In comparing these two groups they found that those labeled "emotionally disturbed" were inferior to "normals" in their ability to generate a number of solutions to hypothetical problem situations. Further, their solutions were frequently inappropriate relative to social norms. Systematic training in personal problem solving was apparently quite effective with this "emotionally disturbed" group (Spivack, Platt, & Shure, 1976).

Problem-solving training has also been used in the treatment of obese adults (Black, 1987). Problem-solving training was added to a weight loss program including nutritional education, exercise, and self-monitoring. Weight loss increased after problem-solving training was begun, and there was a strong relationship between problem-solving ability and weight loss.

# Summary

Behavioral theory and therapy emphasize the observable environmental circumstances controlling the learning and continued presence of behavior and emotions. Social learning theory also emphasizes environmental events but places more stress on the importance of cognitive processes occuring within the individual.

Classical, or respondent, conditioning occurs when a previously neutral stimulus is temporally associated with an unconditioned stimulus that already elicits a specific response. After repeated pairings, the neutral stimulus becomes a conditioned stimulus and elicits the response when presented alone. In Pavlov's classic experiments, the neutral stimulus of a bell was paired with the presentation of the unconditioned stimulus of food. After repeated pairings, presentation of the bell alone led to the response of salivation.

Operant conditioning occurs when a behavior results in consequences making the later emission of that same behavior more or less probable. The addition of positive reinforcers increases the probability of a behavior, whereas the removal of negative reinforcers increases the probability.

Social learning theory emphasizes observational learning, in which a behavior may be learned even though the learner does not emit the behavior or receive direct reinforcement. By observing a model engaged in a behavior the learner may acquire the model's behavior. If the model is positively reinforced, the observer receives vicarious reinforcement and is more likely to perform the acquired behavior. Four features are required for the occurrence of observational learning: attention, retention, reproduction, and motivation. Self-efficacy is the degree to which an individual expects to be able to successfully perform a behavior.

Behavior therapies apply principles from classical, operant, and social learning theory to the treatment of behavioral, psychological, and psychophysiological problems. Systematic desensitization reduces maladaptive anxiety by pairing relaxation with stimuli that are anxiety provoking. Patients visualize anxiety-provoking scenes while relaxed until the scenes no longer elicit anxiety.

Aversive counterconditioning procedures pair unpleasant reactions with previously pleasant, but undesirable, behaviors. In this way the undesirable behavior comes to elicit an unpleasant response and the behavior therefore becomes less likely. The counterconditioning process may be in vivo, such as when nausea is physically induced in response to alcohol. The process may also occur in imagination, such as in covert sensitization. In this procedure, patients imagine distasteful consequences as they visualize themselves in undesirable behavior.

Contingency management alters the consequences of a behavior and thereby increases or decreases the likelihood of the behavior's occurrence. Desirable behaviors may be rewarded, and thus have the probability of occurrence increased. The probability of the occurrence of undesirable behaviors may be reduced by time-out and response-cost procedures. In time-out, the occurrence of undesirable behavior is followed by isolation from social stimulation or activities. In response cost, reinforcers such as money or tokens are withdrawn if a behavior occurs.

Modeling is used to teach new behaviors. Subjects may observe models engaging in desirable behaviors, imitate the behaviors after observing the model, or imagine themselves engaging in the desired behavior. Modeling may be combined with contingency management procedures by reinforcing the subject for successful demonstration of the observed behavior.

Self-control therapies change behavior by emphasizing self-observation and regulation. Stimulus control procedures alter behavior by changing the environmental cues associated with the behavior. Self-monitoring increases self-awareness as subjects keep careful records of behavior. This increased self-awareness may then lead to increased ability to regulate behavior.

Cognitive behavioral therapies stress the interaction of thoughts, emotions, and behavior. These therapies change behavior by changing thoughts, or how patients evaluate their abilities and experiences. Cognitive restructuring therapies change cognitive misperceptions and distortions and thereby attempt to change emotions and behavior. Aaron Beck's treatment approach to depression is an example of a cognitive restructuring therapy.

Rational-emotive therapy attempts to change irrational beliefs. Albert Ellis's ABC model stresses that activating events are not the real cause of maladaptive emotions and behaviors. Instead, the beliefs held about the events are much more important. Irrational beliefs are beliefs that have no basis in objective reality, whereas rational beliefs do have such a basis.

Coping skills therapies teach behaviors that allow for successful coping with stressful situations. Stress-inoculation training teaches patients skills for coping with stressful events and helps them change their self-statements about these same events and their coping abilities. In the final stage of stress-inoculation training, patients practice new coping skills in the face of real or imagined stressors. Problem-solving therapies teach patients more effective procedures for analyzing and solving life problems.

# References

ANANT, S. S. (1968). The use of verbal aversion (negative conditioning) with an alcoholic: A case report. *Behaviour Research and Therapy, 6,* 695–696.

BANDURA, A. (1965). Influence of model's reinforcement contingencies on the acquisition of imitative responses. *Journal of Personality and Social Psychology, 1,* 589–595.

BANDURA, A. (1969). *Principles of behavior modification*. New York: Holt, Rinehart and Winston.

BANDURA, A. (1971). *Social learning theory*. Morristown, NJ: General Learning Press.

BANDURA, A. (1977). *Social learning theory*. Englewood Cliffs, NJ: Prentice-Hall.

BECK, A. T. (1976). *Cognitive therapy and the emotional disorders*. New York; International Universities Press.

BLACK, D. R. (1987). A minimal intervention program and a problem-solving program for weight control. *Cognitive Therapy and Research, 11*, 107–120.

CAUTELA, J. R. (1966). A behavior therapy approach to pervasive anxiety. *Behaviour Research and Therapy, 4*, 99–109.

ELLIOT, R., & TIGHE, T. (1968). Breaking the cigarette habit: Effects of a technique involving threatened loss of money. *Psychological Record, 18*, 503–513.

ELLIS, A. (1970). *The essence of rational psychotherapy: A comprehensive approach to treatment*. New York: Institute for Rational Living.

ELLIS, A. (1974). *Humanistic psychotherapy*. New York: McGraw-Hill.

EVANS, R. I. (1984). A social inoculation strategy to deter smoking in adolescents. In J. D. Matarazzo, S. M. Weiss, J. A. Herd, N. E. Miller, & S. M. Weiss (Eds.), *Behavioral health* (pp. 765–776). New York: Wiley.

FERSTER, C. B., NURNBERGER, J. I., & LEVITT, E. B. (1962). The control of eating. *Journal of Mathetics, 1*, 87–109.

GOLDFRIED, M. R. (1971). Systematic desensitization as training in self-control. *Journal of Consulting and Clinical Psychology, 37*, 228–234.

GRIFFITHS, R. R., BIGELOW,. G., & LIEBSON, I. (1977). Comparison of social time-out and activity time-out procedures in suppressing ethanol self-administration in alcoholics. *Behaviour Research and Therapy, 15*, 329–336.

HOMME, L. E. (1965). Perspectives in psychology: XXIV. Control of coverants, the operants of the mind. *Psychological Record, 15*, 501–511.

JACOBSON, E. (1938). *Progressive relaxation*. Chicago: University of Chicago Press.

JANDA, H. L., & RIMM, D. C. (1972). Covert sensitization in the treatment of obesity. *Journal of Abnormal Psychology, 80*, 37–42.

KAZDIN, A. E. (1972). Response cost: The removal of conditioned reinforcers for therapeutic change. *Behavior Therapy, 3*, 533–546.

MAHONEY, M. J. (1977). Personal science: A cognitive learning therapy. In A. Ellis and R. Grieger (Eds.), *Handbook of rational psychotherapy*. New York: Springer.

MAHONEY, M. J., & ARNKOFF, D. B. (1978). Cognitive and self-control therapies. In S. Garfield, & A. E. Bergin (Eds.), *Handbook of psychotherapy and behavior change: An empirical analysis* (2nd ed.) (pp. 689–722). New York: Wiley.

MAHONEY, M. J., & MAHONEY, L. (1976). *Permanent weight control*. New York: W. W. Norton.

MASTERS, J. C., BURISH, T. G., HOLLON, S. D., & RIMM, D. C. (1987, 1989). *Behavior therapy: Techniques and empirical findings* (3rd ed.). New York: Harcourt, Brace, Jovanovich.

MEICHENBAUM, D. (1977). *Cognitive behavior modification*. New York: Plenum.

SHERRINGTON, C. S. (1906). *Integrative action of the nervous system*. New Haven, CT: Yale University Press.

SIPICH, J. F., RUSSEL, R. K., and TOBIAS, L. L. (1974). A comparison of covert sensitization and "nonspecific" treatment in the modification of smoking behavior. *Journal of Behavior Therapy and Experimental Psychiatry, 5*, 201–203.

SKINNER, B. F. (1953). *Science and human behavior*. New York: Macmillan.

SPIVACK, G., PLATT, J. J., & SHURE M. D. (1976). *The problem-solving approach to adjustment*. San Francisco: Jossey-Bass.

STUART, R. B., (1967). Behavioral control over-eating. *Behaviour Research and Therapy, 5*, 357–365.

SUINN, R. M., & RICHARDSON, F. (1971). Anxiety management training: A nonspecific behavior therapy program for anxiety control. *Behavior Therapy, 2*, 498–510.

TOOLEY, J. T., and PRATT, S. (1967). An experimental procedure for the extinction of smoking behavior. *Psychological Record, 17*, 209–218.

WATSON, J. B., & RAYNER, R. (1920). Conditioned emotional reaction. *Journal of Experimental Psychology, 3*, 1–14.

WOLPE, J. (1958). *Psychotherapy by reciprocal inhibition*. Stanford, CA: Stanford University Press.

WOLPE, J. (1982). *The practice of behavior therapy* (3rd ed.). Oxford, England: Pergamon.

# The Diathesis-Stress Model

The medical model of disease discussed in Chapter 3 attempts to explain illness as the result of biological factors alone. Thus, the medical model does not address the role of behavioral, psychological, and social factors in the onset of and course of illness. In recent years research has demonstrated that behavioral and psychosocial variables make important contributions to many, if not all, diseases. As an alternative to the medical model, the diathesis-stress model of illness proposes that behavioral, psychological, social, environmental, and biological elements should all be considered in the description of disease (Levi, 1974).

According to the diathesis-stress model, biological factors alone cannot explain health and illness. We also need to consider the interaction of stress and diathesis, factors that predispose a person to illness. For example, why do some people who are exposed to a flu virus develop the illness whereas others remain healthy? Although biological factors are important, psychological variables such as stress will also influence the onset and course of illness. Similarly, behavioral, social, and environmental variables help to determine the state of an individual's health.

The *biopsychosocial model*, a model that is very similar to the diathesis-stress model, states that psychological, social, and cultural factors will interact with biological variables to determine the onset, severity, and course of illness. In the original formulation of the biopsychosocial model, Engel (1977) pointed out that biological variables alone are not sufficient to explain disease. He proposed that psychological variables such as stress could interact with biological factors to alter susceptibility to disease. Moreover, he challenged the arbitrary classification of diseases as organic (i.e., a disease with a known biological cause) and psychogenic (i.e., a disease with a psychological cause only). According to both the biopsychosocial and diathesis-stress models, biological and psychological factors are involved in the onset of all diseases.

When individuals develop illnesses, psychological and social factors influence how they experience symptoms and whether or not they seek medical treatment (Engel, 1980). The biopsychosocial and diathesis-stress models also emphasize the importance of psychosocial factors in the relationship between the patient and the physician. Thus, the success or failure of medical treatment will depend on psychological and social as well as biological factors. Similarly, the severity, course, and outcome of an illness will be the result of multiple interacting variables.

This chapter describes several models of stress that have contributed to the development of the diathesis-stress and biopsychosocial models of illness. In addition, behavioral, psychological, and social factors that influence stress are examined. Finally, the use of the diathesis-stress model in health psychology is discussed.

## Selye's Biological Model of Stress

Hans Selye (1936, 1956) was one of the first researchers to systematically study stress. In a series of laboratory experiments, Selye injected rats with toxic substances (e.g., formaldehyde) and observed their physiological responses. He found that a wide variety of toxins produced the same physiological changes: (a) enlargement of the adrenal cortex, (b) atrophy, or shrinking, of the thymus, spleen, and lymph nodes, and (c) bleeding ulcers in the lining of the rats' stomachs. Selye (1956) proposed that these bodily changes were part of a *general adaptation syndrome* (GAS), a nonspecific reaction to any noxious agent. The noxious agent, or *stressor*, usually was a toxic substance or an environmental condition such as excessive heat, cold, or crowding.

According to Selye (1976), all animals, including humans, who are exposed to stressors for an extended time period will demonstrate the GAS. The GAS is composed of three stages that are depicted in Figure 5.1: (a) the alarm reaction, (b) the stage of resistance, and (c) the stage of exhaustion. During the initial *alarm reaction*, a high level of adrenocorticotrophic hormone (ACTH) is secreted by the anterior pituitary gland. The ACTH stimulates the adrenal cortex to release high levels of glucocorticoids. The glucocorticoids are anti-inflammatory hormones that prepare the animal to defend against the threat of the stressor.

During the *stage of resistance*, the second stage of the GAS, the physiological changes of the alarm reaction gradually cease. At this time the animal has strong resistance to the stressor. Any new stressor, however, poses great difficulty for the animal. Moreover, if the original stressor continues, the animal enters the *stage of exhaustion*, the final GAS stage. This phase is characterized by a failure of lymphocyte (white blood cell) production. In addition, the anterior pituitary gland and adrenal cortex lose the capacity to release hormones. As a result of this physiological exhaustion, the animal becomes very susceptible to disease. Selye (1976) proposed that *diseases of adaptation* such as peptic ulcers and hypertension are apt to develop during the stage of exhaustion in animals with biological factors that predispose them to the diseases.

In Selye's model, *stress* is defined as the nonspecific response of the body to any demand (i.e., stressor) placed upon it (Selye, 1974). The three stages of the GAS constitute the nonspecific response. Selye's model has been criticized, however, for its simplicity and nonspecificity. The physiological response to stress appears to be more complicated than the GAS (Mason, 1975). Moreover, different stressors may cause specific patterns of physiological responses (Mason, 1971). Additional problems with Selye's model are that it

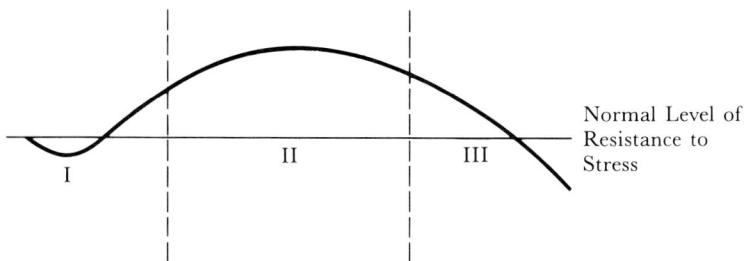

FIGURE 5.1   The three stages of Selye's General Adaptation Syndrome. Stage I is the alarm reaction, stage II is resistance, and stage III is exhaustion.

underestimates the importance of psychological stressors and cognitive factors involved in the appraisal of stressors.

# Lazarus's Psychophysiological Model of Stress

Richard Lazarus and his colleagues have developed a psychophysiological model of stress that includes psychological as well as biological variables (Lazarus, 1966; Lazarus & Folkman, 1984b). Lazarus (1966) pointed out that Selye's definition of a stressor as a noxious agent is inadequate because it does not explain why a stimulus may be a stressor for one person but not for another. For example, taking an organic chemistry exam may be a stressor for one student but not for another. According to Lazarus, the key variable is not the nature of the stressor but the individual's perception that he or she is threatened by the stressor. In Lazarus's three-stage model of stress, he emphasizes the importance of cognitive perceptions or appraisals, as outlined in Figure 5.2. *Stress* is defined as a particular relationship between the person and environment that is appraised by the person as taxing or exceeding his or her resources and endangering his or her well-being (Lazarus & Folkman, 1984b).

## Cognitive Appraisals

The first stage in Lazarus's model, *appraisal*, explains why a stimulus may be noxious for one individual but not for another. When individuals encounter an external stimulus in the environment (e.g., chemistry exam) or an internal stimulus (e.g., physical symptom), they make a *primary appraisal* of the stimulus. This appraisal evaluates the significance of the stimulus in regard to its possible effect on their well-being. They may evaluate the stimulus as irrelevant, benign-positive, or stressful (Lazarus & Folkman, 1984b). If the encounter with the stimulus has no implication for the person's well-being, then the encounter is judged as *irrelevant*. *Benign-positive* appraisals are made if the encounter with the stimulus protects or enhances well-being or promises to do so.

A *stress appraisal* is made if the encounter with the stimulus involves harm/ loss, threat, or challenge. *Harm* or *loss* includes damage to the individual caused by injury, illness, reduced self-esteem, loss of a loved person, and so forth. When the harm or loss is expected in the future, then a *threat* appraisal is made. The third type of stress appraisal, *challenge*, is an evaluation of a stimulus encounter as an opportunity for gain, growth, or mastery. It should be noted that the three types of stresss appraisal are not mutually exclusive. For example, a majority of students facing an important examination reported both threat and challenge appraisals (Folkman & Lazarus, 1985).

When a stress appraisal is made, the individual then makes a *secondary appraisal*, an evaluation of what might and can be done to cope with the stressful encounter (Lazarus & Folkman, 1984b). The person evaluates the different coping strategies available, the possible outcomes of using the strategies, and his or her ability to employ the strategies. The process of secondary appraisal, in combination with primary appraisal, determines the individual's emotional reaction and the degree of stress. For example, if a person makes a threat appraisal and believes that no effective coping strategies are available that will reduce the threat, then the degree of stress will be great. Moreover, the person will probably experience a negative emotion such as anxiety, depression, or anger. In contrast, when a person makes a stress appraisal but feels confident that he or she can use effective coping strategies, then the stress will not be great. Positive emotions such as excitement or eagerness may be experienced, and any negative emotions will probably not be overwhelming.

## Coping

During the process of secondary appraisal, the individual evaluates and selects coping strategies that are implemented in the second or coping stage of Lazarus's model. *Coping* is defined as constantly changing cognitive and be-

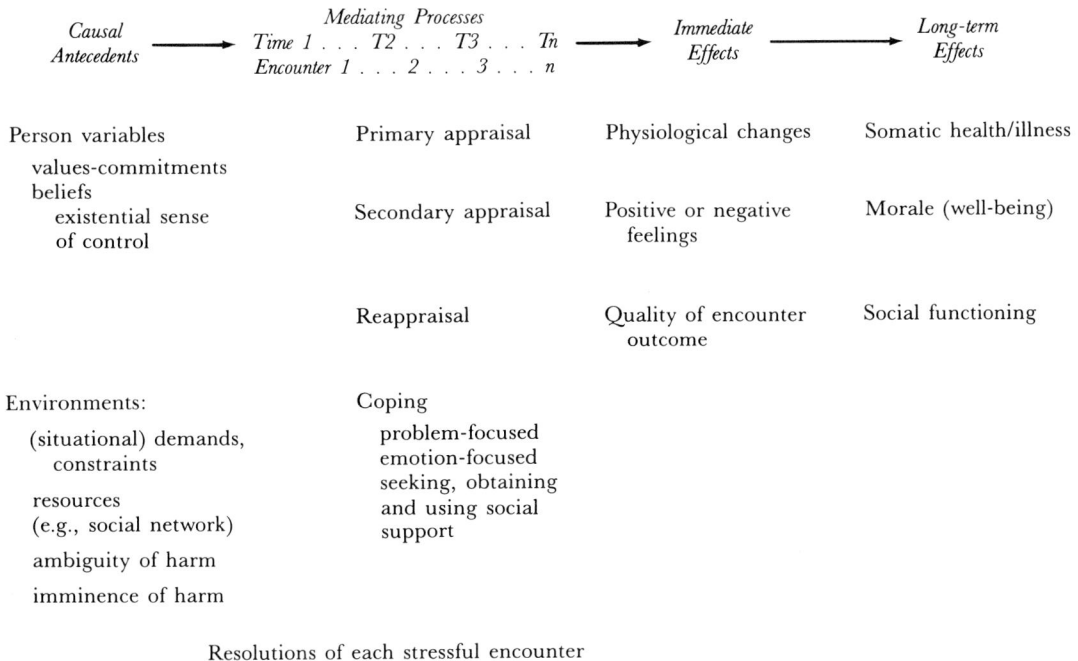

| Causal Antecedents → | Mediating Processes<br>*Time 1 . . . T2 . . . T3 . . . Tn*<br>*Encounter 1 . . . 2 . . . 3 . . . n* → | Immediate Effects → | Long-term Effects |
|---|---|---|---|
| Person variables | Primary appraisal | Physiological changes | Somatic health/illness |
| values-commitments<br>beliefs<br>existential sense<br>of control | Secondary appraisal | Positive or negative feelings | Morale (well-being) |
| | Reappraisal | Quality of encounter outcome | Social functioning |
| Environments: | Coping | | |
| (situational) demands, constraints | problem-focused<br>emotion-focused<br>seeking, obtaining<br>and using social<br>support | | |
| resources<br>(e.g., social network) | | | |
| ambiguity of harm | | | |
| imminence of harm | | | |

Resolutions of each stressful encounter

FIGURE 5.2 Richard Lazarus' model of stress. The model presents a theoretical scheme for understanding stress, coping with it, and adapting to it as a process occurring over time, with immediate and long range health consequences. From *Stress, Appraisal, and Coping* (p. 305) by R. S. Lazarus and S. Folkman, 1984, New York: Springer. Reprinted by permission.

havioral efforts to manage a specific stimulus that is appraised as stressful (Lazarus & Folkman, 1984a). Coping strategies can be divided into problem-focused coping and emotion-focused coping. *Problem-focused coping* attempts to alter or manage the stressful stimulus. Examples of problem-focused coping strategies include studying for an examination and seeking medical care for a physical symptom. *Emotion-focused coping* attempts to alter or manage one's emotional responses to the stressful stimulus. Examples of emotion-focused coping strategies include practicing relaxation exercises and taking tranquilizing drugs to reduce anxiety.

Emotion-focused coping strategies tend to be used when the person's secondary appraisal indicates that nothing can be done to modify the encounter with the stimulus. Problem-focused coping strategies are likely when the secondary appraisal indicates that direct action can change the encounter with the stressful stimulus. Both types of coping strategies, however, may be used at once. The two types may enhance or reduce each other's effectiveness (Lazarus & Folkman, 1984a).

Recent research has identified problem- and emotion-focused coping strategies that are often employed when the stressor is related to health and illness. Individuals who experience a physical symptom or illness may use the emotion-focused strategy of *denial*. Denial allows the individual to cope with the threat of illness by denying or minimizing the meaning or seriousness of physical symptoms. For example, a person who experiences chest pain may deny the possibility that he or she is having a heart attack. The use of denial typically reduces anxiety but may delay medical treatment.

Additional emotion-focused strategies frequently used to cope with the threat of illness are requesting emotional support and reassurance, seeking relevant information regarding the illness or symptoms, and finding a purpose or meaning in the illness. As an example, most patients with spinal cord injuries seek information regarding their rehabilitation and also attempt to explain why they were injured (Bulman & Wortman, 1977).

Problem-focused strategies used to cope with the stress of illness include learning specific illness-related procedures such as measuring blood pressure or giving insulin injections. Similarly, patients with specific illnesses may set concrete goals such as learning to walk again, reducing pain intensity, or losing weight. Individuals who face stressful medical procedures may use the problem-focused strategy of mental rehearsal of the procedure and rehearsal of steps that can be used to deal with the stressor (see Chapter 7).

## Outcome

The effectiveness of the coping strategies chosen and the skill with which they are employed help to determine the *outcome* of the stimulus encounter, the third stage in Lazarus's model of stress. Three kinds of outcomes are influenced by stressful encounters: (1) functioning in work and social living, (2) morale or life satisfaction, and (3) somatic health (Lazarus & Folkman,

1984b). Outcomes are affected by environmental and social variables (e.g., material resources and social support) as well as by the choice of coping strategies. Additionally, constitutional factors such as organs or organ systems that are vulnerable to stress and autonomic nervous system reactivity to stress contribute to the outcomes of stressful encounters.

HEALTH OUTCOMES    Figure 5.3 depicts how an encounter with a stressor may contribute to the development of a specific illness. The person-environment relationship will be influenced by the person's background and personal factors such as intellectual ability and learning history. The individual's physical and social environment (e.g, financial resources, social support) will also affect an encounter with a potential stressor in the environment. If the individual makes a stress appraisal, then he or she will select coping strategies to manage the encounter with the stressor.

Lazarus and Folkman (1984a,b) have proposed that the use of specific coping strategies may contribute to the development of specific illnesses. For example, the strategies used to cope with anger-inducing situations may contribute to the development of hypertension in certain individuals. Harburg, Blakelock, and Roeper (1979) interviewed workers to determine how they coped with work-related anger in response to a difficult boss. Subjects who reported using the coping strategies of "just walking away from the situation," "protesting to the boss," or "reporting the boss to the union" demonstrated higher blood pressures during the interview than subjects who used the coping strategy of "talking to the boss after he had cooled down." Thus, specific coping strategies may contribute to the development of hypertension in susceptible individuals. Genetic and/or externally produced weaknesses of particular organs or organ systems also contribute to the development of specific illnesses. For example, individuals with a family history of hypertension are

**The Specificity Model of Illness**

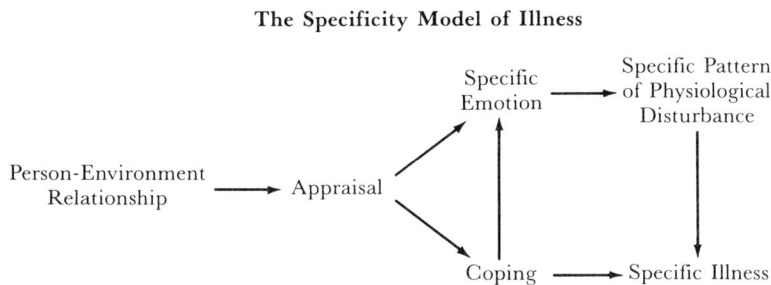

FIGURE 5.3   The specificity model of illness. This model suggests that specific emotions and coping processes may be associated with the development of specific illnesses. From *Stress, Appraisal, and Coping* (p. 219) by R. S. Lazarus and S. Folkman, 1984, New York: Springer. Reprinted by permission.

more vulnerable to the development of this illness than individuals with no family history.

The specific emotions that result from an individual's cognitive appraisal of a potential stressor may also contribute to the development of specific illnesses (Lazarus, 1966; Lazarus & Folkman, 1984b). Individual emotions have been associated with specific patterns of physiological arousal (Mason, 1975). Thus, a chronic negative emotion that is associated with potentially damaging physiological changes (e.g., elevated catecholamine levels) may be a factor involved in the onset of disease. In contrast, positive emotions may produce physiological changes that help to prevent disease and maintain health (Lazarus, Kanner, & Folkman, 1980).

# Factors That Influence Stress

## Behavioral Factors

When an individual encounters a potential stressor in the environment, certain characteristics of the stressor will influence the person's reaction to it. *Duration*, the length of time the person is exposed to a stressor, helps to determine the person's appraisal of the stressor and the outcome of the stressful encounter. In general, stress appraisals and negative outcomes are more likely when the duration of the stressor is long than when the duration is brief. For example, individuals with a chronic illness such as cancer are more likely to perceive their illness as a serious threat and to experience negative reactions (e.g., depression, disability) than individuals with a brief illness such as the flu (Burish & Bradley, 1983).

In some cases, negative outcomes may be less likely when the duration of the stressor is long than when it is brief. For example, subjects exposed to a brief period of noise bursts typically demonstrate impaired performance on cognitive tasks administered immediately after the noise (Glass & Singer, 1972). In contrast, research on the effects of chronic noise suggests that most adults can adapt to a moderate level of chronic noise in their environment (Cohen, Glass, & Phillips, 1978). People's ability to adjust to a chronic stressor is probably related to their cognitive appraisals of the stressor and use of coping strategies as well as to the characteristics of the stressor.

One important characteristic of the stressor that influences reactions to stress is *predictability*. People usually report that they prefer predictable to unpredictable stressors. In one recent study, female subjects were exposed to predictable and unpredictable electric shocks (Katz & Wykes, 1985). The subjects perceived the predictable shocks as less aversive and less distressing than the unpredictable shocks. Moreover, the subjects demonstrated less autonomic nervous system arousal during the brief waiting period before the predictable shocks than during the period before the unpredictable ones.

Although most individuals report a preference for predictable as opposed to unpredictable stressors, several studies have found that subjects demonstrated more autonomic arousal and affective distress before predictable than before unpredictable stressors (e.g., Monat, Averill, & Lazarus, 1972). When the waiting period was longer than a few seconds, subjects facing an unpredictable stressor were able to distract themselves more effectively than subjects who knew when the stressor would occur. Thus, the effective use of distraction or other avoidant-type coping strategies before an unpredictable stressor may help to reduce autonomic arousal and emotional distress.

Other factors besides the efficacy of coping strategies will affect people's reactions to predictable and unpredictable stressors. The type of stressor is important; some stressors are probably easier to cope with when they are predictable. In addition, whether or not individuals can control or change the stressor will influence their reactions to the stressor.

## Psychological Factors

PERCEIVED CONTROL   Perceived control, the belief that one can control a stressor, appears to be an important factor influencing cognitive appraisals of stress, coping, and adaptational outcomes (Lazarus & Folkman, 1984a). Beliefs about control can be general beliefs or situational appraisals of control. A general belief about control indicates the extent to which people think they can control events and outcomes of importance. *Locus of control* orientation (LOC; Rotter, 1966) is a personality dimension that assesses people's general beliefs about control in their lives. Individuals with an *internal LOC* believe that events and outcomes are contingent on their behavior. In contrast, individuals with an *external LOC* believe that events and outcomes depend on fate, luck, chance, or the influence of powerful people.

The results of research examining the influence of LOC on reactions to potential stressors related to health and illness indicate that individuals with an internal LOC tend to demonstrate more effective coping behavior and more positive outcomes than external LOC individuals (Strickland, 1978). For example, external LOC patients with genital herpes had more frequent recurrences of the herpes infection and greater discomfort than internal LOC patients (Silver, Auerbach, Vishniavsky, & Kaplowitz, 1986). In a study of patients hospitalized for spinal cord injuries, patients with an internal LOC had more positive self-concepts and reported less depression than subjects with an external LOC (Dinardo, 1972). Other studies, however, have found no relations between LOC and coping or emotional reactions to illness (e.g., Bulman & Wortman, 1977).

In a review of the research on LOC and health-related behaviors, Strickland (1978) concluded that LOC is only one of a number of complex factors influencing reactions to the stress of illness. The conflicting LOC findings may be related to numerous assessment instruments used to measure LOC.

The Multidimensional Health Locus of Control Scale (Wallston, Wallston, & DeVellis, 1978), an instrument that assesses general beliefs about control over health and illness, may be the most appropriate measure to use in studies of LOC and stress associated with illness.

*Situational control appraisals* refer to the individual's beliefs about the possibilities for control in a particular stressful situation (Folkman, 1984). These appraisals are part of the secondary appraisal process and depend on the individual's analysis of the demands of the situation, coping resources and strategies available, and his or her ability to implement needed coping strategies. Situational appraisals of control are similar to Bandura's concept of self-efficacy (see Chapter 4). Self-efficacy is the belief that one can perform the behavior necessary to produce a desired outcome (Bandura, 1977). Thus, a person with a high level of self-efficacy in a stressful situation probably believes he or she can control the stressor.

Many investigators have assumed that situational appraisals of a high level of control will be stress reducing (Averill, 1973). Most of the research on situational-control appraisals and stress supports this hypothesis. In a classic study of the effects of control on adjustment to a nursing home, patients who were given responsibility for making daily decisions subsequently demonstrated more activity, alertness, and positive affect than patients who were encouraged to allow the staff to make their decisions (Langer & Rodin, 1976). The results of a follow-up study eighteen months later revealed that the patients who were encouraged to control daily decisions had experienced better general health and fewer mortalities than patients who were not encouraged to control decisions (Rodin & Langer, 1977).

Situational beliefs about control may affect the coping and adjustment of patients with chronic illness. In a study of patients with breast cancer, women who reported the belief that they could control their cancer demonstrated better adjustment than women without this belief (Taylor, Lichtman, & Wood, 1984). If a patient believed that she could control her illness, she was asked how she thought she could exert the control. *Cognitive control*, the belief that one has a cognitive strategy available that can reduce the stressfulness of an event, was strongly associated with good adjustment. A frequently reported cognitive strategy was "thinking about life differently." *Behavioral control*, the belief that one has a behavioral strategy available that can reduce the stressfulness of an event, was also significantly correlated with good adjustment. A frequently reported behavioral strategy was "taking more time for leisure activities." Thus, when assessing situational appraisals of control, it is important to determine how individuals believe they can exert control and over what aspects of the stressful situation.

In contexts related to health and illness, people may make situational appraisals of control over information, behaviors, cognitions, emotions, and/or physiological processes. An individual may perceive control over one aspect of a stressful situation but not over other aspects (Folkman, 1984). For example, patients with spinal cord injuries may believe that learning to transfer from a bed to a wheelchair is under their control but that learning to walk is not under their control. In some situations, appraisals of control over multiple factors can increase rather than reduce stress. Mills and Krantz (1979) found that blood donors who were given informational control (i.e., description of procedures and expected sensations involved in donating blood) and behavioral control (i.e., choice of arm to be used) reported more discomfort than donors who were given one type of control.

Perceptions of control that do not match reality may also be stress inducing. For example, patients with rheumatoid arthritis who believe they can control their illness using nontraditional therapies (e.g., copper bracelets) but fail to do so may experience more distress than patients who do not believe in nontraditional treatments. Thus, the context as well as the type of control appraisal must be considered when assessing the effects of perceived control on coping and adaptation.

LEARNED HELPLESSNESS    When individuals are exposed to repeated uncontrollable events, they may experience debilitating consequences. According to the *learned helplessness* theory, learning that important outcomes in one's life are uncontrollable results in motivational, cognitive, and emotional deficits (Seligman, 1975). The *motivational deficit* consists of a reduction in behavioral responses; the individual decides that responding is futile. The *cognitive deficit* consists of difficulty in future learning of behavioral responses that will produce desired outcomes. The *emotional deficit* is the emotional distress that results from learning that the current events are uncontrollable.

The learned helplessness phenomenon was first observed in laboratory animals. Dogs exposed to repeated unavoidable electric shocks seemed to give up and passively accept the shock (Seligman & Maier, 1967). When the shocks became avoidable, the dogs did not learn the escape reponse but demonstrated their emotional distress by whining, lying down, and so forth. The learned helplessness phenomenon has also been demonstrated in humans exposed to uncontrollable events (Seligman, 1975). Critics of the learned helplessness theory, however, have pointed out that people who lack control over desired outcomes do not always develop motivational, cognitive, and emotional deficits (Buchwald, Coyne, & Cole, 1978; Peterson, 1982). In a revision of the original learned helplessness theory, Abramson, Seligman, and Teasdale (1978) proposed that the development of learned helplessness will depend on the *attributions*, or explanations, that individuals make for their lack of control. Learned helplessness is most apt to develop when people attribute the uncontrollability to their global, stable personality factors (e.g., incompetence, lack of intelligence). As noted in the discussion of situational-control appraisals, other cognitive appraisals in addition to attributions will influence the effects of uncontrollability. For example, individuals may perceive control over their emotions and cognitions even when events are uncontrollable.

Although the learned helplessness phenomenon is more complex than its original formulation, the theory appears to have important applications in research on the stress associated with illness. For example, patients with a chronic disease whose cause, course, and cure are unknown may perceive the disease as uncontrollable. This perception of uncontrollability may cause patients to experience the emotional, motivational, and cognitive deficits characteristic of learned helplessness. Patients who perceive their illness as uncontrollable may also demonstrate negative behaviors such as excessive medication intake and nonadherence to treatment regimens. The failure of these patients to cope effectively with their disease may reinforce their perceptions of helplessness and the deficits associated with helplessness.

HARDINESS    Kobasa (1979) has proposed that a personality style called "hardiness" may help to protect individuals from the potentially negative effects of stress. Hardiness is composed of three personality traits: (1) the belief that one can *control*, or influence events in one's life, (2) a sense of *commitment*, involvement, and purpose in daily activities, and (3) the flexibility to adapt to change in the environment as though change is a *challenge* to further personal growth. Thus, "hardy" individuals are characterized by a sense of control, commitment, and challenge. The control dimension is similar to an internal LOC but also includes cognitive control, or the ability to find meaning in stressful situations.

The results of several studies have suggested that individuals with a hardy personality style adapt more effectively to stressful life events than individuals without the personality style. In a five-year study of a large sample of business executives, the subjects periodically reported any stressful life events and illnesses that they experienced (Kobasa, Maddi, & Kahn, 1982). Hardiness was assessed using a questionnaire made up of standardized personality tests, and the executives were divided into high-hardiness and low-hardiness groups. A high level of life stress and low hardiness both were significantly associated with self-report of increased illness. Hardiness, however, appeared to help protect the high-stress subjects from increased illness. The high-stress/high-hardiness executives reported only half as much illness as the high-stress/low-hardiness executives.

Other studies have demonstrated the positive influence of hardiness on the physical and mental health of lawyers, army officers, and college students (Kobasa, 1982a, 1982b; Wiebe & McCallum, 1986). Unfortunately, most of the studies on hardiness have measured self-report of health problems but not actual health. It is not clear whether hardiness influences health or only people's reports of their health (Funk & Houston, 1987).

# Social Factors

LIFE EVENTS    Major life events such as marriage or loss of a job may be powerful social stressors in a persons's life. Many clinical case studies have suggested that stressful life events often precede the onset of illness. In the early 1960s, Holmes, Rahe, and their colleagues studied the case histories of more than 5,000 patients and developed a list of events that often occurred just prior to the onset of illness (Rahe, Meyer, Smith, Kjaer, & Holmes, 1964). From this list, Holmes and Rahe (1967) developed the Social Readjustment Rating Scale (SRRS), an instrument used to measure the stress associated with negative and positive life events (see Figure 5.4).

As can be seen in Figure 5.4, each life event has a point value associated with it. The point values were determined by asking a large sample of people to rate the amount of change and adjustment required by each life event. Holmes and Rahe (1967) assumed that events that produce many life changes and necessitate much adjustment are more stressful than events that are associated with less change and adjustment. The most stressful event, death of a spouse, has the highest number of points, or *life-change units*. Losing a spouse causes many disruptions and adaptations in a person's life. In contrast, a life event such as Christmas is assigned a low number of life-change units because it does not require many life changes and adaptations.

After the life-change units were established using the SRRS, Holmes and Rahe (1967) developed the Schedule of Recent Experiences (SRE), a self-administered questionnaire that contains the events from the SRRS. The SRE asks the subject to check all events that occurred in a given time period (e.g., the past year). In an early study using the SRE, Rahe (1972) asked more than

| Rank | Life Event | Mean Value |
|------|------------|------------|
| 1. | Death of spouse | 100 |
| 2. | Divorce | 73 |
| 3. | Marital separation | 65 |
| 4. | Detention in jail or other institution | 63 |
| 5. | Death of a close family member | 63 |
| 6. | Major personal injury or illness | 53 |
| 7. | Marriage | 50 |
| 8. | Being fired | 47 |
| 9. | Marital reconciliation | 45 |
| 10. | Retirement | 45 |
| 11. | Major change in the health or behavior of a family member | 44 |
| 12. | Pregnancy | 40 |
| 13. | Sexual difficulties | 39 |
| 14. | Gaining a new family member (e.g., through birth, adoption, oldster moving in, etc.) | 39 |
| 15. | Major business readjustment (e.g., merger, reorganization, bankruptcy, etc.) | 39 |
| 16. | Major change in financial state (e.g., a lot worse off or a lot better off than usual) | 38 |
| 17. | Death of a close friend | 37 |
| 18. | Changing to a different line of work | 36 |
| 19. | Major change in the number of arguments with spouse (e.g., either a lot more or a lot less than usual, regarding child-rearing, personal habits, etc.) | 35 |
| 20. | Taking out a mortgage or loan for a major purchase (e.g., for a home, business, etc.) | 31 |

FIGURE 5.4   The first twenty items of the Social Readjustment Rating Scale. From "The Social Readjustment Rating Scale" by T. H. Holmes and R. H. Rahe, 1967, *Journal of Psychosomatic Research, 11,* p. 214. Reprinted by permission.

2,000 navy personnel to report their life events and histories of illness for each of the past ten years. Subjects who reported only a few life-change units for a given year tended to report good health for the following year. When subjects reported many life-change units for a given year, they were also apt to report one or more illnesses during the next year. This correlation between life-change units and subsequent illness was small (about .30) but statistically significant.

In prospective studies using the SRE, the number of life-change units has been used to predict the probability of future illness. For example, the SRE was administered to sailors who were ready to depart on a six-month cruise (Rahe, Mahan, & Arthur, 1970). Life-change units for the six months prior to the cruise were compared with shipboard medical records. The sailors who reported many life-change units experienced significantly more illnesses than sailors who reported few life changes. Thus, scores on the SRE predicted which sailors were apt to become ill.

Other prospective and retrospective studies have found significant associations between life-change units and sudden cardiac death (Rahe, Romo, Bennett, & Siltanen, 1974), abnormal menstrual bleeding (Tudiver, 1989), and athletic injuries (Bramwell, Masuda, Wagner, & Holmes, 1975). Significant correlations have also been found between life-change units and psychiatric symptoms and disorders such as depression (Paykel, Prusoff, & Myers, 1975). In general, people who experience many life changes appear to be more vulnerable to subsequent physical and psychological problems than people who experience few life changes.

Although numerous studies have shown a relationship between life events and illness, the relationship is not a strong one. Life change is only one of many factors that help to explain the onset of illness. Moreover, the SRE has been criticized for multiple flaws (Cohen, 1979; Miller, 1989). As the scale contains more negative than positive events, it may exclude many positive events that are potentially stressful. Similarly, the SRE does not allow individuals to list additional negative or positive events that have occurred. Another problem with the SRE is that some of the life events (e.g., major change in eating habits) may be symptoms of incipient illness rather than stressful events that contribute to the onset of illness.

That the SRE relies on self-report is an additional problem. People may forget some of the life events they have experienced, or they may forget when a specific event occurred. When individuals are asked to report their histories of illness and life events, they may give a biased report. As many people believe that stress contributes to illness, they may make their report of life events correspond to their report of illness. In spite of the problems associated with the SRE, it remains a useful research tool for studying the impact of potentially stressful life events. Similar scales have been developed, however, that have attempted to correct the problems associated with the SRE (Miller, 1989).

The Hassles Scale

Directions: Hassles are irritants that can range from minor annoyances to fairly major pressures, problems, or difficulties. They can occur few or many times. Listed below are a number of ways in which a person can feel hassled. First, circle the hassles that have happened to you in the past month. Then look at the numbers on the right of the items you circled. Indicate how severe each of the circled hassles has been for you in the past month by circling a 1, 2, or 3.

(Severity: 1 = somewhat severe; 2 = moderately severe; 3 = extremely severe.)

|    |    |    |    |    |
|----|----|----|----|----|
| 1. | Misplacing or losing things | 1 | 2 | 3 |
| 2. | Concerns about owing money | 1 | 2 | 3 |
| 3. | Too many responsibilities | 1 | 2 | 3 |
| 4. | Planning meals | 1 | 2 | 3 |
| 5. | Home maintenance (inside) | 1 | 2 | 3 |
| 6. | Having to wait | 1 | 2 | 3 |
| 7. | Not getting enough sleep | 1 | 2 | 3 |
| 8. | Concerns about weight | 1 | 2 | 3 |
| 9. | Not enough time to do the things you need to do | 1 | 2 | 3 |
| 10. | Hassles from boss or supervisor | 1 | 2 | 3 |

FIGURE 5.5  Sample items from the Hassles Scale. From "Comparisons of Two Modes of Stress Measurement: Daily Hassles and Uplifts Versus Major Life Events" by A. D. Kanner, J. C. Coyne, C. Schaefer, and R. S. Lazarus, 1981, *Journal of Behavioral Medicine, 4,* p. 39. Reprinted by permission.

DAILY HASSLES  Several researchers have begun to study the role that minor life events called *daily hassles* may play in the onset of disease. Examples of daily hassles include misplacing or losing things, concerns about weight, having too many things to do, and planning meals. Lazarus and his colleagues have developed the Hassles Scale, an instrument that contains 117 daily hassles (Kanner, Coyne, Schaefer, & Lazarus, 1981). The scale requires subjects to indicate which hassles happened to them in the past month and how severe the hassles were. In addition, subjects may list any additional hassles they have experienced that are not listed in the scale. Figure 5.5 contains an excerpt from the Hassles Scale.

In one study (DeLongis, Coyne, Dakof, Folkman, & Lazarus, 1982), the Hassles Scale was administered once a month for nine months to a sample of middle-aged adults. At the beginning and end of the study, the subjects completed the Life Events Questionnaire, an instrument similar to the SRE, and also reported any illnesses and physical symptoms. The results indicated that scores on the Hassles Scale were more strongly associated with physical health than were scores on the Life Events Questionnaire. Similarly, scores on the Hassles Scale were a better predictor of future physical health than life-event scores.

The presence of daily hassles has also been correlated with psychological symptoms such as anxiety and depression (Kanner et al., 1981). Overall, daily hassles appear to be more strongly related to psychological and physical health than do major life events (Weinberger, Hiner, & Tierney, 1987). Lazarus and his colleagues have suggested that major life events may affect health indirectly by increasing the frequency and intensity of daily hassles (Kanner et al., 1981).

In addition to daily hassles, Lazarus and his colleagues have studied the effects of minor positive events called *daily uplifts* on physical and psychological health (Kanner et al., 1981). Daily uplifts include positive experiences such as completing a task, eating out, spending time with family, and laughing. The Uplifts Scale asks subjects to indicate how often they have experienced a variety of daily uplifts in the past month. The scale also allows subjects to list uplifts not included in the scale that have occurred to them. In the research to date, no consistent relationships have been found between scores on the Uplifts Scale and physical or psychological health (DeLongis et al., 1982).

To summarize, daily hassles appear to have a greater impact on health than major life events. This finding may have important implications for the prevention and treatment of stress-related illness. Teaching people how to change or cope with minor daily hassles may be more effective than trying to modify major life events.

SOCIAL SUPPORT    Another social factor influencing individuals' reactions to stress is social support. *Social support* may be defined as the comfort, assistance, and/or information that a person receives through interactions with individuals or groups (Wallston, Alagna, Devellis, & Devellis, 1983). Social support includes *emotional support*, or the feeling that one is loved and cared about; *tangible support*, or direct aid and services; and *informational support*, or advice and information regarding a potential problem (Schaefer, Coyne, & Lazarus, 1981). A large body of research has examined the effects of social support on people's reactions to stress.

One hypothesis emerging from the research on social support and stress is the *stress buffering hypothesis*. This hypothesis states that social support acts as a buffer to protect individuals from the negative effects of stress (Cobb, 1976). There are several possible stress-buffering functions of social support. To begin with, the social support available to a person influences his or her reaction to a potential stressor in the environment. For example, a family member who encourages an individual to wear a seat belt reduces the risk of an injury in the event of an automobile accident.

When an encounter with a potential stressor occurs, social support may influence the individual's primary appraisal. A threat or harm/loss appraisal may be less likely for individuals with social support than for individuals without support. As an example, a pregnant woman with a supportive husband or partner may perceive childbirth as less threatening than a woman with no partner to coach her during labor and delivery. Similarly, social support may influence secondary appraisals of coping resources available when a stress appraisal is made. In fact, social support itself is an important coping resource that can influence adaptational outcomes (Lazarus & Folkman, 1984a). Finally, social support may facilitate physiological responses to a stressor and thereby help to maintain health and prevent illness (Cohen & Wills, 1985).

The results of a number of studies suggest that social support acts as a buffer when a person experiences a stressful life event. In a study of blue-collar workers who lost their jobs as a result of factory closings, Gore (1978) assessed the men's health status and their perceptions of the support given by wives, friends, and relatives. Men who felt unsupported demonstrated higher serum cholesterol levels, more symptoms of illness, and more depression than men who felt supported. Similarly, a study of young widows one year after their husbands' death found that women who reported positive social relationships demonstrated fewer health problems than women with unsatisfactory relationships (Kraus & Lilienfeld, 1959).

Social support may also help individuals cope with the stress associated with medical procedures and acute or chronic illness. Women whose husbands participated extensively during childbirth reported less pain and required less analgesic medication than women whose husbands participated less extensively (Henneborn & Cogan, 1975). High levels of social support have also been associated with positive adjustment in samples of patients with chronic illness. As an example, patients with heart disease who reported high levels of emotional social support demonstrated less depression after heart surgery than patients with lower levels of support (Coombs, Roberts, Crist, & Miller, 1989).

Although the majority of the research to date suggests that the effects of social support on reactions to stress are positive, several studies found possible negative effects of social support. Men recovering from congestive heart failure who rated their families as very protective were less likely to return to work than men who did not perceive their families as very protective (Lewis, 1966). Possible negative effects of social support were also found in a study of adult cancer patients (Revenson, Wollman, & Felton, 1983). Social support was significantly correlated with poorer adjustment for patients not undergoing chemotherapy or radiation treatments and for patients with many limitations on physical functioning. Revenson et al. concluded that cancer patients who are not experiencing an acute crisis (e.g., chemotherapy) or who are chronically impaired may perceive social support as a reminder of their inability to reciprocate the support. This reminder may precipitate negative emotional reactions.

Thus, when considering the effects of social support on stress, it is important to consider the context and type of stressor as well as the quality and type of social support (Schwarzer & Leppin, 1989). Wide variations in the definition and measurement of stress and social support across studies have contributed to conflicting findings. Overall, the research to date suggests that social support that facilitates effective coping can act as a buffer to protect individuals from the negative effects of some stressors. As relationships with other people often entail responsibilities and demands as well as benefits, the negative effects of social support found in several studies are not surprising.

# *Psychoneuroimmunology*

The material presented thus far has demonstrated how stress and the behavioral, psychological, and social factors that influence stress may play important roles in the prevention, onset, course, and outcome of illness. An exciting new area of research called psychoneuroimmunology is contributing to our understanding of the effects of stress on bodily functioning and the development of illness. *Psychoneuroimmunology* refers to the study of the interactions among the immune system, central nervous system, and endocrine system (Ader, 1981). The *immune, or immunological, system* is the body's defense system against foreign invaders such as bacteria or viruses and abnormal cells such as those found in cancer tumors. The components of the immune system are responsible for identifying and destroying these bodily "enemies."

The results of several recent studies have demonstrated a decline in immune system functioning following stressful life events such as the death of a family member (Schleifer, Keller, Siris, Davis, & Stein, 1984) and school examinations (Halvorsen & Vassend, 1987; Kiecolt-Glaser, Garner, Speicher, Penn, Holliday, & Glaser, 1984). These results suggest that psychological stress may contribute to dysfunction of the body's immune system. Immune dysfunction makes the individual vulnerable to health problems such as infections, allergies, tumor growth, and autoimmune diseases. In *autoimmune diseases* (e.g., rheumatoid arthritis) the body's immune system reacts against the body's own tissues as if they were foreign invaders.

In one recent study of medical students, immune system functioning was assessed using blood samples drawn from the students one month before final examinations and on the last day of the exams (Kiecolt-Glaser, Glaser, Strain, Stout, Tarr, Holliday, & Speicher, 1986). Analyses of different components of the immune system found in the blood samples revealed a decline in immune system functioning from the first sample to the second. For example, natural killer cell activity decreased significantly from the preexam blood sample to the exam sample. *Natural killer cells* are immune cells that protect the body against viruses and tumor growth. The observed decline in natural killer cell activity during the exam period suggested that the psychological stress associated with final exams had negative effects on the students' immune systems.

Although stressful life events can have adverse effects on the immune system, practicing effective coping skills for managing stress appears to improve immune function. In a study of geriatric residents of independent-living facilities (Kiecolt-Glaser, Glaser, Williger, Stout, Messick, Sheppard, Ricker, Romisher, Briner, Bonnell, & Donnerberg, 1985), the elderly subjects were randomly assigned to one of three groups: (1) relaxation training, (2) social contact, or (3) no contact. The geriatric subjects in the relaxation and social contact groups were seen individually three times a week for one month. The subjects in the relaxation training group were taught basic muscle relaxation and imagery techniques, whereas subjects in the social contact group had social interactions with the experimenter. Blood samples were obtained from the subjects prior to the intervention, at posttreatment, and at a one-month follow-up.

At the end of the interventions the relaxation group demonstrated a significant increase in natural killer cell activity. In contrast, the social contact and no contact groups did not show any changes in natural killer cell functioning. These data suggest that relaxation techniques may enhance immune function. However, the natural killer cell activity of the relaxation group had returned to its pretreatment level at the one-month follow-up assessment. This decline in natural killer cell activity at follow-up may have been because most subjects quit practicing the relaxation techniques after treatment ended. Continued practice may be necessary for relaxation to produce long-term positive effects on immune function.

Both the diathesis-stress and biopsychosocial models emphasize the important role of psychological stress in the maintenance of health and the course of disease. Future research in the area of psychoneuroimmunology should help us to understand better how psychological stress affects bodily functioning and how psychological interventions may be used to improve immune system function.

## The Diathesis-Stress Model and Health Psychology

Health psychology focuses on the interplay between factors predisposing a person to illness (diathesis) and that same individual's stressors and coping resources. Health psychology researchers study how biological predispositions, such as genetic background, and psychological tendencies, such as common behavioral and emotional reactions, interact with a person's daily experiences to increase or decrease the probability of health problems. Health psychology practitioners apply the knowledge gained from this research to the treatment and prevention of health problems. Genetic background cannot be changed, but a person with a family history of illness may be helped to alter his or her emotional reactions, behavior patterns, or environment and thereby reduce the risk of the onset or recurrence of illness. The clock cannot be turned back to change the fact that a person had a heart attack, but the patient may be helped to return to a normal life-style and to reduce the risk of future cardiovascular problems.

In order to understand and improve anyone's health status, a health psychologist must attend to the person's current and prior biological status. Traditional medicine evaluates a patient's biological condition and intervenes biologically, such as with medication or surgery. Behavioral or psychological

# The Case of Bill H.

Bill H. is a 20-year-old business management major. He came to the university health center because he experienced shortness of breath and unusually rapid heart rate after running to class. This had happened several times over the last few months and was becoming more frequent as the semester wore on. Although Bill considered himself to be healthy, he knew that at 195 pounds he was a bit overweight. He also knew he probably needed to get more exercise.

Bill had been late to class more than usual because his boss was requiring him to work late with increasing regularity. He found himself falling behind at school because of his work schedule, and his grades were suffering. He always had to study hard because he felt that he had trouble telling exactly what

part of the class material was most important, and his work schedule was making it just that much harder for him to find time to study as much as he needed to. He was beginning to feel angry and frustrated, but the only way he could see to improve his situation was to work harder.

The physician at the health center found no serious illnesses, but he did find that Bill's blood pressure was slightly elevated and his cholesterol levels were high. He told Bill to lose some weight and start getting more regular exercise, and he also suggested that Bill "learn how to relax." If Bill was able to do these three things, he probably would not have to take medication to bring his blood pressure down.

changes may be suggested ("You need to learn to relax" or "Lose weight"), but direct assistance in reaching such goals is provided less frequently. Health psychologists take biological status as the backdrop against which psychological, behavioral, and social factors are evaluated. They then intervene psychologically, with the ultimate goal of seeing psychological and behavioral changes reflected in improved health.

The final section of this chapter uses the case of Bill H. to illustrate how health psychologists apply the diathesis-stress model of health and illness as they work to integrate biological, psychological, behavioral, and social components. Bill's life situation and the symptoms prompting him to seek help are presented in Boxed Highlight 5.1.

## Biological Components

Several biological features suggest that Bill H. is at risk for future cardiovascular disease. First, Bill is male. Males are at higher risk for the development of heart disease than are females (Williams et al., 1980). As we will see later in Chapters 6 and 8, Bill also has several other biological characteristics that increase his risk of heart attack. His cholesterol level and his blood pressure are both high, and he is overweight. There are thus several reasons to be concerned that given the appropriate circumstances, Bill would be a prime candidate for heart disease and/or a heart attack. However, he has one major point in his favor: age. Given that heart disease develops slowly and heart attacks are uncommon among people in their twenties, changes made now may go a long way toward preventing serious heart disease later in life.

## Psychological, Behavioral, and Social Factors

A health psychologist evaluating Bill would immediately be struck by several features. Perhaps most notable would be the way Bill describes his feelings about school and his coworkers at his part-time job. He feels as though his good work in class is not rewarded. He is not getting the grades he thinks he deserves for the work he is doing. He feels that his job is making more and more demands on his time and that he is working more hours than he initially agreed to work. He feels frustrated and angry that neither school nor work is going well. He is not only angry, but he also holds his anger in because he fears that expressing his feelings or expressing his concern at work or school could get him in trouble with his boss or his teachers. The MacDougall, Dembroski, Dimsdale, and Hackett (1985) study discussed in Chapter 2 suggests that Bill may be at higher risk than average for heart disease as a result of his anger-in tendencies and inclination toward feelings of hostility. From the behavioral point of view, Bill overeats, tends to eat a lot of fatty foods as he works and studies late, and says he has little or no time for exercise because he is always working so hard. All of these behaviors contribute to his high blood pressure and high cholesterol, increasing his risk even more.

Bill is thus predisposed biologically to heart disease, and his emotional reactions and behavior are increasing his biological risk. He is also experiencing a significant amount of stress. His description of school is a clear example of a primary threat appraisal, as discussed by Lazarus and Folkman (1984b) and described earlier in this chapter. He is always anticipating the possibility of a loss in the future. What if he is unable to find enough time to study and does poorly on an exam, or what if he loses his temper and is embarrassed? His secondary appraisal of the situation leads him to the conclusion that he can only work harder to reduce his risk of failure, but this is not a very effective coping strategy because there is always another exam coming up and he also does not feel he gets the grades he really deserves. In fact he feels trapped and angry, and feels he has very limited control over his situation. This increases his perceived level of stress.

However, there are some positive features to Bill's psychological and behavioral situation. He has a good social support network at school and at work. He is continuing to try to control and improve his situation and believes that given the chance, he will be successful. He does not feel helpless, and if he can find some more effective coping strategies, he may be able to begin to reduce his sense of distress and change his behavior.

## Treatment Interventions

Bill originally saw his physician because he was experiencing shortness of breath and dizziness when he exerted himself. These symptoms were related to his moderately high blood pressure, so his physician suggested that he lose weight, exercise, and work on relaxing some. If he did these things, he might be able to reduce his blood pressure without the need for medication. Bill began an exercise program by signing up for an aerobics class at school. However, he had more trouble losing weight and feeling more relaxed. After a few months of trying to reach these goals on his own, Bill sought help from a psychologist associated with the campus health center.

The psychologist started Bill on a program of progressive muscle relaxation, as described in Chapter 4. The relaxation provided Bill with an emotion-focused coping technique, and we will see later in Chapter 8 that relaxation has been found to be useful in behavioral blood-pressure reduction programs. The psychologist also asked Bill to self-monitor his eating. Bill had already eliminated his late-night eating, so it appeared that his weight would probably begin to drop if he kept up with the exercise class. As we will see in the next chapter, simply changing the amount eaten may not reduce weight without concurrent changes in activity level because the body may simply adjust to the lower level of calories by reducing metabolic rate.

## Preventive Interventions

Exercise, weight loss, and increased relaxation began to bring Bill's blood pressure down toward the normal range, but the psychologist stressed that the prevention of future problems with cardiovascular disease was the major reason for altering blood pressure. He went on to point out that recent research has suggested that consistent anger is a risk factor for heart disease, and he suggested that Bill try some problem-focused coping techniques to reduce his level of anger and distress at school and in his job. Because Bill was uncertain as to what he might do to improve his grades, the psychologist suggested that he talk to his instructors to try to clarify for himself what their expectations were. Bill's job seemed to be making more and more demands on his time. With some self-monitoring of his schedule Bill discovered that if he consolidated his work hours he could control his schedule and reduce his level of stress and daily hassles. As he began to feel more able to cope with his situation, his primary appraisal changed from one of threat to one of challenge, and Bill's anger reduced significantly.

This case illustrates how a health psychologist might apply the diathesis-stress model to a common health problem. Biological and psychological risk factors predisposing a client to a particular type of disorder are evaluated, and suggestions for behavioral, psychological, and/or social alterations are made. Some risk factors may be altered, such as, in Bill's case, obesity and anger. Other risk factors may be permanent, such as gender or genetic background. The higher the number of permanent risk factors present, the greater the importance of altering malleable variables. Stress levels may also be reduced by the provision of new coping responses, such as, in Bill's case, relaxation and changes at school and work. By altering risk factors and stress levels, it is hoped that ongoing disorders may be treated and the development of other, perhaps more serious, disorders may be prevented.

# Summary

The diathesis-stress model explains illness development and health maintenance as a function of the interaction between predisposition to illness (diathesis) and the stress that an individual experiences. Biological, behavioral, psychological, and social factors are thus all important in understanding health and illness. The biopsychosocial model views illness and health very similarly. It points out that biological factors alone cannot adequately explain health status, but psychological, behavioral, and social factors must also be considered.

Hans Selye defined stress as the nonspecific response of the body to any demand. The general adaptatation syndrome, with its stages of alarm, resistance, and exhaustion, is this nonspecific response. Diseases of adaptation develop during the exhaustion stage in animals predisposed to illness.

Richard Lazarus's model of stress includes psychological and biological variables. Lazarus defines stress as existing when a person appraises the environment as taxing or exceeding coping resources, thus endangering well-being. Primary appraisals evaluate the significance of a stimulus, and secondary appraisals evaluate a person's ability to cope with the stimulus. Primary stress appraisals involve perceptions of harm, loss, threat, or challenge. Coping may be problem focused or emotion focused. Stress appraisals in the absence of effective coping strategies result in high levels of stress. Stressful encounters may result in several outcomes, incuding changes in somatic health.

A person's reaction to stress is influenced by the duration and predictability of the stressor. Perceived control also influences reactions to stress. Some research has suggested that people with an internal locus of control (those who believe that outcomes are the results of personal behavior) cope more effectively. Control may be cognitive, such as changing beliefs, or behavioral, such as changing the situation or personal behavior.

Repeated exposure to uncontrollable events may lead to learned helplessness, a condition in which a person feels unable to control important life outcomes. Learned helplessness results in motivational, cognitive, and emotional deficits. People with a chronic disease of unknown cause or cure may experience learned helplessness and cope with their disease poorly.

Hardiness is a personality style comprising senses of control, commitment, and challenge. Hardiness may reduce the impact of stressful events on health.

Major life events may be powerful stressors. Holmes and Rahe ranked the stressful quality of life events according to the amount of life changes required to adjust to each event. Although there are some problems with the life-event research, there is a low, positive relationship between the occurrence of stressful life events and illness. Daily hassles have also been found to influence health negatively, sometimes more negatively than major life events.

Social support also influences reactions to stress. Support may be emotional, tangible, or informational. Social support that facilitates effective coping may act as a buffer against the harmful effects of stressors.

Psychoneuroimmunology is the study of how the immune system interacts with the central nervous and endocrine systems. Psychological stress may affect the immune system and increase a person's vulnerability to illness. Stress-induced immune system changes may be a primary avenue through which stress is related to illness.

In applying the diathesis-stress model, health psychologists must evaluate multiple variables. Biological, behavioral, and psychological risk factors must be considered. Changes in behavior, cognitions, emotions, and social/environmental status may alter risk factors, reduce stress, and improve health status. The case of Bill H. illustrates how all of these variables may be considered in an individual case. Chapters in this text focusing on specific disease entities follow this same model. Evidence concerning biological, psychological, behavioral, and social components of each condition is reviewed. Psychological and behavioral reactions to the diseases and disorders are summarized, and the available treatments and preventive strategies are presented.

# References

ABRAMSON, L. Y., SELIGMAN, M. E. P., & TEASDALE, J. D. (1978). Learned helplessness in humans: Critique and reformulation. *Journal of Abnormal Psychology 87*, 49–74.

ADER, R. (Ed.) (1981). *Psychoneuroimmunology*. New York: Academic Press.

AVERILL, J. R. (1973). Personal control over aversive stimuli and its relationship to stress. *Psychological Bulletin, 80*, 286–303.

BANDURA, A. (1977). *Social learning theory*. Englewood Cliffs, NJ: Prentice-Hall.

BRAMWELL, S., MASUDA, M., WAGNER, N., & HOLMES, T. (1975). Psychosocial factors in athletic injuries: Development and application of the Social and Athletic Readjustment Scale (SARRS). *Journal of Human Stress, 1*, 6–20.

BUCHWALD, A. M., COYNE, J. C., & COLE, C. S. (1978). A critical evaluation of the learned helplessness model of depression. *Journal of Abnormal Psychology, 87*, 180–193.

BULMAN, R. J., & WORTMAN, C. B. (1977). Attributions of blame and coping in the "real world": Severe accident victims react to their lot. *Journal of Personality and Social Psychology, 35*, 351–363.

BURISH, T. G., & BRADLEY, L. A. (1983). Coping with chronic disease: Definitions and issues. In T. G. Burish & L. A. Bradley (Eds.), *Coping with chronic disease: Research and applications*. New York: Academic Press.

COBB, S. (1976). Social support as a moderator of life stress. *Psychosomatic Medicine, 38*, 300–314.

COHEN, F. (1979). Personality, stress, and the development of physical illness. In G. C. Stone, F. Cohen, & N. E. Adler (Eds.), *Health psychology—a handbook*. San Francisco: Jossey-Bass.

COHEN, S., GLASS, D. C., & PHILLIPS, S. (1978). Environment and health. In H. E. Freeman, S. Levine, & L. G. Reeder (Eds.), *Handbook of medical sociology*. Englewood Cliffs, NJ: Prentice-Hall.

COHEN, S., & WILLS, T. A. (1985). Stress, social support, and the buffering hypothesis. *Psychological Bulletin, 98*, 310–357.

COOMBS, D. W., ROBERTS, R. W., CRIST, D. A., & MILLER, H. L. (1989). Effects of social support on depression following coronary artery bypass graft surgery. *Psychology and Health, 3*, 29–35.

DELONGIS, A., COYNE, J. C., DAKOF, G., FOLKMAN, S., & LAZARUS, R. S. (1982). Relationship of daily hassles, uplifts and major life events to health status. *Health Psychology, 1*, 119–136.

DINARDO, Q. E. (1972). Psychological adjustment to spinal cord injury. *Dissertation Abstracts International, 32*, 4206B–4207B (University Microfilms No. 71-27, 248).

ENGEL, G. L. (1977). The need for a new medical model: A challenge for biomedicine. *Science, 196*, 129–135.

ENGEL, G. L. (1980). The clinical application of the biopsychosocial model. *American Journal of Psychiatry, 137*, 535–544.

FOLKMAN, S. (1984). Personal control and stress and coping processes: A theoretical analysis. *Journal of Personality and Social Psychology, 46*, 839–852.

FUNK, S. C., & HOUSTON, B. K. (1987). A critical analysis of the Hardiness Scale's validity and utility. *Journal of Personality and Social Psychology, 53*, 572–578.

GLASS, D. C., & SINGER, J. E. (1972). *Urban Stress*. New York: Academic Press.

GORE, S. (1978). The effect of social support in moderating the health consequences of unemployment. *Journal of Health and Social Behavior, 19*, 157–165.

HALVORSON, R., & VASSEND, O. (1987). Effects of examination stress on some cellular immunity functions. *Journal of Psychosomatic Research, 31*, 693–701.

HARBURG, E., BLAKELOCK, E. H., JR., & ROEPER, P. J. (1979). Resentful and reflective coping with arbitrary authority and blood pressure: Detroit. *Psychosomatic Medicine, 41*, 189–202.

HENNEBORN, W. J., & COGAN, R. (1975). The effect of husband participation on reported pain and probability of medication during labor and birth. *Journal of Psychosomatic Research, 19*, 215–222.

HOLMES, T. H., & RAHE, R. H. (1967). The Social Readjustment Rating Scale. *Journal of Psychosomatic Research, 11*, 213–218.

KANNER, A. D., COYNE, J. C., SCHAEFER, C., & LAZARUS, R. S. (1981). Comparison of two modes of stress measurement: Daily hassles and uplifts versus major life events. *Journal of Behavioral Medicine, 4*, 1–39.

KATZ, R., & WYKES, T. (1985). The psychological difference between temporally predictable and unpredictable stressful events: Evidence for information control theories. *Journal of Personality and Social Psychology, 48*, 781–790.

KIECOLT-GLASER, J. K., GARNER, W., SPEICHER, C., PENN, G. M., HOLLIDAY, J. E., & GLASER, R. (1984). Psychosocial modifiers of immunocompetence in medical students. *Psychosomatic Medicine, 46,* 7–14.

KIECOLT-GLASER, J. K., GLASER, R., STRAIN, E., C., STOUT, J. C., TARR, K. L., HOLLIDAY, J. E., & SPEICHER, C. E. (1986). Modulation of cellular immunity in medical students. *Journal of Behavioral Medicine, 9,* 5–21.

KIECOLT-GLASER, J. K., GLASER, R., WILLIGER, D., STOUT, J., MESSICK, G., SHEPPARD, S., RICKER, D., ROMISHER, S. C., BRINER, W., BONNELL, G., & DONNERBERG, R. (1985). Psychosocial enhancement of immunocompetence in a geriatric population. *Health Psychology, 4,* 25–41.

KOBASA, S. C. (1979). Stressful life events, personality, and health: An inquiry into hardiness. *Journal of Personality and Social Psychology, 37,* 1–11.

KOBASA, S. C. (1982a). Commitment and coping in stress resistance among lawyers. *Journal of Personality and Social Psychology, 42,* 707–717.

KOBASA, S. C. (1982b). The hardy personality: Towards a social psychology of stress and health. In J. Suls & G. Sanders (Eds.), *Social psychology of health and illness.* Hillsdale, NJ: Erlbaum.

KOBASA, S. C., MADDI, S. R., & KAHN, S. (1982). Hardiness and health: A prospective study. *Journal of Personality and Social Psychology, 42,* 168–177.

KRAUS, A. S., & LILIENFELD, A. M. (1959). Some epidemiological aspects of the high mortality rate in the young widowed group. *Journal of Chronic Disease, 10,* 207–217.

LANGER, E. J., & RODIN, J. (1976). The effects of choice and enhanced personal responsibility for the aged: A field experiment in an institutional setting. *Journal of Personality and Social Psychology, 34,* 191–198.

LAZARUS, R. S. (1966). *Psychological stress and the coping process.* New York: McGraw-Hill.

LAZARUS, R. S., & FOLKMAN, S. (1984a). Coping and adaptation. In W. D. Gentry (Ed.), *The handbook of behavioral medicine.* New York: Guilford.

LAZARUS, R. S., & FOLKMAN, S. (1984b). *Stress, appraisal, and coping.* New York: Springer.

LAZARUS, R. S., & FOLKMAN, S. (1985). If it changes it must be a process: Study of emotion and coping during three stages of a college examination. *Journal of Personality and Social Psychology, 48,* 150–170.

LAZARUS, R. S., KANNER, A. D., & FOLKMAN, S. (1980). Emotions: A cognitive-phenomenological analysis. In R. Plutchik & H. Kellerman (Eds.), *Theories of emotion: Vol. 1. Emotion: Theory, research, and experience.* New York: Academic Press.

LEVI, L. (1974). Psychosocial stress and disease: A conceptual model. In E. K. Gunderson & R. H. Rahe (Eds.), *Life stress and illness.* Springfield, IL: Charles Thomas.

LEWIS, C. E. (1966). Factors influencing the return to work of men with congestive heart failure. *Journal of Chronic Disease, 19,* 1192–1209.

MacDOUGALL, J. M., DEMBROSKI, T. M., DIMSDALE, J. E., & HACKETT, T. P. (1985). Components of Type A, hostility, and anger-in: Further relationships to angiographic findings. *Health Psychology, 4,* 137–152.

MASON, J. W. (1971). A reevaluation of the concept of "non-specificity" in stress theory. *Journal of Psychiatric Research, 8,* 323–333.

MASON, J. W. (1975). A historical view of the stress field: Part I. *Journal of Human Stress, 1,* 6–12.

MILLER, T. W. (Ed.). (1969). *Stressful life events*. Madison, CT: International Universities Press.

MILLS, R. T., & KRANTZ, D. S. (1979). Information, choice, and reactions to stress: A field experiment in a blood bank with laboratory analogue. *Journal of Personality and Social Psychology, 37*, 608–620.

MONAT, A., AVERILL, J. R., & LAZARUS, R. S. (1972). Anticipatory stress and coping reactions under various conditions of uncertainty. *Journal of Personality and Social Psychology, 24*, 237–253.

PAYKEL, E. S., PRUSOFF, B. A., & MYERS, J. K. (1975). Suicide attempts and recent life events. *Archives of General Psychiatry, 32*, 327–333.

PETERSON, C. (1982). Learned helplessness and health psychology. *Health Psychology, 1*, 153–168.

RAHE, R. H. (1972). Subject's recent life changes and their near-future illness reports. *Annals of Clinical Research, 4*, 250–265.

RAHE, R. H., MAHAN, J. L., JR., & ARTHUR, R. J. (1970). Prediction of near-future health changes from subject's preceding life changes. *Journal of Psychosomatic Research, 14*, 401–406.

RAHE, R. H., MEYER, M., SMITH, M., KJAER, G., & HOLMES, T. H. (1964). Social stress and illness onset. *Journal of Psychosomatic Research, 8*, 35–44.

RAHE, R. H., ROMO, M., BENNETT, L., & SILTANEN, P. (1974). Recent life changes, myocardial infarction, and abrupt coronary death. *Archives of Internal Medicine, 133*, 221–228.

REVENSON, T. A., WOLLMAN, C. A., & FELTON, B. J. (1983). Social supports as stress buffers for adult cancer patients. *Psychosomatic Medicine, 45*, 321–331.

RODIN, J., & LANGER, E. J. (1977). Long-term effects of a control-relevant intervention with the institutionalized aged. *Journal of Personality and Social Psychology, 35*, 897–902.

ROTTER, J. B. (1966). Generalized expectancies for internal versus external control of reinforcement. *Psychological Monographs: General and Applied, 80* (Whole No. 609).

SCHAEFER, C., COYNE, J. C., & LAZARUS, R. S. (1981). The health-related functions of social support. *Journal of Behavioral Medicine, 4*, 381–406.

SCHLEIFER, S. J., KELLER, S. E., CAMERINO, M., THORNTON, J. C., & STEIN, M. (1983). Suppression of lymphocyte stimulation after bereavement. *Journal of the American Medical Association, 250*, 374–377.

SCHWARZER, R., & LEPPIN, A. (1989). Social support and health: A meta-analysis. *Psychology and Health, 3*, 1–15.

SELIGMAN, M. E. P. (1975). *Helplessness: On depression, development, and death*. San Francisco: Freeman.

SELIGMAN, M. E. P., & MAIER, S. F. (1967). Failure to escape traumatic shock. *Journal of Experimental Psychology, 74*, 1–9.

SELYE, H. (1936). A syndrome produced by diverse nocuous agents. *Nature, 138*, 32–36.

SELYE, H. (1956). *The stress of life*. New York: McGraw-Hill.

SELYE, H. (1974). *Stress without distress*. Philadelphia: Lippincott

SELYE, H. (1976). *Stress in health and disease*. Reading, MA: Butterworth.

SILVER, P. S., AUERBACH, S. M., VISHNIAVSKY, N., & KAPLOWITZ, L. G. (1986). Psychological factors in recurrent genital herpes infection: Stress, coping style, social support, emotional dysfunction, and symptom recurrence. *Journal of Psychosomatic Research, 30*, 163–171.

STRICKLAND, B. R. (1978). Internal-external expectancies and health related behaviors. *Journal of Consulting and Clinical Psychology, 46*, 1192–1211.

TAYLOR, S. E., LICHTMAN, R. R., & WOOD, J. V. (1984). Attributions, beliefs about control, and adjustment to breast cancer. *Journal of Personality and Social Psychology, 46*, 489–502.

TUDIVER, F. (1989). Dysfunctional uterine bleeding and prior life stress. In T. W. Miller (Ed.), *Stressful life events*. Madison, CT: International Universities Press.

WALLSTON, B. S., ALAGNA, S. W., DEVELLIS. B. M., & DEVELLIS, R. F. (1983). Social support and physical health. *Health Psychology, 2*, 367–391.

WALLSTON, K. A., WALLSTON, B. S., & DEVELLIS, R. (1978). Development of the Multidimensional Health Locus of Control (MHLC) Scales. *Health Education Monographs, 6*, 161–170.

WEINBERGER, M., HINER, S. L., & TIERNEY, W. M. (1987). In support of hassles as a measure of stress in predicting health outcomes. *Journal of Behavioral Medicine, 10*, 19–31.

WIEBE, D. J., & MCCALLUM, D. M. (1986). Health practices and hardiness as mediators in the stress-illness relationship. *Health Psychology, 5*, 425–438.

WILLIAMS, R. B., HANEY, T. L., LEE, K. L., KONG, Y., BLUMENTHAL, J., & WHALEN, R. (1980). Type A behavior hostility, and coronary atherosclerosis. *Psychosomatic Medicine, 242*, 539–549.

# PART III

# Health Psychology's Contributions to the Assessment, Treatment, and Prevention of Illness

CHAPTER 6

# Health-Enhancing and Health-Endangering Behaviors

*CHAPTER OUTLINE*

Behaviors promoting health and illness are of critical interest to health psychologists. The role of behavior in the development of such disorders as obesity, alcoholism, and smoking is unmistakable. The role of behavior in such health-enhancing activities as exercise and compliance with medical instructions, such as taking prescribed medication and keeping medical appointments, is likewise apparent.

The following chapter describes several health-endangering conditions and health-enhancing activities that are of particular interest to the field of health psychology. Epidemiological factors, the health-related consequences, and behavioral treatments applied to promote health-enhancing behaviors are discussed.

# Obesity

Obesity is a major health hazard in our society. A significant portion of the population is overweight, and obese individuals between twenty-five and thirty years of age are twelve times more likely to die than are nonobese people of the same age (Stunkard, 1984).

Obesity is defined best as a surplus of body fat. The normal proportion of body fat is typically thought to be 15%–20% for men and 20%–25% for women. Obesity is considered to be present when a 10%–20% excess of body fat over these values occurs (Kannel, 1983). Mild obesity is present when one is 20%–40% overweight; moderate obesity when 41%–100% overweight; and severe obesity when more than 100% overweight.

Although obesity was one of the first major medical disorders to receive attention in the field of health psychology, the variables contributing to this problem are just now coming to light. The medical complications of obesity, factors contributing to its development, and prospects for the treatment and prevention of this disorder are discussed in the following pages.

## Epidemiology

Although variable estimates of the prevalence of obesity have been made, a prevalence rate as high as 35% of the total population has been reported (Stunkard, 1984). Obesity is found among all age groups. Its prevalence increases with age (at least until middle age), and a greater proportion of women than men are obese. As may be seen in Table 6.1, black women appear to be more likely than white women to have this problem. Particularly in women, it is more prevalent in lower socioeconomic groups (Goldblatt, Moore, & Stunkard, 1965). When obesity has been determined by measuring tricep skinfolds, approximately 10% of men aged twenty to sixty-four, 25% of women aged twenty to forty-four, and 30%–50% of women aged forty-five to sixty-four were found to be obese (Bray, 1979).

TABLE 6.1   Percentage of People 25 to 74 Years of Age in the United States Who Are Overweight

| | All races | | White | | Black | |
|---|---|---|---|---|---|---|
| | 1960–62 | 1976–80 | 1960–62 | 1976–80 | 1960–62 | 1976–80 |
| Both sexes | 27.4 | 28.4 | 26.4 | 27.2 | 35.9 | 41.1 |
| Males | 24.8 | 26.7 | 25.1 | 26.7 | 24.1 | 30.9 |
| Females | 29.6 | 29.8 | 27.3 | 27.5 | 47.3 | 49.5 |

SOURCE:   National Center for Health Statistics (1989). *Health, United States, 1988* (DHHS Publication No. PHS 89–1232). Washington, DC: U.S. Government Printing Office.

## Health-Related Consequences of Obesity

Obesity is considered a significant health hazard because it precipitates or exacerbates certain other diseases, poses a major threat to longevity, and decreases the social and economic quality of life. Obesity has been found to be associated with a wide array of health problems. Participants' weight upon entry to the Framingham study (described in Chapter 2) predicted the development of cardiovascular disease. This was particularly true for women. Weight gain after the young adult years was found to significantly increase the risk of cardiovascular disease. It has been suggested that when obesity is present between the ages of twenty and forty, it may have a greater impact on cardiovascular disease formation than when it occurs after age forty (Rabkin, Mathewson, & Hsu, 1977).

Obesity has also been found to increase the risk of development of kidney stones, gallstones, hypertension, stroke, and diabetes (Larsson, Bjorntorp, & Tibblin, 1981). It has also been found to contribute to problems in respiratory and digestive functioning and pregnancy and has even been implicated as a contributing factor to the development of cancer (Bray, 1986).

The effects of obesity have been found not only to be physical but also to negatively influence social status and self esteem. The emphasis in our society on the value of being thin would, not surprisingly, lead to social rejection or discrimination and consequent heightened depression and low self-esteem. Not only might discrimination result, but educational opportunities may be more limited. Though no differences in level of intelligence or academic grades have been found between thin and obese high school students, obese females have been reported to have only one-third the chance to be admitted to college as do nonobese females. This discrepancy has been suggested to be related to prejudice on the part of admissions interviewers (Canning & Mayer, 1966).

Some research has indicated that many obese people are stigmatized because they are held responsible for their overweightness (DeJong, 1980). It is assumed that they lack self-control and willpower, two characteristics highly prized in our culture. Not only, then, do they possess a physical disability, but others may mistakenly assume that obese people have character problems as well. As Allon (1982) has pointed out, discrimination may not only be based on erroneous grounds, but also may be extreme. "Fat people are viewed as bad or immoral; supposedly, they do not want to change the errors of their ways" (Allon, 1982, p. 131).

# Etiology

Theories describing the etiology of obesity no longer propose a process that is unidimensional. Multiple factors are now thought to play a role in its development. Progress has been made in the identification of these factors and their interrelationships. Psychological theories have typically focused on potential intrapsychic phenonema, psychopathological personality traits, maladaptive eating styles, and/or problematic reactions to food cues as responsible for the development of obesity.

PSYCHODYNAMIC EXPLANATIONS   Striegel-Moore and Rodin (1986) describe psychoanalytic theories as identifying two etiological factors involved in obesity. First, unconscious conflicts have been thought to play a role in overeating. These conflicts may involve intense unmet needs for nurturance or dependency, significant emotional frustration, or problems coping adaptively with stress. Such difficulties are described as arising from traumatic and unresolved experiences in childhood and are manifest by the symptom of overeating. Second, overeating is viewed as a response to emotional distress such as anxiety or depression, a response with the aim of decreasing these negative emotions and/or defending against the experience of them (Kornhaber, 1970; Garetz, 1973).

Much effort has been devoted to uncovering pathological personality traits that relate to obesity. However, the search has largely been unsuccessful. In a review of this research Striegel-Moore and Rodin (1986) report that "current evidence suggests that obese persons do not as a group differ from normal-weight individuals on measures of global psychological adjustment and on standard measures of personality" (p. 102).

EATING STYLE AND OBESITY   The eating styles of obese people and the amounts of food eaten have been studied as possible determinants of obesity. Obese people have been assumed to eat more rapidly, take larger bites, and chew their food less than do normal-weight individuals. However, the majority of data seem to suggest that differences in amount eaten do not correlate with the degree of overweightness or level of weight gain, and research on styles of eating shows no consistent associations between eating style and obesity (Spitzer & Rodin, 1982; Striegel-Moore & Rodin, 1986).

THE EXTERNALITY HYPOTHESIS   Schachter and his colleagues (Schachter, 1968) proposed that the stimulation of eating is different for obese than for normal-weight people. Whereas normal-weight persons are stimulated to eat by internal signals such as hunger pangs or other physiological cues, obese persons are stimulated to eat by external, nonphysiological cues such as the time, taste and sight of food.

Nonobese women have been found to report feeling hunger during periods of gastric motility, whereas obese women report no hunger during these periods (Stunkard, 1959). Thus, it was thought that obese people may be less sensitive to internal, physiological cues of hunger. Schachter suggested that obese individuals may instead be more responsive to external environment food cues, such as the presence of food or the smell of food.

Several speculations have been offered to explain findings supporting the "externality hypothesis" of obesity. Schachter has suggested, for instance, that "externality" may be related to differences in functioning of the ventromedial hypothalamus portion of the brain between obese and nonobese individuals. Such speculations have been derived from the observation that, in studies with animals, this portion of the hypothalamus is key in the regulation and control of hunger. Future research is needed to more clearly uncover the potential physiological mechanisms that may be involved in obesity.

BIOLOGICAL FACTORS   The physiological basis of obesity rests on the premise that energy stores in the body reflect the balance between energy input (from food and drink) and energy expenditure. "Obesity is a condition in which the energy stores of the body (mainly fat) are excessively large" (Garrow, 1986, p. 45).

The "set-point" theory of obesity (Keesey, 1986) is based on the observation that the body weights of obese people, like normal-weight individuals, are maintained at rather stable levels. Some obese individuals are found to regulate their weight at a high set-point such that with modest weight loss there is a large decline in metabolic rate and thus in energy expenditure. This decline is the physiological attempt to resist weight change. Such reductions in metabolic rate are not transitory but persist over long periods of time. This physiological resistance to weight loss may be a key to understanding the chronic nature of obesity and the difficulties obese people experience while attempting to lose weight.

## Behavioral Treatment of Obesity

Most behavioral weight control programs include four basic elements: (1) the behavior to be controlled is fully described and a detailed assessment of this behavior is made; (2) the stimuli that precede eating are identified and controlled; (3) techniques are employed to control the act of eating; and (4) the consequences of eating are modified (Penick, Filion, Fox, & Stunkard, 1971).

1. *Description of the behavior to be controlled.* In order to sensitize patients to the specifics of their eating patterns, methods referred to as self-monitoring techniques are used. Self-monitoring is a form of behavioral assessment that

requires patients to keep very detailed records of their food intake. This sensitizing procedure has been found to be effective in and of itself in curbing overeating. Diaries of food intake are kept that include the time patients eat, the types of food and amounts eaten, and the circumstances under which food is eaten.

2. *Control of the stimuli preceding eating.* An analysis of patients' self-monitoring records usually leads to a better understanding of the factors that customarily precede the eating response. Efforts may then be directed toward reducing the number of stimuli that are associated with eating. These efforts, termed *stimulus control techniques*, are aimed at decreasing the stimuli that generally elicit overeating. To this end, patients are encouraged to eat only at specific times of the day and in certain places. They are also told to restrict themselves during those specified times only to eating rather than performing other activities such as watching television at the same time. Furthermore, the accessibility to high caloric foods is made more limited, and only low calorie foods are kept available.

3. *Development of techniques to control the act of eating.* Patients are taught to engage in eating patterns that increase their awareness of the eating process and decrease aspects of this process that promote overeating. To this end, they are instructed to take large numbers of small mouthfuls of food and to record the number of mouthfuls taken during a meal. They are also told to rest between mouthfuls of food and to focus their attention on the sensory qualities of the particular foods eaten. All of these instructions represent attempts to help individuals adopt eating patterns that reduce their food intake.

4. *Modification of the consequences of eating.* Behavioral treatment programs incorporate procedures designed to increase the incentive to reduce weight. Point systems are often used wherein patients accumulate points for engaging in adaptive eating behaviors. These points are then traded in for more tangible rewards. Changes in eating behavior may be rewarded in ways that are best suited to the individual (e.g., monetary rewards, special activities, etc.).

## THE EFFECTIVENESS OF BEHAVIORAL APPROACHES TO OBESITY

Participants in behavioral treatment programs for obesity often lose weight, but the amount of weight loss and the degree to which it is maintained vary (Brownell & Wadden, 1986). Mahoney (1978) has suggested that poor long-term results are due to several questionable assumptions on which behavioral interventions for obesity are based. First, although many behavioral programs attempt to change the eating patterns of obese people, it is very unlikely that obesity is simply the result of a learning process wherein the individual learns to engage in overeating. You will recall that Keesey (1986) suggested that there is a physiological set-point for the amount of body fat present in any particular organism. The set-point is defended by the body regardless of changes in food intake. Energy-conserving metabolic adaptations that resist weight change will thus diminish the effect of reduced-caloric intake. Second, behavioral programs generally include a stimulus-control component focused on altering the external elements that may precipitate eating. These procedures are designed to counteract the external responsivity of obese people. However, increased external responsivity may not characterize all obese people (Rodin, 1980). Third, the majority of behavioral programs for obesity assume that obese people eat more and eat differently than normal-weight people. We have already seen that these assumptions may be unwarranted (Spitzer & Rodin, 1982; Striegel-Moore & Rodin, 1986). Training obese people to eat differently ("like a normal-weight person") may thus be of little benefit.

## Recent Advances in the Treatment of Obesity

Treatment approaches that involve a large number of therapy and weight-loss techniques have been purported to be more successful than earlier attempts to treat this problem (Brownell & Wadden, 1986). Cognitive restructuring (i.e., helping patients think differently about factors involved in instigating overeating), exercise, and social support interventions are often included in these more recent approaches. However, problems related to the maintenance of weight loss still prevail. Social support from family members or peers promotes weight loss maintenance (Brownell, Heckerman, Westlake, Hayes, & Monti, 1978; Rosenthal, Allen, & Winter, 1980; Perri, McAdoo, Spevak, & Newlin, 1984).

Commercial weight-loss organizations, such as TOPS (Take Off Pounds Sensibly), provide social support to a wide number of people and lead to successful weight loss for many participants. Such groups are typically led by laypeople. The major facets of the program include weekly group meetings that provide social support and at which weigh-ins occur. Unfortunately, these groups seem to have a high dropout, or attrition, rate. High attrition makes the programs difficult to evaluate because people who complete these programs are likely more motivated than those who have dropped out. These approaches, however, do have the advantage of being affordable and accessible to a large number of people (Stunkard, 1986).

In summary, it is clear that obesity is a significant problem in our society, affecting the emotional and physical well-being of a large number of individuals. One of the earliest health-related behaviors to be targeted by health psychology, obesity remains a difficult disorder to treat. Advances have certainly been made, however, in our knowledge of the etiological factors involved in obesity and in the development of successful behavioral and community programs to treat this disorder.

# Alcoholism

Alcohol consumption has been a social custom in society since at least the beginning of recorded history. An awareness of potential problems with alcohol was reflected as early as 1700 B.C., when restrictions were first placed on its sale (Caddy, 1983). Alcohol consumption is an area of critical concern for many reasons. First, alcohol dependence and alcohol-related diseases are thought to account for more than 3 million days of hospitalization (Pardes, 1982). Second, many health problems are thought to be associated with its excessive use. Gastrointestinal diseases, liver disease, neurological disorders, and malnutrition are among the many conditions arising from alcoholism. Third, alcoholism is often a contributing factor in many accidents and injuries. High blood-alcohol concentrations were found among more than one-third of the patients entering a department caring for traumatic injuries, and injuries are among the most common causes for medical consultation in inebriated patients (Pardes, 1982).

Despite the pervasive, health-endangering effects of alcohol, medical care givers often fail to detect problems with alcoholism in many medical and psychiatric patients. Westermeyer, Doheny, and Stone (1978) found that the majority of physicians and nurses in a major medical facility did not even take an adequate alcohol and drug-related history from their patients. Furthermore, when chemical dependency was identified as a medical problem, it was often not identified as a problem to be addressed in the treatment of the patient. Similarly, Kissin and Begleiter (1979) reported that 15%–33% of the patients requesting emergency room medical and surgical treatment were alcoholic, although few of these patients were referred for treatment of this problem.

Two types of alcohol disorders are currently defined in the American Psychiatric Association's *Diagnostic and Statistical Manual of Mental Disorders* (1987). *Alcohol abuse* entails recurrent use of alcohol in physically hazardous situations or continued use despite knowledge that a personal problem is caused or made worse by alcohol. The problem may be social, occupational, psychological, or physical. The second alcohol-related disorder, that is, *alcohol dependence*, involves all of the factors associated with alcohol abuse. However, the disorder is more serious in that the person has impaired contol of his or her drinking. Tolerance or withdrawal may also be present. *Tolerance* is defined as a state in which increasing amounts of alcohol are required to achieve the desired effect. In this state a diminished effect is achieved with regular use of the same dose. *Withdrawal* is identified when symptoms like shakiness or malaise occur after stopping or reducing the amount of alcohol consumed. Such symptoms can be relieved by consuming alcohol.

## Epidemiology

In the past two decades there has been a notable increase in per capita alcohol consumption, with the rate of consumption rising 32% since 1964

(Selzer, 1980). It has been estimated that 8% of the adult U.S. population drinks heavily; heavy drinking is defined as consuming one ounce or more of absolute alcohol per day. In 1985, 14% of U.S. males and 3% of U.S. females were heavy drinkers (National Center for Health Statistics [NCHS], 1989).

It is important to note when considering alcohol consumption patterns that approximately one-tenth of the drinking population consume about half of the alcoholic beverages sold. Approximately 6.5% of the drinking population at the upper end of the consumption curve drink an average of almost sixteen drinks each day (Russell, 1986).

Alcohol problems are common among the young, and are particularly significant in young males. National surveys of the young reveal that in 1985 34% of males 12 to 17 years old and 78% of males 18 to 25 years old had used alcohol during the past month. This compares to 28% and 64% of females in these same age groups (NCHS, 1989).

## Health-Related Consequences of Alcoholism

Alcohol has powerful and toxic effects on virtually all the organ systems of the body. It is transported by the bloodstream and is absorbed by most tissues. It even passes through the blood-brain and placental barriers. The organs with the highest rate of circulation receive the higher concentrations of the substance. In this way they sustain the most damage (Segal & Sisson, 1985). Furthermore, the more highly specialized the tissue, the more susceptible it is to the adverse effects of alcohol. Therefore, organs such as the brain, liver, peripheral nerves, pancreas, and endocrine glands may show early and serious impairment (Segal & Sisson, 1985).

Two distinguishable chronic organic brain syndromes may result from chronic, excessive alcohol use: *alchoholic dementia* and *alcohol amnestic* (memory loss) *syndrome*, also known as Korsakoff's psychosis. Alcoholic dementia is characterized by a global intellectual decline, poor abstract-reasoning ability, poor problem-solving skills, and problems in verbal expression and motor skill. *Korsakoff's psychosis*, on the other hand, does not involve global deficits in cognitive functioning of this nature but, rather, severe and often persistent memory impairment (Butters, 1982). Problems acquiring new information and problems recalling recent events are characteristic of this syndrome. It is suspected that these difficulties may be caused by a nutritional deficiency, such as thiamine (vitamin $B^1$) deficiency, often present in alcoholics.

Because the metabolism of alcohol occurs almost exclusively in the liver, it is not surprising that cirrhosis of the liver is the disease most commonly associated with alcoholism. Cirrhosis is the seventh leading cause of death in the U.S (Russel, 1986).

A multitude of other physical problems result from excessive use of alcohol. When it is consumed most is absorbed into the bloodstream through the small intestine. It is then found to disturb the functioning of the stomach and small intestine. Such conditions as gastritis, involving severe heartburn, pain, nausea and/or vomiting may result. Additionally, alcohol may affect the heart and cardiovascular systems. Alcoholic cardiomyopathy is a disease of the heart muscle caused by excessive alcohol consumption. This condition may be fatal if drinking continues.

The hazardous effects of prenatal alcohol exposure are widely known. Such effects have been found to range from pregnancy complications and low birth weight to a cluster of abnormalities known as *fetal alcohol syndrome* (FAS) in the newborn (DHHS, 1984a). Fetal alcohol syndrome typically involves growth retardation, abnormal head and facial features, central nervous system damage, mental retardation, and eye and ear defects. An estimated 5% of American women between ages eighteen and thirty-four consume an average of two or more drinks per day, or thirteen or more drinks per week. A substantial number of women thus confront the need for behavior change if they become pregnant (Clark & Midanik, 1982).

# Etiology

Numerous factors have been proposed as contributors to the development of alcoholism. Alcoholism has been associated with cultural norms, learning history, personality traits, biological characteristics, and the expectations of the drinker for the effects of alcohol.

CULTURAL FACTORS   The customs and mores of different cultures are thought to influence the use of alcohol. For example, a positive social meaning may be given to drinking in societies that incorporate alcohol into common social practices. Examples of such social practices may be religious ceremonies and rituals, including traditional Christian ceremonies (Galanter, 1983). Additionally, the tone or feeling set by a culture about drinking may have profound effects on actual consumption (Leigh, 1985). Leigh notes, for example, that "integrated drinking" has been used to describe societies that show approval of and widespread participation in alcohol consumption. Not surprisingly, this is often associated with a high rate of alcohol consumption (Leigh, 1985).

LEARNING HISTORY   The development of alcohol use patterns is also affected by the behavior of important people in one's environment. In addition, the reinforcing qualities of the drug itself may assist in the development of drinking. Maladaptive styles of drinking are subject to the same principles of learning by which many other behaviors develop, that is, through vicarious learning, modeling of significant others, and from the positively reinforcing pharmacological effects of alcohol.

Many people take their first drink of alcohol while surrounded by a group of their peers. In this way, peers may serve as models for alcohol consumption patterns (Stumphauser, 1980). The importance of observational learning and modeling is further supported by the fact that the use of drugs by parents has been found to be moderately related to drug use by their children

(Fawzy, Coombs, & Gerber, 1983). Additionally, the presence of a partner or peer who drinks heavily has been found to increase both the amount and rate at which alcohol is consumed (Caudill & Marlatt, 1975; Lied & Marlatt, 1979).

PERSONALITY TRAITS   Personality traits such as impulsivity, antisocial behavior, immaturity, and problems coping with stressful life events have been purported to predict future alcohol abuse (Leigh, 1985). Vaillant (1980), in a follow-up longitudinal study of college freshmen, however, found no associations between such traits and future alcohol abuse. Many of the personality traits identifying alcoholics are also common to other psychiatric groups, thus suggesting that they would not be predictive of this particular manifestation of maladjustment (Leigh, 1985). Depression has also been a commonly cited factor reponsible for alcohol abuse, but can also be viewed as a reaction to alcohol dependence. The personality traits noted, together with psychological disturbances such as depression, may (1) be present prior to using alcohol, (2) develop through the pharmacological effect of the substance itself, or (3) even be due to the social conditions that accompany heavy alcohol use (Leigh, 1985).

BIOLOGICAL FACTORS   Several types of physiological abnormalities stemming from alcohol abuse have been suggested as important factors in alcohol addiction. For example, one such hypothesis suggests that alcohol may produce a morphinelike substance in the brains of certain individuals, thereby increasing the chances of addiction (Bloom, 1982; Davis & Walsh, 1970). As of yet, adequate evidence for this is nonexistent, although it has stimulated further thinking about potential biochemical etiologic factors in alcoholism (Schuckit, 1986).

There is good evidence that genetic factors may contribute to the development of alcoholism. There appears to be a two- to three-fold higher level of concordance for alcoholism in monozygotic than in dizygotic twins (Schuckit, 1983). Furthermore, children of alcoholics separated from their biological parents near birth and raised by foster parents have higher rates of alcoholism than adopted children of nonalcoholic parents (Bohman, 1978; Cadoret, Cain, & Grove, 1980). Such studies strongly suggest that genetic factors play a role in the development of alcoholism.

EXPECTANCY   Expectancy refers to the beliefs held by individuals and society about alcohol and its effects. Research has shown that when the *belief* that one has consumed alcohol exists, this leads to greater aggression (Lang, Goecker, Adesso, & Marlatt, 1975), more sexual interest and arousal (Wilson & Lawson, 1976), and less social anxiety (Wilson & Abrams, 1977), regardless of the actual alcohol content of the beverage. Alcoholics drink faster as well as consume significantly greater amounts and take fewer sips of the beverage when they expect they are drinking alcohol as opposed to tonic-water placebo (Rohsenow & Marlatt, 1981). The drinker's expectations of enjoyable effects may thus be equally, if not more, important as a factor encouraging alcohol abuse.

# Behavioral Treatment of Alcoholism

The treatment of alcoholism has been approached from a number of different vantage points. Some approaches have attempted to tackle the problem of alcohol abuse by decreasing the positive valence that accompanies drinking (aversion therapy). Other approaches have applied not only principles of aversion or punishment, but positive reinforcement and rewards for desired behavior (operant conditioning) and/or techniques for altering cognitions or expectancies associated with drinking (cognitive-behavioral methods).

*Aversion therapy* was probably one of the first behavioral approaches to the problem of alcoholism. This approach stems from Pavlovian conditioning theory, which predicts that the sight, smell, and taste of alcohol will acquire aversive properties if repeatedly paired with noxious stimuli. Alcoholic patients have been exposed to electric shocks while tasting, seeing, and smelling alcohol. They have also been required to drink alcohol after being given the drug *emetine*, which causes nausea and vomiting (Kantorich, 1929; Voegtlin, 1940). Chemical aversion can be effective for employed, married, well-motivated alcoholics, but the effectiveness of electrical aversion is doubtful (Miller & Hester, 1980). When these two aversion procedures were compared, chemical aversion was shown to be more effective than electrical aversion at six months, but this advantage after one year was not significant (Cannon, Baker, & Wehl, 1981).

*Operant approaches* have shown promise in the treatment of alcoholism (Miller & Hester, 1980). These treatment techniques include not only punishments for excessive drinking but also the use of rewards and reinforcements for sobriety. Reinforcements often found to be successful are those that are social in nature. There exists, for example, a community reinforcement procedure in which rewards include such things as the availability of a social club for patients who maintain sobriety (Hunt & Azrin, 1973). This type of program has been found to be very effective in reducing the amount of time spent drinking, as well as the amount of time required for treatment of alcohol-related problems.

Whereas traditional behavioral treatments have focused on the alteration of observable antecedents and consequences of excessive alcohol use, *cognitive-behavioral approaches* have been characterized by the use of interventions designed to alter internal factors—that is, cognitions and expectancies—associated with drinking. Marlatt (1979), for example, suggested that a drinker's alcohol consumption may be related to the presence or absence of a sense of control in challenging situations. Without an adequate coping response, the sense of self-control may diminish in situations posing a challenge to the drinking pattern, such as when a host offers "one for the road" to a party guest who is trying to avoid drinking before driving home. A sense of helplessness may subsequently lead to the occurrence of excessive drinking.

In order to enhance the drinker's sense of control, behavior therapists have stressed the importance of teaching new, adaptive coping skills. One such approach, called *relapse-prevention training*, assists patients in the identification of high-risk situations, or those situations characteristically involved in the drinking response. After developing skill in identifying these situations, patients are taught alternative means of coping with them. Patients who have received relapse-prevention-skills training have been found to have less severe relapse episodes, were more likely to be employed, and attended outpatient treatment sessions more regularly than patients in control groups (Chaney, O'Leary, & Marlatt,1978).

## Moderation or Abstinence?

The viability of drinking in moderation as a goal in the treatment of alcoholism has been a point of controversy. The proposition that alcoholics could be returned to social drinking in moderation was stimulated by findings that a small proportion of treated alcoholics were able to return to moderate drinking without serious problems (Pattison, 1976). Behavioral treatments have also been used effectively for teaching moderation to middle-income, nonalcoholic problem drinkers (Pomerleau, Pertschuk, Adkins, & Brady, 1978). More recent studies have reported that some alcoholics have been able to maintain moderation in drinking for up to twelve months following treatment (Armor, Polich, & Stambul, 1978; Moos, Finney, & Chan, 1981).

A less optimistic view of the viability of drinking in moderation as a treatment goal for alcoholics has been generated by data involving longer follow-up intervals. The relapse rate four years after treatment has been reported to be higher (41%) for patients drinking moderately eighteen months after treatment than for those abstaining at that time (30% relapse rate) (Polich, Armor, & Braiker, 1981). A two-year follow-up of patients treated for alcoholism found that patients drinking moderately six months after treatment were more likely than abstainers to revert to heavy drinking (Finney & Moos, 1981). It is currently unclear whether moderation is a viable treatment goal for many, if any, alcoholics.

In summary, alcoholism is a widespread health-endangering disorder in our country. The cultural, environmental, interpersonal, intrapersonal and biological factors contributing to its development are beginning to be more fully delineated. Numerous behavioral treatment approaches have been applied to this problem with variable success. Research is still needed to clarify the possibility that alcoholics may successfully pursue the goal of drinking in moderation rather than maintaining total abstinence.

# *Smoking*

Between one-quarter and one-third of the U.S. population smoke cigarettes (NCHS, 1989). Although the process by which tobacco use contributes to the development of these diseases has not been definitively determined, there is agreement that smoking increases the risk for lung cancer, cardiovascular disease, and cancers of the throat, stomach, and bladder (Istvan & Matarazzo, 1984).

Tobacco dependence was included in the nomenclature of mental disorders for the first time in 1980 with the publication of the third edition of the *Diagnostic and Statistical Manual of The American Psychiatric Association* (1980). It was defined as the persistent use of tobacco, usually exceeding a half pack of cigarettes a day, in addition to the presence of either of the following: feelings of distress caused by the need to use tobacco repeatedly and/or physiological dependence on nicotine when there exists a serious physical disorder involving its use or it is an apparent causative or exacerbating factor. Tobacco withdrawal was also described in this manual as a syndrome in which the abrupt cessation of significant tobacco use leads to numerous symptoms such as irritability, anxiety, and restlessness.

## Epidemiology

As of 1987, 31.5% of American men and 27% of American women smoked cigarettes. Smoking is becoming less common. In 1965, 52.1% of males and 34.2% of females smoked cigarettes. These declines in smoking rates are likely to continue, because the number of teenage and young adult smokers is decreasing (NCHS, 1989). A large percentage of the population may qualify as being distressed about their tobacco use as indicated by surveys that suggest that at least 80% of smokers indicate the desire to quit, with 75% of them attempting to decrease tobacco use, and 60% of them having tried, but failed, to abstain (Greden, 1985). By 1987, 31.4% of males and 18.9% of females were former smokers (NCHS, 1989).

## Health-Related Consequences of Smoking

Smoking is a major cause of cancer of the lung, larynx, oral cavity, and esophagus and is a contributory factor for cancer of the kidney, urinary bladder, and pancreas (Department of Health & Human Services [DHHS], 1982). Life expectancy at any age is significantly shortened by cigarette smoking. A two-pack-a-day smoker between the ages of thirty and thirty-five has a life expectancy eight to nine years shorter than that of a nonsmoker of the same age (Schwartz, 1987). About 390,000 people die annually as a consequence of smoking. Most of these deaths are due to lung cancer, cardiovascular disease, and chronic obstructive lung disease (DHHS, 1989).

Overall, smokers are ten times more likely to die from lung cancer than are nonsmokers, and heavy smokers are fifteen to twenty-five times more at risk (Schwartz, 1987). Furthermore, an estimated 50%–70% of oral, laryngeal, and esophageal cancer deaths are related to smoking (Schwartz, 1987). Smokers are twice as likely as nonsmokers to die of cancers of the bladder and pancreas. Stopping smoking reduces the risk of cancer substantially.

Smoking has been determined to be a significant risk factor in the development of coronary heart disease (DHHS, 1984b). It acts synergistically with other factors such as hypertension, hypercholesterolemia, and even the use of oral contraceptives in the development of coronary problems. Smokers are found to have greater respiratory problems than nonsmokers, including such difficulties as respiratory infections, emphysema, and bronchitis.

Smoking has been found to have an adverse effect on the developing fetus during pregnancy. Smoking during pregnancy increases the risk of such problems as spontaneous abortion, premature birth, and death of the infant during the first days of life. Respiratory infections are more common among children with parents who smoke than among children with nonsmoking parents (DHHS, 1985).

## Behavioral Treatment of Smoking

Diverse behavioral methods have been applied to the problem of smoking cessation. Oftentimes such treatments have been used alone and, more recently, in combination. Two general approaches to the behavioral treatment of smoking may be identified: (1) aversive procedures, including such techniques as rapid smoking and other smoke-aversion procedures, utilizing an approach of punishment and/or negative reinforcement for smoking; and (2) self-management procedures, including such techniques as self-monitoring, nicotine fading, and self-control programs, focusing on positive reinforcement for smoking cessation.

*Aversion techniques* have probably been the most common procedures applied to smoking. Excessive levels of cigarette smoke and electric shock have been used as noxious stimuli. In such procedures, the aversive stimulus is paired with the target behavior: smoking.

One aversion strategy showing definite promise is a technique developed by Lichtenstein and his colleagues called *rapid smoking*. It involves having patients smoke cigarettes at very rapid rates until they are unable to tolerate additional inhalation. Cigarettes are inhaled once every six seconds for the duration of the cigarette or until the patient is nauseated. This procedure is repeated several times until the individual expresses no desire to smoke. Abstinence rates of 54% three months to six months after treatment and 34% two years to six years after treatment have been reported (Lichtenstein & Rodrigues, 1977).

The rapid-smoking procedure is not without risks, however. Rapid smoking produces significant increases in heart rate, the presence of certain noxious gases in one's system, and heightened blood nicotine levels. Cardiac complications, including cardiovascular irregularities during the procedure, are of major concern. The technique is suggested for use only with healthy young adults in settings in which screening for risk factors can be easily accomplished and medical care is available (Lichtenstein & Mermelstein, 1984).

Electric shock as an aversive stimulus paired with smoking behavior has had limited success. Schwartz (1987) noted that there have been no reports regarding the use of electric shock therapy for smoking cessation since 1977, and those filed before this time showed widely ranging success rates. Quit rates for the early shock studies ranged from 0%–63% (Schwartz, 1987). In reviewing the aversive methods for smoking cessation in general, Schwartz (1987) concluded that techniques such as rapid smoking can eliminate smoking, but he also called for the use of maintenance and reinforcement procedures to continue the behavior change.

*Self-management techniques* include such methods as self-monitoring, nicotine fading, contingency management, and self-control therapy. Self-monitoring is a procedure that requires patients to monitor the number of cigarettes smoked in a certain period of time and to record numerous details of the situation where this behavior occurred. Whereas most behavioral approaches require the recording of the number of cigarettes smoked per day in order to obtain a baseline and estimate of change over time, this procedure entails a rather elaborate recording. Individuals are asked to record such things as their mood when smoking each cigarette, the activity engaged in during this time, events that preceded smoking, and the place where it occurred. Some encouraging results have been reported using self-monitoring, suggesting that it reduces cigarette intake in the short run (Levanthal & Avis, 1976). Typically it is used in conjunction with other behavioral methods. Further investigation of this approach in reducing smoking is required to adequately assess its utility.

*Monitored nicotine fading* is a technique aimed at changing cigarette consumption by reducing the tar and nicotine in the cigarette brand used (Foxx & Brown, 1979). This procedure involves smokers gradually switching to brands that contain progressively less nicotine than their original brand. Smokers also self-monitor the amount of nicotine intake each day. Nicotine fading produces variable results, with quit rates ranging from 7% to 46%, with a median of 25% for one-year trials (Schwartz, 1987). Schwartz concluded that "for those smokers who wish to reduce their dependence on nicotine gradually, nicotine fading offers the opportunity, but it will be necessary to provide maintenance support, including coping strategies and relapse prevention" (p. 84).

*Self-control programs* are based on the assumption that although specific strategies may not, in and of themselves, be useful in promoting smoking cessation, they may be effective when combined with one another. Furthermore, it is assumed that a multiplicity of factors may be involved in the development and maintenance of smoking and that these factors likely vary between individuals. Therefore, self-control programs offer a "package" approach to the problem of smoking, utilizing a variety of smoking-cessation techniques. These programs are generally referred to as *multicomponent* programs.

Self-control procedures, such as self-monitoring and coping-skills training, are often included in multicomponent treatment packages. Some include an aversive treatment component, whereas others do not. Other techniques are frequently employed and include stimulus-control procedures, group support, and learning to engage in behaviors incompatible with smoking. Some of the multicomponent programs have been successful. The median quit rate for seventeen multicomponent programs with one-year follow-ups was 40%, with two-thirds of these reaching medians of 33% (Schwartz, 1987). A recent multicomponent program with only 20 to 30 minutes of individualized training reported one-year abstinence rates near 15% (Windsor & Lowe, 1988). It appears that the "package" approach to smoking cessation may be a fruitful avenue of pursuit.

### THE USE OF NICOTINE CHEWING GUM IN SMOKING CESSATION

Some smokers find it difficult to quit smoking because they have become dependent upon the chemically reinforcing properties of nicotine. Chewing gum containing nicotine has been developed to help these smokers gradually withdraw from nicotine. Patients are encouraged to gradually reduce the amount of gum chewed each day as the urge to smoke fades. Gradually decreasing the amount of nicotine gum chewed allows for the body's physiological adjustment to the absence of nicotine, thus preventing abrupt cessation and consequent withdrawal symptoms.

In a review of the studies on the effectiveness of nicotine gum in smoking cessation, Schwartz (1987) concluded that it can indeed be an effective tool in achieving abstinence from cigarettes, particularly when used in conjunction with some other therapy (such as counseling or behavioral approaches).

Some attempts have been made to identify those individuals who will profit most from the use of nicotine gum. One factor suspected to be important is the degree to which smokers are dependent on nicotine. Nicotine gum has been found to be particularly helpful for those who are highly dependent on nicotine, and perhaps even counterproductive for those who are less dependent (Jarvik & Schneider, 1984; Fagerstrom, 1980). Other factors likely related to the effectiveness of nicotine gum include the adequacy of the information provided individuals pertaining to the instructions for gum use, the provision of supplemental cessation methods to aid in its effectiveness, and a trial consisting of an adequate period of time for the gum to decrease the possibility of relapse.

Further research is necessary to determine the degree to which those who use nicotine gum and achieve abstinence maintain it. Without such information it remains unclear if it is an intervention method that successfully assists individuals in stopping smoking on a long-term basis.

In summary, smoking has been found to be a major cause and/or contributing factor in the development of several fatal, or potentially fatal, illnesses. Numerous behavioral treatment strategies have been applied to this problem with some success. Recent treatment advances have involved programs utilizing several treatment strategies.

# Exercise

In today's society there has been a growing emphasis on the benefits of engaging in regular exercise. Even though its significance in the workplace has decreased due to technological advances, the popularity of exercise as a recreational pastime has soared. In this section the role of exercise as a health-enhancing behavior will be described. The patterns of physical activity in our current life-style, the physical consequences of exercise, and the ramifications of exercise for emotional health will be addressed. Problems related to the adherence to physical fitness programs and interventions aimed at improving this compliance are also presented.

## Patterns of Physical Exercise

Physical activity has become an increasing part of the typical American life-style. The percentage of nonactive adults has declined from 75% in 1961 to 41% in 1978 (Oldridge, 1984). It is still the case, however, that only 15% of adults in the United States participate in recreational activity that results in a significant, health-enhancing energy expenditure of at least 1,500 kcal per week. An energy expenditure of 1,500 kcal per week is accomplished by such exercise patterns as an hour a day of walking at 3.0 to 3.5 miles per hour, a daily twenty- or thirty-minute run at 6.0 miles per hour, or an hour of swimming at 1 mile per hour, five days per week. Although the percentage of active adults has certainly risen over the past several years, a relatively small portion of our society engages in moderate and regular physical activity. This small percentage is echoed in other countries such as Australia, Canada, and Belgium (Oldridge, 1984).

## Physical Consequences of Exercise

There are many popular notions of what constitutes physical fitness, and many claims regarding the health benefits of exercise. To some individuals, the concept of physical fitness may mean the absence of disease. To others, it may mean a trim body, or a certain degree of muscular development. For activities to promote fitness, however, they must involve the heart muscle and improve the efficiency with which other parts of the cardiorespiratory system (heart, lungs, and blood vessels) perform in a physically stressful situation (Insel & Roth, 1977).

Aerobic exercise is thought to achieve the greatest health benefits. It requires the use of large muscles and moving the body weight against gravity or over distance. Aerobic exercise has three benefits:

1. The maintenance of optimal body weight or composition.
2. The prevention of coronary heart disease.
3. The normalization of carbohydrate metabolism. (Haskell, 1984)

Haskell further reports that there is evidence that sedentary individuals may achieve significant health gains from exercise performed at an adequate intensity, duration, and frequency. In one study, for example, forty-three men, aged forty-five to fifty-five years, participated in a jogging program to promote physical functioning. Two-thirds of these subjects were previously sedentary. They all participated for six to ten years in a thrice weekly, thirty- to forty-minute jogging program. At the end of that time, subjects showed consistent decreases in resting heart rate and increases in maximum oxygen consumption (MOC). Maximum oxygen consumption is a measure of cardio- respiratory fitness, and indicates how much oxygen the body can use during strenuous exercise. These results reveal a pattern that is a reversal of the normal decline in MOC associated with age. Sedentary middle-aged men actu- ally reversed the expected age-related decline in physical functioning through participation in a regular exercise program.

## Psychological Consequences of Exercise

A variety of claims have been made regarding the psychological benefits of regular exercise. Physical fitness training has been related to improvements in behavior, self-concept, and mood. However, many of these investigations have been corrrelational in nature, relating participation in an exercise program to psychological changes that occur. It has been difficult to determine from such studies if the psychological changes that are identified are necessarily related to the exercise per se or reflect the individual's choice to engage in an exer- cise program. Those seeking to participate in an exercise program, for in- stance, may be seeking a personal change that is independent from the actual training program (Jasnoski, Holmes, Solomon, & Aguiar, 1981). The actual physical activity may therefore be irrelevant to a psychological change that may already be ongoing.

BEHAVIOR AND SELF-CONCEPT  It has been suggested that participation in physical activity programs may lead to changes in such behaviors as work performance, sleep, and social adjustment. Exercise training has been related to a reduction of absenteeism on the job as well as improvements in work performance and work attitudes (Donoghue, 1977). Although their study did not involve the use of sophisticated measures of sleep behavior, Folkins, Lynch, and Gardner (1972) found that physical fitness training positively af- fected the sleep behavior of college females.

There is some evidence that increased physical fitness levels may corres- pond to positive changes in self-concept (Hughes, 1974). Physical fitness im- provements have also been thought to improve the self-concept of such clini- cal populations as rehabilitation clients (Collingwood, 1972) and obese teen- agers (Collingwood & Willett, 1971).

Folkins and Sime (1981) suggest that the changes in self-concept associated with participation in physical fitness programs may be due to the perception of improved fitness, rather than to actual changes in physical fitness. Partici- pants in an exercise program have been found to feel more confident and able than nonparticipants. However, changes in aerobic capacity were unre- lated to improvements in confidence and ability ratings. It seems likely that the reported changes in self-perceptions may have been due to the personal and social factors related to participating in the program rather than the actual changes that occurred in the subjects' physical fitness (Jasnoski et al., 1981).

MOOD   Studies of the effects of exercise training on mood have primarily focused on anxiety and depression. There is a large body of evidence documenting the idea that exercise of an appropriate level, duration, and frequency has an anxiety-relieving effect. This effect is said to last anywhere from 30 minutes to several hours after exercising. The prescription of exercise in the treatment of clinical depression has likely stemmed from the collection of symptoms often characterizing this disorder. Clinical depression may include feelings of hopelessness, sadness, frequent tearfulness, and low self-esteem. It is often associated with feelings of lethargy and a lack of interest or pleasure in everyday activities. Exercise is thought to combat some of these symptoms because of its very nature as an action-oriented task and because its physical effects, such as weight loss and increased strength may enhance one's self-image. In a review of research on the effect of exercise on depression, Folkins and Sime (1981) found support for the idea that mood improves as a function of exercise. This improvement was particularly notable when subjects' level of depression was higher than normal prior to their engaging in an exercise program.

Several mechanisms have been suggested to account for the changes in depression related to increased exercise (Sime, 1984). One theory suggests that exercise increases cerebral blood flow and oxygenation and in that manner is related to elevations in mood (Kostrubala, 1977). Another theory identifies increases in the catecholamine (neurotransmitter) norepinephrine as accounting for the antidepressant effect of exercise (Howley, 1976). Norepinephrine has been shown to be low in clinically depressed individuals. Other authors have focused on the personal sense of mastery and self-control that may develop in depressed people who engage in regular exercise (Greist, Klein, Eischens, Faris, Gurman, & Morgan, 1978). The results of a recent study suggest that changes in mood are related to improvements in personal satisfaction with physical fitness levels. Improvements in aerobic capacity following a six month exercise program were not found to be related to improvements in anxiety or depression. However, increased satisfaction with personal attributes such as physical shape, appearance, and weight was related to decreases in depression and anxiety (King, Taylor, Haskell, & DeBusk, 1989).

## Interventions to Improve Exercise Compliance

Although the emotional and physical health benefits of exercise are quite significant, a fairly low percentage of U.S. adults participate regularly in recreational physical activity. Furthermore, among those who join health-oriented exercise programs, as many as 50% drop out of the programs after six months (Oldridge, 1984). Thus, one of the major contributions to be made by health psychology may be the development of behavioral strategies to increase motivation to join and adhere to exercise programs and/or regimens.

Social reinforcement in the exercise program and the type of program chosen can positively affect exercise adherence (Oldridge, 1984). Many participants in exercise programs prefer to exercise in groups. Positive reinforcement, when provided by the exercise leader, has also been found to increase exercise adherence (Oldridge, 1977; Heinzelmann & Bagley, 1970). Individuals who set flexible goals are more likely to exercise (Martin & Dubbert, 1982), and social support from spouse and family has been found to increase exercise adherence (Bjurstrom & Alexiou, 1978).

Bélisle, Roskies, and Lévesque (1987) combined self-management and relapse-prevention training with group exercising, and reported that adherence to exercise programs could be significantly increased at a cost of only $3.33 per participant. These costs reflected the time required for a psychologist to train and supervise exercise group leaders. In view of the potential long-term health benefits of regular exercise, this seems a remarkably cost-effective use of professional time. Given the many physical and psychological benefits of regular exercise, further attention to the development of behavioral programs to increase exercise program adherence is certainly called for.

# Compliance

## The Problem of Noncompliance

Cooperation with medical regimens is perhaps one of the most important factors influencing treatment success. The medical profession, and those attempting to be successfully medically treated, face an extremely serious problem in patient noncompliance. Noncompliance results not only in the inefficient use of medical services but causes patients to remain untreated, often exacerbating existing health problems (Sackett & Snow, 1979).

Noncompliance may take many different forms. For example, patients may fail to take medication as appropriately described, e.g., taking too much or too little medicine, failing to follow a prescribed diet and/or exercise regimen, continuing to smoke although ill advised, and/or even failing to follow through with future medical appointments designed to monitor health-progress (DiNicola & DiMatteo, 1984).

From 15% to 94% of patients do not comply with medical recommendations (Davis, 1966). Compliance averages around 30% (Sackett & Haynes, 1976). These percentages are so variable because many factors influence compliance. The complexity of the medical regimen and the degree to which it inconveniences the patient or requires life-style change, the treatment's length of time (Haynes, 1979), and the severity of discomfort of the illness as judged by the patient (Becker & Maiman, 1980), all appear to play a role in the degree to which a patient will comply (DiNicola & DiMatteo, 1984).

# Factors Contributing to Compliance

PATIENT-PHYSICIAN RELATIONSHIP   The patient's relationship to the practitioner has a major effect on compliance (DiNicola & DiMatteo, 1984). The patient's understanding of the instructional component of the physician's communication and the affective (emotional) component of the communication both influence patient compliance. With regard to the "instructional" component, it is certainly understandable that patients are unable to comply with a medical regimen they do not understand. It has been found that only 40% of patients interviewed after a visit with their doctor understand the medical regimen prescribed (Boyd, Covington, Stanaszek, & Coussons, 1974). If one is given information in a fashion that is understandable, the evidence suggests that it will indeed by remembered (Becker & Maiman, 1980).

Although the instructional component of the patient-physician visit must be understood before a patient may comply, the quality of that relationship, or the affective component, is a primary ingredient in compliant behavior (DiNicola & DiMatteo, 1984; Hulka, 1979; Aday & Andersen, 1974, 1975). When patients experience their physician as warm, caring, interested, friendly, and competent, patients are more likely to comply (Becker, Drachman, & Kirscht, 1972; DiMatteo, Prince, & Taranta, 1979). Physician behaviors such as eye contact, smiling, forward leaning, and head nodding create positive perceptions (DiNicola & DiMatteo, 1984). Such perceptions likely affect patients' willingness to trust physicians and their recommendations.

PATIENT CHARACTERISTICS   Demographic variables, such as race and sex, do not appear to be consistently related to compliance (Haynes, Taylor, & Sackett, 1979). As DiNicola and DiMatteo (1984) note, the failure of demographic factors to consistently predict compliance may in part be due to the multitude of varied regimens and disease entities researched. These authors suggest that perhaps the most important patient characteristics influencing compliance to specific regimens include the availability of social support within the patient's social environment and their beliefs and attitudes about health and health-care.

Social support has been thought to be an exceedingly important factor for continued compliance with medical regimens. Such support may include emotional support and acceptance from family and friends, and/or physical assistance and tangible resources like money and time (DiNicola & DiMatteo, 1984; Caplan, 1979). Furthermore, family members may provide helpful reminders to patients of their regimen and provide reinforcement for follow-through with medical regimens. However, DiMatteo and Hays (1981) have noted that family support may have negative consequences for some patients. The nature of the expressions of support from family members may vary in quality and degree. Patients may also differ in their view and experience of support as helpful or harmful. An important goal of future research in this area may be the identification of family interactions involved in compliance and other health-enhancing and health-endangering behaviors.

In summary, noncompliance is one of the most important factors contributing to the failure of medical interventions. The relationship between the patient and physician and certain attributes of patients and their support systems strongly affect compliance. Further development of interventions that promote adherence to medical regimens is sorely needed.

# Summary

About 28% of the U.S. population is overweight. Obesity is defined as a 10%–20% excess of body fat. It is associated with a wide array of health problems, including cardiovascular disease, hypertension, stroke, and diabetes. Because our society values being thin, obese people are at risk for depression and problems with low self-esteem.

Personality does not appear to play a significant role in the development of obesity, and data concerning the relationship between eating habits and obesity are not consistent. The externality hypothesis of obesity suggests that obese people are more responsive to external cues, such as the smell or sight of food, than they are to internal cues, such as hunger. The set-point theory of obesity argues that the metabolism of obese people adjusts to resist weight loss, so reductions in food intake may be counteracted by lower metabolic rates.

Behavioral treatment of obesity relies on careful recording of eating behavior (self-monitoring), control of the stimuli associated with eating (stimulus control), alteration of eating habits, and reinforcement of eating behavior or weight loss. The lack of a reliable relationship between eating habits and obesity may limit the ultimate effectiveness of programs concentrating on the modification of eating behavior. Newer treatment programs incorporate cognitive restructuring, social support, and exercise.

About 8% of the adults in the United States consume one ounce or more of absolute alcohol each day. About one-tenth of drinkers consume half of the alcohol sold in the U.S. Alcohol abuse involves repeated use of alcohol despite knowledge that its use causes or exacerbates a personal problem. Alcohol dependence involves impaired control of drinking. Tolerance is present if increasing amounts of alcohol are required to achieve the desired effect. Withdrawal includes symptoms such as shakiness or malaise when alcohol use is reduced or stopped.

Alcohol affects many organ systems. Chronic, excessive alcohol use may lead to brain disorders such as alcoholic dementia and alcoholic amnestic syndrome (Korsakoff's psychosis). Alcohol use is also associated with cirrhosis of the liver, cardiac disorders, and gastrointestinal problems. Pregnant mothers who continue to drink increase the risk for complications during pregnancy and for their children being born with fetal alcohol syndrome.

Patterns of alcohol use are affected by social customs, an individual's learning history, and by the drinking behavior of parents and peers. Personality factors do not appear to play a significant role in the development of alcoholism, but disturbances such as depression often accompany alcohol abuse and dependence. Twin studies suggest that genetic background may increase the risk for alcoholism. The drinker's expectations regarding the effects of alcohol can influence both drinking behavior and behavioral and emotional reactions to alcohol.

Aversion therapies for alcoholism use nausea-inducing chemicals and electric shock to inhibit alcohol use; chemical aversion is more effective. Operant treatments reinforce sobriety with rewards such as social interaction. Cognitive-behavioral treatments change the cognitions of the drinkers, such as the drinker's sense of a lack of control. Relapse prevention training teaches coping behaviors that the former drinker can use when confronted with the temptation to drink. Although some alcoholics resume moderate drinking after treatment, those who do so are at greater risk for a return to heavy drinking than are those who abstain.

Smoking rates are declining, but between one-quarter and one-third of the United States population still smokes cigarettes. Smoking is associated with the development of many health problems, including lung cancer and heart disease. Smoking during pregnancy increases the risk of spontaneous abortion and premature birth, and the children of smoking parents suffer more respiratory infections than do the children of parents who do not smoke.

Rapid smoking and electric shock aversion therapy have been used to reduce or eliminate smoking. Rapid smoking is more effective than electric shock. Self-management procedures to reduce smoking behavior include self-monitoring, nicotine fading, contingency management, and self-control programs. Nicotine gum allows some smokers to gradually withdraw from nicotine dependence, but use of the gum may be counterproductive for smokers not physically dependent on nicotine.

The percentage of nonactive adults has declined since 1961, but a minority of today's adults participate in regular, moderate physical activity. Aerobic exercise requires the use of large muscles and moves the body's weight against gravity or over distance. Aerobic exercise helps maintain optimal body weight or composition, prevent heart disease, and normalize carbohydrate metabolism.

Improved self-concept has been associated with regular exercise, but the improvements are more closely related to perceptions of improved fitness rather than to actual changes in physical condition. Reduced anxiety and depression may also be consequences of exercise. Reductions in depression may be caused by physiological changes following exercise or to changes in feelings of mastery and control. Adherence to exercise programs may be improved with social reinforcers, such as group exercising and support from family.

Patients often do not comply with medical recommendations; rates of noncompliance range from 15% to 94%. Compliance is lower if medical regimens are complex, inconvenient, and extend over long periods of time. Patients are more likely to comply if they experience discomfort as a result of illness, understand the medical recommendations, and see their care-givers as warm, caring, and competent. Social and family support may also improve compliance.

# *References*

ADAY, L. A., & ANDERSEN, R. (1975). *Access to medical care.* Health Administration Press: Michigan.

ADAY, L. A., & ANDERSEN, R. (1974). A framework for the study of access to medical care. *Health Services Research, 9,* 208–220.

ALLON, N. (1982). The stigma of overweight in everyday life. In B. B. Wolman (Ed.), *Psychological aspects of obesity: A handbook.* (pp. 130–174). New York: Van Nostrand Reinhold.

American Psychiatric Association (1980). *Diagnostic and statistical manual of mental disorders* (3rd ed.). Washington, DC: Author.

American Psychiatric Association (1987). *Diagnostic and statistical manual of mental disorders* (3rd ed. rev.). Washington, DC: Author.

ARMOR, D. J., POLICH, J. M., & STAMBUL, H. B. (1978). *Alcoholism and treatment.* New York: John Wiley and Sons.

BECKER, M. H., & MAIMAN, L. A. (1980). Strategies for enhancing patient compliance. *Journal of Community Health, 6,* 113–135.

BECKER, M. H., DRACHMAN, R. H., & KIRSCHT, J. P. (1972). Predicting mothers' compliance with pediatric medical regimens. *Journal of Pediatrics, 81,* 843–854.

BÉLISLE, M., ROSKIES, E., & LÉVESQUE, J. M. (1987). Improving adherence to physical activity. *Health Psychology, 6,* 159–172.

BJURSTROM, L. A., & ALEXIOU, N. G. (1978). A program of heart disease intervention for public employees. *Journal of Occupational Medicine, 20,* 521–531.

BLOOM, F. E. (1982). A summary of workshop discussions. In F. Bloom (Ed.), *Beta-carbolines and terahydroisiquinolines.* New York: Alan R. Liss.

BOHMAN, M. (1978). Some genetic aspects of alcoholism and criminality. *Archives of General Psychiatry, 35,* 269–276.

BOYD, J. R., COVINGTON, T. R., STANASZEK, W. F., & COUSSONS, R. T. (1974). Drug-defaulting. II. Analysis of noncompliance patterns. *American Journal of Hospital Pharmacy, 31,* 485–491.

BRAY, G. A. (1969). Definition, measurement and classification of the syndromes of obesity. *International Journal of Obesity, 2,* 99–122.

BRAY, G. A. (1986). Effects of obesity on health and happiness. In K. D. Brownell & J. P. Foreyt (Eds.), *Handbook of eating disorders: Physiology, psychology, and treatment of obesity, anorexia, and bulimia* (pp. 3–44). New York: Basic Books, Inc.

BROWNELL, K. D., & WADDEN, T. A. (1986). Behavior therapy for obesity: Modern approaches and better results. In K. D. Brownell & J. P. Foreyt (Eds.), *Handbook of eating disorders: physiology, psychology, and treatment of obesity, anorexia, and bulimia* (pp. 180–197). New York: Basic Books, Inc.

BROWNELL, K. D., HECKERMAN, C. L., WESTLAKE, R. J., HAYES, S. C., & MONTI, P. M. (1978). The effects of couples training and partner cooperativeness in the behavioral treatment of obesity. *Behavior Research and Therapy, 16,* 323–333.

BUTTERS, N. (1982). The Wernicke-Korsakoff syndrome. In National Institute on Alcohol Abuse and Alcoholism, *Biomedical processes and consequences of alcohol use. Alcohol and Health Monograph No. 2.* (DHHS Publication No. ADM 82–1191). Washington, DC: U.S. Government Printing Office.

CADDY, G. R. (1983). Alcohol use and abuse: Historical perspective and present trends. In B. Tabakoff, P. B. Sutker, & C. L. Randall. *Medical and social aspects of alcohol abuse.* New York: Plenum Press.

CADORET, R. J., CAIN, C. A., & GROVE, W. M. (1980). Development of alcoholism in adoptees raised apart from alcoholic biologic relatives. *Archives of General Psychiatry, 37,* 561–563.

CANNING, H., & MAYER, J. (1966). Obesity—its possible effect on college acceptance. *New England Journal of Medicine, 275,* 1172–1174.

CANNON, D. S., BAKER, T. B., & WEHL, C. K. (1981). Emetic and electric shock alcohol aversion therapy: Six and twelve-month follow-up. *Journal of Consulting and Clinical Psychology 49,* 360–368.

CAPLAN, R. D. (1979). Patient, provider and organization: Hypothesized determinants of adherence. In S. J. Cohen (Ed.), *New directions in patient compliance.* Lexington, MA: D. C. Heath.

CAUDILL, B. D., & MARLATT, G. A. (1975). Modeling influences in social drinking: An experimental analogue. *Journal of Consulting and Clinical Psychology, 43,* 405–415.

CHANEY, E., O'LEARY, M., & MARLATT, G. A. (1978). Skill training with alcoholics. *Journal of Consulting and Clinical Psychology, 46,* 1092–1104.

CLARK, W., & MIDANIK, L. (1982). Alcohol use and alcohol problems among U.S. adults. Results of the 1979 national survey. In *National Institute on Alcohol Abuse and Alcoholism. Alcohol and Health Monograph No. 1* (DHHS Publication No. ADM 82–1190). Washington, DC: U.S. Government Printing Office.

COLLINGWOOD, T. (1972). The effects of physical training upon behavior and self-attitudes. *Journal of Clinical Psychology, 28,* 583–585.

COLLINGWOOD, T., & WILLETT, L. (1971). The effects of physical training upon self-concept and body attitudes. *Journal of Clinical Psychology, 27,* 411–412.

DAVIS, J. S. (1966). Variations in patients' compliance with doctors' orders: Analysis of congruence between survey responses and results of empirical investigations. *Journal of Medical Education, 41,* 1037–1048.

DAVIS, V. E., & WALSCH, M. J. (1970). Alcohol, amines, and alkaloids: A possible biochemical basis for alcohol addiction. *Science, 167,* 1005–1007.

DEJONG, W. (1980). The stigma of obesity: The consequences of naive assumptions concerning the causes of physical deviance. *Journal of Health and Social Behavior, 21,* 75–87.

DEPARTMENT OF HEALTH AND HUMAN SERVICES. (1982). *The health consequences of smoking—Cancer, a report of the Surgeon General.* DHHS Publication No. PHS 82–50179. Washington, DC: U.S. Government Printing Office.

DEPARTMENT OF HEALTH AND HUMAN SERVICES. (1984a). *Fifth special report to the U.S. Congress on alcohol and health from the Secretary of Health and Human Services.* DHHS Publication No. ADM 84–1291. Washington, DC: U.S. Government Printing Office.

DEPARTMENT OF HEALTH AND HUMAN SERVICES. (1984b). *The health consequences of smoking—Cardiovascular disease, a report of the Surgeon General.* DHHS Publication No. PHS 84–50204. Washington, DC: U.S. Government Printing Office.

DEPARTMENT OF HEALTH AND HUMAN SERVICES. (1985). *The health consequences of smoking for women, a report of the Surgeon General.* Washington, DC: U.S. Government printing Office.

DEPARTMENT OF HEALTH AND HUMAN SERVICES. (1989). *Reducing the health consequences of smoking—25 years of progress, report to the Surgeon General.* DHHS Publication No. CDC 89–8411. Washington, DC: U.S. Government Printing Office.

DIMATTEO, M. R., & HAYS, R. (1981). Social support and serious illness. In B. Gottlieb (Ed.), *Social networks and social support.* Beverly Hills, CA: Sage.

DIMATTEO, M. R., PRINCE L. M., & TARANTA, A. (1979). Patients' perceptions of physicians' behavior: Determinants of patient commitment to the therapeutic relationship. *Journal of Community Health, 4,* 280–290.

DINICOLA, D. D., & DIMATTEO, M. R. (1984). Practitioners, patients, and compliance with medical regimens: A social psychological prespective. In A. Baum, S. E.

Taylor, & J. E. Singer (Eds.) *Handbook of psychology and health, Vol IV: Social psychological aspects of health* (pp. 55–84). Hillsdale, NJ: Lawrence Erlbaum Associates.

DONOGHUE, S. (1977). The correlation between physical fitness, absenteeism and work performance. *Canadian Journal of Public Health, 68*, 201–203.

FAGERSTROM, K. O. (1980). Physician dependence on nicotine as a determinant of success in smoking cessation. *World Smoking and Health, 5*, 22–23.

FAWZY, F. I., COOMBS, R. H., & GERBER, B. (1983). Generational continuity in the use of substances: the impact of parental substance use on adolescent substance use. *Addictive Behaviors, 8*, 109–114.

FINNEY, J. W., & MOOS, R. H. (1981). Characteristics and prognoses of alcoholics who become moderate drinkers and abstainers after treatment. *Journal of Studies on Alcohol, 42*, 94–105.

FOLKINS, C. H., & SIME, W. E. (1981). Physical fitness training and mental health. *American Psychologist, 36*, 373–389.

FOLKINS, C. H., LYNCH, S., & GARDNER, M. M. (1972). Psychological fitness as a function of physical fitness. *Archives of Physical Medicine and Rehabilitation, 53*, 503–508.

FOXX, R. M., & BROWN, R. A. (1979). Nicotine fading and self-monitoring for cigarette abstinence or controlled smoking. *Journal of Applied Behavior Analysis, 12*, 111–125.

GALANTER, M. (1983). Religious influence and the etiology of substance abuse. In E. Gottheil, K. A. Druley, T. E. Skoloda, & H. M. Waxman (Eds.), *Etiologic aspects of alcohol and drug abuse*. Springfield, IL: Charles C. Thomas.

GARETZ, F. K. (1973). Socio-psychological factors in overeating and dieting with comments on popular reducing methods. *Practitioner, 210*, 671–686.

GARROW, J. S. (1986). Physiological Aspects of Obesity. In K. D. Brownell & J. P. Foreyt (Eds.), *Handbook of eating disorders: Physiology, psychology, and treatment of obesity, anorexia, and bulimia* (pp. 45–62). New York: Basic Books.

GOLDBLATT, P. B., MOORE, M. E., & STUNKARD, A. J. (1965). Social factors in obesity, *Journal of the American Medical Association, 192*, 1039–1044.

GREDEN, J. F. (1985). Caffeine and tobacco dependence. In H. I. Kaplan, & B. J. Sadock (Eds.), *Comprehensive textbook of psychiatry/IV (Vol. 1)*. Baltimore: Williams & Wilkins.

GREIST, J. H., KLEIN, M. H., EISCHENS, R. R., FARIS, J., GURMAN, A. S., & MORGAN, W. P. (1979). Running through your mind, *Journal of Psychosomatic Research, 22*, 259–294.

HASKELL, W. L. (1984). Overview: Health benefits of exercise. In J. D. Matarazzo, S. M. Weiss, J. A. Herd, N. E. Miller, & S. M. Weiss (Eds.), *Behavioral health: A handbook of health enhancement and disease prevention* (pp. 490–423). New York: John Wiley & Sons.

HAYNES, R. B. (1979). Determinants of compliance: The disease and the mechanics of treatment. In R. B. Haynes, D. W. Taylor, & D. Sackett (Eds.), *Compliance in health care*. Baltimore: Johns Hopkins University Press.

HEINZELMANN, F., & BAGLEY, R. W. (1970). Response to physical activity programs and their effects on health behavior. *Public Health Reports, 85*, 905–911.

HOWLEY, E. (1976). The effect of different intensities of exercise on the excretion of epinephrine and norepeinephrine. *Medicine and Science in Sports, 8*, 219–222.

HUGHES, C. A. (1974). A comparison of the effects of teaching techniques of body conditioning on physical fitness and self concept. *Dissertation Abstracts International, 34*, 3957A–3958A. (University Microfilms No. 73–31, 255)

HULKA, B. S. (1979). Patient-clinician interactions and compliance. In R. B. Haynes, D. W. Taylor, & D. L. Sackett (Eds.), *Compliance in health care*. Baltimore: Johns Hopkins University Press.

HUNT, G. A., & AZRIN, N. H. (1973). A community reinforcement approach to alcoholism. *Behavior Research and Therapy, 11*, 91–104.

INSEL, P. M., & ROTH, W. T. (1977). *Health in a changing society: Core concepts.* Palo Alto, CA: Mayfield Publishing Company.

ISTVAN, J., & MATARAZZO J. D. (1984). Tobacco, alcohol and caffeine use: A review of their interrelationships. *Psychological Bulletin, 95*, 301–326.

JARVIK, M. E., & SCHNEIDER, N.G. (1984). Degree of addiction and effectiveness of nicotine gum therapy for smoking. *American Journal of Psychiatry, 141*, 790–791.

JASNOSKI, M. L., HOLMES, D. S., SOLOMON, S., & AGUIAR, C. (1981). Exercise, changes in aerobic capacity and changes is self-perceptions: An experimental investigation. *Journal of Research in Personality, 15*, 460–466.

KANNEL, W. B. (1983). Health and obesity: An overview. In P. T. Kuo, H. I. Conn, & E. A. DeFelice (Eds.), *Health and obesity* (pp. 1–20). New York: Raven Press.

KANTOROVICH, N. V. (1929). An attempt at associative reflex therapy in alcoholism. *Novoye v Reflekologii i Fiziologii Neronoy Sistemy, 3*, 436.

KEESEY, R. E. (1986). A set-point theory of obesity. In K. D. Brownell & J. P. Foreyt, *Handbook of eating disorders: Physiology, psychology, and treatment of obesity, anorexia, and bulimia (pp. 63–87). New York: Basic Books.*

KING, A. C., TAYLOR, G. B., HASKELL, W. L., & DEBUSK, R. F. (1989). Influence of regular aerobic exercise on psychological health: A randomized, controlled trial of healthy middle-aged adults. *Health Psychology, 8*, 305–324.

KISSIN, B., & BEGLEITER, H. (1979). *The biology of alcoholism. Vol. 2. Physiology and behavior.* New York: Plenum Press.

KORNHABER, A. (1970). The stuffing syndrome. *Psychosomatics, 11*, 580–584.

KOSTRUBALA, T. (1977). Jogging and personality change. *Today's Jogger, 1*, 14–15.

LANG, A. R., GOECKNER, D. J., ADESSO, V. J., & MARLATT, G. A. (1975). Effects of alcohol on aggression in male social drinkers. *Journal of Abnormal Psychology, 84*, 508–518.

LARRSON, B., BJORNTORP, P., & TIBBLIN, G. (1981). The health consequences of moderate obesity. *International Journal of Obesity, 5*, 97–116.

LEIGH, G. (1985). Psychosocial factors in the etiology of substance abuse. In T. E. Bratter & G. G. Forrest (Eds.), *Alcoholism and substance abuse: Strategies for clinical intervention.* New York: The Free Press.

LEVANTHAL, H., & AVIS, N. (1976). Pleasure, addiction and habit: Factors in verbal report or factors in smoking behavior? *Journal of Abnormal Psychology, 85*, 478–488.

LICHTENSTEIN, E., & MERMELSTEIN, R. J. (1984). Review of approaches to smoking treatment: Behavior modification strategies. In J. D. Matarazzo, S. M. Weiss, J. A. Weiss, N. E. Miller, & S. M. Weiss (Eds.), *Behavioral health* (pp. 695–712). New York: John Wiley & Sons.

LICHTENSTEIN, E., & RODRIGUES, M-R. P. (1977). Long-term effects of rapid smoking treatment for dependent cigarette smokers. *Addictive Behaviors, 2*, 109–112.

LIED, E. R., & MARLATT, G. A. (1979). Modeling as a determinant of alcohol consumption: Effect of subject sex and prior drinking history. *Addictive Behaviors, 4*, 47–54.

MAHONEY, M. J. (1978). Behavior modification in the treatment of obesity. *Psychiatric Clinics of North America, 1*, 651–660.

MARLATT, G. A. (1979). Alcohol use and problem drinking: A cognitive behavioral analysis. In P. C. Kendall & S. D. Hallon (Eds.), *Cognitive-behavioral interventions: Theory, research and procedures.* New York: Academic Press.

MARTIN, J. E., & DUBBERT, P. M. (1982). Exercise applications and promotion in behavioral medicine: Current states and future directions. *Journal of Consulting and Clinical Psychology, 50,* 1004–1017.

MATARAZZO, J. D. (1982). Behavioral health's challenge to academic, scientific and professional psychology. *American Psychologist, 37,* 1–14.

MILLER, W. R., HESTER, R. K. (1980). Treating the problem drinker: Modern approaches. In W. R. Miller (Ed.), *The addictive behaviors.* New York: Pergamon Press.

MOOS, R. H., FINNEY, J. W., & CHAN, D. A. (1981). The process of recovery from alcoholism. I. Comparing alcoholic patients and matched community controls. *Journal of Studies on Alcohol, 42,* 383–402.

NATIONAL CENTER FOR HEALTH STATISTICS. (1989). *Health, United States, 1988.* DHHS Publication No. PHS 89–1232. Washington, DC: U.S. Government Printing Office.

OLDRIDGE, N. B. (1977). What to look for in an exercise class leader. *Physician and Sports Medicine, 5,* 85–88.

OLDRIDGE, N. B. (1984). Adherence to adult exercise fitness programs. In J. D. Matarazzo, S. M. Weiss, J. A. Herd, N. E. Miller, & S. M. Weiss (Eds.), *Behavioral health: A handbook of health enhancement and disease prevention* (pp. 467–487). New York: John Wiley & Sons.

PARDES, A. (1982). Treatment of alcohol dependence within the health care system. *Psychiatric Annals, 12,* 459.

PATTISON, E. M. (1976). Nonabstinent drinking goals in the treatment of alcoholism: A clinical typology. *Archives of General Psychiatry, 33,* 923–930.

PENICK, S. B., FILION, R., FOX, S., & STUNKARD, A. J. (1970). Behavior modification in the treatment of obesity. *Psychosomatic Medicine, 33,* 49–55.

PERRI, M. G., McADOO, W. G., SPEVAK, P. A., & NEWLIN, D. B. (1984). Effects of a multicomponent maintenance program on long-term weight loss. *Journal of Consulting and Clinical Psychology, 52,* 480–481.

POLICH, J. M., ARMOR, D. J., & BRAIKER, H. B. (1981). *The course of alcoholism: Four years after treatment.* New York: John Wiley and Sons.

POMERLEAU, O. F., PERTSCHUK, M., ADKINS, D, & BRADY, J. P. (1978). A comparison of behavioral and traditional treatment methods for middle-income problem drinkers. *Journal of Behavioral Medicine, 1,* 187–200.

RABKIN, S. W., MATHEWSON, F. A., & HUS, P. H. (1977). Relation of body weight to development of ischemic heart disease in a cohort of young North American men after a 26-year observation period. The Manitoba study. *American Journal of Cardiology, 39,* 452–458.

RODIN, J., RENNERT, K., & SOLOMON, S. K. (1980). Intrinsic motivation for control: Fact or fiction. In A. Baum & J. E. Singer (Eds.), *Advances in environmental psychology: Applications of personal control* (Vol. 2). Hillsdale, NJ: Lawrence Erlbaum Associates.

ROHSENOW, D. J., & MARLATT, G. A. (1981). The balanced placebo design: Methodological considerations. *Addictive Behaviors. 36,* 1508–1531.

ROSENTHAL, B. S., ALLEN, G. J., & WINTER, C. (1980). Husband involvement in the behavioral treatment of overweight women: Initial effects and long-term follow-up. *International Journal of Obesity, 4,* 165–173.

RUSSELL, M. (1986). The epidemiology of alcoholism. In N. J. Estes & M. E. Heinemann, *Alcoholism: Development, consequences, and interventions* (pp. 31–52). St. Louis: C. V. Mosby.

SACKETT, D. L., & SNOW, J. C. (1979). The magnitude of compliance and noncompliance. In R. B. Haynes, D. W. Taylor, & D. L Sackett (Eds.), *Compliance in health care.* Baltimore: Johns Hopkins University Press.

SACKETT, D. L., & HAYES, R. B. (1976). Compliance with therapeutic regimens. Baltimore: Johns Hopkins University Press.

SCHUCKIT, M. A. (1986). Etiologic theories on alcoholism. In N.J. Estes & J. E. Heinemann, *Alcoholism: Development, consequences and interventions* (3rd ed., pp. 15–30). St. Louis: C. V. Mosby.

SCHUCKIT, M. A. (1983). Alcoholism and other psychiatric disorders. *Hospital and Community Psychiatry, 34*, 1022–1027.

SCHWARTZ, J. L. (1987). *Review and evaluation of smoking cessation methods: The United States and Canada, 1978-1985* (NIH Publication No. 87–2940). Washington DC: National Institutes of Health.

SEGAL, R., & SISSON, B. V. (1985). Medical complications associated with alcohol use and the assessment of risk of physical damage. In R. E. Bratter & G. G. Forrest (Eds.), *Alcoholism and substance abuse: Strategies for clinical intervention* (pp. 137–175). New York: The Free Press.

SELZER, M. L. (1980). Alcoholism and Alcoholic Psychoses. In H. I. Kaplan, A. M. Freedman, & B. L. Sadock (Eds.), *Comprehensive textbook of psychiatry/III* (Vol.2). Baltimore: Williams and Wilkins.

SCHACTER, S. (1968). Obesity and eating. *Science, 161*, 751–756.

SIME, W. E. (1984). Psychological benefits of exercise training in the healthy individual. In J. D. Matarazzo, S. M. Weiss, J. A. Herd, N. E. Miller, & S. M. Weiss (Eds.), *Behavioral health: A handbook for health enhancement and disease prevention.* New York: John Wiley and Sons.

SPITZER, L., & RODIN, J. (1981). Human eating behavior: A critical review of studies in normal weight and overweight individuals. *Appetite, 2*, 293–329.

STRIEGEL-MOORE, R., & RODIN, J. (1986). The influence of psycholgical variables in obesity. In K. D. Brownell & J. P. Foreyt (Eds.), *Handbook of eating disorders: Physiology, psychology, and treatment of obesity, anorexia, and bulimia* (pp. 99–121). New York: Basic Books.

STUMPHAUSER, J. S. (1980). Learning to drink: Adolescents and alcohol. *Addictive Behaviors, 5*, 277–283.

STUNKARD, A. (1959). Obesity and the denial of hunger. *Psychosomatic Medicine, 21*, 281–289.

STUNKARD, A. J. (1986). The control of obesity: Social and community perspectives. In K. D. Brownell & J. P. Foreyt (Eds.), *Handbook of eating disorders: Physiology, psychology, and treatment of obesity, anorexia, and bulimia* (pp. 213–228). New York: Basic Books.

STUNKARD, A. J. (1984). The current status of treatment of obesity in adults. In A. J. Stunkard & E. Stellar (Eds.), *Eating and its disorders.* New York: Raven Press.

VAILLANT, G. E. (1980). Natural history of male psychosocial health. Part 7: Antecedents of alcoholism and "orality." *American Journal of Psychiatry, 137*, 181–186.

VOEGTLIN, W. J. (1940). The treatment of alcoholism by establishing a conditioned reflex. *American Journal of Medical Science, 199*, 802–809.

WESTERMEYER, J., DOHENY, S., & STONE, B. 1978). An assessment of hospital care for the alcoholic patient. *Alcoholism, Clinical and Experimental Research, 2*, 53.

WILSON, G. T., & LAWSON, D. M. (1976). Expectancies, alcohol, and sexual arousal in male social drinkers. *Journal of Abnormal Psychology, 85*, 587–594.

WILSON, G. T., & ABRAMS, D. B. (1977). Effects of alcohol on social anxiety and physiological arousal: Cognitive versus pharmacological processes. *Cognitive Therapy & Research, 1*, 195–210.

WINDSOR, R. A., & LOWE, J. B. (1988). The effectiveness of worksite self-help smoking cessation program: A randomized trial. *Journal of Behavioral Medicine, 11*, 407–421.

# CHAPTER 7

# Psychological Preparation for Stressful Medical and Dental Procedures

During the course of a lifetime, most people experience a variety of potentially stressful medical and dental procedures. These procedures can range from routine examinations and diagnostic tests to more complicated medical and dental treatment interventions. Most patients report that invasive medical and dental procedures are particularly stressful. An *invasive procedure* can be defined as a medical or dental technique that requires the penetration of bodily tissue or the invasion of a bodily opening. Such a procedure typically involves the use of instruments and is performed by a health care professional for the purpose of diagnosis, treatment, and/or health maintenance.

Some degree of physical risk is associated with most invasive procedures. For example, surgical patients often face the possibility of suffering pain, bodily changes, or complications of the operation. In addition, patients who are hospitalized for invasive procedures have to cope with the disruption of daily activities and the substitution of complicated, bewildering medical routines. Not surprisingly, patients frequently react to the threats to bodily integrity and to the psychosocial changes with some degree of emotional distress. Prospective surveys have found that the majority of medical and dental patients facing invasive procedures expressed moderate to high levels of anxiety regarding those procedures (Carnevali, 1966; Graham & Conley, 1971; Janis, 1958; O'Hara, Ghoneim, Hinrichs, Mehta, & Wright, 1989; Ryan, 1975; Wolfer & Davis, 1970). Moreover, several studies have found significant negative correlations between preoperative anxiety and postoperative recovery, with high-anxiety patients showing the least favorable outcome on such measures as number of sedatives, analgesics, and days to discharge (Sime, 1976); number of complaints and tranquilizers (Cohen & Lazarus, 1973); self-report of hospital adjustment (Auerbach, 1973); and resumption of employment (Boyd, Yeager, & McMillan, 1973).

The frequent negative correlation between preoperative anxiety and postoperative adjustment suggests that reducing patients' concerns regarding upcoming invasive procedures facilitates their adaptation following these procedures. Using this rationale, psychological techniques designed to prepare patients for invasive procedures have usually attempted to reduce anxiety and psychological stress. *Psychological preparations* are interventions delivered before an invasive procedure in order to facilitate adaptation and recovery. This chapter will summarize the research on the major preparatory treatments in an attempt to evaluate their effectiveness. The large category of invasive procedures will be subdivided into several major types: surgery, diagnostic medical tests, dental procedures, and obstetrical-gynecological procedures. The literature on psychological preparation will be discussed for each subcategory. Methodological problems apparent in the research will also be addressed. Finally, an analysis will be made of the utility of employing various preparation techniques in everyday medical and dental practice.

# Surgery

Surveys of surgical patients have revealed that the majority of patients studied expressed at least some fears about their impending operation (Carnevali, 1966; Ryan, 1975; Salmon et al., 1988). Frequently reported concerns have included (a) fear of pain and discomfort; (b) outcome of the surgery; (c) destruction of body image; (d) the unknown; (e) possibility of cancer; (f) separation from the normal environment; (g) disruption of life plans; (h) loss of control; and (i) death. Psychological preparations have been used to help patients cope with these concerns, either by providing information or by teaching specific coping skills such as relaxation exercises or self-hypnosis. Many preparatory interventions have included more than one of these therapeutic components. In order to facilitate evaluation of their efficacy, the preparations for surgery will be categorized according to their main treatment component: information provision, modeling, behavioral techniques, cognitive-behavioral interventions, and hypnosis.

## Informative Preparations

Survey studies of surgical patients have found that patients who possessed accurate information about their impending operations tended to demonstrate better postoperative adjustment than less well informed patients (Janis, 1958, 1971). Janis (1958) speculated that the realistic information had encouraged patients to develop accurate expectations about their surgery and to reassure themselves that they could cope effectively with the stressful event. The positive correlation between preoperative surgical knowledge and postoperative adjustment has encouraged the development of informative preparations.

Several studies have examined the effects on surgical patients of the provision of *procedural information*. This preparation consists of basic information about presurgical, surgical, and postsurgical procedures. In general, patients receiving procedural information have fared slightly better than control patients on measures of recovery. For example, Chapman (1970) gave patients scheduled for hernia surgery detailed procedural information about their surgery and the events that would occur during their hospital stay. The informed patients did not report any less postoperative anxiety than control patients who received no intervention. The prepared patients, however, required fewer postoperative analgesics and were discharged sooner from the hospital than control subjects. As the control group received routine nursing care only, the effect of extended contact with the nurse who delivered the procedural information was not determined.

In an attempt to improve the effectiveness of informative preparations, a number of investigators have added *sensory information* to their descriptions of basic procedures. Sensory information describes the typical sensations that a patient will feel, hear, smell, taste, and see before, during, and after the invasive procedures. For example, specific sensory and procedural information has been used successfully to prepare patients for minor gynecological surgery (Reading, 1982). The patients were fifty-nine women who were undergoing *laparoscopy*, an exploratory operation in which a small tube and optical system is inserted into the abdomen through a small incision to observe the abdominal organs and detect any abnormalities. The women were randomly assigned to one of three groups. The first group received an informative preparatory interview from a physician. The second group of patients received a placebo interview to control for the effects of contact with a concerned health professional. The patients were asked neutral questions about their hospital experience and medical history. The third group of patients received standard hospital care but no preoperative interview. After the surgery, the three groups reported similar levels of pain intensity and anxiety. Only 10% of the prepared patients, however, requested postoperative analgesic medication, as compared to 38% in the placebo and 45% in the non-treatment control group. The prepared patients also tended to report a more rapid return to full health than placebo and control group patients. Reading (1982) concluded that the preparatory information altered the behavioral response to pain but not the sensory experience of pain.

Sensory and procedural information has not always been an effective preparation. For example, when Langer, Janis, and Wolfer (1975) gave sensory and procedural information to patients scheduled for elective surgery (e.g., hysterectomy, tubal ligation, hernia repair), the results revealed that the informed patients did not differ from control patients on postoperative measures of recovery. The characteristics of the patient sample and the information provided, however, may have limited the effectiveness of the informative approach. Although the sample included patients scheduled for a wide variety of surgical procedures, the same information was given to all subjects in the information group. Individualized information pertaining to a specific invasive procedure might have been more helpful.

Other studies using sensory and procedural information as preparation for surgery have been reported (for reviews see Anderson & Masur, 1983; Kendall & Watson, 1981; Suls & Wan, 1989). Overall, the results are similar to those just described. In some reports, a combination of sensory and procedural information appeared to facilitate adaptation to surgery on several self-report, behavioral, or physiological measures but not on others. Some studies (e.g., Langer et al., 1975), however, demonstrated that preparatory information had no significant effects on outcome following surgery.

INDIVIDUAL DIFFERENCES   It has been suggested that informative preparations will not be beneficial to all patients because of individual differences in personality style (Auerbach, 1989). Thus, inconsistent results among studies using informative interventions may have been related to the personality characteristics of the patients studied. Several investigators have attempted to classify individuals according to their typical response to a stressful event (e.g., surgery). People referred to as *sensitizers*, *copers*, or *monitors* typically prefer to obtain information about a stressful event, whereas people referred to as *repressors*, *avoiders*, or *blunters* usually prefer to avoid such information (Byrne, 1964; Krantz, Baum, & Wideman, 1980; Miller & Mangan, 1983; Peterson & Toler, 1986).

Several studies on preparation for surgery have examined this information-seeking versus information-avoiding coping style (Andrew, 1970; DeLong, 1971; Scott & Clum, 1984). The overall results indicate that patients who prefer to seek information benefit more from preparatory information than patients who prefer to avoid information. For example, DeLong (1971) examined the effects of general and specific information on patients with different coping styles. Overall, patients who received specific information about their surgery had fewer complications and were discharged sooner from the hospital than patients who received general information about the hospital. There were significant interactions of coping style with type of information, however. Avoiders (repressors) typically had slow, complicated recoveries. Avoiders who received specific information, however, voiced more postoperative complaints than avoiders who received the general data. Among the sensitizers, patients in the specific-information group recovered more rapidly than patients in the general-information group.

INFORMATION PLUS EMOTIONAL SUPPORT   A number of early studies with children and their parents examined the effects of interventions consisting of sensory and procedural information plus emotional support and reassurance (e.g., Vaughn, 1957). In a comprehensive review of the early literature on preparing children for hospitalization and invasive procedures, Vernon, Foley, Sipowicz, and Schulman (1965) concluded that a number of methodological problems in these studies left the results open to differing interpretations. Although the experimental groups usually fared better than the control groups, the outcome measures of recovery were limited and often unreliable. Moreover, as each preparation contained multiple treatment components, it could not be determined which components were effective. Another methodological problem was that the control groups received routine hospital care only. Thus, the investigators failed to control for the possible effects of attention and interaction with the experimenter.

Unfortunately, subsequent research with pediatric patients using informative preparations has suffered from similar methodological problems. For example, Wolfer and Visintainer (1975) have developed a very effective preparatory treatment for children and their parents consisting of sensory and procedural information, behavioral rehearsal, play therapy, and emotional support. Children hospitalized for minor surgery who received the preparatory package demonstrated more cooperation, less emotional behavior, lower pulse rates, less resistance to anesthesia induction, reduced postoperative urinary retention, and better postdischarge behavioral adjustment than children who received routine hospital care only. Once again, it cannot be determined which components of the treatment were effective.

Adult patients have also received effective preparatory interventions consisting of information plus emotional support (e.g., Egbert, Battit, Welch, & Bartlett, 1964). As the interventions typically included support, attention, and information, the effect of information alone was not determined.

Although the research on informative preparations for adult and pediatric surgical patients has not produced fully definitive results, several general conclusions can be made. Informative preparations for adult patients that include sensory information appear to be more effective than preparations that contain only procedural data. Individual difference variables, however, may influence whether patients respond favorably to preparatory information. Pediatric patients and their parents have also benefited from preparations that include information. The efficacy of information alone, however, cannot be determined in these pediatric studies (Atkins, 1987).

## Modeling Preparations

*Modeling* preparations are interventions that expose patients to one or more patient models who have undergone the invasive procedure and describe their experiences to the patients. Modeling therapies were originally developed by social learning theorists to treat phobias and other unrealistic fears (Bandura, 1969, 1977). According to social learning theory, the sight of another person approaching a feared stimulus will reduce a subject's avoidance behavior and related anxiety. In recent years, films, videotapes, and other innovative modeling displays have been used to prepare patients for surgery and other invasive procedures.

In one of the first studies to use a modeling preparation, hospitalized children who were scheduled for tonsillectomy, hernia, or urinogenital surgery were shown either a film depicting a seven-year-old boy coping with hospitalization and surgical procedures or a control film that depicted a child on a nature trip (Melamed & Seigel, 1975). The modeling film, entitled *Ethan Has an Operation*, demonstrated events that most children experience when hospitalized for surgery, such as admission procedures, blood tests, anesthesia induction, recovery room procedures, and so on. The film was narrated in part by the patient model, who described his feelings and concerns during the hospital experience.

Subjects who viewed the hospital film demonstrated better preoperative and postoperative adjustment than control subjects on an impressive range of outcome measures. The prepared children showed less sweat-gland activity (an index of autonomic arousal) and fewer anxiety-related behaviors (e.g., crying, stuttering, trembling) than control children. In addition, the prepared children reported fewer medical concerns and fears at both the preoperative and postoperative assessments.

Modeling preparations have also been used with adult patients. In one recent study, male patients were prepared for cardiac surgery by watching a videotape that presented patients who described their experiences with cardiac surgery (Anderson, 1987). The patients in the control group received the standard hospital preparation and were interviewed on hospital-related topics. Patients who received the modeling preparation reported less emotional distress and were rated by nurses as making a better recovery than patients in the control group. The prepared patients also had a lower incidence of postoperative hypertension, a complication that frequently occurs after cardiac surgery.

INDIVIDUAL DIFFERENCES   Several studies have demonstrated that individual difference variables can affect how pediatric surgery patients respond to modeling preparations (Melamed, Dearborn, & Hermecz, 1983; Faust & Melamed, 1984). For example, Melamed et al. (1983) showed patients either an audio-visual presentation of a thirteen-year-old male undergoing minor surgery or a film of a child on a fishing trip. Subjects viewing the patient model were rated as more cooperative in the operating room, used less pain medication, and had fewer postsurgical problems than subjects who viewed the fishing film. The effects of the modeling treatment, however, were not always advantageous. Age and previous surgical experience were two variables that influenced how children reacted to the presentations. Children under the age of eight who had previous surgery were rated as more anxious and reported more medical concerns after seeing a patient model than after a control film. Figure 7.1 depicts the effects of age, previous experience, and type of preparation on observer ratings of anxiety. The authors concluded that young, experienced children might be better prepared using alternative strategies.

A variety of modeling displays have been used effectively to prepare patients for surgery. Variables such as age and previous surgical experience, however, appear to influence the effectiveness of modeling preparations. The timing of the intervention in relation to the surgery and the child's level of cognitive development also appear to be important factors (Faust & Melamed, 1984). In addition, the influence of parents on children's adaptation to surgery must be considered. Personality characteristics of the parents (e.g., anxiety level) and parental behaviors (e.g., reassurance) appear to influence children's reactions to stressful medical procedures (Melamed & Ridley-Johnson, 1988). Furthermore, the efficacy of modeling preparations for pediatric patients may be increased by having a parent present during the preparation (Pinto & Hollandsworth, 1989).

# Behavioral Preparations

*Behavioral preparations* for surgery attempt to teach patients specific behaviors that they can use to facilitate their adaptation and recovery (e.g., postsurgical deep breathing exercises to prevent lung complications). Early studies on be-

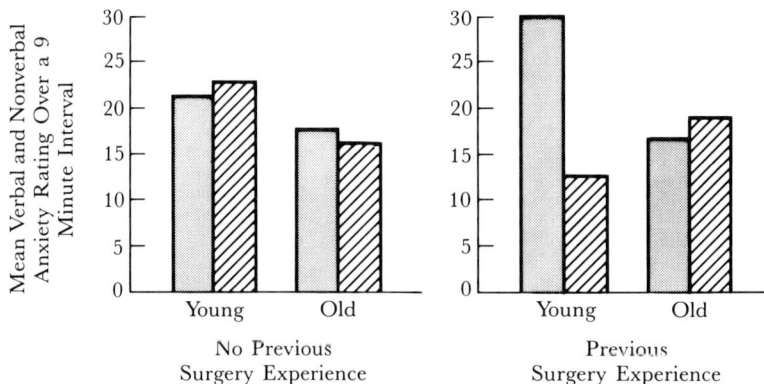

FIGURE 7.1   Anxiety levels of children who watched either a film about a child in the hospital for surgery (shaded columns) or a film of a child on a fishing trip (lined columns). The film about surgery reduced anxiety for most children. However, children under the age of eight who had previously undergone surgery were more anxious after watching the film about surgery. From "Necessary Considerations for Surgery Preparation: Age and Previous Experience" by B.G. Melamed, M. Dearborn, and D.A. Hermecz, 1983, *Psychosomatic Medicine, 45,* p. 520. Reprinted by permission.

havioral instruction in techniques designed to speed physical recovery suffered from a lack of random assignment to groups and inadequate statistical analyses (e.g., Healy, 1968; Lindeman & Aernam, 1971). Studies that have employed randomization and adequate statistical analyses have found positive effects for presurgical preparations consisting of behavioral instruction in breathing, coughing, exercising, and moving (Fortin & Kirouac, 1976; Schmitt & Wooldridge, 1973). In both of these studies, however, the instructional package included procedural information and emotional support. Thus, the effectiveness of the intervention may have been due to several factors, including the attention of the experimenter.

In addition to behavioral instruction, anxiety-reduction techniques adapted from behavior therapy have been used to prepare patients for surgery. Training in muscle relaxation has been evaluated as a preparatory strategy in several studies (Aiken & Henrichs, 1971; Flaherty & Fitzpatrick, 1978; Leserman, Stuart, Mamish, & Benson, 1989; Pickett & Clum, 1982; Scott & Clum, 1984; Wilson, 1981). In one of the studies with an adequate control group, Wilson (1981) gave patients scheduled for abdominal surgery a tape-recorded exercise in muscle relaxation. The exercise focused the patients' attention on individual muscle groups and on how to relax those muscle groups. Patients who received the relaxation training required fewer injections for pain, were discharged sooner from the hospital, and reported less pain as well as more energy and strength than control patients, who received standard hospital care. Patients who received sensory and procedural information were also discharged sooner from the hospital but did not differ from control patients on other outcome measures.

A second study of the effectiveness of relaxation training for surgical patients reported negative results (Pickett & Clum, 1982). One group of gallbladder surgery patients was taught progressive muscular relaxation. A second group was given a typed description of the relaxation instructions. Neither relaxation group reported less pain or anxiety or required fewer analgesic medications than the no-treatment control group. The conflicting results of Wilson (1981) and Pickett and Clum (1982) may be related to differences in their patient samples, assessment techniques, and/or training procedures. For example, whereas Wilson began assessing patients' responses to surgery on the first postoperative day, Pickett and Clum did not measure patients' responses until the fifth postoperative day.

Although behavioral instruction in body mechanics and other physical techniques may facilitate recovery, the research to date is inconclusive. No study has examined the effects of an intervention consisting solely of instructions in physical techniques. Recent research on relaxation training has been methodologically sound but has produced mixed results (Leserman et al., 1989; Pickett & Clum, 1981; Scott & Clum, 1984; Wilson, 1981). In future investigations of behavioral techniques, manipulation checks are needed to determine how often patients practice the techniques. It is possible that the patients who benefit from the training are the individuals who practice regularly. In addition, the possible interaction of individual difference variables and behavioral preparations should be considered. The results of one recent study suggested that sensitizers are more apt to benefit from a relaxation preparation than repressors (Scott & Clum, 1984).

## Cognitive-Behavioral Preparations

Recent developments in cognitive therapies have facilitated the development of *cognitive-behavioral preparations*. Cognitive-behavioral preparations teach patients cognitive and/or behavioral self-control strategies such as distraction and selective attention that they can use to reduce the anxiety and pain associated with invasive procedures. A frequent rationale for cognitive-behavioral preparation is that patients' cognitions about an invasive procedure will help to determine the amount of stress experienced. Thus, modifying maladaptive cognitions is one way to reduce patients' distress (Meichenbaum, 1977).

Langer et al. (1975) developed a cognitive-behavioral strategy based on the cognitive reappraisal of surgery as a stressful event. Patients were taught selective attention to distract themselves from the negative aspects of surgery and to attend to the positive factors (e.g., the surgery would improve their health; their hospital stay was a needed vacation). They were encouraged to focus on the positive factors whenever they felt upset about the unpleasant aspects of the surgical experience. Relative to a control group who had a neutral interview with the psychologist, the cognitively trained subjects were rated by an observer as less anxious and better adjusted prior to surgery. Moreover, the cognitive group requested fewer sedatives and analgesics after surgery than the control group.

An attention-redirection approach employed by Pickett and Clum (1982) consisted of imagined surgical scenes followed by pleasant scenes that directed the patients' attention away from the surgery. Patients who learned this cognitive distraction technique reported less postsurgical anxiety and less severe "pain at its worst" as compared to a no-treatment control group. In addition, the individual difference variable of locus of control orientation appeared to influence patients' reactions to the distraction technique. *Locus of control* orientation (LOC; Rotter, 1966) is a personality dimension that assesses a person's generalized expectancies for control of his or her life. Patients with an internal LOC believe that they have control over the reinforcement that they obtain as a consequence of their behavior. In contrast, patients with an external LOC believe that their reinforcement is determined by factors outside of their control (i.e., fate, luck, chance, or the influence of powerful people). Pickett and Clum found that patients with an internal LOC tended to benefit more from the distraction preparation than patients with an external LOC orientation. The authors concluded that internal LOC subjects benefited from learning a self-control strategy that allowed them to control their reactions to surgery.

Children and their parents also have benefited from cognitive-behavioral preparations. The effectiveness of training in coping skills was compared to information and anxiety reduction preparations in a study of pediatric patients (Zastowny, Kirschenbaum, & Meng, 1986). The preparations were scheduled one week prior to hospitalization for scheduled surgery. The parents and children in all three groups received information describing hospitalization and surgery. Parents in the coping skills group learned how to teach their children coping skills such as deep breathing and relaxation. In the anxiety reduction group parents learned techniques (e.g., relaxation) to reduce their own anxiety levels. The coping skills and anxiety reduction preparations significantly decreased the children's fearfulness and the parents' distress. Children in the coping skills group also demonstrated fewer maladaptive behaviors during hospitalization and at home (prior to admission and after discharge) than children in the other groups (see Figure 7.2).

Cognitive-behavioral preparations for surgery appear to be effective for many pediatric and adult patients. However, in one recent study, a cognitive-behavioral preparation was not effective for a group of adult patients who underwent cardiac surgery (Postlethwaite, Stirling, & Peck, 1986). Future research can determine which cognitive-behavioral techniques are worthwhile for different patient populations. The findings of Pickett and Clum (1982) suggest that individual difference variables will influence the efficacy of cognitive-behavioral preparations.

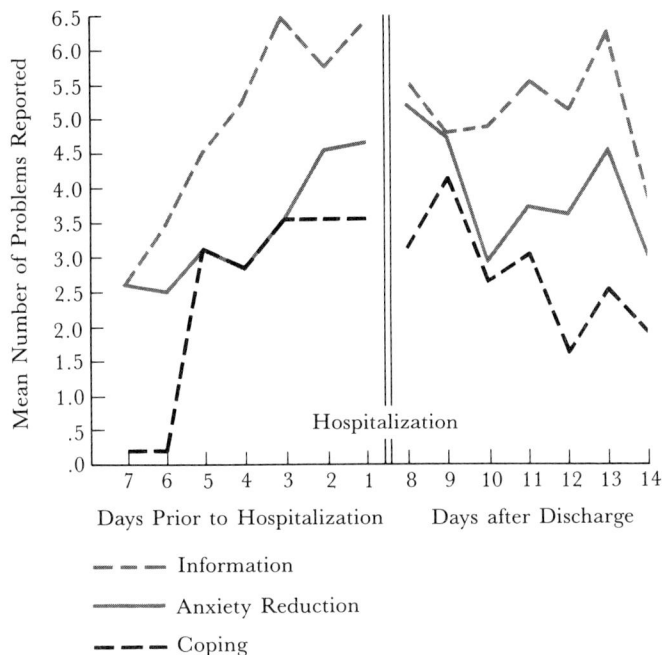

FIGURE 7.2  Mean number of daily problems parents recorded for their children during seven days prior to hospitalization and seven days after hospitalization. Parents trained in how to help their children cope (the coping group on the graph) reported fewer child problems before and after hospitalization than did parents who were instructed to spend an hour each day in one-to-one contact with their child (the information group on the graph). Children of parents trained in anxiety reduction procedures were intermediate in problem frequency between the coping and information groups. From "Coping Skills Training for Children: Effects on Distress Before, During, and After Hospitalization for Surgery" by T. R. Zastowny, D. S. Kirshenbaum, Anne L. Meng, 1986, *Health Psychology*, 5, p. 241. Reprinted by permission.

# Hypnotic Preparations

Hypnosis has been described as an excellent preparation for surgery (Fredericks, 1978). The hypothesized benefits of preoperative hypnosis include reduced anxiety, increased relaxation, less required surgical anesthesia, fewer postoperative sedatives and analgesics, less bleeding, and general facilitation of recovery. Although numerous case studies have described the positive effects of preoperative hypnosis, controlled group research has not unequivocally supported the efficacy of hypnotic preparations.

Field (1974) investigated the effectiveness of a hypnotic tape that included multiple components: suggestions of relaxation, drowsiness, comfort and quick recovery, as well as procedural information about surgery. Patients who listened to the tape prior to orthopedic surgery did not adapt better than control patients who heard a tape describing hospital facilities. Unfortunately, the only outcome measures were retrospective ratings by the surgeons as to patients' nervousness and speed of recovery.

In a study with a broader range of outcome measures, cardiac patients were taught an autohypnotic technique by a psychiatrist, who also corrected any misconceptions about their surgery (Surman, Hackett, Silverberg, & Behrendt, 1974). Relative to control patients who received standard hospital care, the hypnotically trained patients did not differ as to incidence of postoperative delirium, medication requirements, and ratings of anxiety, depression, and pain. As 45% of the trained subjects did not use the autohypnotic techniques, the lack of significant findings is not surprising.

Regular practice and use of hypnosis may be necessary for positive effects to be demonstrated. Wakeman and Kaplan (1978) found that the repeated use of hypnosis was an effective preparation for severely burned patients undergoing surgical debridement procedures that involve the removal of damaged tissues. The patients using self-hypnosis required lower dosages of analgesics than patients who received placebo interviews. It is unfortunate that other outcome measures of adaptation were not obtained.

In summary, the research on preoperative hypnosis has produced mixed results. Regular practice of hypnotic techniques may be necessary for positive effects to be seen. In addition, recent research has indicated that patients who are susceptible to hypnotic induction are more apt to benefit from hypnotic preparations than patients who are not susceptible (Reeves, Redd, Storm, & Minagawa, 1983). The Highlight Box discusses hypnotic susceptibility and its interaction with hypnotic preparation.

## Diagnostic Medical Tests

Many diagnostic medical tests are invasive procedures that involve the pentration of bodily tissue or the invasion of a body orifice. The majority of patients undergoing invasive tests are concerned about possible pain or discomfort as well as about the diagnostic results of the test. Additionally, patients must typically remain awake during the tests to cooperate with their physicians and cannot be given large amounts of sedative or analgesic medications. In recent years, psychological preparations have been developed to improve the adaptation of patients to invasive tests such as cardiac catheterization and gastrointestinal endoscopy. The efficacy of different types of preparations will be examined in the passages that follow.

BOXED HIGHLIGHT 7.1
# Hypnotic Susceptibility and Preparation for Hyperthermia

Radiofrequency-produced *hyperthermia* is an experimental treatment for cancer in which tumors are destroyed by heating them to temperatures above 42°C. Acute pain typically results from hyperthermia and can lead to premature termination of the treatment. Moreover, analgesic medication may not significantly reduce hyperthermia pain. In one recent study, a hypnotic preparation was employed in an attempt to reduce patients' pain during hyperthermia (Reeves, Redd, Storm, & Minagawa, 1983).

Twenty-eight cancer patients who were scheduled for hyperthermia treatment were administered the Stanford Hypnosis Clinical Scale (SHCS; Hilgard & Hilgard, 1965), a standardized procedure for measuring hypnotic susceptibility in patients. In this procedure, patients are hypnotized and then asked to follow specific suggestions of the hypnotist. For example, they are asked to act like a young child in school. The patients' ability to follow each suggestion is scored; their total score provides a measure of susceptibility or responsiveness to hypnosis.

In the Reeves et al. (1983) study, the cancer patients were divided into low- and high-hypnotic susceptibles based on their SHCS scores. Then the patients were randomly assigned to hypnosis or no-treatment control groups until an equal number of low- and high-hypnotic susceptibles were in each group. Patients in the hypnosis group learned a hypnotic pain control procedure called Rapid Induction Analgesia (RIA; Barber, 1977).

In this procedure, the hypnotist first makes suggestions for feelings of deep relaxation, heaviness, enjoyment, and comfort. Next, suggestions for analgesia are provided. Part of the text of RIA is as follows:

> I wonder if you'll notice that you'll feel surprised that your visit here today is so much more pleasant and comfortable than you might have expected. . . . I wonder if you'll notice that surprise . . . that there are no other feelings . . . nothing to bother, nothing to disturb. . . . Whatever you are able to notice . . . everything can be a part of your experience of comfortableness, restfulness, and restfulness and relaxation. . . . Everything you notice can be a part of being absolutely comfortable.

Patients in the hypnosis group received two sessions of RIA training and were instructed to practice the hypnosis prior to and during their next two hyperthermia sessions. Throughout each hyperthermia session, patients in the hypnosis and control groups were asked to rate the intensity of their pain. A total pain-score was derived for each hyperthermia treatment. The results revealed a significant interaction between hypnotic susceptibility and patient group. In the hypnosis group, only the high-hypnotic susceptibles reported a significant decrease in pain intensity across treatment days (see Figure 7.3). High- and low-hypnotic susceptibles in the control group and low suceptibles in the hypnosis group tended to report stable levels of pain intensity across the

*(continued)*

*Boxed Highlight 7.1 (continued)*

treatment days.

Reeves et al. (1983) suggested that their data should be interpreted cautiously because no attention-placebo control group was included. Also, extended hypnotic training might have benfited patients who were low in hypnotic susceptibility. Nonetheless, the results of the study strongly suggest that hypnotic susceptibility is an important individual difference variable that will influence patients' responses to hypnotic preparations.

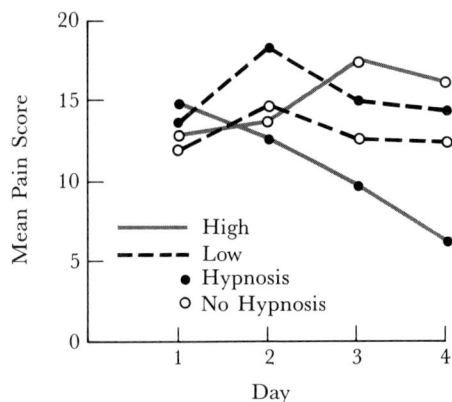

FIGURE 7.3   Mean hyperthermia pain scores for subjects high and low in hypnotic susceptibility. Hypnosis was not used on days one and two. Some subjects were hypnotized on days three and four. As the graph indicates, hypnosis was an effective pain control method only for subjects high in hypnotic suceptibility. From "Hypnosis in the Control of Pain During Hyperthermia Treatment of Cancer" by J. L. Reeves, W. H. Redd, F. K. Storm, and R. Y. Minagawa, in *Advances in Pain Research and Therapy* (vol 5), 1983, J. J. Bonica, U. Lindblom, and A. Iggo (Eds). Reprinted by permisssion.

## Informative Preparations

Johnson and her colleagues have examined the effectiveness of different types of informative preparations for patients undergoing invasive medical tests (Johnson, 1972; Johnson & Leventhal, 1974; Johnson, Morrissey & Leventhal, 1973). Johnson et al. (1973) compared the relative efficacy of sensory and procedural information for patients scheduled for *gastrointestinal endoscopy*, a diagnostic test used when upper gastrointestinal pathology is suspected. The procedure involves the insertion of a flexible fiberoptic tube called an endoscope through the mouth and into the gastrointestinal tract. The physician views the lining of the gastrointestinal tract through the endoscope and can detect abnormalities such as ulcers and tumors. Patients who received a description of the sensations that patients usually experience during the test demonstrated better adjustment during the test than patients who received procedural information alone. The sensory-information group displayed significantly less restlessness and fewer signs of tension in their arms during passage of the tube than the procedural information group. Both information groups, however, required less sedation than a no-treatment control group, a finding that could have been due to their greater contact with the experimenter.

*Cardiac catheterization* is a second diagnostic test for which informative preparations have been used. In this procedure, a small tube called a catheter is inserted into a blood vessel in the arm or leg and guided to the heart of patients with suspected cardiac disease. The cardiologist then inserts dye through the catheter and takes special X-ray pictures of the heart and coronary arteries. These special X-rays called angiograms, are used to detect the presence of coronary artery disease.

In a well-controlled study, Kendall, Williams, Pechacek, Graham, Shisslak, and Herzoff (1979) provided patients scheduled for cardiac catheterization with sensory and procedural information related to heart disease and to the catheterization procedure. Informed patients did report less anxiety during the test and were rated as better adjusted than attention-placebo and no-treatment control groups. The attention-placebo group was given a supportive interview with the experimenter in order to control for the effects of attention and emotional support. On most of the dependent measures, this group did not differ from the no-treatment control group, who received standard hospital procedures.

In summary, informative preparations that include sensory information appear to be beneficial for patients scheduled for endoscopy or cardiac catheterization. Moreover, information may be more effective than emotional support for patients undergoing these invasive tests. Because the research on preparation for surgery has indicated that variables such as coping style will influence patients' reactions to information provision, future studies of diagnostic procedures should consider the possible interaction of individual difference variables and informative preparations (Miller & Mangan, 1983).

## Modeling Preparations

Several studies have employed modeling preparations to prepare patients for invasive diagnostic tests. For example, Shipley and his colleagues prepared patients for their first gastrointestinal endoscopy by showing them a videotape of an anxious male model undergoing the procedure (Shipley, Butt, Horwitz, & Farbry, 1978). Patients who viewed the videotape were rated as less anxious during the endoscopy and reported less postprocedural anxiety than control patients, who viewed a biographical film. In order to explore the effects of repeated exposure to the endoscopy videotape, half of the subjects in the modeling condition viewed the videotape once and half viewed it three times. Although these two groups did not differ on many of the dependent measures, the patients who had three viewings did require less sedation and had lower heart rate increases during the first five minutes of the procedure than patients who viewed the videotape only once.

The investigators also looked at the effect of individual coping styles on patients' responses to the endoscopy videotape. Patients classified as sensitizers who viewed the modeling videotape showed lower heart rate increases during the test than sensitizers who saw the unrelated film. As predicted by their vigilant coping style, sensitizers who saw the videotape three times had lower heart increases than sensitizers who saw it once. For patients classified as repressors, viewing the videotape once was associated with a greater heart rate increase than viewing it three times or not at all. Shipley et al. (1978) concluded that viewing the videotape three times had extinguished the fear of the repressors. Indeed, repressors who repeatedly saw the videotape required less sedation during the test than repressors who saw it once.

Modeling preparations were more effective than informative and cognitive-behavioral interventions in a study of adults undergoing cardiac catheterization (Anderson & Masur, 1989). The modeling intervention consisted of a slide-tape presentation of a middle-aged male who described his experiences with the test. Figure 7.4 shows a slide from the modeling preparation.

In the cognitive-behavioral condition, patients were taught the coping skills of relaxation, distraction, and reframing. First, they learned brief muscle relaxation and breathing exercises. Next, the patients were taught how to reframe negative cognitions about the catheterization into more positive thoughts. For example, instead of thinking that "the equipment in the catheterization laboratory is frightening," patients were encouraged to think that "the equipment is the best machinery available for carefully monitoring a patient's condition during the test." Finally, the patients were taught how to distract themselves from the test by counting, imagining pleasant scenes (e.g., a meadow on a sunny day), or picturing themselves involved in a favorite activity. The infor-

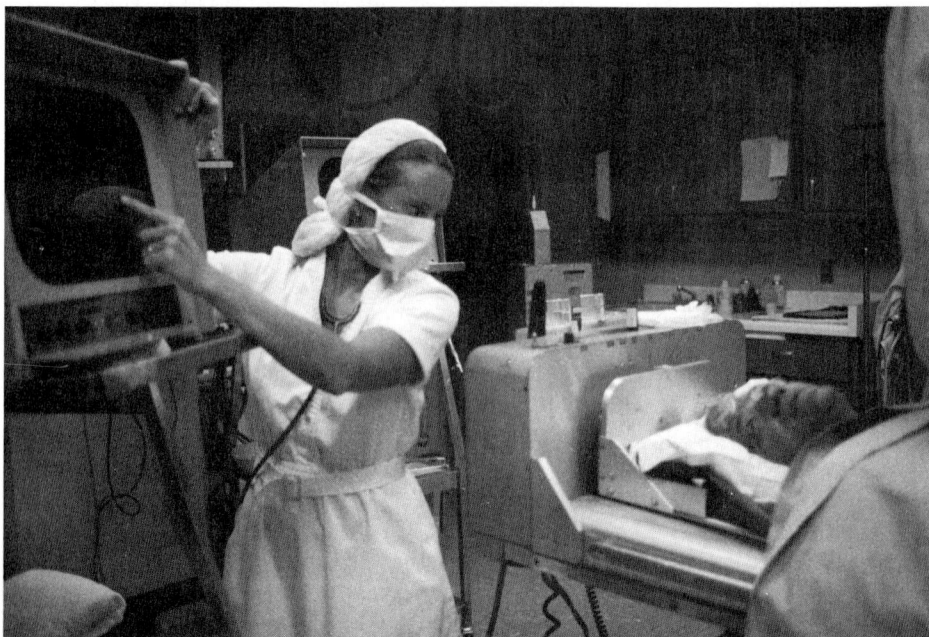

FIGURE 7.4   A scene from the modeling preparation in the Anderson and Masur (1989) study. The middle-aged patient describes his experiences during cardiac catheterization.

mation group patients received sensory and procedural information related to catheterization. An additioanl group of patients received a combination of the modeling and cognitive-behavioral preparations. The results indicated that patients in the two modeling groups had lower levels of physiological arousal and reported less anxiety during and after the test than patients in an attention-placebo control group. Patients in the two modeling groups also demonstrated fewer anxiety-related behaviors and better adjustment during the catheterization than control patients. The addition of the coping skills training did not appear to enhance the effectiveness of the modeling preparation. It should be noted, however, that the training was relatively brief and may not have encouraged subjects to practice the coping skills sufficiently.

Modeling preparations for invasive tests may benefit pediatric as well as adult patients. A puppet show that enacted cardiac catheterization using puppet models and equipment successfully prepared children for the catheterization test (Cassell, 1965). Children in the modeling group were rated as less distressed during the test and expressed more willingness to return to the hospital for further treatment than unprepared children.

In summary, modeling preparations for diagnostic medical tests have been effective for adult and pediatric samples. Additional research is needed to determine what types of modeling displays are most effective for different patient populations. Individual coping styles appear to influence how patients respond to modeling preparations. The results of Shipley et al. (1978) suggest that sensitizers benefit more than repressors from one exposure to a modeling preparation. Repeated exposure to a modeling treatment may prove helpful for repressors who have no previous experience with an invasive test.

## Behavioral and Cognitive-Behavioral Preparations

Behavioral and cognitive-behavioral interventions that teach patients specific coping skills have been used as preparations for invasive tests. Several recent studies have examined the efficacy of variations of *stress-inoculation training* (SIT), a three-phase intervention designed to reduce anxiety and pain (Meichenbaum & Turk, 1976). The first phase of SIT is educational and provides subjects with a rationale for using coping strategies to reduce anxiety and/or pain. The second, or rehearsal, phase exposes subjects to a variety of cognitive and behavioral coping strategies and allows them to choose the techniques they want to employ. Behavioral strategies frequently employed in SIT include relaxation exercises and deep breathing techniques. Cognitive coping strategies usually include the use of positive statements that patients say to themselves during each phase of a stressful event. Figure 7.5 provides examples of coping self-statements rehearsed in SIT for the control of anxiety and pain. The final phase of SIT is an application phase in which subjects are encouraged to practice their coping skills in response to real or imagined stressors.

Preparing for the painful stressor
*What is it you have to do?*
*You can develop a plan to deal with it.*
*Just think about what you have to do.*
*You have lots of different strategies you can call upon.*

Confronting and handling the pain
*You can meet the challenge.*
*One step at a time; you can handle the situation.*
*Just relax, breathe deeply, and use one of the strategies.*
*Don't think about the pain, just do what you have to do.*
*This tenseness can be an ally, a cue to cope.*
*Relax. You're in control; take a slow deep breath. Ah, good.*

Coping with feelings at critical moments
*When pain comes just pause; keep focusing on what you have to do.*
*Don't try to eliminate the pain totally; just keep it under control.*
*Just remember, there are different strategies; they'll help you stay in control.*

Reinforcing self-statements
*Good, you did it.*
*You handled it pretty well.*
*Wait until you tell the trainer about which procedures worked best.*

FIGURE 7.5 Sample coping self-statements for pain control used in stress inoculation training. From "Stress Inoculation in the Management of Clinical Pain" by R. L. Wernick, in *Stress Reduction and Prevention*, 1983, D. Meichenbaum and M. E. Jaremko (Eds), New York: Plenum Press. Reprinted by permission.

In the Kendall et al. (1979) study of cardiac catheterization, one group of patients was taught a variation of SIT. The patients received individual training in the discrimination of stress and anxiety-producing cues and in the application of coping strategies in response to such cues. Based on observer ratings and self-report, patients in the cognitive-behavioral group were better adjusted and less anxious during the test than patients in the attention-placebo and no-treatment control groups. In addition, the cognitive-behavioral patients were rated as better adjusted during and reported less anxiety after the procedure than patients who received the informative preparation.

Positive results for an SIT intervention were reported in a study of preparation for *sigmoidoscopy*, an invasive test that is embarrassing and uncomfortable for most patients (Kaplan, Atkins, & Lenhard, 1982). The test involves the insertion of a small scope into the anal cavity to examine the colon for any abnormalities. Kaplan et al. (1982) compared the effectiveness of SIT and brief relaxation training as preparations for the test. Patients who received the SIT intervention rated themselves as less anxious, had fewer body movements, and made fewer spontaneous verbalizations during the exam than patients in an attention-placebo control group. Training in muscle relaxation and deep breathing also appeared to have positive benefits. Subjects who learned relaxation skills rated themselves as less anxious and made fewer requests to stop the test than patients who did not receive relaxation training.

Relaxation training and a cognitive variation of SIT were beneficial preparations for another invasive test, *clinical electromyographic (EMG) examination* (Kaplan, Metzger, & Jablecki, 1983). The EMG test, a neurological procedure that is employed to diagnose neuromuscular disorders, requires the delivery of multiple electrical shocks to peripheral nerves and insertion of needle electrodes into muscles. The modified SIT group was taught that thoughts about a potentially painful situation can greatly influence the amount of discomfort experienced. The patients were encouraged to focus their attention on positive aspects of the situation. A tape recording of positive, coping self-statements was played to model for the patients the type of thoughts they should use during the test. A patient model narrated the tape, which included statements such as: "When I started to feel some pain, I would say things like 'this does hurt, but I can handle it. . . . One step at a time. . . . Don't think about the pain. . . . Relax.'" After listening to the tape, the patients were asked to close their eyes and to imagine themselves in the examination room. Then they practiced using the positive self-statements. The relaxation group was encouraged to practice progressive muscle relaxation and deep breathing in order to reduce muscle tension and possible pain during the test. A third group of patients was taught both cognitive SIT and relaxation training. The results demonstrated that patients in the three preparation groups adjusted better to the test than patients in an attention-placebo control group. Subjects who learned relaxation skills demonstrated lower heart rates than subjects who received cognitive SIT preparation only. On other dependent measures, however, cognitive SIT and relaxation training produced equivalent positive effects.

In summary, behavioral and cognitive-behavioral interventions appear to be effective preparations for a variety of invasive medical tests. Both SIT and relaxation training have produced positive results in several studies. Future research should examine the possible influence of individual difference variables on patients' responses to behavioral and cognitive-behavioral preparations.

## Hypnotic Preparations

Hypnosis recently has been used with pediatric cancer patients as a preparation for aversive diagnostic tests (Katz, Kellerman, & Ellenberg, 1987; Zelter & LeBaron, 1982). Pediatric cancer patients often undergo *bone marrow aspiration* (BMA), which involves the insertion of a large needle into the hip bone followed by the suctioning of bone marrow cells, to examine the marrow for cancer cells. Children with cancer may also receive *lumbar punctures*, in which a needle is inserted into the spinal canal to withdraw fluid.

Hypnosis was compared with cognitive-behavioral techniques in a study of children and adolescents undergoing BMA and lumbar punctures. The patients in the hypnosis group were taught how to use imagery and fantasy as coping strategies. In addition, an exciting or funny story was told to each patient during the tests. Patients in the cognitive-behavioral group learned deep breathing and distraction techniques. The results indicated that hypnosis was more effective than the cognitive-behavioral preparation for reducing the patients' pain and anxiety during the tests.

In a subsequent study, pediatric cancer patients were randomly assigned to a hypnotic or play therapy preparation. The children were having repeated BMA procedures and had demonstrated anxiety and/or pain during previous BMA tests. The hypnotic preparation included training in imagery, relaxation, and suggestions (e.g., suggestions for coping well). The preparation was provided prior to the BMA. The play therapy preparation consisted of nonmedical play with a therapist. Children in the hypnosis and play therapy groups reported decreases in fear and pain during BMA from pretreatment to post-treatment, with no differences between the two groups. The hypnotic preparation might have been more effective if hypnosis had been induced during the BMA as well as prior to it.

Hypnosis appears to be an effective preparation for pediatric patients prior to aversive diagnostic tests. Future studies should investigate the influence of hypnotic susceptibility on patients' responses to hypnotic preparation.

# Dental Procedures

Fear of dental treatment appears to be widespread in the general population. For example, Janis (1958) found that 60% of adult patients awaiting routine amalgam restorations (fillings) expressed some degree of anxiety. When the dental patients have been children, even higher percentages of subjects have expressed preprocedural concerns (Baldwin, 1966; Klein, 1967; Sonnenburg & Venham, 1977). Simple examinations, restorations, extractions, endodontic treatments, and oral surgical procedures are fairly common dental treatments that can be anxiety arousing for adults and children. Frequent dental fears reported by patients include fear of pain and discomfort; the unknown; damage to the body; use of instruments; anesthesia; bleeding; and inadequate treatment (Morse & Furst, 1978). Unfortunately, dental fears often lead to avoidance of treatment and unnecessary complications. Psychological preparations have been used to reduce the anxiety and discomfort associated with dental procedures and to encourage adherence to subsequent dental treatments.

## Informative Preparations

Many adult dental fears appear to have their origin in aversive childhood experiences with dentists (Kleinknecht & Bernstein, 1978). For this reason, it is particularly important that children be carefully prepared for their early dental visits in order to minimize adverse reactions. Several studies have examined the efficacy of informative preparations for children prior to their first dental visit (Herbertt & Innes, 1979; Siegel & Peterson, 1980). Herbertt and Innes (1979) provided children aged five to eleven with procedural information and a lesson in dental health prior to examination and subsequent treatment. Prepared children did not differ from control-group children on outcome measures of anxiety and cooperation. As the control-group patients were given the dental health lesson in the dental clinic, exposure to the dental treatment situation and general information may have substantially reduced their anxiety levels.

In order for information to benefit children scheduled for dental procedures, sensory information may need to be included in the treatment intervention. Siegel and Peterson (1980) presented preschool children with a description of the typical physical sensations, sights, and sounds they would experience during a dental restoration. For example, they were told that when the dentist put "sleepy water" around their tooth, they would feel a pinch and then a tingling, warm sensation. They also heard a brief tape recording of the noise of a dental drill. The children were told that when the dentist had finished they would have a silver filling and that their mouth would feel big and heavy for a short time. As compared to control children who were read a story, the informed patients exhibited fewer disruptive and more cooperative behaviors during the restoration session. The informed children also were rated as less anxious than control children by the dentist and an independent observer.

A combination of sensory and procedural information also has proven helpful for adult dental patients (Auerbach, Kendall, Cuttler, & Levitt, 1976). Subjects scheduled for tooth extractions were provided with either specific sensory and procedural information on the extraction procedure or general information about the dental clinic. It was found that the effects of the informative preparations varied according to the patients' locus of control orientation. Patients with an internal LOC who received specific information demonstrated better adjustment during the extraction than internals who were given the general information. The converse was true of patients with an external LOC, who responded favorably to the general information. Auerbach et al. concluded that the specific information was consistent with the internal patients' belief that they can control events in their lives. In contrast, the general information was compatible with the external patients' view that events are generally beyond their control.

In summary, informative preparations for dental procedures appear to be beneficial for adults and children when sensory as well as procedural information is included. The effectiveness of the information, however, may be influenced by individual difference variables such as locus of control and preference for information (Auerbach, Martelli, & Mercuri, 1983).

# Modeling Preparations

Filmed modeling preparations have been used with children to reduce the anxiety and uncooperative behavior often associated with dental treatment. In a series of studies, Melamed and her colleagues have shown that children's behavior during dental procedures can be positively affected by viewing a peer model who displays appropriate dental behavior (see Melamed & Siegel, 1980, for a review). For example, inner-city children with no previous dental experience were shown a videotape of an initially fearful child who underwent a typical dental procedure with a sensitive dentist (Melamed, Hawes, Heiby, & Glick, 1975). The child model was verbally reinforced for cooperative behavior. Children who saw the modeling preparation demonstrated significantly fewer disruptive and anxiety-related behaviors during dental restorations than children who saw a film unrelated to dental treatment.

Modeling preparations typically include verbal information and visual stimuli, as well as the patient models. Several studies have attempted to separate the effect of viewing a patient model from the effect of receiving information and viewing stimuli (e.g., electric drill, dentist's office) related to dental procedures (Melamed, Yurcheson, Fleece, Hutcherson, & Hawes, 1978; White, Akers, Green, & Yates, 1974). The results of these studies indicate that viewing a model has beneficial effects that cannot be attributed to information and stimulus exposure alone. In the Melamed et al. (1978) experiment, children scheduled for dental restorative treatment were shown one of four videotaped preparations, which varied as to amount of information presented and presence or absence of a peer model. Amount of information was varied by presenting either the entire restorative procedure or the anesthetic injection alone. The films without a model focused on the demonstration of procedures. After viewing the patient modeling tapes, children demonstrated fewer disruptive behaviors during dental treatment and reported less anxiety than children who viewed the demonstration tapes. These results suggest that modeling preparations are more effective than informative preparations that include stimulus exposure.

A series of recent experiments has examined the relative efficacy of different types of dental patient models (Klorman, Hilpert, Michael, La Gana, & Sveen, 1980). A *coping model* has been defined as a person who initially appears anxious in a fearful situation but who overcomes fear and copes well with the situation (Meichenbaum, 1971). In contrast, a *mastery model* expresses no anxiety and copes well during the entire procedure. Children awaiting dental restorations were shown a videotape of either a mastery model, a coping model, or a child playing a game (Klorman et al., 1980). Patients without previous dental experience who viewed either patient model showed less disruptive behavior during dental treatment than inexperienced patients who saw the control tape. The mastery and coping models appeared to be equally effective for the inexperienced children, with no significant differences on outcome measures between the two modeling groups. For patients with previous dental experience, however, neither modeling preparation affected their adaptation to the restoration. The experienced children were generally more cooperative than inexperienced children.

To summarize, modeling preparations can reduce the disruptive behavior and fear of children undergoing dental treatment. Future research should address the potential benefits of modeling preparations for adult dental patients. Additionally, research is needed to determine what types of modeling preparations can benefit experienced patients. As indicated in the research on surgical preparation, experienced individuals may not benefit as much as inexperienced patients from the modeling preparations used to date.

## Behavioral Preparations

The use of behavior therapy techniques to control anxious or disruptive patients has been widely advocated in the dental literature (e.g., Wright, 1975). Frequently recommended techniques include systematic desensitization, relaxation, positive reinforcement, and shaping of appropriate behavior. Although these approaches appear to have significant clinical utility, there is little research pertaining to their use.

A *systematic desensitization* preparation consists of gradual habituation to a hierarchy of anxiety-producing stimuli through the anxiety-inhibiting response of relaxation. Sawtell, Simon, and Simeonsson (1974) compared the efficacy of systematic desensitization, positive reinforcement, and modeling preparations for children prior to their first dental examination. Subjects in the desensitization group were gradually exposed to a hierarchy of dental equipment and procedures, arranged from least to most stressful. In the reinforcement condition, cooperative behavior was reinforced by the experimenter with verbal praise and other social reinforcers. The modeling group saw a videotape of mastery models undergoing dental treatment. The results indicated no differences between the prepared groups and a control group that received friendly interaction with the dental assistant. Any possible differences between groups may have been obscured by the fact that the children were generally cooperative and did not undergo any restorations.

A second study that compared desensitization and modeling preparations found that children in both conditions demonstrated less negative behavior during dental restorations than control-group subjects (Machen & Johnson, 1974). As the control group had no interaction with the experimenter, the relative effects of preparation and social interaction cannot be determined. The results do suggest, however, that desensitization may be an effective preparation for restorative treatment, a procedure that is probably more stressful than a simple examination.

General relaxation training has been used to prepare adult patients for restorations (Corah, Gale, & Illig, 1979) and an anesthetic injection procedure (McAmmond, Davidson, & Kovitz, 1971). In the Corah et al. (1979) investigation, patients in the relaxation group listened via headphones to a relaxation tape both before and during the restorative procedure. They reported less discomfort and demonstrated less physiological arousal than control-group patients, who received standard dental treatment. Similar brief relaxation training was compared to hypnosis and placebo treatment in a sample of patients who reported excessive dental fear and avoidance of dental treatment (McAmmond et al., 1971). For subjects with initially high levels of physiological arousal, relaxation training and hypnosis both produced significant decreases in skin conductance levels but did not affect pain tolerance and anxiety self-report. For subjects with initially low levels of arousal, there were no positive effects for the relaxation and hypnotic preparations.

In summary, both relaxation and systematic desensitization appear to be promising dental preparations. Future studies, however, need to include control groups who receive as much contact with the experimenter as the treatment groups. The results of Sawtell et al. (1974) suggest that social contact alone may help to prepare children for dental examinations.

## Cognitive-Behavioral Preparations

As dental fear is often accompanied by unrealistic or negative cognitions, cognitive preparations may be particularly appropriate for dental patients. Corah and his colleagues have investigated the effects of several cognitive strategies, including distraction and perceived control (Corah et al., 1979). The perceived-control preparation provided adult patients with a buzzer to communicate with the dentist if they felt a need to temporarily stop the treatment. In the distraction condition, patients were allowed to play a video Ping-Pong game during the restoration. The distracted subjects were rated as more comfortable and reported liking the visit more than standard-procedure control subjects. Patients in the perceived-control group did not adjust to the procedure any better than control-group patients. It should be noted that the experimenters did not assess whether patients in the perceived-control group actually felt more in control of the dental session than patients in the other groups.

Imaginal flooding and rehearsal of coping behavior have been used to prepare fearful adult dental patients (Mathews & Rezin, 1977). In *imaginal flooding*, patients are taught to imagine stressful scenes related to an invasive procedure. The rationale for flooding is that subjects' anxiety levels will fall as they habituate to the stressor. Mathews and Rezin compared low-arousal flooding that consisted of moderately stressful scenes to high-arousal flooding that included severely stressful scenes (e.g., an incompetent dentist mistakenly injects the patient's tongue). Half of the patients in each arousal group were taught to imagine appropriate coping behaviors (e.g., distraction, positive self-statements). The low-arousal preparations, as compared to the high-arousal ones, effectively reduced subjective dental anxiety. Rehearsal of coping behaviors interacted with arousal level to influence subsequent dental attendance. Patients in the high-arousal condition who received coping rehearsal were more likely to complete subsequent dental treatment than high-arousal patients who did not rehearse coping.

Training in cognitive-behavioral coping skills has been an effective dental preparation for children as well as adults. Siegel and Peterson (1980) taught preschool children the self-control coping skills of relaxation, pleasant imagery, and calming self-talk. Children in the coping skills group demonstrated lower levels of anxiety, discomfort, disruptiveness, and physiological arousal during subsequent dental restorations than control children who were read a story. Children who received sensory and procedural information also adapted well to the restoration. There were no differences in the adjustment of the two prepared groups. Impressively, the prepared children continued to exhibit superior adjustment, as compared to control children, at a second dental session approximately one week after preparation (Siegel & Peterson, 1981).

Training in cognitive-behavioral coping skills may be presented in a modeling format. Children who reported moderately high dental fear were shown a videotape of children practicing controlled breathing to induce relaxation and pleasant, distracting imagery during dental treatment (Klingman, Melamed, Cuthbert, & Hermecz, 1984). In the participant-modeling group, children were encouraged to practice the coping techniques. In a symbolic-modeling group, the children were told the techniques might be helpful during dental treatment. Children in the participant-modeling condition reported greater reduction in dental anxiety and were more cooperative during subsequent restorative treatment than children in the symbolic group. Thus, rehearsal of coping techniques may be necessary to facilitate their optimal effectiveness.

Cognitive-behavioral preparations appear to benefit child and adult dental patients. The studies to date suggest that a preparation that teaches patients several coping strategies is a particularly effective treatment (Klingman et al., 1984; Siegel & Peterson, 1980). Future research should consider the possible interaction of individual difference variables (e.g., age, previous dental experience, typical coping style) and preparatory treatment.

## Obstetrical and Gynecological Procedures

Women may experience a variety of invasive gynecological and obstetrical procedures during their lifetime. Routine pelvic examinations, PAP smears to detect cervical cancer, insertion of contraceptive devices, therapeutic abortions, and childbirth are procedures that are potentially anxiety-arousing and painful. Although psychological preparation for chidbirth has been advocated for many years, there is a lack of controlled research on its use. The need for preparation for invasive gynecological procedures has recently been noted, but little research has examined the efficacy of psychological preparations for these procedures. Several studies of preparation for surgery did include women scheduled for hysterectomies (e.g., Langer et al., 1975) and have been reviewed previously. The following section will summarize the literature to date on preparations designed specifically for gynecological and obstetrical procedures.

## Pelvic Examinations

Regular pelvic examinations of women are considered important for disease prevention and health enhancement. Unfortunately, this invasive procedure is often viewed by women as aversive, noxious, or unpleasant (Magee, 1975). Psychological preparation for the pelvic exam may help to reduce its aversiveness and associated discomfort, as well as increase compliance with subsequent exams.

Apparently, only one study has examined psychological preparations for routine pelvic examinations (Fuller, Endress, & Johnson, 1978). Young women who had undergone previous pelvic exams were given sensory and procedural information on the pelvic exam or general information on the importance of routine pelvic and breast examinations. Half of the subjects in each information group were taught abdominal relaxation techniques to be used during the exam. Patients who received the sensory and procedural information demonstrated fewer distress-related behaviors during the exam than patients given general information. Although relaxation training did not appear to influence adaptation, the small number of subjects in each group may have obscured treatment effects. There were nonsignificant tendencies for subjects who received relaxation training and sensory-procedural information to show less physiological arousal and report less anxiety than patients in the other groups.

An invasive procedure similar to the pelvic exam but potentially more painful is insertion of an intrauterine device (IUD). The placement of this contraceptive device in the uterus can precipitate cramping, discomfort, and bleeding. Newton and Reading (1977) prepared women for IUD insertion with sensory and procedural information on the procedure. The preparation also included suggested coping techniques for reducing pain such as distraction and pleasant imagery. Women who received the informative preparation did report less pain during the IUD insertion than women who received no preparation. As the preparation included attention from the experimenter and multiple treatment components, the effective ingredients cannot be determined.

Additional research with larger patient samples and adequate control groups is needed to study preparations for pelvic exams, IUD insertion, and other gynecological procedures. Effective preparations may help to improve compliance with subsequent gynecological procedures and thus contribute to health maintenance.

## Therapeutic Abortions

A therapeutic abortion has the potential to be an extremely stressful and emotionally traumatic procedure. Patients must cope with the termination of a pregnancy as well as with the surgical procedure itself. Moreover, the ethical and legal issues related to abortion continue to be debated. A few research reports have examined psychological preparations for this invasive procedure. High levels of preabortion anxiety have been associated with greater pain and discomfort during the abortion procedure, as compared to moderate levels of preprocedural anxiety (Bracken, 1978). Psychological preparations, therefore, have focused on reducing anxiety and enhancing adaptation.

Several studies have compared the effects of different types of informative preparations for women awaiting abortions (Brockway, Plummer, & Lowe, 1976; Williams, Jones, Workhoven, & Williams, 1975). In the Williams et al. (1975) investigation, the anesthesiologist conducted either a cursory (brief and minimally informative) or supportive (long and informative) preoperative interview. Prior to the interview, all patients completed a self-report measure of anxiety. Anxiety levels on the morning of the abortion were measured by a physiological variable, the number of seconds required for anesthesia induction. For patients who initially were highly anxious, the cursory and supportive interviews produced equivalent, low levels of physiological anxiety prior to the abortion. For patients who initially expressed low levels of anxiety, the cursory interview was followed by elevated levels of physiological arousal, relative to the arousal levels of low anxious patients given a supportive interview. As the informative preparations differed on several dimensions (i.e, amount of information, length of the interview, attitude of the physician), it cannot be determined which components were effective.

In the Brockway et al. (1976) study, the effects of specific, detailed information and general, superficial information were compared. Patients who heard the specific information demonstrated less anxiety prior to the abortion, as measured by vocal stress levels, than patients given general information. As in the Williams et al. (1975) study, the informative preparations differed on several dimensions. The effective components, therefore, cannot be determined. The authors observed that patients who appeared to use denial as a coping strategy did not benefit from specific information. In fact, their anxiety levels tended to increase when they were given detailed preparation. Although these observations were not supported with significant data, they do suggest that individual coping styles may interact with informative preparations.

The importance of individual coping styles was demonstrated empirically in a recent study of preparation for abortion (Kay, 1984). The patients received either a brochure containing a cognitive-behavioral preparation or a brochure describing the importance of Rh factor in pregnancy (placebo). All subjects were given basic sensory and procedural information on the abortion. The cognitive-behavioral brochure taught the women to identify stress-related cues and to mobilize coping strategies they had used successfully in the past in response to these cues. The results revealed that all the patients who received brochures reported decreased anxiety. Overall, patients in the cognitive-behavioral group did not appear to adapt to the abortion more effectively than subjects who received the placebo brochure. When individual coping styles (i.e., sensitizer vs. repressor) were considered, however, interesting differences emerged. Patients classified as sensitizers who received the cognitive-behavioral preparation reported significantly less pain during the abortion than sensitizers in the placebo control group. Thus, a cognitive-behavioral preparation for abortion appears to benefit women with a sensitizing coping style.

# Childbirth

Preparation for childbirth is widely available in the United States in the form of group classes that provide training in the Lamaze techniques (Lamaze, 1958), natural childbirth (Dick-Read, 1933), psychoprophylaxis (Velvovsky, Platonov, Ploticher, & Shugom, 1960), and other preparatory approaches. The prepared childbirth classes typically include several of the preparatory interventions that have been employed prior to other invasive procedures: sensory and procedural information, live and filmed models, relaxation and breathing techniques, distraction, behavioral rehearsal, and reassurance. In addition, the woman's husband or support person typically provides emotional support and coaching in specific coping techniques.

Clinical studies of prepared childbirth have claimed that this training results in physiological, medical, psychological, and behavioral benefits for the mother and child (see Beck & Siegel, 1980, for a review). Unfortunately, methodologically sound studies of prepared childbirth are relatively few. Most of the research reports have lacked random assignment, adequate control groups, and appropriate statistical analyses. Hence, only several of the better-controlled studies will be described.

In a study of women experiencing their first pregnancy, the patients were given five sessions of psychoprophylactic training that included information about labor and delivery, a tour of the delivery rooms, relaxation and breathing techniques, and husband participation (Huttel, Mitchell, Fischer, & Meyer, 1972). Thus, the childbirth training was a combination of sensory and procedural information, systematic desensitization, cognitive-behavioral techniques, and emotional support. As compared to a no-treatment control group, the prepared women were given less analgesic medication, appeared less tense, and offered fewer complaints during labor and delivery. Additionally, the prepared women had more positive attitudes toward future pregnancies and were less depressed following delivery than unprepared women. Although Huttel et al. used random assignment and appropriate statistical tests, it cannot be determined which components of their treatment package, including attention and group support, were effective.

In a study of women undergoing Lamaze training, Zax, Sameroff, and Farnum (1975) compared women in their first pregnancy (primiparas) to those with one or more previous deliveries (multiparas). Following training, the multiparas reported significantly less anxiety than prior to the Lamaze course. The anxiety levels of the primiparas did not vary during the course. Attitudes toward labor, delivery, and the baby improved significantly following training for all the prepared patients. The prepared women required fewer general anesthesias than a control group of women at the same hospital who did not receive Lamaze training. As the patients were not randomly assigned to groups, the prepared and unprepared groups may have differed on important variables (e.g., motivation, initial anxiety level) that influenced the results.

Other studies of prepared childbirth have suggested that preparation decreases pain (Leventhal, Leventhal, Shacham, & Easterling, 1989) and is associated with reduced requests for obstetrical analgesia and anesthesia (Enkin, Smith, Dermer, & Emmett, 1972). The lack of random assignment and appropriate control groups in these studies, however, complicates interpretation of the results. As noted above, women who pursue childbirth preparation may differ in many ways from women who choose not to receive preparation. Ideally, patients would be randomly assigned to treatment or control groups. For ethical reasons, however, it is difficult to withhold treatment from pregnant women in order to have a group of unprepared or minimally prepared women.

In a recent study of preparation for cesarean (surgical) delivery, it was possible to assign the patients randomly to treatment and control groups (Greene, Zeichner, Roberts, Callahan, & Granados, 1989). The patients were receiving routine prenatal care, which included minimal preparation for the possibility of cesarean delivery. Patients in the treatment group viewed an audio-visual program that presented procedural and sensory information on cesarean delivery. The patients in the control group viewed an audio-visual program on infant sensorimotor development. The prepared patients who subsequently delivered by cesarean section had lower blood pressures during the delivery and recovered more quickly and with fewer complications than the unprepared patients. The patients' individual coping styles (sensitizer versus repressor) influenced their response to the preparation treatment. Although both sensitizers and repressors responded positively to the preparation, sensitizers appeared to benefit more than repressors.

## Behavioral Preparations

Prepared childbirth classes typically include behavioral techniques such as relaxation training, breathing exercises, and behavioral rehearsal. A few studies have examined preparations that consisted of specific behavioral interventions. Kondas and Scetnicka (1972) developed a systematic desensitization preparation in order to desensitize women who reported high levels of anxiety to anxiety-arousing stimuli associated with labor and delivery. The pregnant patients were matched for age, education, anxiety level, and parity and then randomly assigned to either desensitization or psychoprophylactic training. Both preparations produced a reduction in self-reported anxiety, but the reduction was greater in the desensitization group. Moreover, the desensitization group had shorter labors and were rated by their obstetricians as less restless and experiencing less pain than the psychoprophylactic group. Although these results are impressive, it remains to be seen whether systematic desensitization is an effective preparation for pregnant women who initially report low to moderate levels of anxiety.

A second behavioral approach to childbirth preparation has consisted of biofeedback-assisted relaxation training (Duchene, 1989; Gregg, 1983; St. James-Roberts, Hutchinson, Haran, & Chamberlain, 1983). In a study of primiparous women taking Lamaze classes, the women were randomly assigned to biofeedback and control groups (Duchene, 1989). The biofeedback group attended six training sessions during which they were taught to relax their abdominal muscles using feedback as to their muscle tension levels. The biofeedback patients also were allowed to use biofeedback equipment during labor. The results indicated that the patients trained in biofeedback reported significantly lower pain levels during labor, delivery, and 24 hours after delivery. Also, women in the biofeedback group were in labor for a significantly shorter period of time and used fewer medications than women in the control group.

The small amount of controlled research to date suggests that preparation for obstetrical-gynecological procedures can benefit patients' overall adaptation. Additional research is obviously needed to determine which preparations are most effective for different samples of women. As has been demonstrated in the research on preparation for other invasive procedures, subjects' typical coping styles and other individual difference variables appear to influence their reactions to preparatory treatments.

The research on preparation for childbirth is plagued by methodological problems that future investigators should attempt to remedy. Although appropriate control groups are difficult to obtain, researchers can systematically vary treatment components across groups and thus determine which components are most effective. Behavioral approaches to childbirth preparation appear promising and certainly warrant further research. Cognitive-behavioral preparations such as SIT that emphasize positive self-statements and appropriate coping strategies might also prove effective for pregnant patients.

## Summary

The research on psychological preparation for invasive medical and dental procedures has demonstrated the potential benefits of preparing patients for surgery, diagnostic tests, dental procedures, and obstetrical-gynecological procedures. Each of the major preparatory approaches has potential and warrants further research attention. The limited amount of research on hypnotic preparations has methodological problems that prevent definitive conclusions. Informative preparations that include sensory information appear to be beneficial for patients who have not previously experienced the invasive procedure. Modeling preparations, however, may be even more effective than information provision for inexperienced patients. Although both informative and modeling preparations contain basic informaion, information presented by a patient model has proven more helpful than information alone (cf. Anderson & Masur, 1989; Melamed et al., 1978).

The research on behavioral and cognitive-behavioral preparations generally supports the efficacy of these interventions. Relaxation training and SIT appear particularly promising. One advantage of SIT is that patients are encouraged to use individualized coping strategies in response to stressful stimuli. Thus, SIT allows for individual differences among patients as to preferred coping strategies. There is some evidence, however, that SIT and relaxation training may not be very useful to individuals who do not carefully practice their use of coping strategies prior to the stressful procedure.

The possible interaction of individual difference variables and preparatory treatments must be considered in future research. Such factors as previous experience with an invasive procedure, age and developmental level, and typical coping style may affect patients' responses to preparation. In addition to considering subjects' typical coping styles, it may be necessary to examine coping responses in specific situations. A recent study of volunteer blood donors demonstrated that subjects will choose coping strategies in specific situations that are not necessarily consistent with their typical coping styles (Kaloupek, White, & Wong, 1984).

Future research should attempt to resolve the methodological problems apparent in past studies. The inclusion of a control group that receives as much attention from the experimenter as the treatment groups is necessary to control for the effects of interaction. As many preparatory treatments have contained multiple variables, the definition of treatment components is another concern. Clearly defined treatment components must be systematically varied across groups before the efficacy of individual components can be determined. Manipulation checks are also needed to determine if a procedure had the intended effect and if it was subsequently utilized by patients.

A broad range of outcome measures is necessary to fully assess the effects of preparatory treatments. Many preparations are designed to alleviate anxiety and pain; yet the outcome measures do not adequately assess the multidimensional nature of these variables. Self-report measures can be supplemented with behavioral and physiological outcome measures. In addition, it would be worthwhile to assess the effects of preparatory treatments on patients' adaptation to subsequent invasive procedures (cf. Siegel & Peterson, 1981).

Because a preparatory procedure must be economically feasible to be utilized by the health care system, future research should address the issue of cost-effectiveness. Several reports found that group treatments were as effective as individual ones (Lindeman, 1972; Schmitt & Wooldridge, 1973). In addition, videotapes, audiotapes, brochures, and other educational materials can be employed as preparatory methods that do not require excessive amounts of staff time. As reduction in length of hospitalization has been a frequent outcome of preparatory interventions, their future development is probably warranted on economic grounds (e.g., Pinto & Hollandsworth, 1989). Moreover, psychological preparation can help to fulfill legal and ethical requirements for obtaining informed consent from the patient. Most state laws advocate providing information on the invasive procedure, the significant risks involved, the probable duration of incapacitation, and any significant alternatives for care and treatment (Ludlam, 1978). Preparatory techniques that include information can help to fulfill these requirements. In addition, psychological preparations can help patients to cope with any distressing information they receive regarding their treatment.

A survey of pediatric hospitals in the United States revealed that the majority of them provided some type of prehospital and/or presurgery preparation for children and their parents (Peterson & Ridley-Johnson, 1980). Preparatory programs for adults appear to be less common. Given the potential benefits of preparation for adults as well as children, the further development of preparatory treatments is expected. It is also anticipated that psychologists will continue to play a major role in the development, testing, and implementation of preparatory programs in hospitals and other health care facilities.

# References

AIKEN L. H, & HENRICHS, T. F. (1971). Systematic relaxation as a nursing intervention technique with open heart surgery patients. *Nursing Research, 20*, 212–217.

ANDERSON, E. A. (1987). Preoperative preparation for cardiac surgery facilitates recovery, reduces psychological distress, and reduces the incidence of acute postoperative hypertension. *Journal of Consulting and Clinical Psychology, 55*, 513–520.

ANDERSON, K. O., & MASUR, F. T. III (1989). Psychologic preparation for cardiac catheterization. *Heart and Lung: The Journal of Critical Care, 18*, 154–163.

ANDERSON, K. O., & MASUR, F. T. III (1983). Psychological preparation for invasive medical and dental procedures. *Journal of Behavioral Medicine, 6*, 1–40.

ANDREW, J. M. (1970). Recovery from surgery, with and without preparatory instruction, for three coping styles. *Journal of Personality and Social Psychology, 15*, 223–226.

ATKINS, D. M. (1987). Evaluation of pediatric preparation program for short-stay surgical patients. *Journal of Pediatric Psychology, 12*, 285–290.

AUERBACH, S. M. (1973). Trait-state anxiety and adjustment to surgery. *Journal of Consulting and Clinical Psychology, 40*, 264–271.

AUERBACH, S. M. (1989). Stress management and coping research in the health care setting: An overview and methodological commentary. *Journal of Consulting and Clinical Psychology, 57*, 388–395.

AUERBACH, S. M., KENDALL, P. C., CUTTLER, H. F., & LEVITT, N. R. (1976). Anxiety, locus of control, type of preparatory information, and adjustment to dental surgery. *Journal of Consulting and Clinical Psychology, 44*, 809–818.

AUERBACH, S. M., MARTELLI, M. F., & MERCURI, L. G. (1983). Anxiety, information, interpersonal impacts, and adjustment to a stressful health care situation. *Journal of Personality and Social Psychology, 44*, 1284–1296.

BALDWIN, D. C. (1966). An investigation of psychological and behavioral responses to dental extraction in children. *Journal of Dental Research, 45*, 1637–1651.

BANDURA, A. (1969). *Principles of behavior modification.* New York: Holt, Rinehart and Winston.

BANDURA, A. (1977). *Social learning theory.* Englewood Cliffs, NJ: Prentice-Hall.

BARBER, J. (1977). Rapid induction analgesia: A clinical report. *American Journal of Clinical Hypnosis, 19*, 138–147.

BECK, N. C., & SIEGEL, L. J. (1980). Preparation for childbirth and contemporary research on pain, anxiety, and stress reduction: Review and critique. *Psychosomatic Medicine, 42*, 429–447.

BOYD, I., YEAGER, M., & McMILLAN, M. (1973). Personality styles in the postoperative course. *Psychosomatic Medicine, 35*, 23–40.

BRACKEN, M. (1978). A causal model of psychosomatic reactions to vacuum aspiration abortion. *Social Psychiatry, 13*, 135–145.

BROCKWAY, B., PLUMMER, O., & LOWE, B. (1976). Effect of nursing reassurance on patient vocal stress levels. *Nursing Research, 25*, 440–446.

BYRNE, D. (1964). The repression-sensitization scale: Rationale, reliability and validity. *Journal of Personality, 29*, 334-349.

CARNEVALI, D. L. (1966). Pre-operative anxiety. *American Journal of Nursing, 66*, 1536–1538.

CASSELL, S. (1965). Effect of brief puppet therapy upon the emotional responses of children undergoing cardiac catheterization. *Journal of Consulting Psychology, 29*, 1–8.

CHAPMAN, J. S. (1970). Effects of different nursing approaches on psychological and physiological responses. *Nursing Research Report, 5*, 1–7.

COHEN, F., & LAZARUS, R. S. (1973). Active coping processes, coping dispositions, and recovery from surgery. *Psychosomatic Medicine, 35*, 375–389.

CORAH, N. L., GALE, E. N., & ILLIG, S. J. (1979). Psychological stress reduction during dental procedures. *Journal of Dental Research, 58*, 1347–1351.

DeLONG, R. D. (1971). Individual differences in patterns of anxiety arousal, stress-relevant information, and recovery from surgery. (Doctoral dissertation, University of California, Los Angeles, 1970.) *Dissertation Abstracts International, 32*, 554B.

DICK-READ, G. (1933). *Natural childbirth*. London: W. Heinemann.

DUCHENE, P. (1989). Effects of biofeedback on childbirth pain. *Journal of Pain and Symptom Management, 4*, 117–123.

EGBERT, L. D., BATTIT, C. D., WELCH, C. E., & BARTLETT, M. K. (1964). Reduction of post-operative pain by encouragement and instruction of patients. *New England Journal of Medicine, 270*, 825–827.

ENKIN, M. W., SMITH, S. L., DERMER, S. W., & EMMETT, J. O. (1972). An adequately controlled study of the effectiveness of P.P.M. training. In N. Morris (Ed.), *Psychosomatic medicine in obstetrics and gynecology*. London: S. Karger.

FAUST, J., & MELAMED, B. G. (1984). Influence of arousal, previous experience, and age on surgery preparation of same day of surgery and in-hospital pediatric patients. *Journal of Consulting and Clinical Psychology, 52*, 359–365.

FIELD, P. B. (1974). Effects of tape-recorded hypnotic preparation for surgery. *International Journal of Clinical and Experimental Hypnosis, 22*, 54–61.

FLAHERTY, G. G., & FITZPATRICK, J. J. (1978). Relaxation technique to increase comfort level of postoperative patients: A preliminary study. *Nursing Research, 27*, 352–355.

FORTIN, F., & KIROUAC, S. (1976). A randomized controlled trial of preoperative patient education. *International Journal of Nursing Studies, 13*, 11–24.

FREDERICKS, L. E. (1978). Teaching of hypnosis in the overall approach to the surgical patient. *The American Journal of Clinical Hypnosis, 20*, 175–183.

FULLER, S. S., ENDRESS, M. P., & JOHNSON, J. E. (1978). The effects of cognitive and behavioral control on coping with an aversive health examination. *Journal of Human Stress, 4,* 18–25.

GRAHAM, L. E., & CONLEY, E. M. (1971). Evaluation of anxiety and fear in adult surgical patients. *Nursing Research, 20,* 113–122.

GREENE, P. G., ZEICHNER, A., ROBERTS, N. L., CALLAHAN, E. J., & GRANADOS, J. L. (1989). Preparation for cesarean delivery: A multicomponent analysis of treatment outcome. *Journal of Consulting and Clinical Psychology, 57,* 484–487.

GREGG, R. H. (1983). Biofeedback and biophysical monitoring during pregnancy and labor. In J. V. Basmajian (Ed.), *Biofeedback: Principles and practice for clinicians.* Baltimore: Williams & Wilkins.

HEALY, K. M. (1968). Does pre-operative instruction make a difference? *American Journal of Nursing, 68,* 62–67.

HERBERTT, R. M., & INNES, J. M. (1979). Familiarization and preparatory information in the reduction of anxiety in child dental patients. *Journal of Dentistry for Children, 46,* 319–323.

HILGARD, E. R., & HILGARD, J. R., (1975). *Hypnosis in the relief of pain.* Los Altos, CA: William Kaufmann.

HUTTEL, F. A., MITCHELL, I., FISCHER, W. M., & MEYER, A. E. (1972). A quantitative evaluation of psychoprophylaxis in childbirth. *Journal of Psychosomatic Research, 16,* 81–92.

JACOBSON, E. (1938). *Progressive relaxation.* Chicago: University of Chicago Press.

JANIS, I. L. (1958). *Psychological stress: Psychoanalytic and behavioral studies of surgical patients.* New York: Wiley.

JANIS, I. L. (1971). *Stress and frustration.* New York: Harcourt Brace Jovanovich.

JOHNSON, J. E. (1972). Effects of structuring patients' expectations on their reactions to threatening events. *Nursing Research, 21,* 499–504.

JOHNSON, J. E., & LEVENTHAL, H. (1974). Effects of accurate expectations and behavioral instructions on reactions during a noxious medical examination. *Journal of Personality and Social Psychology, 29,* 710–718.

JOHNSON, J. E., MORRISSEY, J. F., & LEVENTHAL, H. (1973). Psychological preparation for an endoscopic examination. *Gastrointestinal Endoscopy, 19,* 180–182.

KALOUPEK, D. G., WHITE, H., & WONG, M. (1983). Multiple assessment of coping strategies used by volunteer blood donors: Implications for preparatory training. *Journal of Behavioral Medicine, 7,* 35–60.

KAPLAN, R. M., ATKINS, C. J., & LENHARD, L. (1982). Coping with a stressful sigmoidoscopy: Evaluation of cognitive and relaxation preparations. *Journal of Behavioral Medicine, 5,* 67–82.

KAPLAN, R. M., METZGER, G., & JABLECKI, C. (1983). Brief cognitive and relaxation training increases tolerance for a painful clinical electromyographic examination. *Psychosomatic Medicine, 45,* 155–162.

KATZ, E. R., KELLERMAN, J., & ELLENBERG, L. (1987). Hypnosis in the reduction of acute pain and distress in children with cancer. *Journal of Pediatric Psychology, 12,* 379–394.

KAY, R. (1984). *Psychological preparation for a potentially stressful medical procedure.* Unpublished doctoral dissertation, Fordham University, New York.

KENDALL, P. C., WILLIAMS, L., PECHACEK, T. F., GRAHAM. L. E., SHISSLAK, C., & HERZOFF, N. (1979). Cognitive-behavioral and patient education interventions in cardiac catheterization procedures: The Palo Alto Medical Psychology Project. *Journal of Consulting and Clinical Psychology, 47,* 49–58.

KENDALL, P. C., & WATSON, D. (1981). Psychological preparation for stressful medical procedures. In C. K. Prokop & L. A. Bradley (Eds.), *Medical psychology: Contributions to behavioral medicine.* New York: Academic Press.

KLEIN, H. (1967). Psychological effects of dental treatment in children of different ages. *Journal of Dentistry for Children, 34,* 30–36.

KLEINKNECHT, R., & BERNSTEIN, D. (1978). The assessment of dental fear. *Behavior Therapy, 9,* 626–634.

KLINGMAN, A., MELAMED, B. G., CUTHBERT, M. I., & HERMECZ, D. A. (1984). Effects of participant modeling on information acquisition and skill utilization. *Journal of Consulting and Clinical Psychology, 52,* 414–422.

KLORMAN, R., HILPERT, P. L., MICHAEL, R., LaGANA, C., & SVEEN, O. B. (1980). Effects of coping and mastery modeling on experienced and inexperienced pedodontic patients' disruptiveness. *Behavior Therapy, 11,* 156–168.

KONDAS, O., & SCETNICKA, B. (1972). Systematic desensitization as a method of preparation for childbirth. *Journal of Behavior Therapy and Experimental Psychiatry, 3,* 51–54.

KRANTZ, D. S., BAUM, A., & WIDEMAN, M. (1980). Assessment of preferences for self-treatment and information on health care. *Journal of Personality and Social Psychology, 39,* 979–990.

LAMAZE, F. (1958). *Painless childbirth* (L. R. Celestin, Trans.). London: Burke.

LANGER, E. J., JANIS, I. L., & WOLFER, J. A. (1975). Reduction of psychological stress in surgical patients. *Journal of Experimental Social Psychology, 11,* 155–165.

LESERMAN, J., STUART, E. M., MAMISH, M. E., & BENSON, H. (1989). The efficacy of the relaxation response in preparing for cardiac surgery. *Behavioral Medicine, 15,* 111–117.

LEVENTHAL, E. A., LEVENTHAL, H., SCHACHAM, S., & EASTERLING, D. V. (1989). Active coping reduces reports of pain from childbirth. *Journal of Consulting and Clinical Psychology, 57,* 365–371.

LINDEMAN, C. A. (1972). Nursing intervention with the pre-surgical patient. *Nursing Research, 21,* 196–209.

LINDEMAN, C. A., & AERNAM, B. V. (1971). Nursing intervention with the pre-surgical patient—the effects of structured and unstructured preoperative teaching. *Nursing Research, 20,* 319–332.

LUDLAM, J. E. (1978). *Informed consent.* Chicago: American Hospital Association.

McAMMOND, D. M., DAVIDSON, P. O., & KOVITZ, D. M. (1971). A comparison of the effects of hypnosis and relaxation training on stress reactions in a dental situation. *American Journal of Clinical Hypnosis, 13,* 233–242.

MACHEN, J. B., & JOHNSON, R. (1974). Desensitization, model learning, and the dental behavior of children. *Journal of Dental Research, 53,* 83–87.

MAGEE, J. (1975). The pelvic examination: A view from the other end of the table. *Annals of Internal Medicine, 83,* 563–564.

MATHEWS, A., & REZIN, V. (1977). Treatment of dental fears by imaginal flooding and rehearsal of coping behaviour. *Behaviour Research and Therapy, 15,* 321–328.

MEICHENBAUM, D. H. (1977). *Cognitive behavior modification.* New York: Plenum.

MEICHENBAUM, D. H., & TURK, D. C., (1976). The cognitive-behavioral management of anxiety, anger, and pain. In P. O. Davidson (Ed.), *The behavioral management of anxiety, depression and pain*. New York: Brunner/Mazel.

MELAMED, B. G., DEARBORN, M., & HERMECZ, D. A. (1983). Necessary considerations for surgery preparation: Age and previous experience. *Psychosomatic Medicine, 45,* 517–525.

MELAMED, B. G., HAWES, R. R., HEIBY, E., & GLICK, J. (1975). Use of filmed modeling to reduce uncooperative behavior of children during dental treatment. *Journal of Dental Research, 54,* 797–801.

MELAMED, B. G., & RIDLEY-JOHNSON, R. (1988). Psychological preparation of families for hospitalization. *Developmental and Behavioral Pediatrics, 9,* 96–102.

MELAMED, B. G., & SIEGEL, L. J. (1975). Reduction of anxiety in children facing hospitalization and surgery by use of filmed modeling. *Journal of Consulting and Clinical Psychology, 43,* 511–521.

MELAMED, B. G., & SIEGEL, L. J. (1980). *Behavioral medicine: Practical applications in health care*. New York: Springer.

MELAMED, B. G., YURCHESON, R., FLEECE, L., HUTCHERSON, S., & HAWES, R. (1978). Effects of filmed modeling on the reduction of anxiety-related behaviors in individuals varying in level of previous experience in the stress situation. *Journal of Consulting and Clinical Psychology, 46,* 1357–1367.

MILLER, S. M., & MANGAN, C. E. (1983). Interacting effects of information and coping style in adapting to gynecologic stress: Should the doctor tell all? *Journal of Personality and Social Psychology, 45,* 223–236.

MORSE, D. R., & FURST, M. L. (1978). *Stress and relaxation: Application to dentistry*. Springfield, IL: Charles C. Thomas.

NEWTON, J. R., & READING, A. E. (1977). The effects of psychological preparation on pain at intrauterine device insertion. *Contraception, 16,* 523–532.

O'HARA, M. W., GHONEIM, M. M., HINRICHS, J. V., MEHTA, M. P., & WRIGHT, E. J. (1989). Psychological consequences of surgery. *Psychosomatic Medicine, 51,* 356–370.

PETERSON, L., & RIDLEY-JOHNSON, R. (1980). Pediatric hospital response to survey on prehospital preparation for children. *Journal of Pediatric Psychology, 5,* 1–7.

PETERSON, L., & TOLER, S. M. (1986). An information seeking disposition in child surgery patients. *Health Psychology, 5,* 343–358.

PICKETT, C., & CLUM, G. A. (1982). Comparative treatment strategies and their interaction with locus of control and the reduction of postsurgical pain and anxiety. *Journal of Consulting and Clinical Psychology, 50,* 439–441.

PINTO, R. P., & HOLLANDSWORTH, J. G., JR. (1989). Using videotape modeling to prepare children psychologically for surgery: Influence of parents and costs versus benefits of providing preparation services. *Health Psychology, 8,* 79–95.

POSTLETHWAITE, R., STIRLING, G., & PECK, C. L. (1986). Stress inoculation for acute pain: A clinical trial. *Journal of Behavioral Medicine, 9,* 219–227.

READING, A. E. (1982). The effects of psychological preparation on pain and recovery after minor gynaecological surgery: A preliminary report. *Journal of Clinical Psychology, 38,* 504–512.

REEVES, J. L., REDD, W. H., STORM, F. K., & MINAGAWA, R. Y. (1983). Hypnosis in the control of pain during hyperthermia treatment of cancer. In J. J. Bonica, U. Lindblom, & A. Iggo (Eds.), *Advances in pain research and therapy* (Vol. 5). New York: Raven Press.

ROTTER, J. B. (1966). Generalized expectancies for internal versus external control of reinforcement. *Psychological Monographs, 80* (1, Whole No. 609).

RYAN, D. (1975). A questionnaire survey of pre-operative fears. *British Journal of Clinical Practice, 29,* 3–6.

SALMON, P., PEARCE, S., SMITH, C. C. T., HEYS, A., MANYANDE, A., PETERS, N., & RASHID, J. (1988). The relationship of preoperative distress to endocrine and subjective responses to surgery: Support for Janis' theory. *Journal of Behavioral Medicine, 11,* 599–613.

SAWTELL, R. O., SIMON, J. F., & SIMEONSSON, R. J. (1974). The effects of five preparatory methods upon child behavior during the first dental visit. *Journal of Dentistry for Children, 41,* 367–375.

SCHMITT, F. E., & WOOLDRIDGE, P. J. (1973). Psychological preparation of surgical patients. *Nursing Research, 22,* 108–116.

SCOTT, L. E., & CLUM, G. A. (1984). Examining the interaction effects of coping style and brief interventions in the treatment of postsurgical pain. *Pain, 20,* 279–291.

SHIPLEY, R. H., BUTT, J. H., HORWITZ, B., & FARBRY, J. E. (1978). Preparation for a stressful medical procedure: Effect of stimulus pre-exposure and coping style. *Journal of Consulting and Clinical Psychology, 46,* 499–507.

SIEGEL, L. J., & PETERSON, L. (1980). Stress reduction in young dental patients through coping skills and sensory information. *Journal of Consulting and Clinical Psychology, 48,* 785–787.

SIEGEL, L. J., & PETERSON, L. (1981). Maintenance effects of coping skills and sensory information on young children's response to repeated dental procedures. *Behavior Therapy, 12,* 530–535.

SIME, A. M. (1976). Relationship of pre-operative fear, type of coping, and information received about surgery to recovery from surgery. *Journal of Personality and Social Psychology, 34,* 716–724.

SONNENBERG, E., & VENHAM, L. (1977). Human figure drawings as measure of the child's response to dental visits. *Journal of Dentistry for Children, 44,* 438–442.

ST. JAMES-ROBERTS, I., HUTCHINSON, C., HARAN, F., & CHAMBERLAIN, G. (1983). Biofeedback as an aid to childbirth. *British Journal of Obstetrics and Gynaecology, 90,* 56–60.

SULS, J., & WAN, C. K. (1989). Effects of sensory and procedural information on coping with stressful medical procedures and pain: A meta-analysis. *Journal of Consulting and Clinical Psychology, 57,* 372–379.

SURMAN, O. S., HACKETT, T. P., SILVERBERG, E. L., & BEHRENDT, D. M. (1974). Usefulness of psychiatric intervention in patients undergoing cardiac surgery. *Archives of General Psychiatry, 30,* 830–835.

VAUGHN, G. F. (1957). Children in hospital. *Lancet, 1,* 1117–1120.

VELVOVSKY, I., PLATONOV, K., PLOTICHER, V., & SHUGOM, E. (Eds.) (1960). *Painless childbirth through prophylaxis* (D. A. Myshne, Trans.). Moscow: Foreign Languages Publishing House.

VERNON, D. T., FOLEY, J. M., SIPOWICZ, R. R., & SCHULMAN, J. L. (1965). *The psychological responses of children to hospitalization and illness.* Springfield, IL: Charles Thomas.

WAKEMAN, R. J., & KAPLAN, J. Z. (1978). An experimental study of hypnosis in painful burns. *American Journal of Clinical Hypnosis, 21,* 3–12.

WHITE, W. C., AKERS, J., GREEN, J., & YATES, D. (1974). Use of imitation in the treatment of dental phobia in early childhood: A preliminary report. *Journal of Dentistry for Children, 41,* 106–110.

WILLIAMS, J. G. L., JONES, J. R., WORKHOVEN, M. N., & WILLIAMS, B. (1975). The psychological control of preoperative anxiety. *Psychophysiology, 12,* 50–54.

WILSON, J. F. (1981). Behavioral preparation for surgery: Benefit or harm? *Journal of Behavioral Medicine, 4,* 79–102.

WOLFER, J. A., & DAVIS, C. E. (1970). Assessment of surgical patients' pre-operative emotional condition and post-operative welfare. *Nursing Research, 19,* 402–414.

WOLFER, J. A., & VISINTAINER, M. A. (1975). Pediatric surgical patients' and parents' stress responses and adjustment. *Nursing Research, 24,* 244–255.

WRIGHT, G. F. (1975). *Behavior management in dentistry for children.* Philadelphia: W. B. Saunders.

ZASTOWNY, T. R., KIRSCHENBAUM, D. S., & MENG, A. L. (1986). Coping skills training for children: Effects on distress before, during, and after hospitalization for surgery. *Health Psychology, 5,* 231–247.

ZAX, M., SAMEROFF, A. J., & FARNUM, J. E. (1975). Childbirth education, maternal attitudes, and delivery. *American Journal of Obstetrics and Gynecology, 123,* 185–190.

ZELTZER, L., & LEBARON, S. (1982). Hypnosis and nonhypnotic techniques for reduction of pain and anxiety during painful procedures in children and adolescents with cancer. *The Journal of Pediatrics, 101,* 1032–1035.

# Cardiovascular Disease

*Cardiovascular diseases*, or disorders of the heart and blood vessels, are the major health problem in the United States. Heart disease costs the nation more than $70 billion each year in medical costs, lost income, and productivity; each year, about 1.5 million Americans suffer a heart attack. Despite these grim statistics, there is evidence that cardiovascular disease in the United States is on the decline. After steadily increasing until the 1960s, the death rate from cardiovascular disease has decreased by about 25%.

Medical care for victims of cardiovascular disease has improved significantly during the last 20 to 30 years, but there is evidence that much of the decline in the death rate may be due to life-style changes made in response to increases in knowledge about the behavioral and psychological contributors to cardiovascular disease. The rate of first *myocardial infarction*, or heart attack, declined between the late 1950s and the early 1980s (Pell & Fayerweather, 1985). Improved medical care would be expected to decrease the death rate after a heart attack, but factors other than medical care alone must be responsible for a reduction in the rate of a first heart attack.

This chapter presents an overview of the biological, psychological, and behavioral factors relevant to cardiovascular disease. Heart disease, strokes, and *Raynaud's Phenomenon*, a painful disorder associated with reduced blood flow to the extremities, are discussed. Psychological and behavioral contributors to the development of heart disease are emphasized. Programs designed to alter behavior and emotional-reaction patterns associated with cardiovascular disease are also presented.

# Coronary Heart Disease

## Biological Components

*Coronary heart disease* (CHD) is characterized by blockage of the coronary arteries, the vessels supplying blood to the heart muscle. The heart muscle is typically referred to as the *myocardium*. Normal heart function depends on normal blood supply to the heart; a sufficient reduction in blood supply deprives the myocardium of oxygen and nutrients. If the blood supply is completely blocked, the portion of the heart muscle that has been deprived of blood may die. A temporary reduction in the blood supply is referred to as *ischemia*. If tissue dies as a result of prolonged ischemia, an *infarction* has occurred. Thus, a *myocardial infarction* is death of the heart muscle due to oxygen and nutrient deprivation.

The arterial blockages seen in CHD are typically manifestations of *atherosclerosis*, the most common cause of blood vessel disease in the United States (Herd, 1981). Atherosclerosis involves the accumulation of deposits of cholesterol and other lipids (fats), fibrin (clotting material in the blood), cellular debris, and calcium in the walls of the arteries. These deposits, called *plaques*, damage the cardiovascular system in several ways. Plaques restrict blood flow, and they reduce the ability of the arteries to expand and contract as the deposits harden the artery walls.

Atherosclerosis is a form of *arteriosclerosis*; arteriosclerosis is an impairment in blood supply and/or arterial elasticity due to any cause. Arteriosclerosis increases the risk of myocardial infarction because the restricted blood supply makes less blood available to the heart muscle. The lowered elasticity of the arteries compounds the problem as the vascular system is unable to expand and supply more blood during periods of high demand, such as during exercise. Atherosclerosis also increases the risk of stroke, as will be discussed later in this chapter.

*Hypertension*, or high blood pressure, is a condition in which the blood flowing through the arteries exerts an unusually high level of pressure on the artery walls. As the heart contracts and forces blood through the vascular system, blood pressure increases. As it relaxes between contractions, blood pressure decreases. *Systolic* blood pressure is the amount of pressure on the arterial walls as the heart contracts; *diastolic* blood pressure is the lower level of pressure that is present between contractions. Blood pressure is measured by determining how many millimeters (mm) a column of mercury (Hg) in a glass tube may be raised by the pressure of the blood on the artery walls while a person is at rest.

The level of blood pressure is reported by placing the systolic pressure over the diastolic pressure. Blood pressures of less than 140/90 (140 mm Hg systolic pressure/90 mm Hg diastolic pressure) are considered to be normal. Blood pressures between 140/90 and 160/95 are defined as borderline hypertension, and those of 160/95 and above are definite hypertension.

Hypertension is relevant to CHD for several reasons. First, hypertension increases the risk of developing CHD. Individuals with high blood pressure are two to four times more likely to develop CHD than are persons with normal blood pressure (Jenkins, 1988). In addition, the narrowing of the arteries due to atherosclerosis tends to increase blood pressure. The same amount of blood must be pumped through a smaller space, increasing blood pressure just as the pressure in a water hose increases if you squeeze the hose and thus narrow the tube the water must pass through. The loss of elasticity of the artery walls also increases blood pressure and causes the vessels to be more likely to rupture. An individual with high blood pressure and atherosclerosis may be at particular risk when exercising. Exercise typically increases blood pressure and increases the demand of the heart muscle for blood and oxygen. Not only will the narrowed arteries require the heart to work unusually hard to supply sufficient blood, but the hardened vessels are at an increased risk for rupturing, and the heart muscle is at an increased risk for not receiving adequate oxygen and nutrients.

# Behavioral and Psychological Factors

Lifestyle and emotional status have been found to predict CHD. Cigarette smoking, obesity, and dietary and exercise habits may all contribute to the risk of cardiovascular disease. A cluster of psychological traits referred to as *Type A behavior pattern* has also been implicated as a risk factor for CHD. Chronic hostility and cynicism appear to be especially dangerous.

BEHAVIORAL RISKS   Cigarette smoking has been labeled the most important modifiable risk factor for CHD. The death rate from CHD is 70% greater for cigarette smokers than for nonsmokers. For heavy smokers, the

CHD death rate is 200% greater than for nonsmokers (U. S. Public Health Service, 1983). Smoking twenty or more cigarettes per day may double or triple the risk for heart attack (Kannel, 1983). Pipe and cigar smokers do not have a higher risk for CHD, apparently because they do not inhale (Jarvis, 1984).

Obesity also increases the risk for CHD. This increased risk is primarily because obesity is often associated with high blood pressure and high blood levels of cholesterol and other lipids. Obesity is most profitably viewed as a sign of the presence of several other risk factors, most notably poor dietary and exercise habits. However, even though obesity is not a major independent risk factor for CHD, it has been estimated that the rate of CHD would decline by 25% if everyone were at optimal weight (Kannel & Gordon, 1979).

A diet high in saturated fats, or fats from animal sources, increases blood cholesterol levels. Cholesterol is one of the substances that contributes to plaque formation, therefore high levels of cholesterol increase the risk of atherosclerosis, and thus CHD. Current recommendations are that the level of cholesterol in the bloodstream should be no more than 200 milligrams per deciliter (mg/dl), or one-tenth of a liter (National Institutes of Health, 1984). Cholesterol level is not totally dependent on diet; genetic factors are also important determinants (Blackburn & Jacobs, 1984).

It is important to realize that there are several types of cholesterol. Cholesterol is carried in the bloodstream in the form of *lipoproteins*, or substances formed from lipids (fats) and proteins. High levels of low-density lipoproteins increase the risk of CHD, but high levels of high-density lipoproteins lower CHD risk. Diets high in saturated fats and cholesterol increase low-density lipoproteins. Exercise increases levels of high-density lipoproteins.

A majority of the studies of exercise habits and CHD have found that individuals with a physically active life-style have lower rates of CHD. Regular aerobic exercise for three or more twenty-five minute sessions per week may lead to CHD-risk reduction. Exercise not only increases levels of high-density lipoproteins but can also decrease blood pressure and resting heart rate and increase the amount of blood pumped by a single heart contraction (Haskell, 1984).

Finally, the presence of more than one behavioral risk factor may synergistically increase the probability of CHD. The risk for a major coronary event, such as a heart attack, is between eight and nine times as great for a person who smokes cigarettes, has diastolic blood pressure of 90 mm Hg or greater, and cholesterol levels of 250 mg/dl or greater than it is for a person with none of these three risk factors (Holbrook, Grundy, Hennekens, Kannel, & Strong, 1984).

TYPE A BEHAVIOR PATTERN AND HOSTILITY    During the 1950s two physicians, Meyer Friedman and Ray Rosenman, began to wonder if factors other than diet might be important contributors to high cholesterol levels and CHD. As a result of reviewing the medical literature, speaking to patients and families of patients, and surveying the opinions of physicians and laypeople alike, they concluded that stress associated with meeting deadlines might be an important contributor to coronary disease (Friedman & Ulmer, 1984). However, Friedman and Rosenman were aware that the evidence they had gathered was anecdotal, based as it was on opinion and recollection of stressful time periods, so they set out to design an experimental test of their hypothesis.

Friedman and Rosenman tested cholesterol levels and blood-clotting time in a group of tax accountants every two weeks from January to June of 1957. They also questioned the acccountants about diet and their sense of time urgency associated with meeting deadlines. As you might expect, the accountants' sense of time urgency increased dramatically as the April tax deadline approached and decreased dramatically after the deadline passed. The accountants' diets did not change, but cholesterol levels rose, and blood-clotting time decreased as tax deadlines approached and time urgency increased. Cholesterol decreased and clotting time increased after the deadline passed (Friedman & Rosenman, 1959).

As a result of these observations and the results of other studies, Friedman and Rosenman suggested that a particular behavioral style might be a major risk factor for CHD. They labeled this behavioral style the *Type A behavior pattern (TABP)*. The original conception of the TABP included six primary features, most of them related to a sense of competition and urgency. These characteristics are summarized in Table 8.1. Rosenman pointed out that this package of behaviors creates "an enhanced performance designed to assert and maintain control over the environment when this control is challenged or threatened" (Rosenman, 1986, p. 23).

Many studies of the relationship between TABP and CHD have been conducted since Friedman and Rosenman initially described the syndrome. Although results have not been uniformly positive, the majority of the investigations have supported the contention that TABP is a risk factor for CHD (Booth-Kewley & Friedman, 1987; Chesney, Eagleston, & Rosenman, 1981; Dembroski & Costa, 1987). However, research has begun to examine the nature of TABP more closely, looking particularly at the possibilities that there

TABLE 8.1   Characteristics of the Type A Behavior Pattern

1. A pervasive drive to reach usually poorly defined goals.
2. A powerful desire to compete.
3. An enduring need for recognition and advancement.
4. Constant involvement in varied tasks involving deadlines and time pressure.
5. An enduring tendency to speed up mental and physical tasks.
6. High levels of mental and physical alertness.

SOURCE:   Adapted from Rosenman, R. H. (1986). Current and past history of Type A behavior pattern. In T. H. Schmidt, T. M. Dembroski, & G. Blumchen (Eds.), *Biological and psychological factors in cardiovascular disease* (pp. 15–40). New York: Springer-Verlag.

may be specific aspects of TABP that are more "toxic" than others, or there may be other emotions equally important as CHD risk factors.

Hostility and anger, especially hostile cynicism, may be important psychological risk factors for CHD. Williams et al. (1980) reported that hostility predicted the presence of blocked coronary arteries in patients with the symptoms of CHD better than did TABP, and Barefoot, Dahlstrom, and Williams (1983) found that hostility predicted which medical students were likely to develop heart disease during a twenty-five-year follow-up period. As you may remember from Chapter 2, a multivariate correlational study examining TABP (MacDougall, Dembroski, Dimsdale, & Hackett, 1985) found that potential for hostility and anger-in, the tendency to keep angry feelings to oneself, were significantly correlated with the number of blocked coronary arteries in heart disease patients. In the MacDougall et al. study, a sense of time urgency was associated with a *smaller* number of blocked arteries, and factors related to competition and rapid activity were unrelated to CHD.

Other studies have not found a reliable association between hostility and heart disease. Hearn, Murray, and Luepker (1989) conducted telephone interviews with 1399 men who had enrolled at the University of Minnesota in 1953; the men had completed the Minnesota Multiphasic Personality Inventory (MMPI) at the time of enrollment. If the telephone interview was suggestive of CHD, medical records were obtained and the diagnosis was verified. Hearn et al. reported that hostility was not a significant predictor of CHD for the men in this study. Leon, Finn, Murray, and Bailey (1988) found no relationship between hostility and CHD in a sample of 280 men. The men in this study completed the MMPI at an average age of forty-five, and received periodic medical and psychological evaluations over a thirty-year period.

Despite these negative findings, the authors of these studies did not argue that hostility should not be considered a risk factor for CHD. Hearn et al. (1989) noted that their subjects completed the MMPI at age nineteen, thirty-three years before the telephone interviews were conducted. Substantial changes in hostility and in other psychological characteristics could easily have occurred over this long follow-up period. Hearn et al. also pointed out that the Cook-Medley Scale measures cynical hostility, distrust, and suspicion, and it may be that other measures of hostility are required to completely understand the link between hostility and CHD, if such a link exists. Leon et al. (1988) noted that the strongest associations between hostility and heart disease have been found in studies where the subjects' average levels of hostility have been quite high. Thus, hostility may be a risk factor for CHD only when hostility levels are high.

Current evidence suggests that Type A behavior pattern is a moderate contributor to the development of heart disease. However, other emotions such as chronic hostility and anger, may be more important risk factors. Depression and anxiety have also been suggested as important risk factors, although it is uncertain whether TABP and anger lead to emotional exhaustion (such as depression and anxiety) or whether this emotional exhaustion is an independent risk factor (Friedman & Booth-Kewley, 1988; Krantz, Contrada, Hill, & Friedler, 1988). It is tempting to speculate that the Type A person who is anxious about meeting deadlines and feels in competition with others is at risk for beginning to view the world in a hostile and cynical fashion. He or she may eventually become exhausted by his or her struggle to get ahead. Such a person might be at an increased risk for CHD. In contrast, the person who hurries to meet deadlines because he is interested in the tasks, not because he is competing with others, may be at much less risk for becoming angry and exhausted and at less risk for CHD. In fact, there is evidence that monkeys constantly struggling to maintain a dominant position in an unstable social environment are at greater risk for atherosclerosis than monkeys not perpetually competing for dominance (Manuck, Kaplan, Adams, & Clarkson, 1988). Recalling that Rosenman (1986) saw TABP as a response designed to maintain control in the face of a threatening environment, it may be that the chronic arousal associated with confronting the world as an enemy is the common thread in the proposed psychological risk factors for CHD.

## Psychological Reactions

Receiving a diagnosis of CHD, and particularly experiencing a major coronary event such as a heart attack, is clearly a traumatic event with significant psychological impact. More than half of all heart attack patients die within the first few hours after the infarction and before reaching the hospital, but of those who are treated in the hospital and survive, 80% return to their former life and job. The remaining 20% become disabled (Hartley, 1983). Age and disease severity have a large influence on how well a patient recovers from a myocardial infarction, but psychological factors are also important determinants of eventual outcome.

Denial is a common reaction during the first few hours after a heart attack. Most of us prefer to believe the most benign explanation for physical discomfort, and the person who has just experienced a myocardial infarction is likely to explain his or her discomfort as indigestion, muscle tension, or some other relatively mild condition. This period of denial leads to delayed treatment and is a major contributor to the high death rate during the first few hours after a heart attack. In fact, the American Heart Association has suggested that half of all deaths due to heart attack could be prevented by earlier treatment (Hartley, 1983).

After reaching the hospital, several days of anxiety followed by several days of depression are common. After five or six days in the hospital, anxiety and depression typically subside as the patient begins to adjust to the reality of having survived a life-threatening event. Denial may once again take over, or the patient may accept that the heart attack occurred yet avoid the emotional distress associated with thinking about how near death he or she was and that he or she may be at risk for future life and health problems. Although hospitalized patients may not need formal psychological treatment, they may benefit from the opportunity to discuss their concerns and "get things off their chest" (Blumenthal & Mau, 1987).

Depression and other psychological problems often emerge after a patient leaves the hospital, although emotional distress typically declines during the first one to two years after the infarction. Depression may be related to loss. For instance, some patients must give up their normal daily activities, which may include going to work. Financial and social losses are also possible, and patients may be unable to be as physically active as they once were. Individuals who have suffered an infarction can also become excessively concerned about health. These concerns may lead them to avoid activities in which they are medically able to participate. The term *cardiac neurosis* is sometimes used to describe the condition of a patient who has become extremely anxious and concerned about the risk of another infarction and has become fearful about slight exertion and minor physical symptoms (Blumenthal & Mau, 1987).

On the positive side, some patients may reevaluate the meaning of their life. They may become more interested in others and less heavily focused on material success. They may also review their life to date and decide to pursue opportunities that had previously been neglected (Blumenthal & Mau, 1987).

## Treatment Interventions

Appropriate treatment is obviously dependent on the psychological and physical condition of the postmyocardial infarction patient, but some treatment goals are nearly universal. Most patients undergo a program of *cardiac rehabilitation*. Supervised exercise training is common and begins as soon as is practical after a patient's medical condition is no longer life-threatening. Rapid involvement in physical activity helps to avoid excessive fears regarding exertion and also helps to reduce the risk of other medical complications. Most patients are therefore encouraged to take short walks in the hospital halls or around the room and to attend to their own personal hygiene within the first three days of hospitalization. Exercise frequency and intensity is then gradually increased to the degree practical based on the patient's physical condition (Wagner & Williams, 1987).

Education is also a common feature of cardiac rehabilitation efforts. Many patients have concerns about sexual activity after an infarction. Sexual intercourse actually presents most patients with a relatively low risk for another heart attack, and patients often benefit from counseling about postinfarction sexual activity. Supervised exercise may enhance sexual performance, and this news can increase a patient's enthusiasm for an exercise program. Dietary education is also common, as is encouragement to stop smoking and to otherwise make life-style changes to reduce the risk of another cardiac event (Wagner & Williams, 1987).

Despite knowledge about the association between cigarette smoking and the risk of heart attack, it has been reported that nearly half of all smokers who experience a myocardial infarction resume smoking within five years. Smoking may serve as a way to deal with uncomfortable emotional states, such as anxiety and depression. In addition, patients who resume smoking appear to have a lower level of knowledge about cardiac health in general, even though they are aware of the risks of smoking. Education about CHD and myocardial infarction may thus help to reduce the risk that a patient will return to smoking after suffering a heart attack. This more general education helps patients to better understand the health risks of smoking. It can also reduce anxiety and depression, and thus the urge to smoke, as knowledge about cardiac health has been found to be inversely related to anxiety and depression after a heart attack (Havik & Maeland, 1988).

Patient participation in treatment has also been found to be helpful in reducing the risk of depression and disability after a myocardial infarction. Follick et al. (1988) tested a system that allowed patients to monitor their own heart activity, telephone electrocardiogram information in to the hospital, and inject their own medication when instructed to do so by hospital personnel. After nine months, patients able to participate in their own treatment in this way were less likely to be depressed, more likely to be working, and more confident in their own ability to manage cardiac symptoms than were patients who received the usual hospital-managed care.

Other studies have documented that myocardial infarction patients may be trained to better manage stressful situations and thus reduce their heart rate and blood pressure under stress. For example, Gatchell, Gaffney, & Smith (1986) exposed infarction patients to a program of relaxation training and heart-rate biofeedback. The patients were also given training in how to present and prepare an effective public speech. When these patients were required to present a speech at the end of the program, they showed pulse rates, blood pressures, and anxiety levels equivalent to those of patients who had been given propanolol. Propanolol is a drug commonly prescribed to control heart rate and blood pressure reactivity in heart attack patients. About 10%–20% of heart attack patients are unable to take propanolol because of the existence of other disorders or unwanted side effects. Behavioral interventions may therefore provide a useful treatment alternative for some heart attack patients.

# Prevention of Coronary Heart Disease

Myocardial infarctions and other cardiovascular incidents such as strokes (discussed later in this chapter) are associated with high rates of death and disability. It is therefore clear that if CHD is to be effectively combated, prevention must be the primary weapon. A variety of prevention programs have evolved, most commonly focusing on the behavioral modification of CHD risk factors such as dietary and exercise habits, smoking, and/or Type A Behavior Pattern. Some preventive efforts have been targeted at individuals at risk for CHD, while others have attempted to modify the risk of CHD on a communitywide basis.

INDIVIDUAL PREVENTION PROGRAMS    Individually targeted prevention programs typically screen subjects for the presence of CHD risk factors. If risk factors are present, subjects are offered the opportunity to participate in a program to reduce the risk of CHD. Dietary modifications, exercise programs, aid in reducing smoking, stress management and relaxation training are frequent program components.

Otherwise healthy people at risk for CHD have been able to reduce their CHD risk by up to 41% by participating in a program emphasizing training in, and application of, behavioral change principles. In one project, subjects received education about CHD, their own risk for its development, and training in behavior modification procedures to facilitate life-style changes. Services were delivered in group and individual sessions over a period of six months. The treatment sessions went beyond simple education. They included group reinforcement for positive changes, individual goal-setting exercises, and physical assessments as well. Reduced blood pressure and increased exercise capacity were present as long as one year after treatment, and cholesterol levels were reduced six months after treatment. (Cholesterol levels were not tested one year after treatment.) In addition, 28% of the cigarette smokers had stopped smoking one year after treatment ended (Lovibond, Birrell, & Langeluddecke, 1986).

Other individual prevention programs have focused on reducing single-risk factors. Patel (1984) developed a multifaceted program to reduce blood pressure and thus reduce CHD risk. His program includes health education on stress and blood pressure, breathing exercises, muscle relaxation, meditation, galvanic skin-response biofeedback, and suggestions for how to use these relaxation skills in stressful situations. Patel has reported significant reductions in systolic and diastolic blood pressure with this program: up to 26 mm Hg systolic and 15 mm Hg diastolic in one study (Patel, 1984). A less complex program has also been reported to successfully reduce blood pressure. Crowther (1983) trained twenty-four hypertensive patients in relaxation procedures or relaxation plus stress management training, and found that whereas eighteen of the twenty-four trained patients had normal blood pressure after eight weeks of treatment, only one of the ten control subjects, who received only weekly blood pressure checks, had normal blood pressure. Half of the subjects receiving training maintained normal blood pressure six months after treatment.

Stress management training has also been found to lead to significant reductions in systolic blood pressure in a sample of mildly to moderately hypertensive male patients (Bosley & Allen, 1989). The stress management training in the Bosley and Allen study emphasized awareness of behavioral, physiological, and cognitive responses to stress. After the hypertensive patients were aware of their reactions to stress, they were trained to modify their appraisal of stressful situations and thereby reduce the level of stress they experienced. Patients receiving stress management training showed significantly greater gains in coping skills than did patients who received either standard medical treatment for high blood pressure or patients who simply met with a therapist and discussed stressful situations. The use of the coping skills taught in the stress management training was significantly correlated with systolic blood pressure; patients who most often used these strategies showed the greatest reductions in blood pressure. The results of this study led Bosley and Allen to conclude that stress management training is a useful supplement to the medical treatment of high blood pressure.

Type A behavior and hostility have also been targets for change. The Montreal Type A Intervention Project (Roskies et al., 1986) exposed 107 Type A men to three different treatment programs, each lasting ten weeks. Some men received aerobic exercise training, others received weight training, and others received stress management training. The stress management training was directed toward helping subjects better identify and plan for stressful situations, monitor their own stress reactions, and apply new coping skills. TABP was reduced significantly more for the stress management group than for either exercise group. However, no groups showed significant improvement in heart rate or blood pressure measures at the end of treatment. It is thus important to recognize that changes in Type A behavior, or even exercise program participation, may not always lead to immediately observable changes in physiological measures (Roskies et al., 1986).

Although the modification of hostility has not as yet been experimentally studied, Redford Williams, a physician at Duke University Medical Center, has developed a program to help people begin to change their hostile habits. He suggests a twelve-step program that includes practice in monitoring cynical thoughts; stopping hostile thoughts; learning to laugh at yourself; learning to relax; and learning to trust, forgive, and listen to others (Williams, 1989). In view of the previously mentioned evidence suggesting that hostility may be an important risk factor for CHD, it will be interesting to watch for future reports concerning the ability of hostility modification programs such as this to actually modify CHD risk or the incidence of heart attack.

COMMUNITY-BASED PROGRAMS    Individually targeted programs may only affect a limited number of people: subjects who have been identified as being at risk for CHD and who are able to attend individual or group treatment meetings. Community-based programs attempt to modify CHD risk on a larger scale by exposing as many people as possible to information about CHD and to suggestions about how to lower the risk of developing CHD.

The North Karelia Project (Puska, 1984) was the first large-scale community-based program to attempt CHD risk modification. North Karelia is a predominantly rural county in Finland, selected for the project because of the county's unusually high level of deaths from cardiovascular disease. Information about cardiovascular disease, risk factors such as diet and smoking, and available programs to help citizens make positive life-style changes was disseminated through the mass media. Specific dietary changes were suggested, cooking skills emphasizing healthy diets were taught in housewife organizations, and stop-smoking groups were formed wherever possible. Antismoking signs were displayed prominently throughout the community, and the use of food processors was encouraged to produce low-fat products.

Ten years after the program began, cholesterol and blood pressure levels of community residents had been significantly lowered. The risk estimate for CHD had declined significantly for the community as well. More important, cardiovascular disability payments had declined in North Karelia, as had the death rate from CHD (Puska, 1984). In sum, the project had a significant impact on the cardiovascular health of the community.

A similar project has been conducted in the United States under the auspices of Stanford University. The Stanford Three Community Study (Farquhar, 1983) surveyed the citizens of three northern California towns over two years for CHD risk factors and knowledge and attitudes about CHD. Two of the towns were exposed to mass media educational campaigns providing information about CHD and suggestions for changing risk factors. In one of these two towns, high-risk citizens also received face-to-face contact designed to encourage life-style changes. A third town served as a control group.

The media campaigns alone changed body weight, blood pressure, and cholesterol levels enough to reduce the risk of CHD in community residents by 24%. Smoking was more difficult to change: the control town and the media-only town were essentially equivalent in smoking rates. However, 50% of the smokers in the media plus personal contact town stopped smoking, whereas only 15% of the citizens of the control town stopped.

The Stanford Three Community Study and the North Karelia Project demonstrated that it is possible to change CHD risk (and at least in the North Karelia Project, CHD mortality and costs) on a communitywide basis. These efforts are particularly encouraging in view of the major human and economic costs of CHD. The studies suggest that relatively inexpensive public efforts may lead to broad-scale changes in personal behavior and thus to improved community health and reduced medical and social expense. Community interventions may be directed at citizens of all ages, without regard to current CHD risk factor status. Thus, such programs may not only impact on a larger segment of the population than individual programs, but they may also be a cost-effective way to reduce the risk of CHD in persons who could not otherwise receive help and information regarding CHD prevention.

# Cerebrovascular Accidents

A *cerebrovascular accident* (CVA), often referred to as a stroke, is a physiological event involving an abnormality in the blood supply to one or more regions of the brain. This abnormality may be due to a variety of causes, but regardless of the cause it leads to permanent tissue damage to, or temporary impairment in the functioning of, the affected region in the brain. Each year, about 400,000 persons in the United States are discharged from hospitals after treatment for a stroke, and 5% of people over 65 years old have had a stroke at some time during their lives (Kistler, Ropper, & Martin, 1987). Strokes occur with approximately equal frequency in males and females (Sharpless, 1982).

Treatment of stroke patients has improved significantly, but a stroke is still a very serious medical event. Stroke is the third leading cause of death in the United States; dependent on the nature of the stroke, death rates after the first stroke range from 20% to 50%. Although many people who survive a first stroke may experience another stroke as well, the most significant risk to life for stroke survivors is cardiovascular disease (McDowell, 1979), discussed previously in this chapter. The initial treatment following a CVA naturally emphasizes the medical stabilization of the patient, but an extended recovery time after the acute phase is common. The greatest degree of recovery is commonly seen in the first six months after a stroke, although improvement may be seen for up to two years. During recovery, treatment typically concentrates on the rehabilitation of any physical losses the patient may have experienced, and there is beginning to be an increasing emphasis on the psychological and intellectual rehabilitation of the patient as well. The exact symptoms that a person may experience after a CVA vary with the type and location of the stroke. They include paralysis or other impairments in motor ability, sensory and perceptual losses, intellectual impairments, and psychological symptoms such as depression.

## Biological Components

Cerebrovascular accidents may be categorized in a variety of ways, depending on the type of disruption in the blood flow that has occurred, the location of the tissue damage, and the length of time that the disruption in blood flow has lasted. Some strokes involve an *intracranial hemorrhage*, in which a blood vessel in the brain bursts or leaks. Although the blood is gradually reabsorbed after the bleeding stops, the brain has often been damaged by the pressure of the blood on the brain tissue or through direct physical contact with the blood. Other strokes are caused by *cerebral ischemia*. In the case of cerebral ischemia the supply of blood is restricted or totally blocked, causing tissue to die or its function to be temporarily impaired as a result of blood and oxygen deficiency. You will remember from earlier in this chapter that tissue death from ischemia is referred to as infarction. Just as heart tissue dies in a myocardial infarction, brain tissue may also die as a result of ischemia. Infarcts are about four times more common than hemorrhages (Mohr, Kase, & Adams, 1983).

Ischemia often results from the formation of a blood clot in an artery in the brain. If the blood clot is stationary, that is, it remains in the location in which it formed, it is referred to as a *thrombus*. However, a clot may form in one region, break off and flow through the circulatory system, and eventually lodge in a small blood vessel in a different location. Such a migrating blood clot is referred to as an *embolus*. Thus, ischemic strokes may result not only from the formation of blood clots in the brain but also from clots that form in other locations, such as the leg, and then travel to the brain following a blow to the body or some other event that dislodges all or a part of the clot.

Although the brain is dependent on a continous supply of blood and oxygen for normal functioning, a brief disruption in the blood supply may not result in permanent tissue damage or neurological deficit. If blood flow totally ceases, brain tissue will die within three minutes. If blood flow is reduced but not totally stopped, brain tissue can survive for an indeterminate period (Kistler et al., 1987). A temporary disruption of the blood supply to the brain is referred to as a *transient ischemic attack* (TIA). The symptoms of a TIA may include dizziness, fainting, vision problems, and weakness and/or sensory loss (Heyman, Burch, Rosati, Haynes, & Utley, 1979). Ischemic episodes of longer duration lead to infarction of the cerebral tissue; this increases the risk of more severe and longer-lasting impairments.

## Behavioral, Psychological, and Social Factors

The risk factors for cerebrovascular accidents are essentially the same as those for coronary heart disease. TIAs due to atherosclerosis have been found to be predictors of serious cardiac disease and cerebral infarction (Heyman et al., 1984). There is also some evidence that alcohol abuse, particularly recent, heavy drinking, increases the risk of experiencing a CVA. Stroke patients have been found to be more likely to have been drinking during the twenty-four hours prior to hospital admission than hospital patients with other diagnoses, even with equivalent rates of alcoholism in stroke patients and other patients (Taylor, Combs-Orme, Anderson, Taylor, & Koppenol, 1984). Acute,

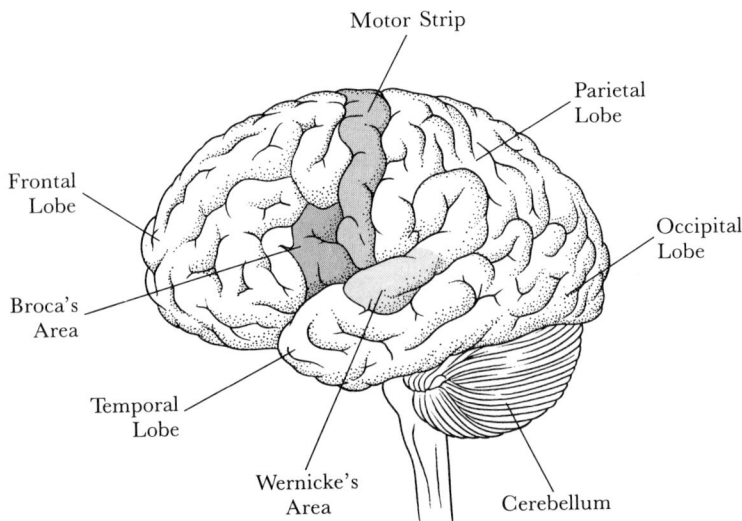

FIGURE 8.1   The major regions of the cortex of the human brain.

heavy drinking has been found to be especially associated with stroke in adolescents and young adults, a group with a very low overall risk for stroke (Hillborn & Kaste, 1981).

# Psychological and Behavioral Reactions

The symptoms an individual may exhibit after suffering a stroke vary a great deal, ranging from coma and paralysis to neurological disorders so minor that they may not disturb normal functioning (Mohr, Kase, & Adams, 1983). The specific symptoms are related to the size and location of the affected area in the brain. If only one side, or hemisphere, of the brain is affected, whether it is the left or right hemisphere that is damaged will have a significant impact on the symptoms experienced. Figure 8.1 contains an illustration of the human brain and the major regions of the cortex. The possible consequences of brain damage due to CVA are summarized in Table 8.2 and discussed in more detail below.

MOTORIC AND PERCEPTUAL IMPAIRMENT    The effect of a CVA that is perhaps most familiar is loss or reduction in the ability to control muscle movements. Such losses are referred to as impairments in *motor control*. The left hemisphere of the brain controls the voluntary muscle movements of the right side of the body, and the right hemisphere controls the left side of the body. Therefore, the side of the body *contralateral*, or opposite, to the side of the brain that is damaged may evidence difficulties with muscle control. The degree of impairment varies with the magnitude and location of the damage. Damage to the *motor strip* is particularly likely to result in deficits in motor control. Impaired coordination is often experienced when the cerebellum has been damaged. See Figure 8.1 for the location of both of these brain areas. In some cases, *hemiparesis* (weakness or partial paralysis of one side of the body) may be present; in others, *hemiplegia* (total paralysis of one side of the body) may occur.

Perceptual impairments may also follow a CVA. For example, visual difficulties involving *field cuts* may result when the occipital lobe is damaged. A

TABLE 8.2   Abilities likely to be impaired by strokes damaging the left or right hemisphere.

| Left Hemisphere Damage | Right Hemisphere Damage |
| --- | --- |
| Verbal learning and memory | Visual learning and memory |
| Language abilities | Spatial abilities |
| Right-sided motor skills | Left-sided motor skills |
| Right-sided sensation | Left-sided sensation |
| Arithmetic skills | Left-sided neglect |
| Vision to right side | Vision to left side |
| Depression | Indifference or inattention |

person suffering from a visual field cut is likely to be unable to see stimuli in one area of their visual field. For example, right occipital damage might cause an individual to experience difficulties driving or walking due to a neglect of the objects to their left. To get a feeling for the difficulties a person with a left visual field cut would experience, close or cover your left eye and notice how much more you must turn your head in order to see all of the objects around you. Reach out and try to grab something a little more than arm's length away. You will probably have difficulty judging distance because depth perception depends on vision in both eyes. Imagine the problems you would face if you had to drive a car or if you tried to play a sport such as baseball.

Similarly, the ability to perceive tactile or auditory stimulation on the right side of the body may be impaired with left-hemisphere damage, whereas the ability to perceive left-sided tactile or auditory stimulation and patterns in acoustic or tactile stimuli may be impaired with right-hemisphere damage (Sharpless, 1982).

COGNITIVE IMPAIRMENT   The ability to think, learn, and communicate effectively is often impaired folowing a stroke and can be the cause of significant frustration for the stroke victim. Imagine for yourself the reactions you would have if you suddenly found yourself unable to solve problems that were easy for you before and unable to find the words to express your thoughts, feelings, and desires. Damage to the temporal lobes of the brain is likely to impair memory and learning ability, with damage to the right anterior temporal lobe impairing memory and learning for visual material and damage to the left anterior temporal lobe impairing learning and memory for verbal material. Left-hemisphere damage may also impair arithmetic skills.

A stroke affecting the left hemisphere is much more likely to impair verbal abilities than one affecting the right hemisphere. Language skills are located in the left hemisphere in about 95% of right-handed normals and 70% of left-handed normals. Language skills are localized to the right hemisphere in approximately 5% of right-handed normals and 15% of left-handed normals; the remaining 15% of left-handers appear to have bilateral control of language (Bloom, Lazerson, & Hofstadter, 1985).

*Aphasia* is the name given to a broad class of disorders involving deficits in language. Receptive language may be impaired, such that a person has difficulty understanding language. Expressive language ability may also be impaired. In these cases an individual has difficulty finding words and expressing him- or herself. However, these two varieties of aphasia often occur together, and most aphasics have difficulty with both expressive and receptive language abilities (Sharpless, 1982). Aphasia may result from impairment in several aspects of language functioning, but it is important to remember that it is distinct from communication impairment due to sensory or motor problems. Thus, an aphasic individual may be able to hear quite clearly but be unable to understand the words he or she can hear. Obviously, it is not helpful in such a case for the speaker to raise his or her voice, for the problem does not lie in hearing, but in understanding. Some people suffering from aphasia may have difficulty finding the word that they want to say, so they may describe the object they are trying to name in order to communicate. For example, instead of saying, "Give me the pencil," they might say, "Give me the thing that I can write with." This style of communication, in which a word is "talked around" instead of directly expressed is referred to as *circumlocution*.

Two major types of aphasia are *Broca's aphasia* and *Wernicke's aphasia*. Broca's area and Wernicke's area are noted in Figure 8.1. In Broca's aphasia, an individual's speech is slow, halting, and limited. Sentences are likely to be telegraphic, lacking grammatical structure and connecting words. If a Broca's aphasia patient were asked to describe a picture of a boy hiding, a broken window, and a girl apparently being blamed for the accident, he or she might say "'Window ... break. Boy, man, anger ... girl what, boy hide, do it'" (Bradshaw & Nettleton, 1983, p.37).

In Wernicke's aphasia the ability to comprehend speech is severely impaired. The sufferer's speech is fluent and effortless, but it does not make sense. Instead, it is composed of nonsense jargon. An example of Wernicke's aphasia in a 72-year old right-handed male who suffered a right hemisphere infarct was reported by Sweet, Panis, & Levine (1984). When asked to describe a picture showing a cookie being stolen, he said, "'Well, let's say wa ... trellin, may, what are there? May ... charteress, chit. Va ... va, she did some bulb there, I guess'" (p. 476). Thinking back to the data concerning the lateralization of language abilities, you will note that this case is highly unusual in that the infarct in this man occurred in the right hemisphere, yet Wernicke's aphasia resulted. It has been estimated that aphasia following right-hemisphere damage occurs in only 0.4% to 3.5% of right-handed persons (Sweet ei al., 1984).

PSYCHOLOGICAL IMPAIRMENT  A major medical disorder such as a stroke would be expected to carry with it a risk for depression as the affected individual struggles with his or her symptoms and adjusts to any necessary changes in life-style. Estimates of the incidence of depression following stroke have varied, dependent on the nature of the stroke and the time since the stroke that the patient was assessed. In a study of ninety-one stroke patients, Feibel and Springer (1982) reported that nurses rated 26% of stroke patients as depressed six months after the occurrence of their stroke. However, Robinson, Starr, & Price (1984) found depression to be a more common phenomenon in a sample of sixty-one stroke patients. These investigators measured depression while the patients were in the hospital immediately following the stroke and at three and six months poststroke. They found that 60% of the patients had been depressed at some time during the six-month period.

The nature of the psychological symptoms experienced by stroke patients may be related to the hemisphere damaged by the CVA. Persons with left-hemisphere damage have been reported to be more depressed than persons with right-hemisphere damage, whereas those with right-hemisphere damage have been reported to be more likely to be cheerful but apathetic or indifferent to their losses (Gainotti, 1972; Robinson & Price, 1982). Denial of and indifference to physical limitations has been found to be more common in those with right-hemisphere damage than in those with left-hemisphere damage by ratios ranging from 3:1 to 16:1. It has been suggested that this difference may be due to the possibility that right-hemisphere damage interferes with the ability to synthesize and integrate sensory stimuli. Thus, a person with right-hemisphere damage may be unaware of the degree of their impairment, and in extreme cases may totally neglect their impaired extremities. This condition has been referred to as the *hemi-inattention syndrome* (Sharpless, 1982).

However, a consistent relationship between emotional reactions to stroke and the hemisphere that is damaged has not always been found (Feibel & Springer, 1982; Robinson, Starr, Kubos, & Price, 1983). Instead, the depressive symptoms noted in CVA patients have been suggested to be due to psychosocial factors such as grief over lost functioning, concerns regarding loss of control due to disability, changes in body image, and the loneliness and isolation that serious illness often brings (Feibel & Springer, 1982). As might be expected, the degree of depression experienced has sometimes been found to be related to the degree of physical and cognitive impairment resulting from the stroke. Robinson, Starr, Kubos, and Price (1983) found significant correlations, ranging from .22 to .38, between impairment and depression in 103 stroke patients interviewed two weeks after their stroke.

Impairment subsequent to CVA does not appear to be the only factor determining the presence or severity of depression. Feibel and Springer (1982) found that depression in their sample of ninety-one stroke patients was unrelated to cognitive impairment or independence in activities of daily living but instead was correlated with a failure to resume social activities. It will be remembered that Feibel and Springer assessed patients six months after their stroke, whereas Robinson et al. (1983) conducted their assessment two weeks poststroke. It may be that depression is more related to the degree of disability in the initial phases of recovery than during later phases, after the stroke victim has had an opportunity to begin to accept and adjust to his or her limitations. Even if no neurological symptoms remain after a stroke, many individuals may decrease their activities and withdraw from social interaction for no apparent medical reason. This tendency has been found to be more common in the aftermath of stroke than that of other medical disorders, and it has been suggested that stroke survivors may be more likely to perceive their illnesss as a social stigma than are survivors of other serious medical problems (Labi, Phillips, & Gresham, 1980). These investigators reported that there was some relationship between the degree of neurological impairment and decrease in activities, but 25% to 40% of long-term stroke survivors with no neurological deficit decreased their social activities inside and outside the home and also reduced their involvement in hobbies and other interests.

Depression may also be a problem for the family members of a stroke victim. Depressive symptoms are two to three times more common among primary support persons of stroke victims than they are for the general population (Tompkins, Schulz, & Rau, 1988). Support persons at greatest risk for depression have been found to be the spouses of younger, more seriously impaired stroke patients. Support persons with low household income, low levels of optimism, and a small network of friends who were visited frequently prior to the patient's stroke are also at risk for depression (Tompkins et al., 1988).

As noted, some CVA patients do not experience depression and indeed may appear indifferent to their symptoms or to deny the presence of any difficulties. It has been suggested that these people may have seen illness as a weakness or disgrace prior to suffering a stroke and thus resist acknowledging the presence of physical stroke-related limitations because disability and illness are inconsistent with their self-image (Weinstein & Friedland, 1977). It may also be that the depression that is sometimes reported by observers of stroke victims at least partially represents a projection of the observers' concerns and feelings rather than an objective perception of the patient's emotional state. Alexy and Bracy (1983) have argued that patients involved in an active rehabilitation program are not as depressed as it is sometimes assumed. In a survey of the daily moods of sixty-two stroke and head injury patients, they found that the patients consistently rated their moods on the positive side of neutral and tended to base their mood ratings on perceptions of achievement and performance in the rehabilitation program. No differences were found between head injury and stroke patients or between patients with left- as opposed to right-hemisphere CVAs.

## Treatment Approaches

The areas of potential impairment due to stroke are quite varied; thus, the treatment of poststroke symptoms is ideally a multidisciplinary endeavor focusing on a wide array of problem areas. Physical disability is commonly treated with therapy involving exercises designed to increase strength, range of motion, and motor control. There has also begun to be an increasing trend toward the use of biofeedback as another means of rehabilitating physical disability. Cognitive deficits and aphasia are typically approached by means of training programs that attempt to help the patient to relearn lost knowledge and skills; computer-directed programs are beginning to become available for cognitive rehabilitation efforts. The treatment of psychosocial difficulties following stroke has employed individual, group, and family modalities.

REHABILITATION OF PHYSICAL LIMITATIONS   The rehabilitation of physical disability following stroke is typically oriented toward returning the patient to the highest level of independent functioning possible. Initial goals are often quite basic, such as bathing, dressing, and eating without assistance. Later in the rehabilitation program more complex activities such as independent walking or driving may be concentrated on until a patient is able to reenter as many of his or her prestroke activities as possible. It is quite difficult to separate the results of treatment from the spontaneous recovery of function that is commonly seen after a CVA, particularly the rapid improvement that occurs in the first six months. Indeed, Lind (1982) reviewed seven studies of stroke rehabilitation and concluded that most of the improvement in functional ability seen in stroke patients resulted from spontaneous recovery and "improvements which are attributable to comprehensive rehabilitation programs are so slight as to escape reliable measurement" (p. 148). However, Lind also noted that some patients do appear to benefit from the rehabilitation effort, and even a slight improvement in the ability to independently perform the normal activities of daily living may allow a person to avoid institutionalization.

Electromyographic (EMG) biofeedback has been used at an increasing rate in rehabilitation efforts. *Neuromuscular reeducation* using biofeedback relies on the principle that the provision of immediate feedback concerning muscle contractions may help the patient regain muscle control. Small contractions may be below the threshold of awareness, but EMG feedback may bring these contractions into the patient's awareness and thus allow for increased control over the contractions. An example of such a treatment program was presented by Burnside, Tobias, and Bursill (1982). Eleven stroke patients were treated with biofeedback plus typical exercise therapy and eleven matched control patients were treated with exercise therapy alone. All patients exhibited foot-drop, in which the ability to raise the foot is impaired due to paralysis of the anterior-tibialis muscle in the front of the calf of the leg. After six weeks of twice-weekly sessions, the patients receiving the combined treatment showed more improvement in muscle strength than the controls. Although both groups of patients showed initial improvement in range of motion and gait, only the biofeedback group maintained the improvement at a six-week follow-up test.

One of the most impressive features of this study is that spontaneous recovery was highly unlikely to be a significant factor in the improvement. The biofeedback patients had suffered their strokes an average of 4.45 years ago, and the exercise-only patients were an average of 5.2 years poststroke. Burnside et al. (1982) suggested that biofeedback may have enhanced the compliance of the patients with the exercise program by indicating that muscle activity was occurring in presumably "paralyzed" muscles. Thus, biofeedback may have acted as a motivating factor in the treatment program by allowing the patients to see that some change in muscle strength might be possible because the muscles were not completely inactive.

A variety of explanations have been advanced to account for the physiological mechanism underlying this apparent recovery of function in muscles previously thought to be out of the patient's control. It has been suggested that biofeedback may activate neural synapses previously used for functions other than motor commands and/or allow for the development of new movement strategies (Wolf, 1983). Despite the uncertainty as to the mechanism by which biofeedback may improve muscle control, it does appear that EMG biofeedback may make a significant addition to physical-therapy programs for neuromuscular reeducation.

COGNITIVE RETRAINING   Attempts to remediate the cognitive deficits of stroke patients are relatively recent developments. In fact, Diller and Gordon (1981) compared the state of the art to that of aviation pioneers in the early twentieth century, when the major goal was to demonstrate the possibility of flight rather than its cost-effectiveness or speed. Similarly, many cognitive retraining programs are in their infancy and therefore focus more on demonstrating that it is possible to improve cognitive functioning than on specification of the exact methods used or their mechanisms of action. However, a common strategy is to modify the manner in which the stroke victim performs a task so that intact abilities may be substituted for damaged ones.

It would be expected that patients who had suffered a left hemisphere CVA, and thus experienced difficulty with language skills, might be better able to learn new material if they were trained in the use of visual imagery techniques as a substitute for the verbal skills they previously employed. In a test of this hypothesis, Giasparrini and Satz (1979) found that left hemisphere stroke patients with visual imagery training showed a greater improvement in memory ability than similar patients who practiced their memory skills without such training. Similarly, in an early study Fordyce and Jones (1966) reported that patients with left hemisphere damage were better able to learn from pantomime instructions, whereas those with right hemisphere damage were better able to learn from verbal instructions.

A second approach to cognitive retraining has been to encourage patients to use cues to guide performance so they might minimize errors. Impaired visual scanning is particularly amenable to this treatment model. A simple version of this type of program is to have a patient who neglects the right side of the visual field draw a red line down the right margin of a page before reading. The red line may then be used as a cue that the complete line has been read, and comprehension errors due to visual neglect may thus be reduced (Sharpless, 1982).

Another approach to visual deficits involves training individuals in specific scanning patterns in order to minimize their risk of neglecting a portion of their stimulus world. Webster, Jones, Blanton, Gross, Beissel, and Wofford (1984) trained three stroke victims suffering from left-visual-field deficits to consistently scan from left to right and thus decrease their neglect of the stimuli on the left side of their visual field. A moving target and two rows of colored lights were mounted on a large board. The patients were then trained to follow the left to right motion of the moving target with their eyes, then to attend to the patterns in which the colored lights on the board were illuminated. Verbal cues such as "Anchor left" were also included to encourage consistent left to right scanning. Finally, the patients practiced estimating when they passed objects while using their wheelchair, particularly emphasizing objects on the left. Immediate reinforcement was provided in the form of verbal encouragement and discussion of effective and ineffective scanning techniques. Although there were differences between patients in the degree of improvement, improved wheelchair ability and improved visual scanning ability was reported.

Computers have come into increasing use in cognitive retraining programs, particularly because of their advantages in consistency and the opportunity they create for self-paced work at home by patients. Initial case studies have reported significant gains in scores on IQ tests following computer-assisted retraining programs (Bracy, 1983). Computerized treatment programs for aphasia can provide training in identifying the functions of objects and the meaning of words in context, arithmetic skills, and comprehension of paragraphs, among other skills (Katz & Nagy, 1984). Although the computer can offer the opportunity for increased independence, it is important to emphasize that computer-based approaches are dependent on a therapist able to guide and appropriately encourage the patient in counseling sessions during the training program. A summary of a stroke patient's experiences with such a treatment program is presented in Boxed Highlight 8.1. Note the effect of the field cut on both psychological and perceptual functioning and the importance of the interaction between the therapist and patient during a computer-assisted retraining program.

TREATMENT OF PSYCHOSOCIAL PROBLEMS    Although depression and withdrawal from activities is frequently seen after a CVA, the treatment of depression has been referred to as one of the major unmet needs of stroke survivors (Feibel, Berk, & Joynt, 1979). In the study previously noted by Robinson et al. (1984), the investigators did not alter the "usual course of hospital or outpatient treatment" (p. 261). None of the sixty-one stroke patients studied were treated for depression, even though more than 60% had been depressed at some time during the six months of the study.

Because depression in stroke patients has been associated with not returning to normal social activities (Feibel & Springer, 1982), and stroke patients do appear at particular risk for social disability (Labi et al., 1980), a profitable focus for intervention would appear to be attempts to encourage the resumption of normal social activities as soon as practical and to the greatest extent possible in view of any permanent disability. Group treatment, in which stroke patients may get together and share experiences and emotions, has been used for this purpose, but there is relatively little controlled data concerning the effectiveness of these programs (Imes, 1984).

Family relationships may play an important role in the return of a stroke victim to normal social interaction patterns. It has been found that patients living alone were more likely to resume normal activities outside the home than were those living with family members. This relatively surprising finding may be because there is a natural tendency for family members to become overprotective after another member experiences a stroke and thus make it difficult for the patient to return to normal social interactions (Labi et al.,

# A first-person account of a cognitive retraining program

It has been six months since I have cleared the mists from my mind and joined the real world. It is a strange statement, but it is very true. It has been six months since my thinking has become clear enough that I have become a real person again. When I first finished rehabilitation after my stroke, at age twenty-eight, I was told that what I had regained up to that point was all that I would ever have. I could stand with support, but depended upon a wheelchair for mobility. I could not do math, read, or write. It seemed that the whole world was filled with "could nots" and very few "coulds." Although I did not believe this was the way it had to be, no one shared my dreams until I met my therapist who worked with me on Cognitive Retraining.

When I was first tested prior to starting this new type of therapy, I did not believe the test results. I could not comprehend that I was as impaired as the tests showed. Somehow I must have done something wrong, had a bad day, or the technician who gave me the tests must have marked the answers wrong. . . .

. . . When I received my first set of programs, it never occurred to me that they were simple or basic, because to me they were difficult and at times almost impossible to perform. . . . I learned to do the maze and keep the cube within the box. I learned to react to the right light at the right time as fast as I could. I went at it with such great enthusiasm that, at times, I ate only one meal. When my concentration gave out I would lay down

on the floor in front of the T.V. and take a nap. . . .

As my vision and perception slowly improved, the skills began to cross over into the real world. Because things had always been difficult to deal with since my stroke, I had trained to fix my gaze on my knees or my shoes and on absolutely nothing else. Someone would talk to me or the room could catch fire and I would not move my gaze. Yet now things began to look different to me and new things began to intrude into my vision. At that time, it did not occur to me that I was seeing things better or that I had learned to overcome the field cut and was taking more in. That is the way getting better was. At times it did not seem like getting better was better. The more I could do, the more would be expected of me by the people around me and by myself. At times I was not able to cope with this. I was not ready to accept the responsibility. Without the support of my therapist, who answered every call as promptly as possible, always talked calmly, and always reassured me, I do not think I would have made it through this period. He was very patient and never told me I was wrong. He explained how I was not perceiving quite accurately yet and that I was simply misinterpreting my perceptions. It made things easier to accept because now I was being told and I was willing to believe that there were other people who had gone through the same things that I was going through. . . .

Although I cannot pinpoint a specific

*(continued)*

time when things really changed, I found myself wanting to get out more and be a part of the world again. . . .

It was about this time that things really changed. I cannot describe any particulars that happened, it just seemed like all of a sudden I was happy after being sad for so long. For so long I had felt like a person in limbo, like a little girl in a room with adults floating all around her—chattering, moving here and there and ignoring her as she sat placidly in the corner waiting to grow up and be one of them. And all at once I was one of them. There was no particular skill that gave me this confidence. It was just that things had begun to come together. The work, the

time, all began to pay off. I seemed to have all sorts of energy to meet new people and get out. I explored the stores and began to do all my own grocery shopping. I wanted more and more independence. . . .

. . . Without the therapy I am sure that I would be in a nursing home by this time. No matter how determined I was I would not have been able to keep things straight and in order and to keep my mind working logically. People with strokes and other brain injuries do not have to be left in an altered state. I know, I have been there and I remember!

SOURCE: Adapted from "From the patient's point of view" by S. Graham, 1983, *Cognitive Rehabilitation, 1,* pp. 11–12. Copyright © 1983 by B & B Publishing Company. Reprinted by permission.

---

1980). One possible approach to this problem is to work with the family members in family therapy. The family members may then be helped to see that their efforts to "help" the stroke victim may in fact be intensifying the patient's perception that disability prevents a return to being a responsible, independent human being. Watzlawick and Coyne (1980) described a therapy program with one family following this procedure and reported that a formerly inactive and depressed husband returned to much more normal functioning as the family began to reduce its efforts to do everything for the patient.

Another important aspect of the treatment of depression in impaired persons involves helping a patient to see that although she or he may be impaired in some ways, her or his identity as a worthwhile human being includes much more than the lost functioning. It is easy for a paralyzed person to believe that all of his or her being has been rendered useless or destroyed by physical impairment, and psychotherapy stressing that a person is more than physical functioning alone may be helpful. This procedure has been referred to as "containment of the loss" and operates by stressing the limits of the lost functioning and increasing awareness of remaining skills (Dembo, Levitan, & Wright, 1975; Diller & Gordon, 1981).

## Prevention

"Once a thrombotic stroke has developed fully, no therapy so far devised is of any value in restoring the cerebral tissue or its function. *To be effective, therapy must be preventive*" (Mohr et al., 1983, p. 2040, italics in original). As this quotation indicates, the destruction of brain tissue in a stroke is permanent, and although the natural recovery process in conjunction with the therapeutic procedures previously described may result in a return of functioning, this is not a return of the brain tissue to normal. Prevention in CVAs may thus be said to have two levels; the first encompasses prevention of the CVA itself and its consequent damage to the cerebral tissue. Preventive techniques at this level are essentially the same as the preventive techniques for cardiovascular disease in general.

The second stage of prevention involves the avoidance of unnecessary disability and psychosocial deficits following a stroke. Efforts to return stroke victims to independent and active social functioning are thus preventive efforts as well as treatment or rehabilitation efforts. If depression is related to a withdrawal from social interactions, as suggested by the research discussed earlier, then returning an individual to normal activity as quickly as possible may be viewed as a means of preventing the appearance of depressive symptoms. Involvement in an active rehabilitation program may also be a preventive effort. It will be remembered that Alexy and Bracy (1983) reported that the mood ratings of the patients in an active program at a comprehensive rehabilitation center were on the positive side of neutral, and were often attributed to feelings about the rehabilitation program. This contrasts with the 60% frequency of depression reported by Robinson et al. (1984) in patients involved in hospital and outpatient treatment but apparently not in a specialized rehabilitation service. Finally, consider that Gainotti (1972) noted that the depressive reactions they observed in left hemisphere stroke victims were seen chiefly in patients with severe aphasia. Gainotti attributed this depression to the repeated failures in communication the aphasia sufferers experienced. This suggests that cognitive and aphasia retraining programs may also be viewed as preventive efforts as well. Indeed, the case history previously presented clearly indicates the potential effect of improved cognitive functioning on psychosocial well-being.

# Raynaud's Phenomenon

*Raynaud's phenomenon* is a disorder of the cardiovascular system characterized by episodic constriction of the small blood vessels in the hands, feet, and/or the face. As a result of the reduced blood flow, the patient's affected areas feel cold to the touch, often produce pain, and in the most severe cases can become gangrenous (Spittell, 1984). Medical treatment for Raynaud's phenomenon has often proven unsatisfactory (Surwit, Williams, & Shapiro, 1982). However, several self-control strategies developed by psychologists appear to be promising approaches to treatment.

# Biological and Psychophysiological Components

BIOLOGICAL COMPONENTS    The term *Raynaud's disease* refers to the primary form of Raynaud's phenomenon, in which no underlying disease process can be identified (Spittell, 1980). Although the etiology of Raynaud's disease is unknown, it has been suggested that overactivity of the sympathetic nervous system or hypersensitivity to cold in the blood vessels of the extremities are possible causes (Porter & Rivers, 1984). Among patients with Raynaud's disease, the ratio of women to men is approximately 5:1 (Spittell, 1980). The high incidence of Raynaud's disease among women may be related to hormonal factors. Attacks in female patients tend to be more frequent during menstruation and after menopause (Spittell, 1984).

Raynaud's phenomenon may also occur as the result of a variety of medical conditions, including chronic disease (e.g., rheumatoid arthritis, connective tissue disease), injury or operation, and medication side effects (Spittell, 1980). *Secondary Raynaud's phenomenon* is the term used to describe the disorder when an underlying disease or other condition can be identified as the cause. For example, *scleroderma* is a progressive disease affecting the skin and internal organs and involves thickening of the body's connective tissues. Approximately 95% of patients with scleroderma report symptoms of Raynaud's phenomenon (Rodnan, 1979).

During an attack of primary or secondary Raynaud's phenomenon, the arteries, arterioles, and/or capillaries in the affected area constrict and produce a three-stage color change: (1) pallor or a white color of the skin caused by reduced blood flow; (2) cyanosis, a blue color believed to be related to stagnant or slow-moving blood in the vessels; and (3) a red color of the skin due to a rebound state of dilation of the blood vessels (Abramson, 1978). A vasospastic attack may last from minutes to hours and is typically accompanied by unpleasant sensations such as numbness, tingling, tightness, burning, and/or pain (Spittell, 1980). The affected areas usually feel extremely cold and may be slightly swollen. Exposure to cold and/or emotional stress are generally considered to be the factors that precipitate attacks (Surwit et al., 1982).

In advanced stages of Raynaud's phenomenon (primary and secondary), gangrenous ulcers sometimes develop on the tips of the digits (fingers or toes). These lesions may become infected, and amputation of parts of the infected digits may be necessary (Spittell, 1980).

PSYCHOPHYSIOLOGICAL COMPONENTS    Several early studies of patients with Raynaud's phenomenon suggested that emotional factors could precipitate attacks. For example, Mittelmann and Wolff (1939) demonstrated that emotional stress was associated with decreases in the digital (i.e., finger) skin temperatures of normal subjects and patients with Raynaud's phenomenon. Emotional stress was induced by asking subjects to solve cognitive problems, read horrifying literature, or discuss current problems in their life. Mittelmann and Wolff concluded that emotional stress produced an increase in sympathetic nervous system activity that resulted in the finger temperature decreases. In the Raynaud's phenomenon patients, the temperature decreases associated with stress were accompanied by the color changes and pain typical of the disorder. The temperature of the laboratory was also varied in order to see if environmental temperature changes could induce vasospastic attacks in patients with Raynaud's phenomenon. Attacks of the disorder occurred most frequently when both low room temperature and emotional stress were induced. In a subsequent study, Freedman and Ianni (1985) found that both patients with Raynaud's disease and healthy subjects reacted to an imagined stressful scene (being late for an engagement) with decreased finger temperature. However, only the subjects with Raynaud's disease reacted to an imagined snowstorm scene with decreased finger temperature.

# Behavioral, Psychological, and Social Factors

BEHAVIORAL FACTORS   Clinical evidence suggests that several patient behaviors are associated with increased frequency of attacks of primary and secondary Raynaud's phenomenon. Smoking produces vasoconstriction of the arterioles in the extremities and may contribute to the onset of an attack (Abramson, 1978). Patients who are unable to abstain from smoking are typically advised not to smoke in cold environments. The combination of exposure to cold temperatures and smoking may produce severe spasms of peripheral blood vessels in patients with Raynaud's phenomenon.

Exposure to cold temperatures is considered the major precipitant of episodes of primary and secondary Raynaud's phenomenon (Holti, 1982). Patients frequently get attacks when they go outdoors in the cold winter months. Although the frequency of attacks is usually lower in the summer, patients may experience vasoconstrictive episodes even in warm weather when the temperature decreases. Attacks of Raynaud's phenomenon may also occur when patients are exposed to air conditioning, open refrigerators and freezers, or other cold environments.

PSYCHOLOGICAL FACTORS   It has been estimated that a significant percentage of episodes of Raynaud's phenomenon are related to emotional stress (Hunt, 1936). However, only a few investigators have attempted to study this relationship in controlled research. In addition to the early study of Mittelmann and Wolff (1939), Freedman and Ianni (1983) have examined the roles of emotional stress and cold as precipitating factors. Ambulatory monitoring equipment was used to record environmental and finger temperatures and electrocardiograms (EKGs) of patients with Raynaud's disease and patients with Raynaud's phenomenon secondary to scleroderma. All of the subjects wore on their belts cassette players that recorded the physiological data but allowed them to perform their usual daily activities. In addition, the subjects completed ratings of subjective emotional stress every hour. Whenever a Raynaud's attack occurred, they estimated the amount of stress that they were experiencing just before the attack.

The results indicated that significant declines in finger and environmental temperatures accompanied attacks in both groups of patients. About one-third of the attacks of Raynaud's disease, however, were not associated with declines in environmental temperatures. These attacks typically were accompanied by increased stress ratings and rapid heart rates. In contrast, cold environmental temperature alone appeared to provoke most of the attacks of secondary Raynaud's phenomenon. Although the scleroderma patients reported continually elevated stress ratings, their ratings did not tend to increase prior to attacks. Significant increases in heart rate during the majority of attacks were demonstrated by scleroderma patients. Figure 8.2 illustrates these results graphically. Freedman and Ianni (1983) concluded that the vasospastic attacks of Raynaud's disease are precipitated by cold or emotional stress or both. For patients with Raynaud's phenomenon secondary to scleroderma, exposure to cold may be the only precipitating factor for the majority of attacks.

SOCIAL FACTORS   Several sociodemographic variables have been associated with an increased incidence of Raynaud's disease and phenomenon. As discussed previously, Raynaud's disease occurs more often in women than in men. In addition to sex, age appears to be related to the onset of Raynaud's disease. It has been estimated that this disorder in its mildest forms affects approximately 15%–20% of samples of young people (Lewis, 1949; Holti, 1982). Moreover, the disorder tends to begin in the first and second decades of life, with most cases developing before age 40. Cases that develop in the fifth or sixth decade of life tend to be cases of Raynaud's phenomenon associated with chronic disease or other medical conditions (Spittell, 1980).

Certain occupations appear to put people at risk for the development of secondary Raynaud's phenomenon. *Occupational Raynaud's phenomenon* has occurred among workers who regularly use pneumatic and vibrating tools or whose jobs require frequent squeezing or hand pressure on tools, machines, or other objects (Spittell, 1980; Taylor, 1974). Mechanics, chain-saw operators, farmers, typists, and pianists are some of the workers who may be affected by occupational Raynaud's phenomenon. Repetitive vibration and percussion appear to be factors related to the onset of the disorder in these workers.

## Psychological and Behavioral Reactions

Raynaud's phenomenon may produce negative psychological and behavioral reactions in patients' lives. The sensory changes (e.g., numbness, tingling) and pain associated with the vasospastic attacks are anxiety arousing for many patients. They may worry about the meaning of the symptoms and the possibility of developing complications of the disorder (Spittell, 1980). Indeed,

Scleroderma          Raynaud's disease

———— Finger            ———— Finger

— — — Ambient          — — — Ambient

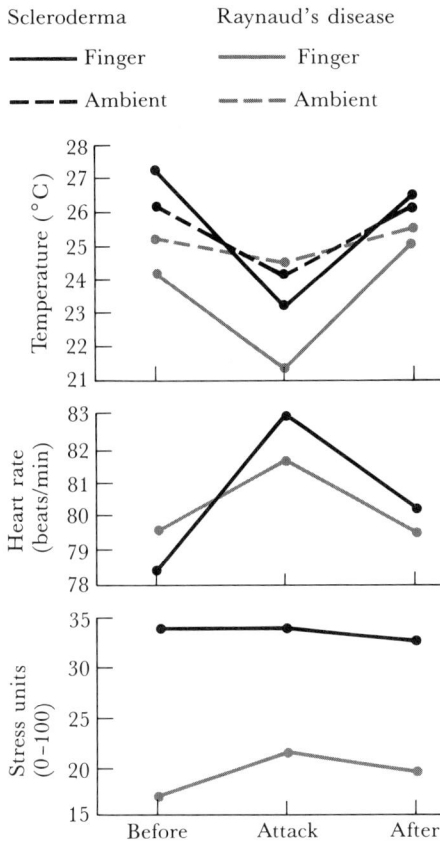

FIGURE 8.2   Finger temperature, ambient temperature, heart rate, and stress ratings for scleroderma and Raynaud's disease patients. Measurements were taken before, during, and after vasospastic attacks. The data suggest that vasospastic effects for Raynaud's patients may be precipitated by cold and/or emotional stress, whereas attacks in scleroderma patients are precipitated only by cold. From "Role of Cold and Emotional Stress in Raynaud's Disease and Scleroderma" by R. R. Freedman and P. Ianni, 1983, *British Medical Journal, 287* p. 1501. Reprinted by permission.

Freedman and Ianni (1983) found that patients with primary and secondary Raynaud's phenomenon reported higher levels of daily stress than normal subjects. Moreover, when the fingers are involved, patients may have difficulty performing simple tasks with the hands during an attack (Wise, Delp, & Willis, 1983). In short, the discomfort, anxiety, and decreased manual dexterity associated with Raynaud's attacks can disrupt patients' lives.

The need to avoid cold environments can also interfere with patients' daily activities and produce behavioral changes. Patients may be reluctant to go outside in cold weather and often need to wear warm clothing even in mild climates. Some patients even have to wear gloves or mittens prior to opening freezers or refrigerators. Patients with advanced cases of Raynaud's phenomenon may be advised to move to a warm climate (Abramson, 1978). This geographical cure is not always successful, however. Decreases in environmental temperature, as well as emotional stress, can precipitate attacks even in warm climates.

Patients with advanced cases of primary or secondary Raynaud's phenomenon face the possibility of developing ulcers and/or gangrene in affected areas. These lesions can be very painful and, in extreme cases, may lead to amputation of parts of fingers or toes (Spittell, 1980). Patients who require amputations may react to the loss and the change in body image with feelings of depression, anxiety, and/or reduced self-esteem.

In cases of occupational Raynaud's phenomenon, patients may be forced to quit their jobs and seek alternative employment (Taylor, 1974). Such job changes can be psychologically as well as financially stressful and require considerable adjustment. Patients with Raynaud's phenomenon secondary to chronic diseases such as scleroderma or rheumatoid arthritis face adjustment problems related to their chronic diseases as well as to the Raynaud's attacks (see Chapter 12).

## Treatment Interventions

Medical treatment for Raynaud's phenomenon is often based on the use of vasodilator drugs to prevent constriction of blood vessels in the affected areas (Surwit et al., 1982). Unfortunately, these drugs frequently have negative side effects (e.g., gastrointestinal disturbance) and may not reduce the frequency of vasospastic attacks (Holti, 1982). In recent years, psychological treatments such as biofeedback and autogenic training have been employed successfully with Raynaud's phenomenon patients.

In *biofeedback therapy*, patients receive information about bodily processes and learn how to control these processes. As research with normal subjects has demonstrated that biofeedback therapy can be used to teach control of peripheral blood flow (e.g., Keefe, 1978), a number of investigators have used biofeedback to teach patients with Raynaud's phenomenon to control peripheral blood flow in affected areas. Patients with primary or secondary Raynaud's phenomenon have received feedback about skin temperature or blood volume in order to learn how to increase blood flow in the affected areas.

In addition to biofeedback therapy, autogenic training and relaxation therapy have been used to treat patients with Raynaud's phenomenon. *Autogenic training* is a psychophysiologic therapy in which the patient passively concentrates on autogenic formulas or phrases (e.g., "I am calm and quiet; my heartbeat is calm and regular"). Through this passive concentration, the patient experiences a state of relaxation and attempts to regulate bodily functions such as heart rate (Schultz & Luthe, 1959). Autogenic training has been used to reduce excessive sympathetic nervous system activity associated with stress-related disorders (Brenneke, 1981). With Raynaud's patients, autogenic formulas that suggest feelings of heaviness and warmth have been used in an attempt to increase blood flow to the affected areas. Relaxation therapy with Raynaud's patients has usually consisted of a modified form of Jacobson's (1964) progressive relaxation exercises. Relaxation training has been employed in order to reduce sympathetic nervous system activity that may be related to the onset of vasospastic attacks (Surwit et al., 1982).

Early case studies with Raynaud's disease patients suggested that finger-temperature or blood-volume biofeedback could help to reduce the frequency and severity of patients' attacks (e.g., Blanchard & Haynes, 1975). In one of the first controlled group studies with Raynaud's disease patients, Keefe, Surwit, and Pilon (1980) compared the effectiveness of autogenic training, a combination of autogenic training and finger-temperature biofeedback, and progressive muscle relaxation. Patients in the autogenic and autogenic plus biofeedback groups were given a cassette of tape-recorded autogenic suggestions focusing on feelings of heaviness and warmth. Patients in the autogenic plus biofeedback group were also given portable temperature-biofeedback units that provided audio and visual feedback of skin temperature changes as small as .01°C. The patients were instructed to use the units to monitor finger temperature during daily home practice sessions with the autogenic cassette tape. In the progressive relaxation training group, the patients received training in progressive muscle relaxation exercises. They were given a cassette tape containing the relaxation instructions and were asked to practice regularly at home.

The effectiveness of the self-control therapies was evaluated with laboratory cold-stress tests during which patients were instructed to maintain finger temperature while the temperature of the laboratory was gradually decreased. The cold-stress tests were given prior to treatment and during the first, third, and fifth weeks of training. The results indicated that patients in all three groups significantly improved their ability to maintain finger temperature during the cold-stress test by the fifth week of treatment. There were no significant differences between groups in their temperature-control skills.

During the study, patients kept home records of the number of vasospastic attacks per day. Analysis of these self-report data revealed that patients in the autogenic and relaxation training groups reported a significant decrease in the frequency of attacks from pre- to posttreatment that was maintained at a four-week follow-up. Patients in the autogenic plus biofeedback group also reported a reduction in the frequency of attacks that failed to reach statistical significance. However, these patients reported fewer attacks at pretreatment than patients in the autogenic and relaxation training groups. Thus, the low frequency of attacks at pretreatment in the autogenic plus biofeedback group made it difficult for this group to demonstrate a significant reduction in the frequency of attacks following treatment. Keefe et al. (1980) concluded that autogenic and relaxation training are simple, economical techniques that are as effective as biofeedback therapy in the treatment of Raynaud's disease.

Recent work by Freedman and colleagues (Freedman, Ianni, & Wenig, 1983), however, has suggested that skin-temperature biofeedback treatment alone (i.e., not in combination with autogenic training) may be more beneficial for Raynaud's disease patients than other self-control therapies. Thirty-two patients with Raynaud's disease were randomly assigned to one of four groups: (1) finger-temperature biofeedback (2) finger-temperature biofeedback under cold stress, (3) frontalis electromyographic (EMG) biofeedback, and (4) autogenic training. All patients received ten training sessions. Patients in the two temperature biofeedback groups were taught to raise the skin temperature of the middle finger of their dominant hands using audio feedback.

In the last five training sessions, patients in the biofeedback under cold stress group were asked to maintain finger temperature while their middle fingers rested on a cold stimulus. In the EMG biofeedback group, subjects were taught to lower muscle tension levels in the frontalis muscle using audio feedback. The autogenic training subjects listened to tape-recorded instructions similar to those of Keefe et al. (1980).

Patients in the finger-temperature biofeedback group demonstrated significant finger temperature increases during training sessions. Although patients in the biofeedback under cold stress group did not raise the temperature of the middle finger that was exposed to the cold stimulus, they did significantly raise the temperature of the nondominant hand during training. In contrast, the finger temperatures of the autogenic and EMG biofeedback groups tended to decline during training sessions. In a posttreatment voluntary control session during which subjects were asked to increase finger temperature without feedback, only the finger-temperature biofeedback group could significantly increase finger temperature.

In a voluntary follow-up control test one year after treatment, both the finger-temperature biofeedback and biofeedback under cold stress groups demonstrated significant finger-temperature increases whereas the EMG and autogenic groups showed significant temperature declines. Figure 8.3 shows that the biofeedback under cold stress group produced a greater finger-temperature increase than that of the finger-temperature biofeedback group. The temperature-control skills of the temperature biofeedback groups were associated with significant reductions in the frequency of vasospastic attacks. As compared to pretreatment, the two temperature biofeedback groups reported significantly fewer attacks during the five coldest months of the one-year follow-up period. Moreover, the biofeedback under cold stress group demonstrated a greater reduction in the frequency of attacks than the temperature biofeedback group. In contrast, the autogenic and EMG groups reported significantly fewer attacks as compared to pretreatment only during the month of October. During an additional two-year follow-up period, the two temperature biofeedback groups continued to report a reduced frequency of attacks (Freedman, Ianni, & Wenig, 1985).

Freedman et al. (1983) concluded that temperature biofeedback is a more effective treatment for Raynaud's disease patients than autogenic training or EMG biofeedback. Moreover, the addition of training under cold stress to temperature biofeedback appeared to improve patients' retention of their temperature-control skills. The efficacy of the temperature biofeedback training could not be attributed to decreased sympathetic nervous system activity because patients in the temperature biofeedback groups demonstrated significant increases in heart rate during training sessions. Freedman et al. (1988) indicated that a vasodilating mechanism in the finger activated by temperature biofeedback may explain increased digital blood flow in the absence of the decreased sympathetic activity associated with relaxation and autogenic training.

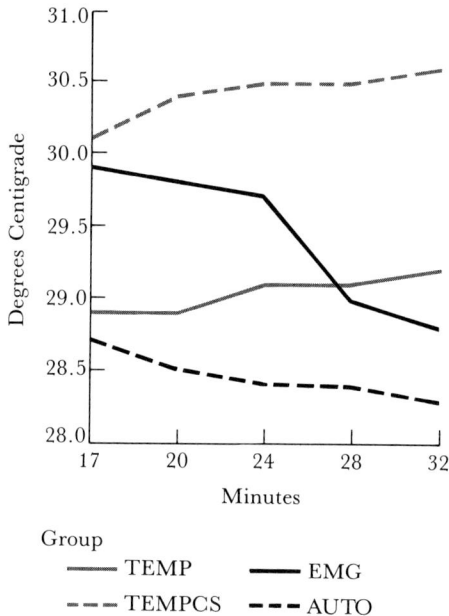

FIGURE 8.3  Finger temperatures of Raynaud's patients during a voluntary control test one year after treatment. The patients who were treated with finger temperature biofeedback while under cold stress were best able to increase finger temperatures. From "Behavioral Treatment of Raynaud's Disease" by R. R. Freedman, P. Ianni, and P. Wenig, 1983. *Journal of Consulting and Clinical Psychology. 51,* p. 544. Copyright (1983) by the America Psychological Association. Reprinted by permission.

*Classical conditioning therapy* also has been used as an effective treatment for Raynaud's disease (Jobe, Sampson, Roberts, & Kelly, 1986). This therapy consists of frequent immersions of both hands in warm water coupled with whole-body exposure to cold air in the treatment room. The warm water is the unconditioned stimulus leading to the unconditioned response of vasodilation in the hands. After repeated trials, the cold air in the room becomes the conditioned stimulus that will produce the conditioned response of vasodilation in the hands (see Chapter 4 for further discussion of classical conditioning). In a recent study, classical conditioning was compared to biofeedback therapy as a treatment for Raynaud's disease (Jobe et al., 1986). The results demonstrated that both treatments significantly increased finger temperature response to cold, with no major differences between treatment groups. As the biofeedback treatment included relaxation training, the effects of biofeedback alone were not determined.

Skin-temperature biofeedback has also been used to treat Raynaud's phenomenon secondary to chronic disease. Several case studies have demonstrated that patients with secondary Raynaud's phenomenon can learn to increase finger temperature and subsequently have fewer vasospastic attacks (Adair & Theobald, 1978: Keefe, Surwit, & Pilon, 1981; Stambrook, Hamel, & Carter, 1988). In one controlled study, patients with Raynaud's phenomenon secondary to scleroderma were randomly assigned to either finger-temperature biofeedback, EMG biofeedback, or autogenic training groups (Freedman, Ianni, & Wenig, 1984). The treatment procedures were identical to those used in the study with Raynaud's disease patients discussed previously (Freedman et al., 1983). Only the patients receiving finger-temperature biofeedback demonstrated significant increases in finger temperature during training and during a posttraining test of voluntary control without feedback. Unfortunately, none of the three treatment groups reported significant decreases in the frequency of vasospastic attacks during the year following treatment. Thus, alternative treatment procedures may be necessary for many patients with secondary Raynaud's phenomenon. One study demonstrated that a combination of vasodilator medication and autogenic training successfully reduced the frequency of reported vasospastic attacks in scleroderma patients (Surwit, Allen, Gilgor, & Duvic, 1982).

# *Summary*

Coronary heart disease most commonly results from atherosclerosis. Atherosclerosis is a form of arteriosclerosis and involves a reduction in blood flow and a decrease in the elasticity of artery walls as a result of plaque formation. A heart attack, or myocardial infarction, occurs when blood flow to the myocardium is totally blocked and heart muscle dies.

Risk factors for coronary heart disease include hypertension (blood pressure greater than 140/90 mm Hg), high levels of cholesterol (greater than 200 mg/dl), and cigarette smoking. Diet and exercise can improve blood pressure and cholesterol status. The Type A behavior pattern, a consistent form of behavior involving high levels of competition and time pressure related to attempts to maintain control, has been associated with CHD. Hostility, anger, and other negative emotions are also risk factors for CHD and may be the emotional states underlying TABP that carry the greatest risk for the development of heart disease.

Reactions to a myocardial infarction include depression and denial, and some patients experience cardiac neurosis, or an excessive fear of another heart attack. These reactions may be dealt with through psychological counseling. Cardiac rehabilitation programs, including exercise, education about CHD, and suggestions for life-style changes such as dietary changes and stopping smoking, may also be helpful. Programs in which patients participate in their own treatment as much as possible appear particularly promising.

CHD risk factors have been modified in individual programs that include education and behavior modification. Blood pressure has been lowered with relaxation training, and some programs have modified Type A behavior by training patients in stress management techniques. Suggestions for reducing hostility and anger are also available, although they have not as yet been experimentally tested. Community-based projects have successfully altered risk for CHD on a large scale by relying on mass media campaigns and community activities for education and behavior-change suggestions.

Cerebrovascular accidents are serious medical events resulting from abnormalities in blood flow in the brain. Although more stroke victims are surviving as a result of improved medical treatment, stroke still ranks as the third leading cause of death in the United States. Some degree of disability is frequently seen following a stroke; the disability may include sensory, perceptual, motor, language, and/or psychological functioning, dependent on the location and magnitude of the brain damage the stroke causes.

Treatment of the aftereffects of a CVA varies according to the nature of the dysfunction seen. Physical therapy, sometimes assisted by EMG biofeedback, may be employed to treat motor difficulties. Language and cognitive impairment are receiving increasing attention in cognitive retraining programs, sometimes employing computer assistance. Depression is not always related to degree of neurological damage, but it is sometimes related to social withdrawal and has been approached with group and family therapy. Persons receiving comprehensive rehabilitation may suffer less from depression than those receiving only standard medical intervention. Some stroke victims may deny the presence of physical disability or totally neglect impaired extremities.

The prevention of strokes and other cardiovascular diseases is essentially identical. However, the rehabilitation of the disabling aftereffects of stroke may be viewed as efforts to prevent continuing disability and psychological distress. Many rehabilitation approaches are still quite new and require additional research to demonstrate their effectiveness and to specify their active ingredients. However, psychological preventive and treatment efforts hold particular promise in the areas of life-style change for prevention of cardiovascular disease, neuromuscular reeducation, cognitive retraining, and the treatment of psychosocial impairment following stroke.

Raynaud's phenomenon is a disorder of the cardiovascular system characterized by episodic spasms of the small blood vessels in the hands, feet, and/or the face. Raynaud's disease is the primary form of Raynaud's phenomenon in which no underlying disease or etiology for the disorder can be found. In secondary Raynaud's phenomenon, an underlying disease or other condition is the cause of the disorder. Exposure to cold temperatures is the major precipitant of episodes of primary and secondary Raynaud's phenomenon. Several studies have demonstrated that emotional stress also can precipitate attacks of primary Raynaud's phenomenon. Cigarette smoking has been associated with increased frequency of episodes of primary and secondary Raynaud's phenomenon.

Psychological treatments such as temperature biofeedback, autogenic training, relaxation therapy, and classical conditioning appear to be beneficial treatments for Raynaud's disease patients. There is some evidence that skin temperature biofeedback is more effective than autogenic training and EMG biofeedback in reducing the long-term frequency of attacks in Raynaud's disease. For most patients with secondary Raynaud's phenomenon, a combination of pharmacologic and self-control therapies may be necessary to significantly affect the vasospastic symptoms.

# References

ABRAMSON, D. I. (1978). *Circulatory diseases of the limbs: A primer*. New York: Grune & Stratton.

ADAIR, J. R., & THEOBALD, D. E. (1978). Raynaud's phenomenon: Treatment of a severe case with biofeedback. *Journal of the Indiana State Medical Association, 71*, 990–993.

ALEXY, W., & BRACY, O. (1983). Mood self-ratings and attributions among physical rehabilitation inpatients. *Cognitive Rehabilitation, 1*, 12–17.

BAREFOOT, J. C., DAHLSTROM, W. G., & WILLIAMS, R. B. (1983). Hostility, CHD incidence, and total mortality: A 25-year follow-up study of 255 physicians. *Psychosomatic Medicine, 245*, 59–63.

BLACKBURN, H., & JACOBS, D. (1984). Sources of the diet-heart controversy: Confusion over population vs. individual correlations. *Circulation, 70*, 775–780.

BLANCHARD, E. B., & HAYNES, M. R. (1975). Biofeedback treatment of a case of Raynaud's disease. *Journal of Behavior Therapy and Experimental Psychiatry, 6*, 230–234.

BLOOM, F. E., LAZERSON, A., & HOFSTADTER, L. (1985). *Brain, mind, and behavior*. New York: Freeman.

BLUMENTHAL, J. A., & MAU, H. S. (1987). Psychologic considerations in coronary artery disease. In K. G. Andreoli, D. P. Zipes, A. G. Wallace, M. R. Kinney, & V. K. Fowkes (Eds.), *Comprehensive cardiac care* (6th ed.) (pp. 385-398). St. Louis: Mosby.

BOOTH-KEWLEY, S., & FRIEDMAN, H. S. (1987). Psychological predictors of heart disease: A quantitative review. *Psychological Bulletin, 101*, 343-362.

BOSLEY, F., & ALLEN, T. W. (1989). Stress management training for hypertensives: Cognitive and physiological effects. *Journal of Behavioral Medicine, 12*, 77–90.

BRACY, O. (1983). Computer based cognitive rehabilitation. *Cognitive Rehabilitation, 1*, 7–8, 18.

BRADSHAW, J. L., & NETTLETON, N. C. (1983). *Human cerebral asymmetry*. Englewood Cliffs, NJ: Prentice-Hall.

BRENNEKE, H. F. (1981). Autogenic training. In R. J. Corsini (Ed.), *Handbook of innovative psychotherapies*. New York: Wiley.

BURNSIDE, I. G., TOBIAS, H. S., & BURSILL, D. (1982). Electromyographic feedback in the remobilization of stroke patients: A controlled trial. *Archives of Physical Medicine and Rehabilitation, 63*, 217–222.

CHESNEY, M. A., EAGLESTON, J. R., & ROSENMAN, R. H. (1981). Type A behavior: Assessment and intervention. In C. K. Prokop & L. A. Bradley ( Eds.), *Medical psychology: Contributions to behavioral medicine* (pp. 19–36). New York: Academic Press.

CROWTHER, J. H. (1983). Stress management training and relaxation imagery in the treatment of essential hypertension. *Journal of Behavioral Medicine, 6*, 169–187.

DEMBO, T., LEVITAN, G., & WRIGHT, B. (1975). Adjustment to misfortune—A problem of social psychological rehabilitation. *Rehabilitation Psychology, 22*, 1–100.

DEMBROSKI, T. M., & COSTA, P. T., JR. (1987). Coronary prone behavior. Components of the Type A pattern and hostility. *Journal of Personality, 55*, 211–236.

DILLER, L., & GORDON, W. A. (1981). Interventions for cognitive deficits in brain-injured adults. *Journal of Consulting and Clinical Psychology, 49*, 822–834.

FARQUHAR, J. W. (1983). Community approaches to risk factor reduction: The Stanford project. In J. A. Herd & S. M. Weiss (Eds.), *Behavior and arteriosclerosis* (pp. 143–148). New York: Plenum.

FEIBEL, J. A., BERK, S., & JOYNT, R. M. (1979). The unmet needs of stroke survivors. *Neurology, 29,* 592.

FEIBEL, J. A., & SPRINGER, C. J. (1982). Depression and failure to resume social activities after stroke. *Archives of Physical Medicine and Rehabilitation, 63,* 276–278.

FOLLICK, M. J., GORKIN, L., SMITH, T. W., CAPONE, R. J., VISCO, J., & STABLEIN, D. (1988). Quality of life post-myocardial infarction: Effects of a transtelephonic coronary intervention system. *Health Psychology, 7,* 169–182.

FORDYCE, W. E., & JONES, R. H. (1966). The efficacy of oral and pantomime instructions for hemiplegic patients. *Archives of Physical Medicine and Rehabilitation, 47,* 676–682.

FREEDMAN, R. R., & IANNI, P. (1983). Role of cold and emotional stress in Raynaud's disease and scleroderma. *British Medical Journal, 287,* 1499–1502.

FREEDMAN, R. R., & IANNI, P. (1985). Effects of general and thematically relevant stressors in Raynaud's disease. *Journal of Psychosomatic Research, 29,* 275–280.

FREEDMAN, R. R., IANNI, P., & WENIG, P. (1983). Behavioral treatment of Raynaud's disease. *Journal of Consulting and Clinical Psychology, 51,* 539–549.

FREEDMAN, R. R., IANNI, P., & WENIG, P. (1984). Behavioral treatment of Raynaud's phenomenon in scleroderma. *Journal of Behavioral Medicine, 7,* 341–351.

FREEDMAN, R. R., IANNI, P., & WENIG, P. (1985). Behavioral treatment of Raynaud's disease. Long-term follow-up. *Journal of Consulting and Clinical Psychology, 53,* 136.

FREEDMAN, R. R., SABHARWAL, S., IANNI, P., DESAI, N., WENIG, P., & MAYES, M. (1988). Non-neural beta-adrenergic vasodilating mechanism in temperature biofeedback. *Psychosomatic Medicine, 50,* 394–401.

FRIEDMAN, H. S., & BOOTH-KEWLEY, S. (1988). Validity of the Type A construct: A reprise. *Psychological Bulletin, 104,* 381–384.

FRIEDMAN, M., & ROSENMAN, R. H. (1959). Association of a specific overt behavior pattern with increases in blood cholesterol, blood clotting time, incidence of arcus senilis and clinical coronary artery disease. *Journal of the American Medical Association, 2169,* 1286–1296.

FRIEDMAN, M., & ULMER, D. (1984). *Treating Type A behavior—and your heart.* New York: Knopf

GAINOTTI, G. (1972). Emotional behavior and hemispheric side of the lesion. *Cortex, 8,* 41–55.

GATCHEL, R. J., GAFFNEY, F. A., & SMITH, J. E. (1986). Comparative efficacy of behavioral stress management versus propanolol in reducing psychophysiological reactivity in post-myocardial infarction patients. *Journal of Behavioral Medicine, 9,* 503–513.

GIASPARRINI, B., & SATZ, P. (1979). A treatment for memory problems in left hemisphere CVA patients. *Journal of Clinical Neuropsychology, 1,* 137–151.

GRAHAM, S. (1983). From the patient's point of view. *Cognitive Rehabilitation, 1,* 11–12.

HARTLEY, L. H. (1983). Post myocardial infarction. In J. A. Herd & S. M. Weiss (Eds.), *Behavior and arteriosclerosis* (pp. 111–116). New York: Plenum.

HASKELL, W. L. (1984). Overview: Health benefits of exercise. In J. D. Matarazzo, Sharlene M. Weiss, J. A. Herd, N. E. Miller, & Stephen M. Weiss (Eds.), *Behavioral health* (pp. 409–423). New York: Wiley.

HAVIK, O. E., & MAELAND, J. G. (1988). Changes in smoking behavior after a myocardial infarction. *Health Psychology, 7,* 403–420.

HEARN, M. D., MURRAY, D. M., & LUEPKER, R. V. (1989). Hostility, coronary heart disease, and total mortality: A 33-year follow-up study of university students. *Journal of Behavioral Medicine, 12,* 105–121.

HERD, J. A. (1981). Treatment of cardiovascular disorders. In C. K. Prokop & L. A. Bradley (Eds.), *Medical psychology: Contributions to behavioral medicine* (pp. 141–156). New York: Academic Press.

HEYMAN, A., BURCH, J. G., ROSATI, R., HAYNES, C., & UTLEY, C. (1979). Use of a computerized information system in the management of patients with transient cerebral ischemia. *Neurology, 29,* 214–221.

HEYMAN, A., WILKINSON, W. E., HURWITZ, B. J., HAYNES, C. S., UTLEY, C. M., ROSATI, R. A., BURCH, J. G., & GORE, T. B. (1984). Risk of ischemic heart disease in patients with TIA. *Neurology, 34,* 626–630.

HILLBORN, M., & KASTE, M. (1981). Ethanol intoxication: A risk factor for ischemic brain infarction in adolescents and young adults. *Stroke, 12,* 422–425.

HOLBROOK, J. H., GRUNDY, S. M., HENNEKENS, C. H., KANNEL, W. B., & STRONG, J. P. (1984). Cigarette smoking and cardiovascular diseases. *Circulation, 70,* 1114A–1117A.

HOLTI, G. (1982). Raynaud's phenomenon. *Advances in Microcirculation, 10,* 1–16.

HUNT, J. H. (1936). The Raynaud phenomena: A critical review. *Quarterly Journal of Medicine, 5,* 399–444.

IMES, C. (1984). Interventions with stroke patients: EMG biofeedback, group activities, cognitive retraining. *Cognitive Rehabilitation, 2,* 4–17.

JACOBSON, E. (1964). *Anxiety and tension control: A physiologic approach.* Philadelphia: Lippincott.

JARVIS, M. (1984). Gender and smoking: Do women really find it harder to give up? *British Journal of Addiction, 79,* 383–387.

JENKINS, C. D. (1988). Epidemiology of cardiovascular diseases. *Journal of Consulting and Clinical Psychology, 56,* 324–332.

JOBE, J. B., SAMPSON, J. B., ROBERTS, D. E., & KELLY, J. A. (1986). Comparison of behavioral treatments for Raynaud's disease. *Journal of Behavioral Medicine, 9,* 89–96.

KANNEL, W. B. (1983). An overview of the risk factors for cardiovascular disease. In N. M. Kaplan & J. Stamler (Eds.), *Prevention of coronary heart disease: Practical management of the risk factors* (pp. 1–19). Philadelphia: Saunders.

KANNEL, W. B., & GORDON, T. (1979). Physiological and medical concomitants of obesity: The Framingham study. In G. A. Bray (Ed.), *Obesity in America* (pp. 125–153) (DHEW Publication No. NIH 79-359). Washington, DC: U. S. Government Printing Office.

KATZ, R., & NAGY, V. T. (1984). CATS: Computerized aphasia treatment system. *Cognitive Rehabilitation, 2,* 8–11.

KEEFE, F. J. (1978). Biofeedback vs. instructional control of skin temperature. *Journal of Behavioral Medicine, 1,* 323–335.

KEEFE, F. J., SURWIT, R. S., & PILON, R. N. (1980). Biofeedback, autogenic training, and progressive relaxation in the treatment of Raynaud's disease: A comparative study. *Journal of Applied Behavior Analysis, 13,* 3–11.

KEEFE, F. J., SURWIT, R. S., & PILON, R. N. (1981). Collagen vascular disease: Can behavior therapy help? *Journal of Behavior Therapy and Experimental Psychiatry, 12,* 171–175.

KISTLER, J. P., ROPPER, A. H., & MARTIN, J. B. (1987). Cerebrovascular accidents. In E. Braunwald, K. J. Isselbacher, R. G. Petersdorf, J. D. Wilson, J. B. Martin, & A. S. Fauci (Eds.), *Harrison's principles of internal medicine* (11th ed.) (pp. 1930–1960). New York: McGraw-Hill.

KRANTZ, D. S., CONTRADA, R. J., HILL, R. D., & FRIEDLER, E. (1988). Environmental stress and biobehavioral antecedents of coronary heart disease. *Journal of Consulting and Clinical Psychology, 56,* 333–341.

LABI, M. L. C., PHILLIPS, T. F., & GRESHAM, G. E. (1980). Psychosocial disability in physically restored long-term stroke survivors. *Archives of Physical Medicine and Rehabilitation, 61,* 561–565.

LEON, G. R., FINN, S. E., MURRAY, D., & BAILEY, J. M. (1988). Inability to predict cardiovascular disease from hostility scores or MMPI items related to Type A behavior. *Journal of Consulting and Clinical Psychology, 56,* 597–600.

LEWIS, T. (1949). *Vascular disorders of the limbs: Described for practitioners and students.* London: Macmillan.

LIND, K. (1982). A synthesis of studies on stroke rehabilitation. *Journal of Chronic Disease, 35,* 133–149.

LOVIBOND, S. H., BIRRELL, P. C., & LANGELUDDECKE, P. (1986). Changing coronary heart disease risk factor status: The effects of three behavioral programs. *Journal of Behavioral Medicine, 9,* 415–438.

MacDOUGALL, J. M., DEMBROSKI, T. M., DIMSDALE, J. E., & HACKETT, T. P. (1985). Components of Type A, hostility, and anger-in: Further relationships to angiographic findings. *Health Psychology, 4,* 137–152.

McDOWELL, F. H. (1979). Cerebrovascular diseases. In P. B. Beeson, W. McDermott, & J. B. Wyngaarden (Eds.), *Cecil textbook of medicine* (15th ed.) (pp. 777–801). Philadelphia: Saunders.

MANUCK, S. B., KAPLAN, J. R., ADAMS, M. R., & CLARKSON, T. B. (1988). Studies of psychosocial influences on coronary artery atherogenesis in cynomolgus monkeys. *Health Psychology, 7,* 113–125.

MITTELMANN, B., & WOLFF, H. G. (1939). Affective states and skin temperature: Experimental study of subjects with "cold hands" and Raynaud's syndrome. *Psychosomatic Medicine, 1,* 271–292.

MOHR, J. P., KASE, C. S., & ADAMS, R. D. (1983). Cerebrovascular disease, In R. G. Petersdorf, R. D. Adams, E. Braunwald, K. J. Isselbacher, J. B. Martin, & J. D. Wilson (Eds.), *Harrison's principles of internal medicine* (10th ed.) (pp. 2028–2060). New York: McGraw-Hill.

NATIONAL INSTITUTES OF HEALTH. (1984). Lowering blood cholesterol: National Institutes of Health Consensus Development Statement. *Journal of the American Dietetic Association, 85,* 586–588.

PATEL, C. (1984). A relaxation-centered behavioral package for reducing hypertension. In J. D. Matarazzo, Sharlene M. Weiss, J. A. Herd, N. E. Miller, & Stephen M. Weiss (Eds.), *Behavioral health* (pp. 846–861). New York: Wiley.

PELL, S., & FAYERWEATHER, W. E. (1985). Trends in the incidence of myocardial infarction and associated mortality and morbidity in a large employed population, 1957–1983. *New England Journal of Medicine, 312,* 1005–1011.

PORTER, J. M., & RIVERS, S. P. (1984). Management of Raynaud's syndrome. In J. J. Bergan & J. S. T. Yao (Eds.), *Evaluation and treatment of upper and lower extremity circulatory disorders.* Orlando, FL: Grune & Stratton.

PUSKA, P. (1984). Community based prevention of cardiovascular disease: The North Karelia Project. In J. D. Matarazzo, Sharlene M. Weiss, J. A. Herd, N. E. Miller, & Stephen M. Weiss, (Eds.), *Behavioral health* (pp. 1140–1147). New York: Wiley.

ROBINSON, R. G., & PRICE, T. R. (1982). Post-stroke depressive disorders: A follow-up study of 103 patients. *Stroke, 13,* 635–641.

ROBINSON, R. G., STARR, L. B., KUBOS, K. L., & PRICE, T. R. (1983). A two-year longitudinal study of post-stroke mood disorders: Findings during the initial evaluation. *Stroke, 14,* 736–741.

ROBINSON, R. G., STARR, L. B., & PRICE, T. R. (1984). A two year longitudinal study of mood disorders following stroke: Prevalence and duration at six months follow-up. *British Journal of Psychiatry, 144,* 256–262.

RODNAN, G. (1979). Progressive systemic sclerosis (scleroderma). In D. McCarty (Ed.), *Arthritis and allied conditions.* Philadelphia: Lea and Febiger.

ROSENMAN, R. H. (1986). Current and past history of Type A behavior pattern. In T. H. Schmidt, T. M. Dembroski, & G. Blumchen (Eds.), *Biological and psychological factors in cardiovascular disease* (pp. 15–40). New York: Springer-Verlag.

ROSKIES, E., SERAGANIAN, P., OSEASOHN, R., HANLEY, J. A., COLLU, R., MARTIN, N., & SMILGA, C. (1986). The Montreal Type A Intervention Project: Major findings. *Health Psychology, 5,* 45–70.

SHARPLESS, J. W. (1982). *Mossman's a problem-oriented approach to stroke rehabilitation* (2nd ed). Springfield, IL: Charles Thomas.

SCHULTZ, J. H., & LUTHE, W. (1959). *Autogenic methods.* New York: Grune & Stratton.

SPITTELL, J. A., JR. (1980). Raynaud's phenomenon and allied vasospastic disorders. In J. L. Juergens, J. A. Spittell, J. F. Fairbairn (Eds.), *Allen-Barker-Hines Peripheral Vascular Diseases* (5th ed.). Philadelphia: Saunders.

SPITTELL, J. A., JR. (1984). The vasospastic disorders. *Current Problems in Cardiology, 8,* 1–27.

STAMBROOK, M., HAMEL, E. R., & CARTER, S. A. (1988). Training to vasodilate in a cooling environment: A valid treatment for Raynaud's phenomenon? *Biofeedback and Self-Regulation, 13,* 9–23.

SURWIT, R. S., ALLEN, L. M., GILGOR, R. S., & DUVIC, M. (1982). The combined effect of prazosin and autogenic training on cold reactivity in Raynaud's phenomenon. *Biofeedback and Self-Regulation, 7,* 537–544.

SURWIT, R. S., WILLIAMS, R. B., JR., & SHAPIRO, D. (1982). *Behavioral approaches to cardiovascular disease.* New York: Academic Press.

SWEET, E. W., PANIS, W., & LEVINE, D. N. (1984). Crossed Wernicke's aphasia. *Neurology, 34,* 475–479.

TAYLOR, J. R., COMBS-ORNE, T., ANDERSON, D., TAYLOR, D. A., & KOPPENOL, C. (1984). Alcohol, hypertension, & stroke. *Alcoholism: Clinical and Experimental Research, 8,* 283–286.

TAYLOR, W. (1974). *The vibration syndrome.* London: Academic Press.

TOMPKINS, C., SCHULZ, R., & RAU, M. (1988). Post-stroke depression in primary support persons: Predicting those at risk. *Journal of Consulting and Clinical Psychology, 56,* 502–508.

U. S. PUBLIC HEALTH SERVICE. (1983). *The health consequences of smoking: Cardiovascular disease. A report of the Surgeon General* (DHHS Publication No. PHS 84-50204). Rockville, Md: U. S. Department of Health and Human Services, Office on Smoking and Health.

WAGNER, E., & WILLIAMS, R. S. (1987). Rehabilitation after myocardial infarction. In K. G. Andreoli, D. P. Zipes, A. G. Wallace, M. R. Kinney, & V. K. Fowkes (Eds.), *Comprehensive cardiac care* (6th ed.) (pp. 399–410). St. Louis: Mosby.

WATZLAWICK, P., & COYNE, J. C. (1980). Depression following stroke: Brief, problem-focused family treatment. *Family Process, 19,* 13–18.

WEBSTER, J. S., JONES, S., BLANTON, P., GROSS, R., BEISSEL, G. F., & WOFFORD, J. D. (1984). Visual scanning with stroke patients. *Behavior Therapy, 15,* 129–143.

WEINSTEIN, E. A., & FRIEDLAND, R. P. (1977). Behavioral disorders associated with hemi-inattention. In E. A. Weinstein & R. P. Friedland (Eds.), *Advances in neurology, vol. 18: Hemi-inattention and hemisphere specialization.* New York: Raven.

WILLIAMS, R. B. (1989). *The trusting heart: Great news about Type A behavior.* New York: Random House.

WILLIAMS, R. B., HANEY, T. L., LEE, K. L., KONG, Y., BLUMENTHAL J., & WHALEN, R. (1980). Type A behavior hostility and coronary atherosclerosis. *Psychosomatic Medicine, 242,* 539–549.

WISE, C. M., DELP, H. L., & WILLIS, H. E. (1983). Raynaud's phenomenon: Functional assessment and response to nifedipine. *Clinical Research, 31,* 657A (Abstract).

WOLF, S. L. (1983). Electromyographic biofeedback applications to stroke patients. *Physical Therapy, 63,* 1448–1459.

# Cancer

Cancer is a large group of diseases that are characterized by the uncontrolled growth and spread of abnormal cells that, if not checked or arrested, will lead to death. Cancer can strike at any age. It kills more children aged three to fourteen than any other disease, and it occurs with even greater frequency in adult populations. About 30%, or more than 75 million Americans, will eventually develop cancer. Approximately 75% of all families will have at least one member with cancer. Each year almost a million new cases of cancer are diagnosed. Overall, cancer ranks as second only to heart disease as a cause of death in the United States.[1]

Unfortunately, although cancer ranks second as a cause of death, it ranks first as the most feared of all diseases. A survey of British women indicated that they found cancer more alarming than coronary heart disease, mental illness, bronchitis, or tuberculosis (Knopf, 1976). When American medical students were asked to fill out some psychological tests as if they were cancer patients, most exhibited serious levels of depression and hopelessness (Cassileth & Egan, 1979). In a national sample of 1,500 Americans, 49% agreed with the statement "The word *cancer* itself scares me" (American Cancer Society, 1980).

In point of fact, much of the alarm over cancer is out of proportion with reality. Some types of cancer can be prevented, and almost all types of cancer can be treated, with the treatments resulting in cure in about 40% of the cases and a prolonged or less painful life in many of the others. In addition, there are several effective techniques for preventing or reducing much of the emotional distress that is caused by cancer or its treatment. In each of these areas—prevention, treatment, and dealing with the psychosocial consequences of the disease—psychologists and other behavioral scientists are playing important and increasingly active roles.

## Biological and Psychophysiological Components

Cancer is a disease of the cells, and as such it occurs in all living things, including plants, animals, and humans. It has existed since the beginning of recorded history. However, because most cancers affect people who are 40 or more years old, it has only been in the last 100 years or so—since the average life span in many parts of the world has climbed above 40—that cancer has gained widespread attention.

Contrary to popular opinion, cancer is not one disease but rather a complex group of more than 250 diseases that can involve all the organs of the body. All cancers have in common the abnormal reproduction of cells. To better understand what cancer is and how it develops, it is helpful to understand something about normal cell growth.

All human cells, at least at some point in their life span, have the inherent capacity to divide, to reproduce. But just as important, cells also have the capacity to stop reproducing. Within a mature, healthy living organism, a steady state eventually has to be reached such that cell birth = cell death. That is, cells multiply only as needed to replace dead cells. If this were not the case, for example, you would never stop growing: you would just get taller and taller, your arms would get longer and longer, your feet would grow bigger

---

[1] Unless otherwise noted, all statistical references to cancer incidence, prevalence, and treatment outcomes are taken from the American Cancer Society's *Cancer Facts and Figures: 1989*.

and bigger, and so on. Unlike normal cells, cancer cells no longer cease multiplying when they reach a critical mass. This uncontrolled growth can eventually lead to the death of normal cells, and if it is allowed to continue unchecked, to the death of the organism. Figure 9.1 shows normal cell growth and cancer cell growth.

What causes a cell to become a cancer cell is not fully understood. Recently a lot of attention has been given to cancer genes, or *oncogenes*. Genes are located on large molecules, known as deoxyribonucleic acid (DNA), in the nucleus of each body cell. During cell reproduction, this DNA splits into two identical segments, with each segment becoming a new cell. Oncogenes are special kinds of genes that are apparently present in normal cells in order to regulate when and how fast cells will reproduce. When abnormalities develop in these genes, cancer may arise. Research on how oncogenes might contribute to the development of cancer is very recent, and much more work needs to be done before we will fully understand the process. Based on what we know now, we think the process may work as follows, at least in some situations. Normally functioning oncogenes may develop abnormalities as a result of mutations, or changes, in the gene structure. Some of these mutations may occur spontaneously, whereas many others probably result from exposure to foreign substances called *carcinogens*, which means substances "capable of causing cancer." Some of the chemicals in cigarette smoke are good examples

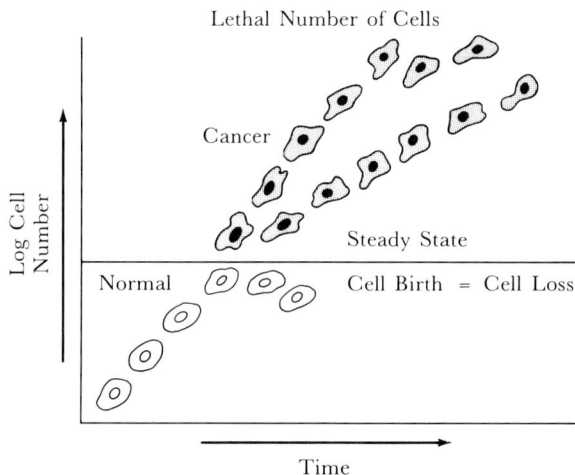

FIGURE 9.1   Growth rates of normal cells versus cancer cells. Normal cell growth rate slows down and stops as we approach adulthood whereas the cancer cell growth rate continues unabated. Adapted from U.S. Department of Health and Human Services. (1982). *Medicine for the Layman: Cancer Treatment.* (NIH Publication No. 82–1807), Washington, D.C.: U.S. Government Printing Office.

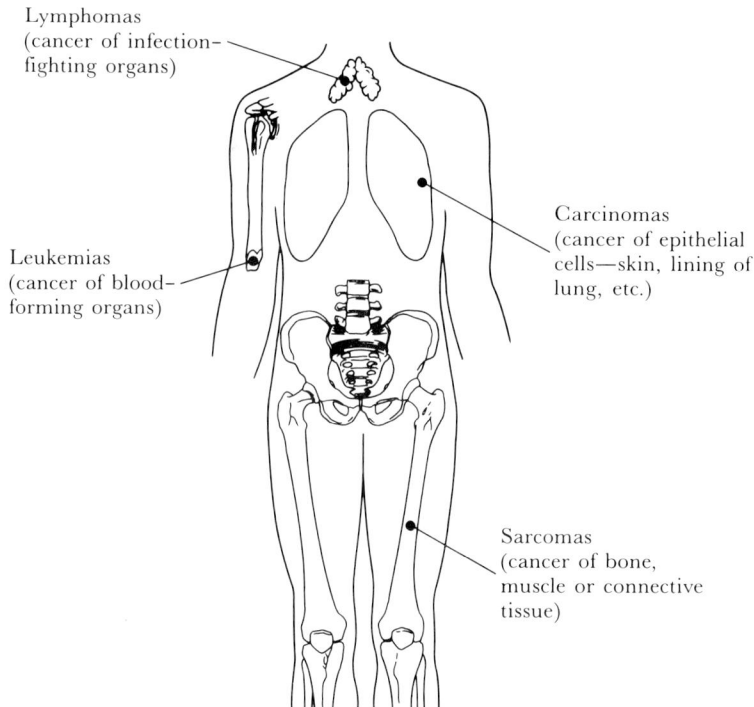

Lymphomas
(cancer of infection-
fighting organs)

Leukemias
(cancer of blood-
forming organs)

Carcinomas
(cancer of epithelial
cells—skin, lining of
lung, etc.)

Sarcomas
(cancer of bone,
muscle or connective
tissue)

Classification of the types of cancer has resulted from
examination of cancer tissues under the light microscope.

FIGURE 9.2   Classification of four different types of cancer. Adapted
from the National Cancer Institute. (1970). *Progress Against Cancer, 1970.*

of carcinogens. There appear to be at least three stages involved in the process by which carcinogens can lead to cancer. These stages are shown in Figure 9.2.

The first stage is called *activation*. Usually the body's own natural defenses
will kill or detoxify alien substances, including some carcinogens, thereby rendering them harmless. However, this natural defense process can go awry,
and instead the carcinogen can be altered so that it more easily enters the
cell's nucleus and attaches to the genetic material. Activation refers to the
modification of the carcinogen in this fasion.

The second stage is called *initiation*. Even most activated carcinogens are
usually destroyed by the natural defenses of the body. But sometimes an activated carcinogen makes it to the cell nucleus and attaches (or binds) to the
DNA. If this mutated or abnormal cell then divides, the new cells will inherit
the mutation, as will all the other cells resulting from future cell divisions.
The development of this first mutation is called *initiation*. Most research suggests that a single mutation will not by itself lead to cancer—one or often
many more mutations must occur, and in the same cell where the first mutation occurred, in order for cancer to develop. Because there are billions of

cells, the odds of this happening are terribly small. But obviously it does occur, and with considerable regularity. The reason for this has to do with the third stage.

The third stage is called *promotion*. Somehow, the first mutation on the cell can change the cell so that it is unusually sensitive to certain substances called promoters. These promoters allow the mutant cell to proliferate more frequently than normal or nonmutant cells, which can eventually result in a growing mass of mutant cells relative to the other tissue. Thus, promotion increases beyond normal proportions the number of cells that carry the single mutation. As the number of these cells steadily increases so do the odds that one of these mutant cells will be hit by a second carcinogen that causes a mutation. This process of mutation and promotion can be repeated several times until eventually the right combination of altered genes occurs to produce a tumor.

Contrary to what has been commonly assumed by many, these tumor cells do not divide faster than normal tissue, but rather they simply do not know when to stop dividing. Thus, instead of the normal equation in adults of cell birth = cell death, in cancer patients cell birth > cell death.

It should be kept in mind at this point that not all tumors are cancerous. Tumors are usually divided into two types: *benign* and *malignant*. Benign tumors are usually self-contained, or largely so, and thus constitute a growing mass of tissue. This mass may push into healthy tissue, or it may grow into and block important openings, such as in the colon or in a blood vessel. If found early enough, these tumors can often be removed surgically, and the person can be completely cured. Cancerous tumors, in contrast, are malignant in nature. Malignant cells do not simply multiply in a self-contained lump; rather, they invade and choke out adjacent normal tissue. This reaching-out-and-choking-off process apparently reminded Hippocrates, who is sometimes referred to as the "father of medicine," of the claws of a crab. He named these malignant growths *cancer*, after the Latin word for crab.

In addition to being malignant, cancer tumors have one more attribute that enables them to kill an organism and that often makes it difficult to treat the disease. When a tumor begins to develop, it is usually confined to a specific region of the body and is said to be localized. Cancers can shed cells from the original tumor. These cells produce enzymes that allow them to enter the bloodstream and the lymphatic channels throughout the body and thus to spread to new locations. Here they can take up additional residences and produce more tumors. This spread of the cancer cells is referred to as *metastasis*. Metastasis can be regional, that is, confined to one region of the body, or can spread throughout the body. When the latter occurs, the cancer is said to be advanced and usually results in death. Often, but not always, an analysis of a metastasized tumor will enable a scientist to tell where the original tumor began. The specific name given to the cancer usually depends on where the cancer originated. Although there are more than 250 specific types of cancers, most are subsumed under one of four basic categories, depending on what part of the body is involved: (1) *carcinomas*, which are cancers of the epithelial cells (e.g., skin); (2) *sarcomas*, which develop from fat, bone, muscle, or other connective tissues; (3) *lymphomas*, which develop in the lymph system; and (4) *leukemias*, which are cancers of the blood-forming organs.

In summary, all cancer cells, regardless of type, have three major characteristics: (1) they reproduce uncontrollably, (2) they invade normal tissues, and (3) they can metastasize to sites in the body far removed from the original tumors.

If left unchecked, cancer cells eventually destroy, crush, block, or choke off the tissue of important organs such as the lungs, colon, or brain. This is what eventually kills a patient with cancer. Before death occurs, however, there are usually a number of symptoms that are readily detected, although in some cases the symptoms do not occur until the cancer is very large and often difficult to treat. For example, a cancer in the large intestine may partially obstruct the passage of fecal material through the bowel resulting in constipation and/or diarrhea. Cancerous growth in the brain can cause increasing intracranial pressure, resulting in headaches, nausea, and vomiting. Sometimes a tumor grows beyond its capacity to obtain nutrients, resulting in some of the cells—usually in the central areas—dying. This process can result in bleeding, and this unexplained bleeding can also be a symptom of cancer.

As complex as the process of cancer genesis is, some researchers believe that cancer develops in most and maybe all people but that our natural defense, or immune, system destroys these cells before they can cause any damage. If one or both of two processes occur, this natural defense system will fail to keep cancer cells in check. First, because our natural defense system is designed to handle only a small number of cancer cells, an unusually large number of cancer cells may overpower the immune system and render it ineffective. For example, overexposure to carcinogens can contribute to the development of a very large number of cancer cells in the body. Second, if something weakens the body's natural defense system so that it does not operate at full capacity, then even a relatively small number of cancer cells might overpower it, take hold, and proliferate freely. As we will see in the next section, a variety of behavioral and life-style factors can affect both of these processes and thus can directly influence whether or not we develop cancer.

# *Behavioral, Psychological, and Social Factors*

Behavioral, psychological, and social factors can play a major role in the etiology, course, and severity of cancer. In recent years there has been a considerable amount of research published in this area. In order to organize this material, we will use a schema similar to that suggested by S. M. Levy (1983; 1985) and displayed in Table 9.1. This table divides the research in this area into two broad areas based on whether the behavioral, psychological, and social factors in question are thought to directly or indirectly contribute to the initiation and/or promotion of cancer. Some factors could be placed in both

TABLE 9.1    Behavioral, Psychological, and Social Factors Affecting Cancer

| *Factors having direct effects* | *Factors having indirect effects* |
|---|---|
| EXAMPLES | EXAMPLES |
| 1. Tobacco | 1. Dietary factors |
| 2. Occupational carcinogens | 2. Stress |
| 3. Alcohol | 3. Personality factors |
| 4. Ultraviolet light exposure (sunbathing) | 4. Noncompliance |
| 5. Certain sexual behaviors | 5. Screening/detection behaviors |

SOURCE:   Adapted from Levy, S. M. (1983). Host differences in neoplastic risk: Behavioral and social contributors to disease, *Health Psychology, 2,* 21–44.

categories, but for ease of presentation, all factors are described in one or the other category.

## Direct Effects in Initiating and Promoting Cancer

Cancer, like several other chronic diseases we have discussed, is in large part a disease of our life-style. What we eat, how much we drink, and whether or not we smoke are all behavioral factors that can play a direct role in whether or not we develop cancer. It is because of this fact that psychologists and other behavioral scientists can play a major role in preventing cancer, for they are perhaps the best trained of all professionals for helping people alter their health-related behaviors.

SMOKING    Probably the best-known behavioral precursor of cancer is tobacco use, especially cigarette smoking. More than twenty-five years of biomedical and epidemiological research clearly has shown that smoking increases the risk of several types of cancers including cancer of the lung, mouth, esophagus, pancreas, and bladder. As we saw in Chapters 6 and 8, smoking also increases the risk of other diseases, such as cardiovascular disease and pulmonary disease. A 1985 study by the U.S. Congress Office of Technology Assessment (see American Cancer Society, 1989) suggests that cigarette smoking costs Americans a total of about $65 billion per year in lost productivity and the treatment of smoking-related disease. It is thus not surprising that tobacco use is regarded as the single most important preventable behavioral factor contributing to illness, disability, and premature death in the United States (U.S. Department of Health and Human Services, 1986).

Cigarette smoke contains carcinogenic substances, such as nicotine and various tars, that can act as both initiators and promoters of cancer cells. Thus, smoking can directly lead to the development of cancer. And the more one smokes, the greater the risk of cancer. For example, someone who smokes one pack of cigarettes a day is ten times as likely to die of lung cancer as a nonsmoker. Someone who smokes two or more packs a day is fifteen to twenty-five times as likely (American Cancer Society, 1989). Overall, smoking is responsible for approximately 30% of all cancer deaths (American Cancer Society, 1989). It should also be emphasized that breathing in cigarette smoke from someone else, sometimes referred to as involuntary smoking, also increases the risk of cancer. For example, one group of researchers found that nonsmoking women who were married to men who smoked a pack or more of cigarettes a day were more than twice as likely to develop colorectal cancer (Garfinkel et al., 1985). In another study (Sandler et al., 1985), researchers found that children whose fathers smoked cigarettes, as opposed to those whose fathers did not, had a 50 percent increase in their risk of developing cancer as adults. Thus, the important variable is breathing in cigarette smoke—whether it's yours or someone else's.

Table 9.2 summarizes the natural history of smoking behavior for most people. As the table indicates, people begin smoking for many reasons, ranging from curiosity to peer pressure. Research suggests that most smokers began to smoke in their teenage years. Once smoking becomes a habit, it is hard to stop, even if the original reasons for taking up the practice are no longer relevant. This is because the nicotine in the smoke can lead to physiological dependence, making withdrawal very unpleasant. Smoking can become psychologically addicting as well, and it can become a standard way of responding to stress or a familiar component of a pleasurable experience. For example, having a cigarette is, to many smokers, the ideal way to complete a fine meal.

Because of the tremendous health costs associated with smoking and the difficulty for many of quitting once the habit is formed, government and private sources have devoted tremendous attention and resources toward smoking prevention and cessation programs. These efforts have had three

TABLE 9.2  The Natural History of Smoking

| Starting: Psychosocial | Continuing: Physiological and psychosocial | Stopping: Psychosocial | Resuming: Psychosocial and physiological |
|---|---|---|---|
| Availability | Nicotine | Health | Withdrawal symptoms |
| Curiosity | Immediate positive | Expense | Stress and frustration |
| Rebelliousness | consequences | Social support | Social pressure |
| Anticipation of | Signals (cues) in | Self-mastery | Alcohol consumption |
| adulthood | environs | Aesthetics | Abstinence violation |
| Social confidence | Avoiding negative | Examples to | effect |
| Social pressure/ | effects | others | |
| modeling: Peers, | (withdrawal) | | |
| siblings, parents | | | |
| and media | | | |

SOURCE: Adapted from Lichtenstein, E., & Brown, R.A. (1982). Smoking cessation methods: Review and recommendations, In W.R. Miller (Ed.), *The addictive behaviors: Treatment of alcoholism, drug abuse, smoking, and obesity*. Oxford: Pergamon Press.

major components. First, they have had an educational focus, informing people of all ages about the dangers of smoking. Survey data suggest that these educational programs have been effective: most Americans, including those who smoke, are aware of the health risks associated with smoking. A second component has been the establishment of policies that restrict smoking in public places and the enforcement of other policies, such as increased taxation on tobacco and restrictions on the advertisement of tobacco products, aimed at decreasing smoking. The rationale behind restricted smoking policies is that people who smoke in public places force involuntary smoking by nonsmokers. These efforts have been successful and resulted, for example, in restrictions on smoking on airlines, in restaurants, and even in many public buildings. Finally, considerable effort has been aimed at developing effective smoking-cessation programs. Smokers who wish to quit can find a variety of programs to help them, including brochures on how to quit on one's own, pharmacological aids such as nicotine gum and behavior modification programs. These educational, policy, and intervention efforts have had a major effect on the smoking behavior of Americans: the per capita number of cigarettes smoked per year has been decreasing continually in recent years (see Figure 9.3). However, there are still subgroups of individuals, such as those with less than a high school education and young females, in which smoking shows little decrease or even an increase.

OTHER DIRECT CAUSES    Although cigarette smoking is probably the major behavioral cause of cancer, there are several other important causes. For example, work-related exposure to certain substances can increase the occupational risks of cancer. Many agents or chemical compounds are known to increase the risk of cancer, and hundreds of other agents are suspected of being either initiators or promoters of cancer (Levy, 1983). Examples of known carcinogens include asbestos, coal dust, cotton dust, and the fumes of various paints and cleaning agents. Reducing or eliminating direct contact with these substances, for instance by using protective masks when working with carcinogenic fumes, can help considerably in reducing cancer risks.

Alcohol consumption is also related to some types of cancers. For example, research on Veteran's Administration (VA) populations suggests that heavy drinking, especially of wine and beer, is associated with increased risks of oral cancers and head and neck cancers. Research also shows that the risk of cancer from alcohol consumption increases dramatically if a person also smokes. For example, the risk of oral cancer for people who consume 1.6 ounces or more of alcohol per day and smoke about two packs or more of cigarettes a day is more than fifteen times the risk of people who neither drink nor smoke (Levy, 1983). Smoking and alcohol consumption are synergistic in terms of cancer: the risk of engaging in both together is greater than the sum of the risks of engaging in either one alone.

Sunbathing also falls into the category of carcinogenic behavior. Sunlight, or more specifically ultraviolet radiation, is the most potent natural carcinogen in the environment. It is the primary cause of skin cancer, which will

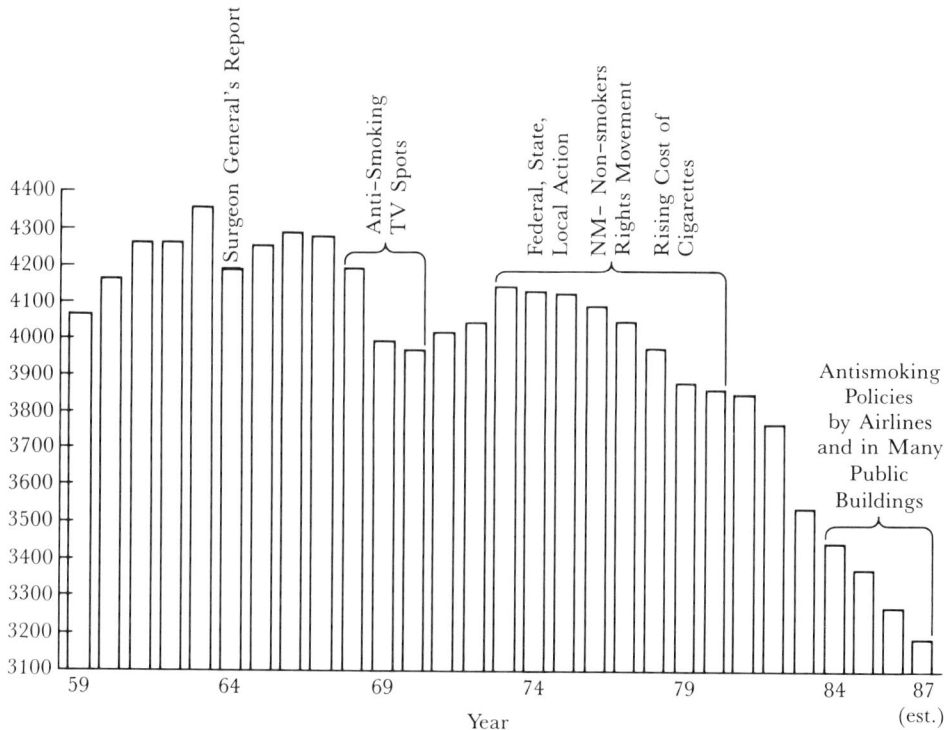

Annual United States per capital consumption of cigarettes by people 18 and older. The labels on the chart are: Surgeon General's Report; Anti-Smoking TV Spots; Federal, State, Local Action; NM— Non-smokers Rights Movement; Rising Cost of Cigarettes; Antismoking Policies by Airlines and in Many Public Buildings. The y-axis ranges from 3100 to 4400, and the x-axis shows Year from 59 to 87 (est.).

FIGURE 9.3   Annual United States per capital consumption of cigarettes by people 18 and older. From the U.S. Department of Agriculture, 1983 estimate by OSH, DHHS, and "The Health Consequences of Smoking: A Report of the Surgeon General, 1988."

eventually strike one of every seven Americans. Fortunately, most skin cancer is benign, can be successfully removed by surgery, and is usually not even counted as cancer in official records of cancer statistics. However, sunlight can also contribute to more serious forms of cancer such as melanoma, a type of cancer that begins with skin cells but can soon invade adjacent tissue and metastasize throughout the body. The ultraviolet radiation from sunlight can penetrate deeply into skin and can cause mutations of the DNA. Skin pigment protects against ultraviolet light, and therefore people with the least skin pigment (light-skinned people, especially blonds) are the most susceptible. Sunlamps and tanning beds also can cause DNA damage. In fact, some research suggests that for equal reddening of the skin, some sunlamps cause seven times as much damage as sunlight (Reif, 1981). Animal studies further suggest that the risk of skin cancer is the greatest if the skin is exposed to both sunlight and to sunlamps (Faivelson, 1988).

Finally, as if it were not enough that cigarette smoking, drinking alcohol, and sunbathing are all possible contributors to cancer, research also suggests that even sex, under certain circumstances, can increase the risk of cancer. Specifically, the data suggest that there is a rather strong relationship between cervical cancer and factors such as age at first intercourse and number of sexual partners. For example, Harris and his colleagues (1980) studied women with (a) cervical cancer, (b) severe dysplasia (*dysplasia* refers to the presence of a type of abnormal cell in the cervix, a condition that is often regarded as a precursor of cancer), (c) mild dysplasia, and (d) no cervical abnormalities. The researchers found a linear trend indicating that the more sexual partners a woman had, the greater her risk of cancer or dysplasia. For example, the risk of having cervical cancer in women with six or more sex partners was more than seven times greater than in women with one partner; the risk for women with even two partners was at least double that of women with one partner. An even more important predictor of cervical cancer appears to be age at first intercourse. In general, research suggests that intercourse before age twenty, and especially before age seventeen, is significantly associated with increased cervical cancer risk. In fact, after reviewing several studies on this topic, Sadehgi and his colleagues (1984) concluded that early sexual intercourse is "the most important factor in the development of cervical neoplasia" (p.726). Interestingly, in support of this conclusion, the data also suggest that cervical cancer is almost nonexistent in virgins and nuns (e.g., Rotkin, 1973).

However, prolonged chastity also has its risks, at least for women. Research suggests that not having children, or not having children until later in life, can also increase the risk of certain types of cancer. For example, never having children or having a first child after age thirty is associated with an increased risk of breast cancer in women. Women who have never had children, as opposed to those who have, are twice as likely to be diagnosed as having ovarian cancer (American Cancer Society, 1989). Overall, therefore, the age at which one first has intercourse, the number of sexual partners one has, and whether or not intercourse leads to childbearing are risk factors that are related to cancer incidence.

## Indirect Effects in Initiating and Promoting Cancer

Behavioral, psychological, and social factors can indirectly affect the initiation and promotion of cancer by serving as mediating variables that influence factors that can directly cause or promote cancer. Because of the extra step in the causal chain, the evidence linking indirect factors to the etiology or promotion of cancer is generally weaker than that for direct factors. The three indirect factors that have been given the most attention recently are diet, stress, and personality variables. In each of these areas the evidence should be regarded as suggestive rather than conclusive.

DIET    Both the American Cancer Society and the National Cancer Institute have suggested that several aspects of the average diet of Westerners can increase the risk of cancer. Unfortunately, research does not suggest that if you follow a certain diet you can be guaranteed of not developing cancer.

Several studies have suggested that high levels of dietary fat can increase the risk of developing cancers of the breast, prostate, and colon. The most widely held theory is that fat does not cause cancer directly but promotes its development by somehow altering the metabolism of normal cells so that they are more susceptible to other carcinogens (Levy, 1982). Americans consume, on the average, about 40% of their calories as fats. It is recommended that we change our eating habits so as to reduce the total fat intake to 30% or less of our daily calories.

Obesity, perhaps in part due to increased fat intake, has also been linked to cancer. For example, a twelve-year study supported by the American Cancer Society found that there was a marked increase of cancers of the uterus, gallbladder, kidney, stomach, colon, and breast in obese as opposed to normal-weight individuals. When people were grossly obese, defined as 40% or more overweight, the increased cancer rate was 55% for women and 33% for men.

Some foods appear to be able to block the development of cancer. For example, it is thought that cruciferous vegetables (so named because the flowers of these plants are shaped like small crosses) such as broccoli, cabbage, Brussels sprouts, turnips, and cauliflower decrease the risk of cancer because one of their metabolic by-products contains chemicals called *retenoids* that appear to block the promoter activity of some carcinogenic substances. It has also been suggested that dietary fiber can reduce the risk of cancer, especially colon cancer. Fiber is usually regarded as the residue of the digestive process, that is, fiber is what remains in your stomach and intestines after your meal has been digested. One theory holds that fiber may chemically bind to carcinogenic substances, rendering them less potent (Willett & MacMahon, 1984). Even some who are skeptical of this theory recommend an increase in dietary fiber because most fiber foods are low in calories, thus a diet that is high in fiber may lead to a decline in obesity or dietary fat intake.

STRESS  Psychological stress, or the failure to cope adequately with it, is becoming increasingly suspected of being a possible contributor to cancer. Most of the human studies in this area can be divided into one of two types: retrospective and prospective.

*Retrospective studies* are those in which people who already have cancer are asked to think back, or "retrospect," about the stresses in their lives before they developed cancer. Most studies linking stress to cancer are of this type. For example, Jacobs and Charles (1980) asked the parents of twenty-five children with cancer and the parents of twenty-five matched children without cancer to complete the Holmes and Rahe Schedule of Recent Events, a scale that measures various life stresses such as divorce, loss of a loved one, and illness. Parents were to complete the form according to the family stresses that occurred during the year prior to the apparent onset of the disease. The results indicated that families of the cancer children had significantly more stress during the year prior to the onset of cancer than families of the non-cancer children, suggesting that stress may be related to the development of cancer. In a more recent study, Cheang and Cooper (1985) interviewed 121 patients who were admitted to a hospital for a biopsy to determine whether the lumps they found on their breasts were cancerous or not. The patients were interviewed and administered a stressful-life-events scale designed by the authors before the biopsy was made. As it turned out, forty-six patients were found to have breast cancer and seventy-five had a benign breast disease. The authors also gave the same stressful-life-events scale to forty-two healthy women with no probable breast lumps. The results showed that the women with cancer had undergone significantly more stressful life events in the two years that proceeded the diagnosis of cancer than patients in either of the other two groups, who did not differ from each other. Many other studies have reported similar findings.

Although the retrospective study suggests a relationship between stress and cancer, there are many methodological problems with retrospective research that lead most researchers to regard their results as tentative at best. For example, cancer cells are present in a person and are having an effect on that person long before they are diagnosed by a physician. In fact, sometimes a cancer tumor exists for several years before it is discovered. Thus, the stressful life events that occur the year or two before the "apparent" onset of cancer may be an effect as much as a cause of cancer. Also, people's memory of how stressful certain events were before the cancer, or how well they coped with them, can be greatly influenced by the cancer experience and by a variety of other factors. Such recall simply cannot be counted on as being accurate.

Because of these and other problems with retrospective research, some investigators have conducted *prospective studies*. In this type of research investigators begin with a large number of subjects who have not been diagnosed as having cancer, and then they follow them to see who eventually is diagnosed as having cancer and who is not. They can then compare those with cancer to those without it across a variety of variables. In general, the results of prospective studies also support the link between stress and cancer. For example, Horne and Picard (1979) found that subjects who develop cancer, as compared to those who develop benign lung tumors, are more likely to report the loss of a significant relationship within the preceding five years and poorer job stability.

Neither retrospective nor prospective studies are ideal from a methodological point of view. The most rigorous test of the relationship between stress and cancer would be an experimental study in which stresses thought to be associated with cancer were given to one group of subjects but not to another and then the subjects were observed to see which ones develop cancer. Obviously, this type of research cannot be conducted with humans, but experimental work has been done with animals. For example, a large group of rats can be "given" enough cancer cells so that under normal conditions, about half of the animals will be able to fight the cancer cells and not develop "clinical cancer" whereas the other half will develop malignant tumors and eventually die from them. Another group of rats is not given any cancer cells. Then, half of the animals in each group are stressed (for example, by being given electric shocks or by being forced to run on an exercise wheel for long

Exposed to Stress

Yes                    No

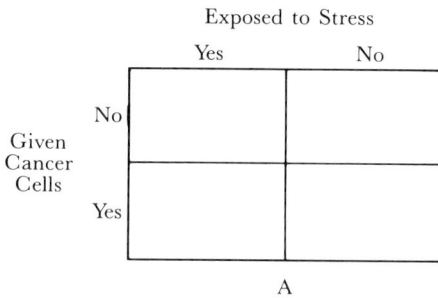

A

FIGURE 9.4a   Design of a typical animal experiment on stress and cancer. Half the animals receive cancer cells while half do not, and half are exposed to stress while half are not, forming four groups in a 2 × 2 factorial design.

During              After
Stress              Stress

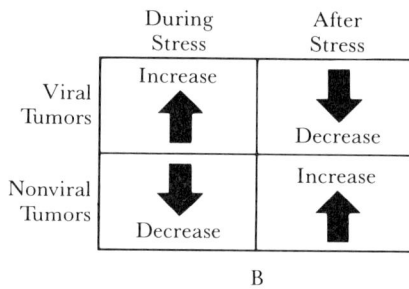

B

FIGURE 9.4b   Hypothesized effects of stress on viral and nonviral tumor growth both during the application of stress and after the stress is removed. Adapted from Justice, 1985. Copyright (1985) by the American Psychological Association. Adopted by permission.

periods), whereas the other half are not. This type of experimental design is sometimes referred to as 2 (cancer, no cancer) × 2 (stress, no stress) factorial (see Figure 9.4a). When such research is done, the data suggest that under certain conditions, (e.g., with certain kinds of stressors, in the absence of adequate means to cope with the stresses, etc.), the group that received both the cancer cells and the stress will develop significantly more malignant tumors than the animals in any of the other conditions (see Figure 9.4b). Overall, the data on stress and cancer are quite strong in suggesting that under certain circumstances, high levels of stress can be associated with an increased likelihood of developing cancer.

It should also be noted, however, that under other circumstances, the data are clear in suggesting that stress can *reduce* the risk of cancer. These contradictory data have given rise to considerable confusion and, to some, heated arguments over the relationship of stress and cancer. In a review of this literature, Justice (1985) has posited that the confusion can largely be resolved by determining the type of cancer tumor in question and whether the measurements of tumor growth were taken during the administration of the stress or shortly after the stress was terminated. Specifically, Justice suggested that exposure to stress, whether it be chronic or acute in nature, can promote the development of viral tumors (i.e., cancer tumors caused by viruses) but often slows down the growth of nonviral tumors. In contrast, the physiological "rebound effects" that naturally occur after stress is terminated can slow down the growth of viral tumors but often facilitate the growth of nonviral tumors. Thus, stress can help or hurt cancer development, depending on the type of cancer and the exact time when one assesses the stress effects. Justice's conclusions are summarized in Figure 9.4b. Although it is too early to tell whether Justice's explanation for the effects of stress on cancer will hold up after rigorous experimental testing, this explanation does appear to be the most comprehensive theory available and to resolve better than any other a large amount of previously confusing data.

What is the mechanism by which stress might in some circumstances contribute to the initiation or promotion of cancer? Many different theories have been offered but most suggest that the bottom line is that stress not adequately coped with can weaken the immune system, thus decreasing the body's own natural ability to destroy cancer cells. For example, Locke and his associates (1978, as reported by Levy, 1983) studied college-aged students who reported a large number of stressful life events over the preceding year and who did or did not show psychiatric symptoms—a presumed index of relative ability to cope or not cope with stress. In testing blood samples from both groups, the researchers found that subjects with the psychiatric symptoms had lower levels of natural killer (NK) cell activity than did subjects who did not have psychiatric symptoms (NK cells are part of the immune system's arsenal of agents that can fight cancer cells). The data suggest that inability to cope with stress was associated with decreased ability to fight the cancer cells.

What is the mechanism by which stress can weaken the immune system? Again, research in this area is relatively new and few scientists are ready yet to unabashedly embrace the answer. One of the most promising notions at present is that stress leads to a considerable change in the levels of various hormones, including corticosteroids, and that these changes can impair immunologic functioning. As new, highly sensitive techniques for measuring hormones are being developed, a host of additional hormones that are sensitive to stress and are associated with immune functioning are being identified. This is indeed an exciting area of investigation that is likely to lead to many new findings in the years to come.

In their review of all the human and animal literature in the area, Sklar and Anisman (1981) reached the following conclusion about the relationship of stress to cancer:

> Essentially, under ideal conditions the organisms' natural defenses might be able to contend with the presence of a few malignant cells. Under less than ideal conditions, however, created by failures to cope with acute stress, the defenses might be inadequate to prevent cell proliferation, and hence the progress of the tumor. (p. 395)

This theory of how stress can contribute to the initiation and progression of cancer has lead many clinicians to suggest that reducing stress in one's life or learning to cope more adequately with it might reduce the risk of cancer. To date, there is little research directly testing this notion. However, even if it is true, as well it may be, it should be kept in mind that the reduction of stress presumably would lead to a reduction in cancer only in a person whose

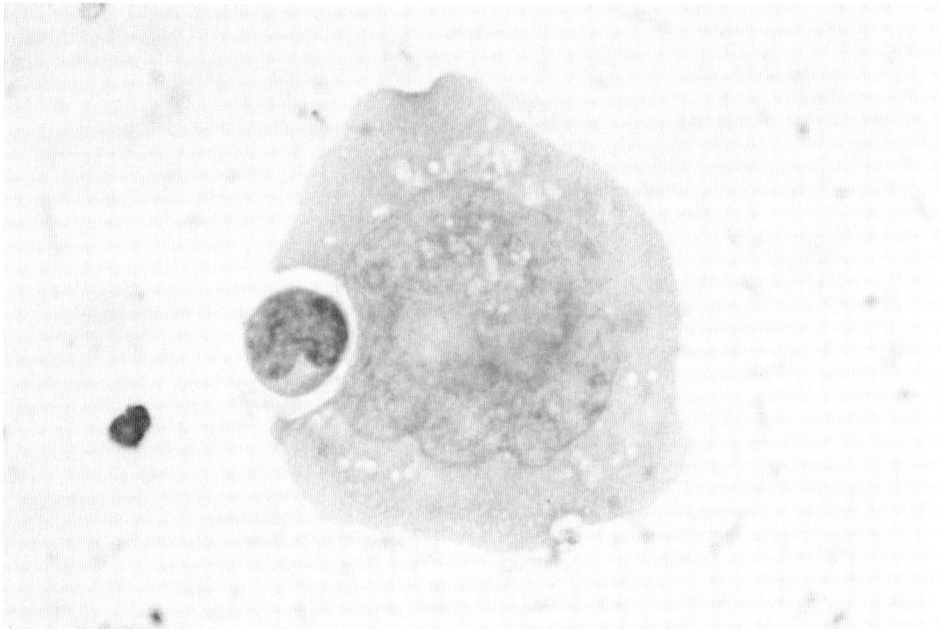

FIGURE 9.4c   This micrograph shows an immune cell called a lymphocyte attacking a larger cancer cell. After several hours, the lymphocyte will destroy the cancer cell.

immune system would otherwise be adequate to protect him or her from the growth of any existing cancer cells. In persons with compromised or weakened immune systems, as is often the case in older individuals, stress-reduction procedures may have considerably less anticancer effect.

CANCER-PRONE PERSONALITY   For many years it has been suggested that certain personality characteristics may predispose people to the development of cancer. The second century AD physician Galen suggested that women with melancholic dispositions were more likely to develop breast cancer than women who were more sanguine. In 1701, Gendron wrote that depressed and anxious women were more prone to develop cancer. Today, questionnaires in the Sunday newspaper or in various magazines purport to tell you immediately whether or not you have a cancer-prone personality. Are there data to support these long-standing claims?

The literature on personality factors in cancer is very similar to the human literature on stress and cancer. In fact, the two bodies of literature are sometimes considered to be variations of the same theme. Most studies on personality and cancer involve retrospective assessments made on people who already have cancer, aimed at determining what these people's personalities were like before they had cancer. The "premorbid" (that is, prior-to-cancer) personalities of the cancer patients are then compared to the personalities of a group of similar people without cancer. Many of these studies suggest that cancer patients either experience significantly greater emotional loss prior to developing cancer, or are distressed more by such losses, than people without cancer. One of the pioneer researchers in this area, Lawrence LeShan, has suggested that a personality orientation marked by feelings of hopelessness may be a necessary factor in predisposing a person to cancer.

A growing number of prospective studies have also supported the relationship between various personality characteristics and cancer. For example, Schmale and Iker (1971) gave the Minnesota Multiphasic Personality Inventory (MMPI) and an interview to women who had suspicious-looking cells in their cervix. Then, before the tests were done to determine whether or not the cells were cancerous, Schmale and Iker tried to predict who did or did not have cancer. Based in part on their hypothesis that high levels of hopelessness would predispose patients to cancer, the authors correctly predicted the occurrence of cancer in thirty-six of the fifty-one cases. Shekelle and his colleagues (1981) found that psychological depression, as assessed by the MMPI, in a group of more than 2,000 healthy males was associated with a two-fold increase in cancer during the seventeen years he followed these patients after the initial testing.

In addition to finding a relationship between personality factors and the diagnosis of cancer, some researchers have suggested that personality and other psychological factors can influence how long people will survive once they have developed cancer. For example, in a retrospective study, Derogatis and his colleagues (1979) gave a battery of personality tests to thirty-five women with metastatic breast cancer and then followed them until they died. The authors found that women who lived more than a year after the testing, compared to those who lived less than a year, scored higher on measures of anxiety, alienation, and dysphoric mood (e.g., depression). In contrast, short-term survivors were less hostile and had higher levels of positive mood. Prospective studies have also suggested that personality factors can affect longevity in cancer patients. For example, Pettingale and his colleagues (1977, 1984) found that breast cancer patients who reacted to their cancer by denial or who had a "fighting spirit" were more likely to be disease free ten years after their treatment than were women characterized by stoic acceptance of their disease or by feelings of helplessness and hopelessness.

Although these findings may appear impressive, many scholars working in this area remain quite skeptical about any relationship between cancer and personality factors. Why? There are several reasons, among the most important being the following. First there is a tremendous amount of inconsistency in the research in this area. Some studies find that bottling up one's emotions is associated with cancer, whereas other studies find the opposite, that is, that cancer is more common in outgoing, extroverted individuals (see Watson & Schuld, 1977). Some research suggests that cancer is more common in depressed individuals (e.g., Shekelle et al., 1981), whereas other research finds no differences in premorbid depression levels between cancer patients and noncancer patients. For example, in a large-scale prospective study, Zonderman and his colleagues (1989) for 15 years followed individuals who, as part of a National Health and Nutrition Examination Survey, completed two well-accepted scales of depression. Approximately 6,000 people completed the first test, the General Well-Being Schedule, and approximately 2,500 completed both the first test and second test, the Center for Epidemiologic Studies Depression Scale, making this one of the largest studies of its kind. The participants were divided into depressed or nondepressed groups, and then the incidence of cancer in each group was determined. After conducting a careful and thorough series of analyses, and after controlling for factors that could have confounded any differences between groups such as history of smoking, age, sex, marital status, and family history of cancer, the authors concluded there was no relationship between depression and cancer. Finally, some research has found no relationship of any type between cancer and a variety of personality variables. For example, in a highly publicized study, Cassileth and her colleagues (1985) measured a variety of personality and other psychosocial variables (including job satisfaction, feelings of helplessness, and adjustment to their illness) in more than 350 cancer patients. The researchers then followed these patients until death (group one) or until they relapsed (group two). The results indicated that none of the personality or other psychosocial factors were significantly related to relapse or to length of survival.

Second, there are a host of methodological problems with much of the research. Many of the studies are retrospective in nature, and as we saw earlier, this type of research has several methodological weaknesses. Many prospective studies are also problematic; for example, the measures of personality could actually have been taken following the onset of cancer but prior to its diagnosis, making it impossible to tell if the reported personality differences were a cause or an effect of cancer. Other studies lack adequate control groups. For example, Dattore and his colleagues (1980) initially reported a study in which there were significant differences on the MMPI between VA patients who later developed cancer and those who did not. However, in a paper published the next year, Greenberg and Dattore (1981) reported that when patients who developed cancer were compared to patients who developed hypertension, ulcers, or even benign tumors, there were no significant differences among the groups. Thus, there did not appear to be any cancer-specific personality differences.

Finally, even if certain personality characteristics are associated with some types of cancer, there may be simpler explanations for the relationship than that the personality characteristics caused the cancer. For example, epidemiologic research suggests that factors such as age, age at first sexual intercourse, number of sexual partners at an early age, engaging in occupations that carry increased exposure to carcinogens, diet, social class, and alcohol intake, among other things, are related to cancer. These factors alone may account for much of the difference in performance on personality tests among various people. Thus, it may be that these factors, not more global "personality differences," account in part for the cancer. Yet rarely are these other factors controlled for in cancer-personality research.

All of these factors make it very difficult to reach a conclusion about the relationship of personality factors and cancer. However, the data do suggest that this is a complex area and that if any relationship does exist, it is likely to be specific as opposed to general in nature. That is, it seems unlikely that any personality factors are so robust that they will be shown to increase the risk of all types of cancer or decrease the length of survival in all people with cancer. Rather, it may be that under certain circumstances, certain types of personality characteristics might be associated with increased risk for certain types of cancers in certain types of people (e.g., those with a physiological predisposition for developing cancer). Clearly, this is an area where there are presently a lot more questions than there are answers.

COMPLIANCE WITH TREATMENT    A major behavior variable affecting the progression of cancer is whether or not patients comply with or adhere to the recommendations of their medical staff. Research in most areas of chronic disease, as we already have seen, suggests that compliance behavior is surprisingly poor among most patients. Patients miss appointments, fail to take their medicines, go off their diets, and avoid prescribed physical therapy or exercise with regularity. There is a surprising paucity of compliance research in the cancer area, perhaps because it has been assumed by many that with the stakes as high as they often are for cancer patients, compliance would not be a problem. The research that has been done suggests otherwise. For example, Smith and his colleagues (1979) measured urine levels of some drugs to determine whether or not a group of children with cancer were taking their medicines. The researchers found that about 33% of the patients were not taking their medicines as prescribed, which in a child population often means that the parents were not giving them the drugs. Among adolescents, the noncompliance rate was more than 50%. It also appears that noncompliance is a problem in adult populations (Levy, 1983).

Why are cancer patients (or their parents) noncompliant when the results of not following a recommended treatment plan can be so devastating? There are many potential behavioral, psychological, and social factors that can influence compliance behavior. Two of these factors should be highlighted because they may be more relevant to cancer patients than to patients with most other diseases. First, as we will see later in this chapter, many cancer treatments are debilitating and have unpleasant side effects. For example, if leukemia patients follow the physician's instructions and take their antibiotic medicines, they may have to ingest as many as three different medicines, six times a day, and experience a prolonged, unpleasant aftertaste each time. The side effects of cancer chemotherapy can be devastating. One cancer patient who received an especially aggressive chemotherapy protocol described her experience as follows:

> Recall the last time you had the flu. Remember especially the worst 10 minutes of that flu episode, when you were hovering over a toilet or basket as you threw up whatever was in your stomach; after that was gone, you just continued to

retch without control. You felt tired. Your muscles ached. You were always cold and shivering. You did not like how you felt, the way you looked, or the putrid odor of vomit you could never get rid of. Then, multiply that experience by 50 or 100 times so that it lasts 8 to 16 hours in a row without much let up. (Burish & Carey, 1984, pp. 147–148)

Second, some cancer patients are not strongly inclined to comply because they are not convinced that the cancer treatment—and all the suffering and hardship it may cause—will cure their cancer or even extend their life. Although this may be true in a few situations, in the majority of cases early cancer treatment can produce complete cures or markedly extended life spans.

Increasing patient compliance is a major area of clinical and research emphasis in health psychology. In the cancer area, increasing patient compliance can be especially important because the nature of cancer is such that if the disease is not stopped or eradicated, it continues to grow until, in many cases, treatment is no longer likely to have much of an effect. Much more research is needed in this area.

EARLY DETECTION AND EXAMINATION PRACTICES    A final area in which behavioral, psychological, and social factors can indirectly affect cancer progression concerns both the regular practice of early-detection behaviors that allow one to discover a cancer in its preliminary stages and the immediate seeking of a medical examination as soon as one suspects that a cancerous lesion may be present. The reason that these behaviors are so important is that for several types of cancer, the chances for cure and/or extended life is significantly greater if the cancer is discovered and treated early than if it is treated late. For example, Levy (1982) reported research on melanoma patients that showed that 83% of the patients who delayed seven months or more in seeing a physician after they noticed signs of the disease were diagnosed as being at high risk of a poor treatment outcome. The percentage dropped to 41% for patients who saw the physician within four to six months after noting symptoms, and to 29% for patients seeing the physician in three months or less.

Perhaps the area that has received the most attention recently is the performance of breast self-examinations (BSE) by women. Although little is known about how to prevent breast cancer, it is generally agreed that the early detection and treatment of the disease can prolong life and increase the chances of cure.

Although BSE is relatively easy to perform (see Figure 9.5), costs nothing, is not time consuming, is not painful, and that large-scale public awareness campaigns have been conducted (in several studies the overwhelming majority of women said they were aware of BSE, e.g., Howe, 1981a, 1981b), the National Cancer Institute (1980) estimates that only 24% of the adult women in the United States practice BSE regularly. A number of strategies have been

Follow These Simple Steps:

Lie down. Put one hand behind your head. With the other hand, fingers flattened, gently feel your breast. Press ever so lightly. Now examine the other breast.

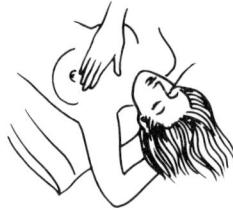

This illustration shows you how to check each breast. Begin where you see the *A* and follow the arrows, feeling gently for a lump or thickening. Remember to feel all parts of each breast.

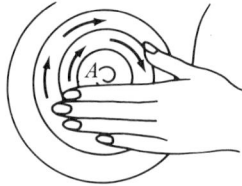

Now repeat the same procedure sitting up, with the hand still behind your head.

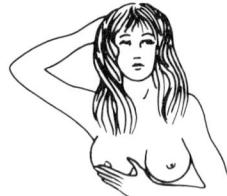

FIGURE 9.5   How to do a breast self-examination. If you find a lump or thickening, see your physician immediately. Most breast lumps are not caused by cancer, but only a physician can make the diagnosis. From "Breast Self-Examination and the Nurse," 1976, by the American Cancer Society, Inc.

tried to increase BSE among adult women. For example, Grady (1984) gave 189 women a private session with a lay instructor on how to conduct BSE and provided a set of written instructions on BSE to take home. The women were then divided into one of four groups formed by a 2 (self-management, no self-management) × 2 (postcard, no postcard) design. Women who received the self-management manipulation had a calendar printed on the back of their instruction sheet and were told to mark a date on each month to do BSE. They were also given 12 stickers that said "mark your calendar" or "do a BSE" to put around the house in places that would remind them. Compliance with specific interventions varied from 19% (using stickers) to 62% (using calendars), with 64% of the women indicating that they used at least one part of the self-management package. Women who received the postcard manipulation were sent postcards once a month for six months to remind them to do the BSE. The results of the study suggested that about 15% of the women in all four conditions never did a BSE and that, on the average, the other 85% of the women practiced BSE about 60% of the time. However, whether or not a woman performed a BSE each month was significantly affected by what group she was in: about 15% of the women in the control group (no self-management, no postcard), 22% in the self-management-only group, 33% in the postcard-only group, and 41% in the self-management-plus-postcard group did a BSE each month. There was an understandable decrease in BSE practice in the postcard groups when the postcard reminders were stopped. In a follow-up study (Grady, Goodenow, & Borkin, 1988), the investigators showed that BSE rates could be increased further by providing an external reward, namely a $1 lottery ticket or $1 in cash, each time the BSE was performed. However, when the reward was withdrawn, the BSE rates decreased sharply. Women who were instructed to "self-reward" themselves for practicing BSE usually did not do so; however, if they did, they showed an increase in BSE comparable to that of women who received an external reward.

There are other early-detection behaviors that people can do and inexpensive tests they can have performed in order to detect many cancers in their early stages; for example, testicular self-examinations and mail-in tests for colon cancer. As biomedical research continues to uncover other means for the early detection of cancer or precancer conditions, it will become increasingly important for health psychologists to devise practical and effective strategies for increasing the use of these procedures by at-risk populations.

# Psychological and Behavioral Reactions

For many people, learning that they have cancer is a traumatic experience. They respond to the diagnosis as if it were a life sentence for pain, disfigurement, and eventually death. Even physically healthy people fear cancer, and some develop a phobia for the disease. Given these attitudes by the public and even some health professionals, it is not surprising that there can be a variety of negative psychological and behavioral reactions associated with cancer.

## Psychiatric Problems

Are psychological reactions to cancer so severe that they can lead to psychiatric dysfunctions? A good deal of research has been conducted on this question.

One of the most comprehensive studies of psychiatric problems among cancer patients was conducted by Derogatis and his colleagues (1983). These investigators administered a battery of psychological tests and a standardized psychiatric interview to 250 randomly selected cancer patients who were new admissions to one of three major cancer centers. After collecting all the information on the patients, the researchers matched what they found to the psychiatric categories listed in the American Psychiatric Association's *Diagnostic and Statistical Manual-Revised*, Third Edition (DSM-III-R) to determine whether a psychiatric diagnosis was appropriate. The results indicated that 47% of the patients had a psychiatric problem. Although this percentage might appear to suggest that almost half of all cancer patients have major emotional or behavioral problems, a closer inspection of the data suggests a somewhat different interpretation. Table 9.3 shows the breakdown of the specific diagnoses given to patients. As the table indicates, more than two-thirds of all the patients who received a psychiatric diagnosis were assigned the label "adjustment disorder." This type of disorder is generally regarded as being transient, due to an obvious environmental stressor (such as cancer), and responsive to psychological interventions. In other words, for most people the dysfunction will remit in a fairly short amount of time, though some patients may need professional help in resolving the problem.

In a study by Bukberg, Pennman, and Holland (1984), sixty-two hospitalized cancer patients were also given psychological tests and a psychiatric interview, and then these data were inspected to determine whether the patients should be given psychiatric diagnoses. The investigators concluded that 42% of the patients were psychiatrically depressed—a much higher percentage than Derogatis and his colleagues reported. However, upon further analysis of the data, Bukberg and her colleagues found that there was a significant relationship between the amount of depression a patient had and the degree of his or her physical disability: depression was more prevalent in patients who had become considerably disabled. Moreover, in patients who did have comparatively high levels of physical disability, depression was more likely to occur if the patient was in pain, had poor social supports (e.g., little support from his or her family), and had a relatively high amount of recent stress in his or her life—all factors that are associated with depression in persons whether or not they have cancer.

In interpreting the data on psychiatric diagnosis and cancer, it also should be kept in mind that, as we will discuss in more detail shortly, it is common and considered "normal" for cancer patients to have some increase in their anxiety and depression. Given the life circumstances of these patients, the aversiveness of the treatments they may be receiving, and the uncertainty of their future, it would be considered "abnormal" by many if they did not have an increase in anxiety and depression. It can be quite arbitrary and difficult to tell when this increase is appropriate versus when it is abnormal and dysfunctional. Overall, then, there does appear to be an increase in psychiatric symptoms among cancer patients, but many of these symptoms are "normal" responses to stress, are temporary, and are due to factors such as physical disability rather than to cancer per se.

## Nonpsychiatric Responses to Cancer

Even if a patient does not exhibit psychiatric symptomology after a diagnosis of cancer, he or she will most likely exhibit some type of psychological or behavioral reaction. These reactions may be caused by the treatments patients receive for their cancer rather than to the disease per se. Also, often these reactions are transitory and are characterized by "islands of significant life disruption" (Ander-

TABLE 9.3   Rates of DSM-III Psychiatric Disorders Observed in Cancer Patients from Three Cancer Centers*

| Diagnostic Category | DSM-III code | Specific category, no. % | Diagnostic class, no. % | % of psychiatric diagnosis |
|---|---|---|---|---|
| Organic mental disorders | | | | |
| Presenile dementia | 290.10 | 1(0.5) | 8(4) | 8 |
| Dementia with depression | 290.21 | 1(0.5) | | |
| Organic affective syndrome | 293.83 | 2(1.0) | | |
| Dementia | 294.10 | 1(1.0) | | |
| Atypical organic brain syndrome | 294.80 | 2(1.0) | | |
| Organic personality syndrome | 310.10 | 1(0.5) | | |
| Major affective disorders | | | | |
| Major affective disorder–unipolar depression | 296.20 | 8(4.0) | 13(6) | 13 |
| Major affective disorder–bipolar depression | 296.50 | 1(0.5) | | |
| Major affective disorder–atypical depression | 296.82 | 3(1.5) | | |
| Dysthmic disorder | 300.40 | 1(0.5) | | |
| Adjustment disorders | | | | |
| Adjustment disorder with depressed mood | 309.00 | 26(12.0) | 69(32) | 68 |
| Adjustment disorder with mixed emotional features | 309.28 | 29(13.0) | | |
| Adjustment disorder with anxious mood | 309.24 | 12(6.0) | | |
| Adjustment disorder with mixed disturbance of emotion and conduct | 309.40 | 2(1.0) | | |
| Anxiety disorders | | | | |
| General anxiety disorder | 300.02 | 1(0.5) | 4(2) | 4 |
| Simple phobia | 300.29 | 1(0.5) | | |
| Obsessive-compulsive disorder | 300.30 | 2(1.0) | | |
| Personality disorders | | | | |
| Schizoid personality disorder | 301.20 | 1(0.5) | 7(3) | 7 |
| Compulsive personality disorder | 301.40 | 2(1.0) | | |
| Histrionic personality disorder | 301.50 | 1(0.5) | | |
| Dependent personality disorder | 301.60 | 1(0.5) | | |
| Other personality disorder | 301.89 | 1(0.5) | | |
| Alcohol abuse (in remission) | 305.03 | 1(0.5) | | |
| Total psychiatric diagnoses | . . . | . . . | 101(47) | . . . |
| Psychiatric diagnosis absent | . . . | . . . | 114(53) | . . . |

*Rates given are for principal diagnoses only.

SOURCE:   From Derogotis et al. (1983). The prevalence of psychiatric disorders among cancer patients. *Journal of the American Medical Association.* 249, 751-757.

sen, Anderson, & deProsse, 1989) rather than by long-lasting global problems in adjustment or psychological functioning. As we will see in a later section, many of these problems can be addressed by psychological intervention.

EMOTIONAL DISTRESS    Emotional responses to cancer are often first seen during the time of diagnosis. This period can be divided into three stages. The first is the discovery, usually by the person or by a health professional, of possible signs or symptoms of cancer. For example, a woman may feel a small lump in her breast that she has never before noticed, or a man whose father was diagnosed as having colon cancer shortly after complaining of prolonged constipation may become quite anxious upon realizing that he, too, has been experiencing constipation off and on for several weeks.

The second stage is the undergoing of an examination and/or of diagnostic tests to confirm or rule out the presence of cancer. The period of time between the administration of these tests and when the results are available is, according to some patients, one of the most stressful times in the whole cancer experience. One's energies and attention during this period are often consumed by the fear that the vigil will end with the diagnosis of cancer.

Finally, if the tests are positive, a formal diagnosis of cancer is made. Prior to the 1960s, many physicians did not tell patients that they had cancer, apparently in large part to spare the patient the emotional anguish that usually accompanies the diagnosis (Oken, 1961). Today, however, virtually all physicians tell cancer patients of their diagnosis immediately upon confirmation. The most common response to the news that one has cancer is a feeling of shock or disbelief. After this initial period of shock, and sometimes also after additional tests or trips to other physicians to confirm the diagnosis, the patient usually accepts that he or she has cancer. Typically, at this stage patients experience some or all of a number of unpleasant emotions, including anxiety, depression, hopelessness, anger, and guilt. When the patient is a child, these responses are often more characteristic of the parents than of the patient, although many children—depending on their age—will eventually come to share these feelings and, in addition, may feel guilty about causing them in their parents.

A newly diagnosed cancer patient's emotional response to his or her disease can be affected radically by the specific treatment given. For example, the disfiguring results of surgery, including the loss of a breast, the reshaping of a face, or the creation of an opening, or stoma, in the abdomen through which fecal material empties, can result in loss of self-esteem, fear of rejection, and despondency. Some chemotherapy regimens can produce hair loss, prolonged nausea and vomiting, and a loss of energy and stamina. These side effects can result in considerable emotional distress. In addition, there is evidence that some chemotherapy drugs can directly produce feelings of depression by their effects on the neurotransmitter substances in the brain. Thus, it is sometimes difficult to tell whether a patient's emotional response is due to the diagnosis, the treatment, or both.

Although the specific emotional responses to the diagnosis and treatment of cancer can vary considerably in composition and intensity from patient to patient depending on a variety of factors, research suggests that six general types of emotional responses predominate.

First, *anxiety* is a common response to cancer at almost all stages. It has been associated with the development of unexpected symptoms, initiation of treatment, concern over pain, and the inevitability of death. Researchers have found that some patients who experience considerable discomfort during prolonged cancer treatments such as chemotherapy will become very anxious upon the termination of treatment, apparently because they fear that once the treatment has stopped the tumor may grow again. On the other hand, anxiety can also cause patients to refuse treatments that have been recommended to them or to elect alternate and usually less effective forms of treatment. Fear of pain, disfigurement, needle sticks, and confinement to a hospital has led some patients to choose a hastened death or unproved forms of treatment (e.g., laetrile or megavitamins) rather than traditional forms of surgery, radiation, or chemotherapy.

Second, almost all cancer patients feel *depressed* at some point during their illness or treatment. As we saw earlier, in some patients this depression can become sufficiently severe to warrant a psychiatric diagnosis. But in most patients the depression is more temporary and less severe, although it can be very unpleasant. The signs of depression in cancer patients include sadness; tearfulness; guilt; impaired concentration; suicidal ideation; feelings of hopelessness, helplessness, or worthlessness; sleep disturbances; and decreased sex drive, energy, or appetite. Of course, any of these symptoms can also result from the direct physical effects of the cancer or its treatment. It is important to remember that there is a relationship between how disabling the cancer is and how depressed the patient becomes. In this sense, cancer patients react like most other people: the more their sexual, occupational, social, and recreational activities are taken away from them or interfered with, the greater the sense of loss and sadness. That is the reason why some clinicians regard depression in cancer patients as normal and to be expected.

A third common problem for cancer patients is a *feeling of loss of control*. Most people prefer to feel that they have some control over important aspects of their life, or over "reinforcers" as behavioral psychologists are fond of saying. For example, people prefer to believe that to some extent their behavior will determine whether they pass an examination (e.g., by studying), are successful at their jobs (e.g., by working hard), and whether they will prevent or recover from illness (e.g., by avoiding close contact with the people who have contagious diseases or by taking their medicine as prescribed). Unfortunately, once a person has cancer, there is little that he or she can do personally to gain mastery or control over the disease. Unlike patients with many other kinds of chronic diseases who can help themselves by altering their diets or beginning exercise programs or at least being responsible for taking their medicine every day, cancer patients often can do little to help themselves. Surgery, radiation, and most forms of chemotherapy are handled by medical staff. The patient simply comes in for treatment and goes home to wait for the next treatment. The sense of loss of control that results from this situation can lead to feelings of anxiety, depression, helplessness, and hopelessness. Some researchers (e.g., Silberfarb & Greer, 1982) have suggested that the increased popularity of a number of unorthodox cancer treatments is due in part to people's need to do something to help themselves — whether it be following a macrobiotic diet or visually imaging the demise of their cancer cells. It is perhaps significant that the proponents of some unproven cancer treatments explicitly claim that cancer patients can and should take control over their own healing. Research has also suggested that one of the ways in which some patients with chronic diseases adapt to their illness is by reducing their desire to have control over their environment, preferring instead to allow others (such as the medical staff) to exert control (Nagy & Wolfe, 1983).

A fourth common consequence of cancer and the treatments for cancer is *cognitive, or "mental status," impairment.* This category of symptoms is very broad and can include confusion, disorientation, out-of-character behavior such as increased irritability or poor judgment, decreased attention span, and inability to remember or recall information. These symptoms are sometimes transitory and sometimes long lasting, but they are almost always distressing to the patient and to the patient's family. They interfere with the person's ability to work, perform routine household tasks, or even carry on a conversation. There are many potential causes of such cognitive impairment. For example, metastatic spread of the cancer to the central nervous system (sometimes referred to as "CNS involvement"), some types of chemotherapy drugs, and radiation to the head can all cause confusion or other cognitive impairments. Sometimes the impairments are due to ancillary problems such as high fevers or metabolic disorders.

One of the most disturbing findings of recent research is the increased presence of long-term cognitive impairments, including decreased IQs, in some children who are treated for leukemia. Many years ago, childhood leukemia was treated primarily with chemotherapy drugs that killed the cancer cells in the blood-related organs from which they arose (e.g., the bone marrow). However, in approximately 50%–75% of the patients, the disease eventually would spread to the central nervous system and the patient could die as a result. In response to this problem, physicians began to anticipate the probable spread of the cancer to the CNS and routinely treated the patient as if there were CNS involvement, often by using radiation to the skull area. This type of therapy is referred to as "CNS prophylaxis." It has proven to be very effective for children with acute lymphoblastic leukemia (ALL), which is the most common type of leukemia, producing complete cure in the majority of these children. But it now appears that this CNS prophylactic treatment may have detrimental effects on brain development and function, especially if the children are relatively young (less than eight years of age) and therefore presumably undergoing continuous brain development at the time of the treatment. Specifically, research has shown that some children receiving CNS prophylaxis show significantly lower IQ scores (Stehbens & Kisker, 1984) and attention deficits such as longer reaction times to a stimulus (Brouwers, Riccardi, Poplack, & Fedio, 1984). Research is now being undertaken to identify more precisely the nature of these problems and to develop learning techniques that might compensate for or prevent them.

*Sexual dysfunctions* represent a fifth problem that is common among cancer patients. Andersen (1985) has suggested that for the most common types of cancer, problems in sexual functioning occur for up to 90 percent of patients, although in some cases the problems are short-lived and not unlike those that occur with other diseases. They include difficulties with having orgasms, sterility, pain during intercourse, or inability to perform intercourse at all or in common positions. Patients become so embarrassed or develop such poor self-concept due to their sexual difficulties that they will be reluctant to let other persons see them unclothed or to have others touch or get physically close to them. Because healthy sexual functioning is an important source of personal pleasure and self-esteem for many adults, the loss of this ability can result in depression, strained relationships, and feelings of isolation.

Andrykowski and Redd (1987), after reviewing the literature on sexual dysfunctions that occur in cancer patients, suggested that these dysfunctions usually stem from one of four major sources. First, the physical impact of cancer or cancer treatments can directly affect sexual functioning. For example, surgery for cancer of the penis or prostate cancer can make erection impossible, and radiation treatment for cervical cancer can produce atrophy of cervical tissue or actual narrowing of the cervical opening. Second, cancer and its treatment, like many other illnesses and their treatments, can cause fatigue, weakness, pain, nausea, depression, and other states that reduce sexual desire, enjoyment, or performance. Third, people's psychological reactions to the cosmetic changes caused by cancer can significantly interfere with sexual activity. For example, some researchers have found that women who have undergone a mastectomy feel ugly, defeminized, and sexually unacceptable. Men who have had much of their penis or scrotum removed may feel similarly. Patients with cancer of the head, neck, and genitalia are at considerable risk for developing body-image disturbances. It is not surprising that a person who feels unattractive or repulsive is likely to have problems in maintaining a healthy sex life. Finally, some sexual problems in cancer patients are due to their sexual partners' attitudes towards them. A partner may withdraw from a cancer patient for fear that he or she will also contract cancer, because of repulsion from surgical scars or deformity, from false impressions that the patient wants to be left alone, or from a fear of hurting the patient. Thus, at a time when most cancer patients need and long for extra support and reassurance, they may receive from their partner even less affection than usual.

Finally, a common response by most cancer patients to their situation is the use of *denial*. Denial involves disavowing some aspect of reality that one is presumed to be aware of at some level of consciousness. For example, a patient who is informed that he or she has terminal cancer may deny that the disease is terminal, insisting that modern science will come up with a cure and that he or she will eventually recover. Research suggests that most cancer patients, at least to some extent, will deny their diagnosis, the seriousness of their illness, the adversiveness of the side effects, or their fears and concerns about the effect of the disease on their life. In many cases this denial can be effective in reducing the patient's distress. For example, M. Watson and her colleagues (1984) assessed the extent to which twenty-four breast cancer patients were using denial within the first week following a mastectomy. The results indicated that patients who denied their first diagnosis or the likelihood of future problems were significantly less dysphoric than patients who did not deny. It is important to note that patients who used denial did not seem to have any negative consequences as a result of disavowing the reality of their situation.

The realization that denial can have a positive value in cancer patients and individuals with other types of chronic disease is a recent and controversial finding. In the traditional literature of psychopathology dating back to Freud, denial is usually considered to be a clear sign of abnormality. The psychoanalytic view and that of several other schools of psychology is that an accurate appraisal of reality is a hallmark of mental health. To deny reality under almost any circumstance is considered a maladaptive and primitive attempt at coping. Research with cancer patients suggests that this is not necessarily so: denying the hopelessness of a situation can uplift one's spirit and outlook and as a result can actually reduce the likelihood of developing psychiatric problems.

This is not to say that denial is effective in all cases: there are clearly adaptive and maladaptive uses of denial. For example, denying that a persistent sore or a small lump in one's breast might be cancerous can be maladaptive if it leads to a delay in seeking medical attention. Similarly, refusal to take recommended chemotherapy treatments because a person denies that he or she has cancer can have obviously negative consequences. It also is important to realize that sometimes cancer patients only appear to be denying. A patient may be fully aware of the nature and seriousness of the disease but may prefer not to talk about these things or even outwardly acknowledge them in order to put up a good front in the presence of family and friends. Terms such as *denial*, *avoidance*, and *suppression* have all been used to refer to such behavior. To some extent, whether or not a person is denying can therefore simply be a matter of semantics. But whatever one calls it, it is clearly common among cancer patients and often remarkably adaptive.

# Treatment Interventions: Medical

Over the past decades significant progress has been made in the medical treatment of cancer. In the 1930s, fewer that 20% of all cancer patients survived five years after treatment. In the 1950s, it was 25%. In the 1960s, it was 30%. Today, approximately 40% of all cancer patients will be alive at least five years after treatment. The great majority of cancer treatments fall into one of three basic categories: surgery, radiation, or chemotherapy. These treatments can be used alone or in combination and are usually initiated for one of three reasons: prevention, cure, or palliation. The specific type of treatment used will depend on a variety of factors, including the type and size of the cancer tumor, the severity of the disease, whether metastasis has occurred, and so forth. A cancer is usually considered cured if a person survives five years after treatment with no sign of disease. Even if treatments do not cure cancer, however, they can lengthen a patient's life or reduce the discomfort caused by the disease.

# Surgery

Surgery, which is one of the oldest treatments for cancer, involves removing as much of the cancerous tissue as possible while leaving intact as much of the normal tissue as possible. Surgery is usually most effective when two conditions are present. First, surgery tends to be most effective when the tumor is localized and there is limited or no metastasis. Under these circumstances it may be possible to cut out all of the cancer before it spreads to other parts of the body. To be safe, in some cases surgeons will remove not only the tumor but also a margin of the normal-looking tissue surrounding the tumor in order to remove any cancer cells that might have spread to this adjacent tissue. Chemotherapy or radiation therapy also may be used after surgery to kill any remaining cancer cells. The second important requirement for surgery to be effective is that the site of the cancer must be such that the surgeon does not have to destroy life-sustaining normal tissue to get at the cancer. Some cancers are rendered inoperable because to get to them the surgeon would have to destroy so much normal tissue that the person could not survive. In some cases the surgical removal of the cancer destroys important normal tissues, but these tissues or their functions can be compensated for by additional surgery. For example, sometimes a person has part of a bowel or intestine removed, causing problems for the important process of waste elimination. Additional surgery, called ostomy, solves this problem by creating a new stoma, or opening, in the wall of the abdomen for the draining of fecal material, thus restoring this vital function.

Surgery can be used in some cases to prevent cancer. For example, by removing the precancerous lesions such as leukoplakia of the labia or vulva, polyps in the large intestine, or heavily pigmented moles on the skin, a surgeon can significantly reduce the likelihood that these minor conditions will lead to cancer. Surgery is sometimes used to completely cure already existing cancers, for example, colorectal cancer and breast cancer. Finally, surgery is sometimes used primarily to palliate. For example, surgical removal of a primary tumor may reduce pain even though metastasized cells are still present throughout the body. Bypass surgery can sometimes lengthen survival, as with the construction of a gastrostoma (a new opening into the stomach) in a patient whose cancer of the esophagus makes normal ingestion of food difficult or impossible.

# Radiation

Radiation therapy, also known as radiotherapy, X-ray therapy, cobalt treatment, or irradiation, refers to the use of high-energy rays to interrupt cell division and growth. Most cancer cells are more sensitive to X rays and radioactive substances than are normal cells, and thus the X rays will often kill the cancer cells before they do irreparable harm to normal tissue. There are basically two types of radiation: *X rays*, which are generated from a machine that uses a cathode ray, and *gamma rays*, which come from natural sources of radiation such as cobalt or cesium. Both types have basically the same properties. Radiation can be administered in one of two general ways. *External radiation*, which is the most common route of administration, involves the use of a beam of ionizing radiation administered from a large machine (e.g., a betatron or linear accelerator) external to the person. Typically, the beam is directed at the tumor to destroy it. *Internal radiation* involves implanting small amounts of radioactive material on or near the cancer cells. For example, radioactive material is often inserted into the upper vagina or uterus corpus to treat cervical cancer. Because patients are radioactive while the implant is in place, patients receiving internal radiation are hospitalized during the treatment. In contrast, most external-beam radiation is conducted on an outpatient basis.

Three points should be kept in mind about radiation therapy. First, like surgery, radiation is used primarily with localized tumors. Although it would be possible technically to radiate the entire body in order to kill metastasized cells, this procedure is uncommon, in part because the doses of radiation that would have to be used in order not to kill the person would be so low that usually they would have little effect on the cancer. Second, radiation usually kills some normal tissue and can therefore produce a variety of side effects or complications. For example, radiation to the head and neck areas can reduce saliva flow by destroying the glands that secrete saliva. Because one of the roles of saliva is to cleanse the mouth and teeth, which helps to prevent tooth decay and gum problems, decreased saliva flow can result in a variety of oral hygiene problems, decreased saliva flow can result in a variety of oral hygiene problems. However, radiation does not involve the disfiguring effects that some surgical procedures entail. Finally, radiation can be used with curative intent (e.g., localized cancer of the cervix), palliative intent (i.e., to reduce pain), or, less commonly, for preventive reasons (because X rays themselves can be carcinogenic, they are used as sparingly as possible with normal tissue).

# Chemotherapy

Chemotherapy involves the administration of drugs (chemicals) aimed at killing cancerous cells or stopping their reproduction. It is the newest of the three major types of cancer treatments, with most advances in the area coming since the 1950s, when Congress gave the National Cancer Institute $5 million to start a cancer-drug-development program. Today, chemotherapy is probably the most commonly used cancer treatment.

Most chemotherapeutic agents work by disrupting cell reproduction, usually by affecting the DNA. Chemotherapy drugs cannot tell the difference between cancer and noncancer cells. However, because cancer cells are usually reproducing more frequently than any other cells in the body, they are affected more than the other cells. Obviously, however, chemotherapy will interfere with some normal cells, especially with those that reproduce the most frequently, such as with cells that make up the skin, the lining of the gastrointestinal tract, hair follicles, and the blood cells. As a result, it is not uncommon for chemotherapy to produce a variety of negative side effects such as discoloration of the skin, nausea and vomiting, mouth sores, hair loss, and problems associated with the reductions in various blood cells, such as anemia and decreased resistance to infectious diseases. Because in children many cells are dividing frequently, additional side effects may occur. As we discussed earlier, for example, there are some data that suggest that chemotherapy treatments for leukemia may have detrimental results on brain cell maturation, resulting in mild decrements in intellectual performance.

Chemotherapy often is used in combination with surgery or radiation treatment. For example, one type of chemotherapy, called *adjuvant chemotherapy*, is used after surgery in order to kill any cancer cells that might have metastasized from the original tumor before it was removed. In this preventive use of chemotherapy, patients are often given the treatments immediately after surgery, even if no further signs of cancer exist, rather than waiting until any shed cancer cells have had time to grow into additional tumors.

Chemotherapy drugs also are used with curative intent. For example, chemotherapy often is used to cure some forms of leukemia, Hodgkin's disease, and testicular cancer. Even when chemotherapy cannot cure the cancer, it may prolong life by slowing the growth of cancer cells. In addition, chemotherapy can be used to reduce pain and for other palliative reasons.

## Additional Treatments

In addition to surgery, radiation, and chemotherapy, other forms of cancer treatments have been developed. Most of these are still used on an experimental basis and often in conjunction with one of the more traditional treatments rather than as a sole treatment approach.

One of the most promising of the new treatment approaches is *immunotherapy*, sometimes referred to as the use of biologicals or biological-response modifiers. The basic aim of immunotherapy is to augment the person's own natural defenses against cancer cells. For example, a person might be given substances aimed at stimulating a greater immune response to the cancer cells, or they might be injected directly with antibodies capable of fighting cancer cells. Immunotherapy also can increase a person's ability to tolerate the side effects of other treatments such as chemotherapy, and as a result might prove to be a useful adjunct to other kinds of cancer treatment.

Another new treatment approach is *hyperthermia* or the use of high levels of heat. This heat may be applied to small areas of the body where the cancer is concentrated, or to large areas by putting the person into a whole-body hyperthermia apparatus. High temperatures are lethal to cancer cells, and they also can potentiate the effects of radiation therapy and chemotherapy. Thus, hyperthermia may be used as an adjunct treatment with some of the more traditional forms of anticancer approaches.

# Treatment Interventions: Psychological

As we have just seen, in recent years medical treatments have become increasingly effective in curing patients or at least in prolonging their life. As a result, there are now more people living with cancer as well as with the remnants of their cancer treatment (such as the loss of a breast or with stoma through which bodily wastes are eliminated) than ever before. This fact has given rise to a new emphasis among patients and health professionals alike on the *quality* of the life that is being prolonged. This fact was stated clearly several years ago by several researchers who were studying the effects of colostomy on cancer patients:

> Society has determined that life must be saved at all costs, and the skill of the surgeon is directed toward this end. We have shown that it is now time to look more closely at the costs and those who bear them. For more emphasis must now be placed on the quality of the life saved. . . . [There is an] immense price paid by the patient for his cure from cancer—a price paid in physical discomfort and in psychological and social trauma. (Devlin, Plant, & Griffin, 1971, p. 418)

This emphasis on quality of life has made behavioral scientists and clinicians increasingly important members of the cancer-treatment team. The scope and nature of the work done by psychologists and other health care professionals who treat cancer patients have varied widely, ranging from controversial treatments aimed at curing cancer to more well accepted interventions for reducing the distress of specific types of problems such as pain or nausea and vomiting. In general, psychological interventions can be divided into four major categories: (1) interventions aimed at altering the disease process, (2) interventions for improving general psychosocial adjustment, (3) interventions for specific problems, and (4) patient self-help programs.

## Psychological Interventions Aimed at Altering the Disease Process

The most well known—and controversial—psychological intervention for altering the disease process is the so-called Simonton approach, named after its originators, Carl Simonton, a physician and radiologist by training, and Stephanie Matthews-Simonton. The Simonton approach emphasizes that, to a

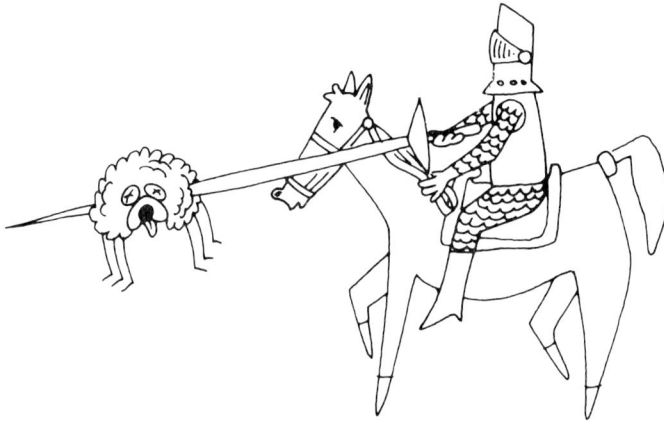

FIGURE 9.6 Patient drawing of a knight (a white blood cell) stabbing an armadillo (a cancer cell). Adapted from Achterberg, J. & Lawlis, G. F. (1978). *Imagery of Cancer.* Savoy, IL: Institute for Personality and Ability Testing.

large degree, people can control their own health. This approach suggests that people who have not effectively managed their own health, and as a result have developed a disease such as cancer, can be taught mental control of basic physiological processes and as a result can promote their own healing. The Simonton treatment program is multimodal in nature, involving relaxation training, physical exercise, and dietary changes, in addition to whatever standard medical treatment the physician prescribes for the patient. The component that has received the most public attention, however, is imagery. The Simontons suggest that imagining the demise of cancer cells at the hands of the body's natural defense system can actually promote disease regression to such an extent that the person is considered cured of his or her cancer. The following case history illustrates this point. The patient was a male with cancer of the pancreas—a type of cancer that is usually fatal.

> [The patient] initially described his cancer cells as armadillos and his white blood cells as white knights [see Figure 9.6]. The knights had a daily quota of creatures they needed to spear on their lancets.... At one time during his therapy he observed that many of his white knights were dropping off or disappearing. He was subsequently informed that his white blood cell count was dropping. Fearing that he would be taken off chemotherapy [chemotherapy itself can decrease the white blood cell count], he was determined to "peg" the number of white blood cells. After making this decision, the white blood cell count stabilized, and the chemotherapy continued. Sometime later, he experienced difficulty with the white knights meeting their daily quota. They were beating the bushes to find armadillos. Shortly after, he had ultrasound diagnosis and there was no evidence of tumor. (Lenard, 1981, p. 62)

Unfortunately, neither the Simontons nor any other group has ever published a scientifically acceptable study supporting the claim that imagery can help cure cancer. Whereas some regard this lack of evidence as only temporary, others view it as a more telling indictment of the Simonton approach. In 1982, the American Cancer Society published an influential paper in which they described their reasons for putting the Simonton approach on their infamous list of "unproven method of cancer management." The authors of this paper emphasized that the approach does have some potentially positive attributes, such as promoting feelings of self-control and teaching effective psychological techniques for reducing distress. However, they also noted that the approach could increase guilt feelings by making patients feel responsible for the progression of their disease. And most important, they concluded that there is no evidence that the use of the Simonton approach can alter in any way the natural course of cancer.

Although the Simontons have developed perhaps the most well articulated psychological intervention for cancer, several other individuals have promoted similar concepts. For example, Bernie S. Siegel, a surgeon and Professor at Yale University, published a best-selling book in 1986 entitled *Love, Medicine, and Miracles*. Siegel, like the Simontons, did not suggest that cancer patients should forgo traditional medical treatment, but rather emphasized the relationship between illness and attitude or belief, and suggested that every person has a "healing potential" within that can be facilitated by love, therapeutic confrontation, and one's attitude. It is the ability of a patient to develop this healing power that, according to Siegel, results in some patients surviving cancer and others succumbing to it, or some patients showing relatively few side effects from their treatment and others becoming very ill. Siegel created Exceptional Cancer Patients, a specialized form of individual and group therapy, to facilitate healing within each person. Although it is likely that this therapy, like the Simontons', improves the quality of life for some patients, there is also no scientific support for the claim that it can increase the quality of life or cure cancer altogether.

Recently, however, a scientifically rigorous study was published suggesting that a more traditional type of psychological intervention can affect the longevity of cancer patients. David Spiegel and his colleagues (1989) assigned 86 women with metastatic breast cancer either to a group that received weekly supportive group therapy for a year or to a control group that did not receive psychological intervention. Each group therapy session lasted approximately ninety minutes, was led by a psychiatrist or social worker with a cotherapist who had breast cancer in remission, and focused on strategies for coping with cancer and for increasing social support. Patients were not led to believe that the intervention would in any way affect the course of their disease. The researchers then followed the women for ten years, by which time all but three had died. The results of the study were striking: the survival time for patients in the treatment group was significantly longer—about eighteen months—than that of patients in the control group, suggesting that psychological intervention can indeed increase the survival time of metastatic breast cancer patients. Although this is not the first study to make such a claim, it is the first methodologically rigorous study to do so. For example, unlike other research in the area, in this study patients were randomly assigned to groups and a large number of possible alternative explanations for the differences between the groups, such as age, type or severity of cancer at the beginning of treatment, type of medical treatment received, and many others, were statistically ruled out.

The Spiegel study provides the first scientifically acceptable support for the claim that psychological intervention, when used as an adjunct with traditional medical treatment, can extend the lives of some cancer patients. This is a major finding that has had a major impact on the field. However, it is important to emphasize what the Spiegel et al. study does not do. First, it does not suggest that the Simonton or Siegel approach, both of which differ markedly from the one used by the Spiegel group, also extend life. Second, it does not suggest why a fairly standard psychological intervention package might extend the life of select cancer patients. The authors suggest that perhaps the therapy produced better compliance with medical treatment, or perhaps the treated patients were less depressed and more active physically, which helped to extend life. But in the end, the authors admit that they do not know the mechanism that produced their results. Finally, the Spiegel et al. study does not answer the question of whether psychological interventions can cure cancer. As suggested earlier in the chapter, there is some evidence that psychological stress can affect disease progression, and it may be that coping adequately with stress can therefore counter such progression. And, as discussed in other chapters, the mind and body are clearly interactive. Emotions can affect physiological functioning and vice versa. Thus, it is conceivable that psychological factors may exert some influence on disease initiation and progression. Whether this influence is large enough to reverse disease progression and overcome cancer entirely, rather than extend life without curing the disease, is not known at this time. Perhaps some people, with certain types of cancer, receiving specific types of medical treatments, will be more likely to be cured of their cancer if they also receive psychological interventions. Perhaps not. Regardless of the eventual answer, this is a critically important question for cancer patients, with major implications for all of health psychology, and one that can only be answered with carefully conducted experimental research.

## Psychological Interventions for Improving General Psychological Functioning

A second general category of psychological interventions consists of techniques that are used to help cancer patients of all types to cope adaptively with the many psychosocial and physical stressors that they may experience as a result of their disease and the treatments they receive. The premise underlying this type of intervention is that the stress of cancer is often of greater proportions than persons can handle adequately with their own resources. The data reviewed earlier on psychiatric disturbances in cancer patients is often marshalled in support of this premise.

One of the most comprehensive and well controlled studies evaluating the impact of a psychosocial intervention on the quality of life of cancer patients was conducted by Gordon and his associates (1980) on more than 300 patients with breast cancer, lung cancer, or melanoma. These patients either did or did not receive, in addition to their standard medical treatment, a comprehensive, individually tailored psychosocial intervention consisting of three major components. First, patients in the intervention group were *educated* about factors that could be helpful in understanding and living with their disease (for example, information about the medical system and their specific diagnosis). Second, patients received *counseling* focused on exploring their reactions to and feelings about their disease. Finally, patients in the intervention condition were given *additional referrals and consultations* with hospital staff and community agencies that might be helpful in meeting any particular needs of the patient. This intervention package was administered by a multidisciplinary team consisting of psychologists, social workers, and a psychiatric nurse and was provided during the patient's initial hospitalization for treatment and on an outpatient basis for up to six months posthospitalization. The results of this study showed that patients who received the psychosocial intervention package showed some improvement over control patients, including a more rapid decline in negative emotional states (e.g., anxiety and depression) and a tendency to be more likely to return to their precancer vocational status. Overall, however, given the tremendous time investment and cost of the intervention, the results were somewhat disappointing.

Why were the results of the Gordon et al. (1980) not stronger? One possibility is that there were many patients in both the intervention and control groups who were coping adequately on their own and did not need or were unlikely to benefit from a formal psychological intervention. If a large number of patients were coping well prior to the beginning of the intervention, it would have been difficult to show a difference between the control group and the intervention group after the intervention was completed. This point was made perhaps most clearly in the well-known Omega Project conducted for several years at Massachusetts General Hospital by Avery Weisman, J. William Worden, Harry Sobel, and their associates. This group of researchers suggested not only that many cancer patients do not need formal psychological interventions to cope adequately, but also that those patients who do need such interventions can be identified early in the course of their illness.

In an initial attempt to test this hypothesis, the investigators gave the MMPI to 133 newly diagnosed cancer patients and then evaluated their coping and distress at five follow-up periods over the next six months (Sobel & Worden, 1979). The data indicated that based on the initial MMPI, the investigators could correctly predict 75% of the time whether patients would subsequently

show high or low distress to their disease and treatment. After several more
years of research, the investigators devised a more accurate assessment instrument that could correctly identify 86% of the patients who would show high
or low levels of distress (Worden, 1983). This instrument measured twenty
different items: (1) church attendance, (2) marital status, (3) living arrange-
ments, (4) family members, (5) socioeconomic status, (6) current symptoms,
(7) history of alcohol problems, (8) history of depressed moods, (9) mental-
health history, (10) history of illness, (11) optimism and pessimism, (12) past
regrets, (13) anatomical staging (a measure of the degree to which their
cancer has progressed), (14) health concerns, (15) religious concerns, (16)
work/finance concerns, (17) family concerns, (18) existential concerns, (19)
friendship concerns, and (20) self-esteem concerns. The general approach
taken by the Omega Project staff also was used by another group of investigators (Mages et al., 1981). These investigators suggested that three global
factors that are made up of many of the same specific items used by the
Project Omega staff—(1) severity of illness, (2) psychological stability, (3) social supports available—are significantly related to whether or not cancer patients will cope adaptively. The point is that several studies now suggest that
it is possible to predict, with considerable accuracy, how well a patient will
cope psychologically with cancer.

After the Project Omega investigators determined that cancer patients most
in need of psychological intervention to improve coping can be identified at
the time of diagnosis, they next investigated whether the high-risk patients
would profit from such an intervention (Worden & Weisman, 1984). In this
study, the refined assessment instrument was given to 381 patients, and from
this number 125 high-risk and 256 low-risk patients were identified. The
high-risk patients then were assigned to one of two different intervention
groups. In addition, a no-treatment control group consisting of high-risk patients
participating in an earlier phase of the Omega Project was included in the study
design. The first intervention used a patient-centered, problem-oriented approach that was aimed at facilitating the expression of emotions, identifying
what problems the patient was experiencing, and exploring in a nondirective
way various approaches to solving the problems. The second intervention had
similar goals to the first but took a more didactic approach. Patients were
taught a specific step-by-step problem-solving strategy that included progressive body relaxation and the use of a series of pictorial drawings illustrating
various problems. Both interventions were designed to be short term in nature, as they were fully administered within four sessions. The results of this
study indicated that patients who received the interventions, as opposed to
those who did not, reported significantly lower levels of emotional distress,
fatigue, and confusion; reported increased feelings of vigor; and produced
higher scores on a scale measuring how well they solved their problems.
There were no significant differences between the two intervention conditions, with each being as effective as the other. These rather strong effects
after only four treatment sessions were attributed in part by the authors to

the fact that all the patients who received the treatments were at risk and there-fore were likely to need and make good use of the interventions offered. Overall, the data from the studies described above and from several others suggest that some people will have a harder time coping with cancer and its treatment than will others, many of these people can be identified in advance by various assessment instruments, and psychosocial interventions can help people who need additional aid to cope more adaptively with their problems.

## Psychological Interventions for Specific Disease-Related or Treatment-Related Problems

In addition to broad-based interventions designed to be effective across a large spectrum of problems experienced by cancer patients, behavioral scientists have developed a number of more limited or focused treatments that are designed to prevent or ameliorate very specific types of problems that some cancer patients experience. For the most part these treatments have incorporated behavioral techniques and methodologies that have been developed in other areas. However, these techniques and methodologies have been refined and adapted for use in cancer-specific situations.

The specific symptoms that have received perhaps the most attention by behavioral scientists are chemotherapy-related side effects, especially nausea and vomiting. As we have already discussed, chemotherapy affects not only cancer cells but also normal cells, producing a wide variety of side effects. From the patients' point of view, among the most distressing of the side effects are the nausea and vomiting produced by the chemotherapy drugs. The nausea and vomiting can be either of two types. The first type is called *pharmacological* nausea and vomiting because it is due directly to the pharmacological properties of the chemotherapeutic agents. The second type is called *conditioned* nausea and vomiting because it is thought to arise from an associative learning process that works as follows. After several courses of chemotherapy, an association is established between the pharmacologically induced nausea and vomiting caused by the chemotherapy and the various sights, smells, and even thoughts associated with the chemotherapy setting. As a result of this association, the neutral stimuli themselves begin to elicit nausea and vomiting (see Figure 9.7). For example, the sight of the chemotherapy nurse, the smell of the drugs, or even the thought of getting chemotherapy can cause nausea and vomiting. Conditioned nausea and vomiting can occur before the chemotherapy is given, in which case it is usually referred to as anticipatory nausea and vomiting. It can also occur during or after chemotherapy but in these situations it is hard to differentiate conditioned nausea and vomiting from pharmacologically caused nausea and vomiting. Approximately 45% of all cancer chemotherapy patients develop conditioned nausea and vomiting (Burish & Carey, 1986).

Several behavioral treatments, including progressive muscle relaxation training with guided relaxation imagery, hypnosis, and systematic desensitization have

```
┌─────────────────────────────────────────────────────────────────┐
│          Before Association in Chemotherapy Context               │
│                                                                   │
│   Conditioned Stimulus        ──────▶   No Response or            │
│   (Sight of Nurse)                      Irrelevant Response        │
│                                                                   │
│   Unconditioned Stimulus      ──────▶   Unconditioned Response    │
│   (Chemotherapy Drugs)                  (Nausea, Vomiting)         │
└─────────────────────────────────────────────────────────────────┘
```

```
┌─────────────────────────────────────────────────────────────────┐
│          After Association in Chemotherapy Context                │
│                                                                   │
│   Conditioned Stimulus        ──────▶   Conditioned Response      │
│   (Sight of Nurse)                      (Nausea, Vomiting)         │
└─────────────────────────────────────────────────────────────────┘
```

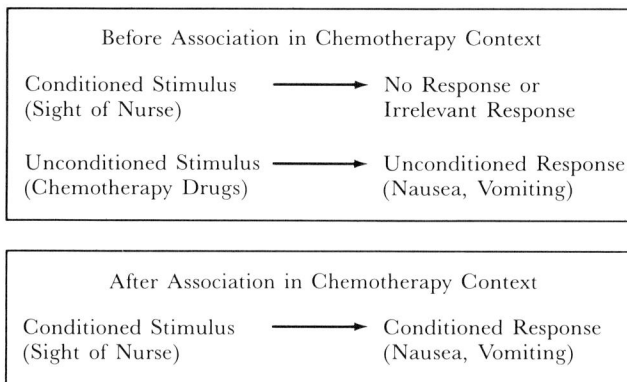

FIGURE 9.7   Example of associative learning in cancer chemotherapy. Previously neutral stimuli (such as the sight of the attending nurse) elicit, because of their association with chemotherapy, the side effects of nausea and vomiting. From Burish & Carey (1984), Conditioned responses to cancer chemotherapy: Etiology and treatment. In B. H. Fox & B. H. Newberry (Ed.), *Impact of psychoendocrine systems in cancer and immunity.* New York: C. J. Hogrefe.

been shown to be highly effective in reducing or preventing conditioned responses. For example, Burish and his colleagues (1987) equated twenty-four cancer chemotherapy patients on the types of drugs they were receiving and then randomly assigned them to either a group that received progressive muscle relaxation training plus guided relaxation imagery or to a no-treatment control group. Each patient in the relaxation training group received from one to three relaxation training sessions during the days preceding the start of chemotherapy treatment (depending on the amount of time available) and also during each of their first three chemotherapy sessions. Patients were instructed to practice the relaxation training at home daily between their chemotherapy sessions. All patients were followed through their first five chemotherapy sessions. The results indicated that patients who received relaxation training had significantly less nausea and vomiting and significantly lower blood pressures, pulse rates, and dysphoria, especially anxiety, than did patients in the control group. Some of these results are shown in Figure 9.8. Results similar to these have been reported in several other studies.

A second example of a problem-specific intervention is a package developed by Jay and her colleagues (1987) to reduce the distress of children with leukemia who undergo frequent bone marrow aspirations. A bone marrow aspiration is a painful procedure that consists of several steps. First, a nurse (or physician) determines the site of the puncture (usually the posterior ileal crest), cleanses the area, and injects a local anesthetic. After a couple of

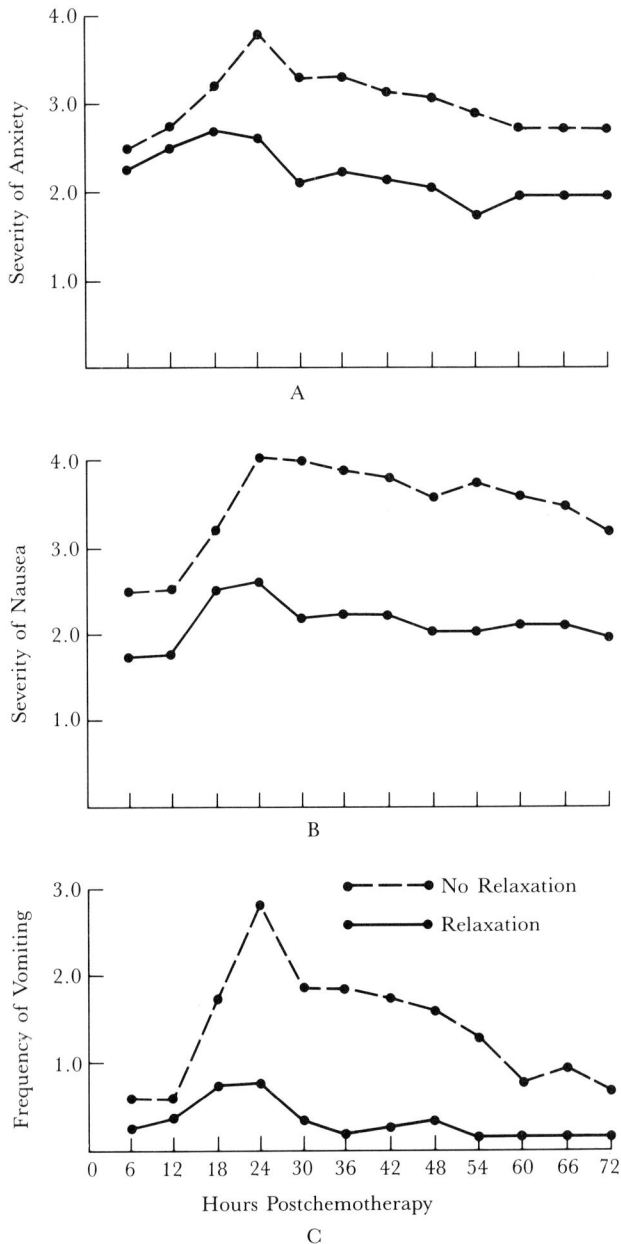

FIGURE 9.8   Patients who received relaxation training and guided imagery reported significantly less anxiety (Panel A), nausea (Panel B), and vomiting (Panel C) during the three days following chemotherapy than patients in the control group. From Burish et al. (1987). Copyright (1987) by American Psychological Association. Reprinted by permission of the publisher.

minutes to allow the anesthetic to take effect, a large needle is inserted through the skin and directly into the pelvic bone. Marrow from inside the bone is then sucked up with an aspiration needle. Although the needle insertion into the bone is painful, most patients find the aspiration even more distressing, producing a sharp pain or cramp that can run all the way down the leg. After the marrow is extracted, the needle is withdrawn and the site is cleansed again. The marrow is then examined to determine if it contains any cancer cells. Young children's reactions to this procedure typically include crying and pleading for help or fighting to avoid the needle stick. Often they must be physically restrained in order to complete the procedure. As one might imagine, the pain and fear that is obvious in the child's face and behavior can also cause great distress to the parents, making the situation very unpleasant for the whole family.

The intervention package used by Jay and her associates contains five components: (1) a film of a child modeling cooperation and good coping behavior during a bone marrow aspiration procedure; (2) the use of breathing exercises and (3) imagery to promote relaxation and provide a source of distraction; (4) verbal reinforcement throughout the procedure for appropriate behavior and a reward (e.g., a favorite toy or a trophy) at the end of the procedure if the child cooperated adequately; (5) behavioral rehearsal of the entire procedure several times prior to the actual bone marrow aspiration. During the first rehearsal the patient might pretend to be the nurse, using a doll as the patient. During a final rehearsal the psychologist might pretend to be the nurse, with the patient performing all of the specific skills (e.g., the breathing exercises, imagery, etc.) just as he or she would during an actual bone marrow aspiration. The emphasis throughout Jay's procedure is on effective coping, not on mastery. The goal is to help the child to tolerate the procedure and cooperate with the medical staff.

In a well controlled test of their cognitive-behavioral intervention, Jay and colleagues (1987) gave three different intervention packages, in a randomized order, to fifty-six leukemic children undergoing bone marrow aspirations: (1) the cognitive behavioral intervention; (2) a standard pharmacological intervention, namely oral Valium; and (3) an attention-control procedure in which children watched cartoons. The results indicated that the cognitive-behavioral intervention significantly reduced behavioral distress, pain ratings, and pulse rates as compared to the attention-control procedure. The Valium treatment was not significantly different from the cognitive-behavioral treatment except that it produced significantly lower diastolic blood pressures. These results suggest not only that the cognitive-behavioral intervention was highly effective, but also that its impact was equivalent to being given tranquilizing medication but without the associated risks.

A final example of a situation-specific behavioral intervention involves a treatment of an operantly developed problem. Redd (1982) reported the case of a sixty-four-year-old terminal-cancer patient who complained of pain and distress. He was given various nonnarcotic drugs (e.g., Valium), backrubs, and a lot of support from his family and the nursing staff, with little apparent effect. He even reported little relief after being given the maximal safe dose of constant intravenous morphine. Soon the patient was spending as much as 60% of his waking hours crying, moaning, and yelling. His cries were so loud that they could be heard in six adjacent rooms and were beginning to cause considerable distress to at least a dozen other patients.

Redd had raters sit outside the patient's room twenty-four hours a day, recording the amount of crying the patient did and the conditions under which the crying occurred. It was discovered that the patient cried mainly when others (nursing staff and family) were present, apparently in order to get attention and support. With the full cooperation of the patient's family and the medical staff, a time-out differential reinforcement procedure was initiated whereby staff and friends were asked to interact with the patient only when he was not crying and to leave the room if he began to cry (nursing staff were to check the patient first to insure that the crying was not the result of some physical problem that should be attended to). The results were dramatic. In less than two weeks the patient's crying and moaning behavior had all but disappeared, and the amount of time he spent conversing with family increased substantially. Not surprisingly, the amount of time his family came to visit him also increased. Overall, this straightforward behavioral intervention thus appeared to improve considerably the quality of life for the patient and those close to him.

## Patient Self-help Interventions

An increasingly popular source of support for cancer patients involves patient self-help interventions. These interventions are composed of and sometimes are organized and run by cancer patients themselves. They are usually focused on providing information and social support to patients, not to providing professional interventions or to dealing with medical or psychiatric problems. Some of the groups are designed for patients with a specific problem (e.g., there are special groups for patients with ostomies or laryngectomies), whereas others are designed to be of more general interest to all cancer patients. Patient self-help programs appear to be based on two premises. The first is that such programs can provide an important source of information and social support. Social support is assumed to help buffer patients against many of the stressors they will experience and to help create a positive emotional state. Unfortunately, as we have noted earlier, cancer patients often find that their friends visit less and include them less in various activities after the former are diagnosed as having cancer, and as a result some of their usual sources of social support decrease at precisely the time some patients have a greater need for such support. Patient self-help interventions can go a long way toward replacing this loss.

Second, patient self-help programs appear to be based on the belief that those who share a common problem can provide a unique and important kind of help and support to each other. Cancer patients know what it is like to face the possibility of an imminent death, to be in pain, to be stared at or treated awkwardly by others, to undergo chemotherapy, or to be surgically disfigured. Patients who have undergone specific types of surgery or experienced specific problems can presumably understand and help each other in ways that people who have not undergone the same experiences cannot. For example, breast cancer patients who have undergone mastectomies can talk to each other knowledgeably and supportively about changes in self-concept and body image and can help each other with problems that most people never think about or have experience with, such as finding an acceptable swimsuit or a comfortable prosthesis. Thus, not only do self-help programs provide considerable information and social support, but the quality and nature of that information and support may be unique and unavailable elsewhere.

One example of a self-help group aimed at a specific subset of patients is Reach to Recovery. Reach to Recovery began in 1952 as an independent, self-help group for mastectomy patients and in 1969 became supported by and promoted formally through the American Cancer Society. The program involves having volunteers who have had a mastectomy visit new mastectomy patients. The visits are always made with the consent of the new patient's physician. The volunteers bring the patient a booklet that discusses ways of coping with various problems and illustrates various exercises that might be helpful, and they also give the patients a temporary breast form (prosthesis) to use under their clothing. The volunteers encourage patients to talk about their concerns and to ask questions. The most comprehensive assessment of the program conducted to date was reported by Rogers, Bauman, and Metzger (1985). The researchers interviewed more than 650 patients who either did or did not participate in the Reach to Recovery Program. The results indicated that almost all of the patients who saw a Reach to Recovery volunteer evaluated the visit as helpful regardless of age, level of education, employment status, the availability of emotional support from their family, or whether they had also talked with friends or relatives who had undergone a mastectomy. The authors found no evidence that the program was harmful in any way. Regarding the reasons for the program's success, the authors offer the following explanation.

> The bond of common experience appears to be the key. As a role model, the volunteer reduces the stigma and isolation that patients feel after breast surgery. She can give the patient information, both practical, and emotional, and because she has gone through the same difficult experience, this information has a special validity. (p. 122)

Other patient self-help programs include Lost Cord Club (a support group for patients with laryngectomies, with hospital visits to new patients as part of the program); Ostomy Club ( a similar group for patients with various types of ostomies); Cansourmount (a one-on-one support system for patients who wish to talk to someone who has the same problem or is undergoing the same treatment they are); I Can Cope (an information and support group for cancer patients and their families); and Candlelighters (an information and support group for parents of children with cancer). Additional information on these and other self-help groups is usually available from the nearest chapter of the American Cancer Society. Unfortunately, little controlled research has been conducted on any of these programs, although their widespread popularity and the favorable reports by a large number of their participants suggest that they provide an important resource for many cancer patients.

# Summary

Cancer is the second leading cause of death in the United States, striking approximately one in three persons and 75% of all families. Yet, to a large degree, cancer is an avoidable disease. Lifestyle factors play a major role in determining whether or not one develops cancer, and if one does, the course and nature of the disease. These lifestyle factors can be divided into those that have direct and indirect effects in either initiating or promoting the disease.

The factor that has the largest direct impact on the initiation or promotion of cancer is tobacco use, especially cigarette smoking. Tobacco use is the single most preventable behavioral factor contributing to illness, disability, and premature death in the United States. It increases the risk of lung cancer alone up to 25 times above that of a nonsmoker, and also is a risk factor for several other types of cancer. Considerable attention has been given to reducing tobacco use through educational, policy, and intervention efforts, and to a large extent these efforts have been successful. However, smoking still remains a problem for select subgroups of individuals, including poorly educated and young females.

In addition to tobacco use, exposure to other chemical carcinogens, alcohol consumption, especially when combined with cigarette smoking, and ultraviolet radiation also can directly affect the development of cancer. In each of theses cases, the degree of exposure, rather than the simple presence or absence of exposure, is the major factor associated with increased risk.

Behavioral, psychological, and social factors can also indirectly affect the development of cancer by serving as mediating variables influencing factors that can cause or prevent cancer. For example, high-fat diets are associated with increased risk for breast, prostate, and colon cancer. Obesity, perhaps partly as a function of increased fat intake, is also associated with an increased cancer risk. On the other hand, certain foods may help to prevent cancer, such as foods with high dietary fiber and cruciferous vegetables.

Inadequately coping with increased stress and certain personality dispositions, such as feelings of hopelessness and passive acceptance of aversive situations, have also been associated with an increased risk of cancer. However, research on stress and personality factors is highly controversial, with studies available to support almost any position. At this time, the preponderance of data suggest that under certain conditions, some types of stress may play an adjunctive role in some individuals in the development of select cancers. The mechanism by which stress or other emotional factors may be linked to cancer is likely to involve impairment of the body's natural ability to fight disease.

Finally, whether or not one engages in early cancer detection behaviors such as breast examinations, testicular self-examinations, and regular examinations by a physician can affect the likelihood of developing cancer or successfully treating it. Some precancerous conditions, such as cervical dysplasia, are detectable by certain tests. Early treatment of these conditions can prevent the development of cancer. In other cases cancers cannot be identified in a precancerous state, but their early detection and treatment can mean the difference between full recovery and certain death. Once one develops cancer, whether or not one complies with treatment recommendations can have a major impact on the likelihood of recovery. Overall, therefore, one's behavior can play a major role in the development and course of cancer.

If a person is diagnosed as having cancer, he or she is likely to find that the experience is highly distressing and to display a variety of emotional responses, including increased feelings of anxiety, depression, and loss of control; cognitive impairment such as confusion and decreased attention span; sexual impairment; and the use of denial. In many cases these problems are transient and can be considered normal responses to a highly traumatic situation. In some cases, however, they reflect more serious psychiatric problems and require professional intervention.

Cancer is usually treated medically by surgery, radiation, chemotherapy, or a combination of these approaches. Newer treatments, such as immunotherapy and hypothermia, are also used with increasing frequency. Because these treatments are not always effective and because they can produce aversive side effects, a number of alternative therapies have been promoted over the years, including several psychological treatments. To date, however, there is no evidence that any psychological treatment can cure cancer. On the other hand, data have been reported that suggest that psychological interventions, used as adjuncts to traditional treatments, might prolong the lives of some types of cancer patients. How this effect is accomplished, however, is not yet known.

Although psychological treatments cannot cure cancer, they can help to reduce the distress caused by the disease and improve the overall quality of life of the cancer patient. These treatments include a variety of different approaches, ranging from supportive counseling to behavioral approaches for reducing specific side effects resulting from cancer treatments. Patient self-help groups are also a popular and widely available source of support.

# *References*

AMERICAN CANCER SOCIETY. (1975). *Teaching about cancer.* New York: American Cancer Society.

AMERICAN CANCER SOCIETY. (1980). *Public attitudes toward cancer and cancer tests. CA-A Journal for Clinicians, 30,* 92–98.

AMERICAN CANCER SOCIETY. (1982). Unproven methods of cancer management. *CA-A Journal for Clinicians, 32*, 58–61.

AMERICAN CANCER SOCIETY. (1989). *1989 Cancer facts and figures.* New York: American Cancer Society.

ANDERSEN, B. L. (1985). Sexual functioning morbidity among cancer survivors: Present status and future research directions. *Cancer, 55*, 1835–1842.

ANDERSEN, B. L., ANDERSON, B., & dePROSSE, C. (1989). Controlled prospective longitudinal study of women with cancer: II. Psychological outcomes. *Journal of Consulting and Clinical Psychology, 57*, 692–697.

ANDRYKOWSKI, M. A., & REDD, W. H. (1987). Life-threatening disease: Biopsychosocial dimensions of cancer care. In R. L. Morrison & A. S. Bellack (Eds.), *Medical factors and psychological disorders: A handbook for psychologists.* New York: Plenum.

BROUWERS, P., RICCARDI, R., POPLACK, D., & FEDIO, P. (1984). Attentional deficits in long-term survivors of childhood acute lymphoblastic leukemia (ALL). *Journal of Clinical Neuropsychology, 6*, 325–336.

BUKBERG, J., PENMAN, D., & HOLLAND, J. C. (1984). Depression in hospitalized cancer patients. *Psychosomatic Medicine, 46*, 199–211.

BURISH, T. G., & CAREY, M. P. (1986). Conditioned aversive responses in cancer chemotherapy patients: Theoretical and developmental analysis. *Journal of Consulting and Clinical Psychology, 54*, 593–600.

BURISH, T. G., CAREY, M. P., KROZELY, M. G., & GRECO, F. A. (1987). Conditioned side effects induced by cancer chemotherapy: Prevention through behavioral treatment. *Journal of Consulting and Clinical Psychology, 55*, 42–48.

CASSILETH, B. R., & EGAN, T. A. (1979). Modification of student perceptions of the cancer experience. *Journal of Medical Education, 54*, 797–802.

CASSILETH, B. R., LUSK, E. J., MILLER, D. S., BROWN, L. L., & MILLER, C. (1985). Psychosocial correlates of survival in malignant disease. *New England Journal of Medicine, 312*, 1551–1555.

CHEANG, A., & COOPER, C. L. (1985). Psychosocial factors in breast cancer. *Stress Medicine, 1*, 61–66.

DATTORE, P. J., SHONTZ, F. C., & COYNE, L. (1980). Premorbid personality differentiation of cancer and noncancer groups: A test of the hypothesis of cancer proneness. *Journal of Consulting and Clinical Psychology, 48*, 388–394.

DEROGATIS, L. R., ABELOFF, M. D., & MELISARATOS, N. (1979). Psychological coping mechanisms and survival time in metastatic breast cancer. *Journal of the American Medical Association, 242,* 1504–1508.

DEROGATIS, L. R., MORROW, G. R., FETTING, J., PENMAN, D., PIASETSKY, S., SCHMALE, A. M., HENRICHS, M., & CARNICKE, C. L. M. (1983). The prevalence of psychiatric disorders among cancer patients. *Journal of the American Medical Association, 249*, 751–757.

DEVLIN, H. B., PLANT, J. A., & GRIFFIN, M. (1971). Aftermath of surgery for anorectal cancer. *British Medical Journal, iii*, 413–418.

FAIVELSON, S. (1988). The dark truth about tanning salons. *American Health*, January/February, 88–89.

GARFINKEL, L., AUERBACH, O., & JOUBERT, L. (1985). Involuntary smoking and lung cancer: A case-control study. *Journal of the National Cancer Institute, 75*, 463–469.

GENDRON, D. Enquiries into the nature, knowledge, and cure of cancer. London, 1701, as cited in Bahnson, C. B. (1980). Stress and cancer: The state of art. *Psychosomatics, 21,* 975–981.

GILLUM, R., LEAN, G. R., KAMP, J., & ALDAMA, J. B. (1980). Prediction of cardiovascular and other disease onset and mortality from 30-year longitudinal MMPI data. *Journal of Consulting and Clinical Psychology, 48,* 405–406.

GORDON, W. A., FREIDENBERGS, I., DILLER, L., HIBBARD, M., WOLF, C., LEVINE, L., LIPKINS, R., EZRACHI, O., & LUCIDO, D. (1980). Efficacy of psychosocial intervention with cancer patients. *Journal of Consulting and Clinical Psychology, 48,* 743–759.

GRADY, K. E. (1984). Cue enhancement and the long-term practice of breast self-examination. *Journal of Behavioral Medicine, 7,* 191–204.

GRADY, K. E., GOODENOW, L., & BORKIN, J. R. (1988). The effect of reward on compliance with breast self-examination. *Journal of Behavioral Medicine, 11,* 43–57.

GREENBERG, R. P., & DATTORE, P. J. (1981). The relationship between dependency and the development of cancer. *Psychosomatic Medicine, 43,* 35–43

HARRIS, R. W. C., BRINTON, L. A., COWDELL, R. H., SKAGGS, D. G., SMITH, P. G., VESSEY, M. P., & DOLL, R. (1980). Characteristics of women with dysplasia or carcinoma *in situ* of the cervix uteri. *British Journal of Cancer, 42,* 359–369.

HORNE, R. L., & PICARD, R. S. (1979). Psychosocial risk factors for lung cancer. *Psychosomatic Medicine, 41,* 503–514.

HOWE, H. (1981a). Social factors associated with breast self-examination among high risk women. *American Journal of Public Health, 71,* 251–255.

HOWE, H. (1981b). Enhancing the effectiveness of media messages promoting regular breast self-examination. *Public Health Reports, 96,* 134–142.

JACOBS, T. J., & CHARLES, E. (1980). Life events and the occurrence of cancer in children. *Psychosomatic Medicine, 42,* 11–24.

JAY, S. M., ELLIOT, C. H., KATZ, E., & SIEGEL, S. E. (1987). Cognitive-behavioral and pharmacologic interventions for children's distress during painful medical procedures. *Journal of Consulting and Clinical Psychology, 55,* 860–865.

JEMMOT, J. B., & LOCKE, S. E. (1984). Psychosocial factors, immunologic mediation, and human susceptibility to infectious diseases: How much do we know? *Psychological Bulletin, 95,* 78–108.

JUSTICE, A. (1985). Review of the effects of stress on cancer in laboratory animals: Importance of time of stress application and types of tumor. *Psychological Bulletin, 98,* 108–138.

KNOPF, A. (1976). Changes in women's opinions about cancer. *Social Science and Medicine, 10,* 191–195.

LENARD, L. (1981, April). Visions that vanquish cancer. *Science Digest,* pp. 59–62, 110–111.

LEVY, S. M. (1982). Biobehavioral interventions in behavioral medicine: An overview. *Cancer, 50* (9, supplement), 1928–1935.

LEVY, S. M. (1983). Host differences in neoplastic risk: Behavioral and social contributors to disease. *Health Psychology, 2,* 21–44.

LEVY, S. M. (1985). *Behavior and cancer.* San Francisco: Jossey-Bass.

MAGES, N. L., CASTRO, J. R., FOBAIR, P., HALL, J., HARRISON, I., MENDELSOHN, G., & WOLFSON, A. (1981). Patterns of psychosocial response to cancer: Can effective adaptation be predicted? *International Journal of Radiation Oncology, Biology, Physics, 7,* 385–392.

NAGY, V. T., & WOLFE, G. R. (1983). Chronic illness and health locus of control beliefs. *Journal of Social and Clinical Psychology, 1,* 58–65.

NATIONAL CANCER INSTITUTE (1980). *Breast cancer: A measure of progress in public understanding.* (DHHS Publication No. 81–2306). Washington, DC: U.S. Government Printing Office.

OKEN, D. (1961). What to tell cancer patients: A study of medical attitudes. *Journal of the American Medical Association, 175,* 1120–1128.

PERRY, C., KILLEN, J., TELCH, M., SLINKARD, L. A., & DANAHER, B. G. (1980). Modifying smoking behavior of teenagers: A school-based intervention. *American Journal of Public Health, 70,* 722–725.

PETTINGALE, K. W. (1984). Coping and cancer prognosis. *Journal of Psychosomatic Research, 28,* 363–364.

PETTINGALE, K. W., GREER, S., & TEE, D. E. H. (1977). Serum IgA and emotional expression in breast cancer patients. *Journal of Psychosomatic Research, 21,* 395–399.

REDD, W. H. (1982). Treatment of excessive crying in a terminal cancer patient: A time-series analysis. *Behavioral Medicine, 5,* 225–236.

REIF, A. E. (1981). The causes of cancer. *American Scientist, 69,* 437–446.

ROGERS, T. F., BAUMAN, L. J., & METZGER, L. (1985). An assessment of the Reach to Recover program. *CA-A Journal for Clinicians, 35,* 116–124.

ROTKIN, I. D. (1973). A comparison review of key epidemiological studies in cervical cancer related to current searches for transmissible agents. *Cancer Research, 33,* 1353–1367.

SADEGHI, S. B., HSIEH, E. W., & GUNN, S. W. (1984). Prevalence of cervical intra-epithelial neoplasia in sexually active teenagers and young adults. *American Journal of Obstetrics and Gynecology, 148,* 726–729.

SANDLER, D. P., EVERSON, R. B., WILCOX, A. J., & BROWDER, J. P. (1985). Cancer risk in adulthood from early life exposure to parents' smoking. *American Journal of Public Health, 75,* 487–492.

SCHMALE, A. H., & IKER, H. P. (1971). Hopelessness as a predictor of cervical cancer. *Social Science Medicine, 5,* 95–100.

SHEKELLE, R. B., RAYNOR, W. J., OSTFELD, A. M., GARRON, D. C. BIELIAUSKAS, L. A., LIU, S. C., MALIZA, C., & PAUL, O. (1981). Psychological depression and 17-year risk of death from cancer. *Psychosomatic Medicine, 43,* 117–125.

SIEGEL, B. S. (1986). *Love, medicine, and miracles.* New York: Harper & Row.

SILBERFARB, P. M., & GREER, S. (1982). Psychological concomitants of cancer: Clinical aspects. *American Journal of Psychotherapy, 36,* 470–478.

SKLAR, L. S., & ANISMAN, H. (1981). Stress and cancer. *Psychological Bulletin, 89,* 369–406.

SMITH, S. D., RASEN, D., TRUEWORTHY, R. C., & LOWMAN, J. T. (1979). A reliable method for evaluating drug compliance in children with cancer. *Cancer, 43,* 169–173.

SOBEL, H. J., & WORDEN, J. W. (1979). The MMPI as a predictor of psychosocial adaptation to cancer. *Journal of Consulting and Clinical Psychology, 47,* 716–724.

SPIEGEL, D., BLOOM, J. R., KRAEMER, H. C., & GOTTHEIL, E. (1989). Effect of psychosocial treatment on survival of patients with metastatic breast cancer. *Lancet,* October 14, 888-891.

STEHBENS, J. A., & KISKER, C. T. (1984). Intelligence and achievement testing in childhood cancer: Three years postdiagnosis. *Developmental and Behavioral Pediatrics, 5*, 184–188.

U.S. DEPARTMENT OF HEALTH AND HUMAN SERVICES (1986). *Smoking and health: A national status report.* (Publication No. HHS/PHS/CDC 87-8396). Washington, D.C.: U.S. Government Printing Office.

WATSON, C. G., & SCHULD, G. (1977). Psychosomatic factors in the etiology of neoplasms. *Journal of Consulting and Clinical Psychology, 45*, 455–461.

WATSON, M., GREER, S., BLAKE, S., & SHRAPNELL, K. (1984). Reaction to a diagnosis of breast cancer: Relationships between denial, delay, and rates of psychological morbidity. *Cancer, 53*, 2008–2012.

WILLET, W. C., & MacMAHON, B. (1984). Diet and cancer—an overview. *New England Journal of Medicine, 310*, 697–703.

WORDEN, J. W. (1983). Psychosocial screening of cancer patients. *Journal of Psychosocial Oncology, 1*, 1–10.

WORDEN, J. W., & WEISMAN, A. D. (1984). Preventive psychosocial intervention with newly diagnosed cancer patients. *General Hospital Psychiatry, 6*, 243–249.

ZONDERMAN, A. B., COSTA, P. T., & McCRAE, R. R. (1989). Depression as a risk for cancer morbidity and mortality in a nationally representative sample. *Journal of the American Medical Association, 262*, 1191–1195.

# Diabetes Mellitus

*Diabetes mellitus*, one of the most common chronic diseases in the United States, is an endocrine disorder characterized by high levels of glucose in the blood. This disorder affects approximately 5% of the population of the United States, with an estimated 5 million diagnosed and 5 million undiagnosed cases (USDHHS, 1985). Moreover, as the incidence of diabetes is increasing, it is estimated that the size of the diabetic population will double within fifteen years (Davidson, 1981). At least 37,000 deaths per year are attributed directly to diabetes, making it the tenth leading cause of death in the United States (USDHHS, 1984). In addition, diabetes is a major cause of other serious health problems such as blindness, renal failure, and cardiovascular disease.

Many physicians believe that the early mortality and complications caused by diabetes can be avoided by careful management of the disease (Santiago, 1984). However, medical treatment of diabetes involves a complex regimen of medication, diet, and exercise. In order to adhere to this regimen, patients are required to assume much responsibility for their own treatment and to make major behavioral changes (e.g., losing weight). Health psychologists can play an important role in the treatment of diabetes by helping patients to make and maintain these behavioral changes (Surwit, Feinglos, & Scovern, 1983). The effects of stress on diabetic patients is another research area to which psychologists can make valuable contributions. As the behavioral and physiological effects of stress can interfere with the management of diabetes, psychological interventions designed to reduce stress may prove beneficial for diabetic patients.

# Biological and Psychophysiological Components

## Biological Components

*Hyperglycemia*, the high level of blood glucose found in diabetic patients, results from a lack of effective insulin action. *Insulin*, a hormone produced by the beta cells of the pancreas, allows the body to use glucose for energy. As diabetic patients lack adequate insulin, glucose cannot be metabolized by the body's cells and therefore accumulates in the bloodstream. Some of the excess glucose in diabetic patients may be excreted in the urine, causing frequent urination and possible dehydration. Other physical symptoms associated with untreated diabetes are excessive fatigue, hunger, thirst, and weight loss (Davidson, 1981).

When the body cannot utilize glucose due to inadequate insulin, it metabolizes the body's energy reserves of fat and protein. Unfortunately, these reserves cannot meet the body's energy needs. Moreover, metabolism of fat produces substances called *ketone bodies* (e.g., acetone). When ketone bodies accumulate in diabetic patients, they cause the blood and other body fluids to become acidic, a condition called *ketoacidosis* (Davidson, 1981). If untreated, ketoacidosis can lead to unconsciousness and death.

The two major types of diabetes mellitus are *Type I*, insulin-dependent diabetes mellitus (IDDM), and *Type II*, non-insulin-dependent diabetes mellitus (NIDDM). Less common types of diabetes also have been identified but will not be discussed in this chapter. In Type I diabetes, the beta cells of the pancreas produce little or no insulin (Harris, 1982). Thus the patient is dependent on daily insulin injections for survival. As Type I diabetes tends to develop in childhood or adolescence, it is sometimes called *juvenile diabetes*. However, IDDM may begin at any age and cannot be diagnosed based on age of onset alone.

In Type II diabetes, or NIDDM, the beta cells of the pancreas continue to secrete a significant amount of insulin. However, *insulin resistance* develops in the body's cells, and the insulin is not used efficiently to metabolize glucose (Harris, 1982). Hyperglycemia is the result of the insulin resistance. In response to the elevated blood glucose levels, the beta cells attempt to produce more insulin but cannot meet the body's needs. However, most Type II diabetic patients do not require insulin injections in order to survive. Oral medications may be used to increase the effectiveness of the body's own insulin.

The etiologies of Type I and Type II diabetes are unknown. Genetic and environmental factors probably play a role in the onset of both types. Thus, individuals who inherit a genetic susceptibility may develop diabetes after exposure to precipitating factors in the environment (Pohl, Gonder-Frederick, & Cox, 1984). Viral infection, dysfunction of the body's immune system triggered by an infectious agent, and psychological stress have been named as factors that may be involved in the onset of Type I diabetes (Marble, 1971).

In Type II diabetes, genetic factors may play a more important role than in Type I (Pyke 1981). A major precipitating factor for most cases of Type II diabetes appears to be obesity. The chronic overeating associated with obesity stimulates excessive insulin production by pancreas (Bloom & Ireland, 1980). The elevated levels of insulin in the blood cause insulin resistance in the body's cells. In addition, the beta cells of the pancreas probably become exhausted or damaged due to the demands for insulin production and subsequently produce less insulin. Thus, the hyperglycemia results from insufficient insulin and/or insulin resistance.

Both Type I and Type II diabetes are associated with long-term complications due to damage to blood vessels and nerves. It is thought that chronic hyperglycemia is the main factor responsible for complications such as retinopathy, nephropathy, cardiovascular disease, and neuropathy (Skyler, 1979). *Diabetic retinopathy* is a disease of the retina, the innermost, light-sensitive covering of the eye. Damage to the small blood vessels supplying the eye causes the retinopathy, which may lead to visual impairment or blindness (O'Grady, 1980). Although blindness occurs in only a small percentage of diabetics, diabetic retinopathy is the leading cause of new blindness in the United States (Lipsett, 1980). *Diabetic nephropathy* is a degenerative kidney disease caused by damage to renal blood vessels (Balodimos, 1971). Many diabetics develop nephropathy and eventually require renal dialysis or kidney transplants. Diabetic patients are also at risk for the development of cardiac and vascular disease, including heart attacks, strokes, and impaired circulation of the extremities (Davidson, 1981).

*Neuropathy*, a disease of the nervous system, is another complication of diabetes. Damage to nerves in the extremities cause *peripheral neuropathy*, a condition that typically produces pain and eventual loss of tactile sensation in the feet or hands (Faerman, Jadzinsky, & Podolsky, 1980). Damage to nerves in the autonomic nervous system causes *autonomic neuropathy*, a disorder that may affect any organ regulated by the autonomic nervous system (Faerman et al.,

1980). Symptoms of autonomic neuropathy may include diarrhea, nausea, urinary incontinence, and sexual impotence in males. Another serious health problem related to diabetes is the development of complications during labor, pregnancy, and delivery. The babies of diabetic women are three times more likely to have birth defects than babies of nondiabetic women (Metzger, 1980).

It should be noted that not all diabetic patients develop complications from their disease. Patients with poorly controlled diabetes of long duration are the diabetics most likely to develop complications (Skyler, 1979). However, the severity and range of potential medical complications points out the importance of maintaining good control of the disease. Optimal medical control of diabetes is the maintenance of normal blood glucose levels or *euglycemia* (Seltzer, 1980). A recently developed measure of long-term diabetic control is *glycosylated hemoglobin $A_1$* (HbA$_1$). As normal hemoglobin A will combine with glucose to form HbA$_1$, the proportion of HbA$_1$ in the blood reflects the amount of glucose in circulation. Because the half-life of hemoglobin is about eight weeks, the level of HbA$_1$ measures the degree of diabetic control during such a period (Bunn, 1981).

## Psychophysiological Components

Stress is an important factor affecting diabetic control. In both normal and diabetic individuals, exposure to stress can trigger an increase in sympathetic nervous system activity and the production of stress hormones (e.g., catecholamines, cortisol). In normal individuals, these hormones reduce insulin production and increase blood levels of glucose and free fatty acids, substances available as energy sources during stress (Efendic, Cerasi, & Luft, 1974). When the stress is reduced, normal individuals demonstrate a substantial increase in insulin production and a subsequent return to normal blood glucose levels.

In diabetic individuals, the psychophysiological response to stress is not well understood. However, it has been suggested that it is difficult for diabetic patients to counteract the effects of the stress hormones (Surwit & Feinglos, 1988). In particular, their inability to produce adequate insulin following stress may make them vulnerable to increased levels of glucose and free fatty acids in the blood.

In an early study, Hinkle and Wolf (1952) examined the effects of emotional stress on metabolic control in Type I and II diabetic patients and in normal subjects. They followed sixty-four diabetics over a three-year period in order to determine if fluctuations in diabetic control were related to stressful life events. Patients for whom a relationship between a specific event and a change in metabolic control could be identified were interviewed while in a fasting state. Following a discussion of neutral topics, the issue of the stressful life event was introduced abruptly. At the end of the interview, the patient was given emotional support and reassurance. Urinary output and blood samples were obtained throughout the interview. During the discussion of stressful life events, the diabetic patients demonstrated increases in urinary volume and excretion of ketones, as well as fluctuations in blood and urine glucose levels. Figure 10.1 shows the physiological changes demonstrated by a 15-year-old patient. The normal subjects demonstrated similar metabolic changes during stressful interviews; however, their changes were less extreme and required less time to return to baseline values. Unfortunately, no statistical analyses of the changes were performed.

Subsequent studies have used stressors such as public speaking, mental arithmetic, noise, and video games to examine the effects of stress on metabolic control in Type I and II diabetic patients (Carter, Gonder-Frederick, Cox, Clarke, & Scott, 1985; Gilbert, Johnson, Silverstein, & Malone, 1989; Kemmer et al., 1986; Naliboff, Cohen, & Sowers, 1985). Overall, the results have not demonstrated significant, consistent changes in blood glucose levels among groups of diabetic subjects in response to brief laboratory stressors. Some individual patients, however, appeared to experience increases in blood glucose levels in response to stress, whereas other patients experienced decreases or no change (Carter et al., 1985). Thus, individual differences among patients may help to account for the inconsistent results across studies (Goetsch, 1989).

# Behavioral, Psychological, and Social Factors

## Behavioral Factors

DIABETIC REGIMEN   Medical management of diabetes involves a complex behavioral regimen of diet, medication, frequent monitoring of blood or urine glucose levels, and exercise. In order to adhere to this regimen, diabetic patients and their families may have to make major behavioral changes in their daily lives. To begin with, diet plays an important role in the regimen of patients with Type I and Type II diabetes. Most diabetics are advised to follow a diet low in fat and simple sugars but moderately high in complex carbohydrates and fiber (Wing, Epstein, Nowalk, & Hyg, 1984). Patients who take insulin injections must eat regular meals of specified amounts of food. Their caloric intake must be carefully balanced against their insulin intake in order to avoid *hypoglycemia*, or low blood glucose levels. In addition, both Type I and Type II diabetics are advised to achieve and maintain normal body weight (Wing et al., 1984). Thus, the dietary management of diabetes typically requires patients to change their dietary habits and to carefully monitor their food intake.

Diabetic patients who need insulin injections must learn complex behaviors related to their self-care. One or more daily hypodermic injections are usually self-administered by patients who are at least twelve years old. Parents or other family members have to administer injections to younger diabetics. In order to determine insulin dosage and coordinate insulin with food intake,

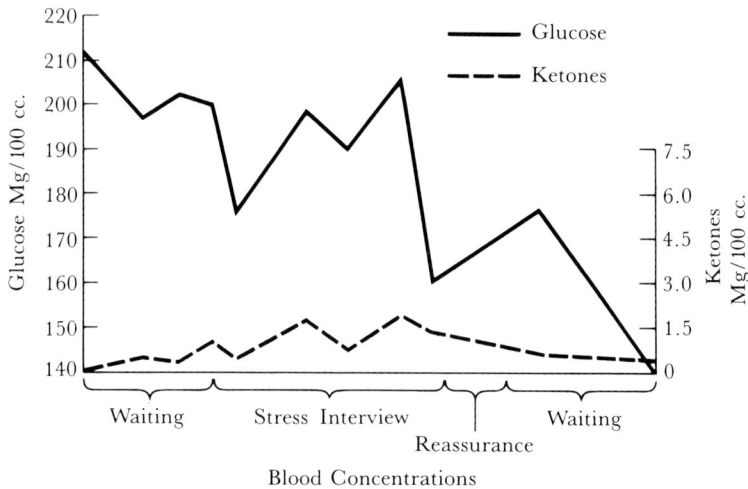

FIGURE 10.1    Blood glucose and ketone concentrations in a fifteen-year-old diabetic boy who became anxious during a discussion of his conflict with his father. From "Importance of Life Stress in Course and Management of Diabetes Mellitus" by L. E. Hinkle, Jr., and S. Wolf, 1952, *JAMA, 148*, p. 516. Reprinted by permission.

diabetic patients or their family members have to monitor urine or blood glucose levels several times each day. Urine testing usually involves dipping a chemically treated strip of paper or tablet into a sample of urine and observing the color change. The final color of the strip or solution is matched with a color chart to determine the glucose level in the urine. Unfortunately, urine glucose levels do not consistently reflect blood glucose levels (Morris, McGee, & Kitabchi, 1981).

Recent technological advances have enabled diabetic patients to directly monitor blood glucose levels. In order to determine a blood glucose level, the patient obtains a blood sample with a finger prick and places the blood on a chemically treated strip. The subsequent color change of the strip reveals the blood glucose level (Gonder-Frederick, Cox, Pohl, & Carter, 1984).

Another important behavior in the diabetic regimen is exercise. Most diabetic patients are advised to follow regular exercise programs. In Type I and Type II diabetes, exercise can have a beneficial effect of lowering blood glucose levels (Zinman, 1984). However, Type I diabetics must carefully coordinate exercise, food intake, and insulin dosage in order to avoid exercise-induced hypoglycemia.

NONADHERENCE    As described, the diabetic regimen is a complex, demanding set of behaviors that may require patients and their families to learn and monitor new behaviors, as well as to alter old behavioral patterns. It is not surprising, therefore, that many diabetic patients are nonadherent to their treatment regimens. When Type I diabetic adults were observed at home, it was found that 80% of the patients made errors in insulin administration (Watkins, Williams, Martin, Hogan, & Anderson, 1967). Moreover, only one-third of the patients tested their urine samples correctly. In a study of the dietary regimens of adult Type I and Type II diabetics, 75% of the patients demonstrated significant dietary errors (Williams, Anderson, Watkins, & Coyle, 1967). Low-adherence rates have also been reported in samples of children with Type I diabetes. When children over the age of 8 were asked to demonstrate their blood glucose testing skills, only 58% of their reported blood glucose levels were even close to the actual levels (Wing et al., 1985).

A number of explanations have been advanced to explain the nonadherence of diabetic patients. Speers and Turk (1982) have suggested that four factors must be present for adherence to occur: (1) knowledge and skills, (2) appropriate beliefs, (3) motivation (i.e., reinforcement for adherence), and (4) correct actions (behaviors). Unfortunately, the results of recent research indicate that many diabetic patients lack one or more of these factors. For example, several studies have found that many diabetic patients do not have the knowledge and skills necessary for adherence (Epstein, Figueroa, Farkas, & Beck, 1981; Johnson et al., 1982).

In part, the knowledge and skills deficits of diabetic patients may be related to ineffective doctor-patient communication. A study of Type II diabetics found that on the average patients understood and remembered about two-thirds of their physicians' instructions (Hulka, Kupper, Cassel, & Mayo, 1975). When patients did understand physician instructions, adherence rates were good. Thus, although knowledge alone does not guarantee adherence, basic understanding of the diabetic regimen is necessary for adherence to occur.

The knowledge and skills deficits associated with nonadherence in diabetic children may be related to their developmental level. Several authors have suggested that children under the age of twelve lack the cognitive development necessary to fully understand the diabetic regimen (Etzwiler, 1962; Johnson et al., 1982). Moreover, children often lack the problem-solving skills required to cope with situations such as glucose in the urine. Given the limited cognitive skills of young diabetic children, parents or other adults must assume responsibility for the management of the diabetic regimen. Unfortunately, the knowledge and problem-solving abilities of parents are often deficient also (Johnson et al., 1982). Moreover, knowledge and skills alone do not insure adherence (Graber, Christman, Algona, & Davidson, 1977).

In addition to knowledge and skills, specific health beliefs may facilitate adherence in diabetic patients. It has been hypothesized that the extent to which diabetic patients perceive their illness as controllable will influence their adherence to the diabetic regimen (Alogna, 1980). The Multidimensional Health Locus of Control (MHLC) scale has been used to measure the degree to which patients believe that their overall health is controlled internally (i.e., by they themselves) and/or the extent to which they believe it is controlled by external factors such as chance or powerful other people (Wallston, Wallston, & DeVellis, 1978). Several studies have found a positive relationship between greater internality on the MHLC scale and adherence in Type I and Type II diabetic patients (Alogna, 1980; Schlenk & Hart, 1984). Although the correlations between a belief in internal control and adherence were not large, the significant relationships suggest that the perception of control is an important factor associated with adherence.

According to Speers and Turk (1982), another factor that will promote adherence to the diabetic regimen is motivation or reinforcement. Unfortunately, performing most of the behaviors in the diabetic regimen does not provide immediate positive reinforcement. In fact, some of the behaviors may be perceived as punishing (e.g., self-injections of insulin). Speers and Turk have suggested that patients need to reinforce themselves with positive self-statements when they adhere to the diabetic regimen. External reinforcement from family members and health care providers can also help to promote adherence (Carney, Schechter, & Davis, 1983).

A final factor necessary for adherence is the performance of specific behaviors in the diabetic regimen. In order to perform the behaviors correctly, patients must retrieve knowledge from memory, utilize skills, and make appropriate evaluations and judgments in different situations (Speers & Turk, 1982). Moreover, patients must attend to internal cues (e.g., weakness) that may indicate a certain behavior should be performed (e.g., eating). If patients cannot retrieve knowledge, utilize skills, or make appropriate judgments, then they cannot perform the behaviors correctly.

To summarize, nonadherence to the diabetic regimen is a serious problem that can interfere with optimal medical treatment. Factors that have been associated with nonadherence are knowledge and skills deficits, maladaptive health beliefs, and a lack of reinforcement. In addition, Speers and Turk (1982) have suggested that diabetic patients must perform the behaviors in the diabetic regimen correctly in order for adherence to occur. An additional factor that may influence the adherence of diabetic patients is psychological stress. A survey of diabetic patients revealed that 26% of their dietary violations (e.g., overeating) were attributed to negative emotions and conflicts related to stressful situations (Kirkley, 1982).

## Psychological Factors

Psychological stress has been related both to the etiology and course of diabetes. It has been suggested that emotional stress may precipitate the disease in individuals who have a genetic or physiological susceptibility (Menninger, 1935). Adult and adolescent diabetic patients have reported a high incidence of major losses (e.g., death of family member, loss of job) and stressful life events (Robinson & Fuller, 1985) prior to the onset of diabetes (Slawson, Flynn, & Kellar, 1963; Stein & Charles, 1971). Unfortunately, these studies have been based on retrospective reports of losses that may have occurred many years before diabetes onset. Several reviews have concluded that there is no convincing evidence that psychological factors play an important role in the etiology of diabetes (Fisher, Delamater, Bertelson, & Kirkley, 1982; Turk & Speers, 1983).

Psychological factors do appear to play an important role in the course of the disorder. As noted previously, the physiological effects of stress may disrupt diabetic control in some patients (Hinkle & Wolf, 1952). Indeed, emotional stress may be a significant precipitant of episodes of ketoacidosis. A review of seventy-three hospitalizations of diabetic patients for ketoacidosis revealed that emotional factors appeared to precipitate the loss of metabolic control in at least 15% of the cases (Cohen, Vance, Runyan, & Hurwitz, 1960). It should be noted that emotional stress may affect diabetic control in at least two ways: directly, through physiological changes, and indirectly, through nonadherence to the diabetic regimen.

Direct and indirect effects of stress may be produced by recent stressful life events such as a job change or divorce. Holmes and Rahe's development of the Social Readjustment Rating Scale (SRRS; Holmes & Rahe, 1967) has enabled researchers to study the relationship of stressful life events and diabetic control. Several studies have found significant correlations between life stress scores and diabetic control (Bradley, 1979; Chase & Jackson, 1981). For example, when an age-appropriate form of the SRRS was administered to Type I diabetics aged six to eighteen, significant, positive correlations were found between life stress scores and both $HbA_1$ levels and blood glucose concentrations (Chase & Jackson, 1981). Patients in poor metabolic control reported more recent life stress than patients in good control. However, an analysis of different age groups revealed that the correlations between stress scores and diabetic control were significant only for the fifteen-to-eighteen-year-old group.

The stress caused by day-to-day hassles and frustrations may affect some diabetic patients more than the stress related to major life events. In a study of the relationship between daily stress and diabetic control, Cox and his associates administered the Hassles Scale (see Chapter 5) to a sample of sixty adult Type I diabetic patients (Cox, Taylor, Nowacek, Holley-Wilcox, Pohl, & Guthrow, 1984). The Hassles Scale (Kanner, Coyne, Schaefer, & Lazarus, 1981) is a self-report measure that assesses recent day-to-day hassles and frustrations in patients' lives (e.g., too many things to do, misplacing or losing things). At the time the Hassles Scale was completed, blood samples were drawn for analysis of patients' $HbA_1$ levels. Analysis of the results revealed that scores on the Hassles Scale correlated significantly with $HbA_1$ values. Patients who reported more recent hassles demonstrated poorer metabolic control than patients who reported fewer hassles.

In a related study, Cox et al. (1984) asked a large sample of Type I diabetics who used blood glucose self-monitoring to rate on a 100-mm scale their perceptions of how stress affected their blood glucose values. As depicted in Figure 10.2, the majority of patients reported that stress had a significant

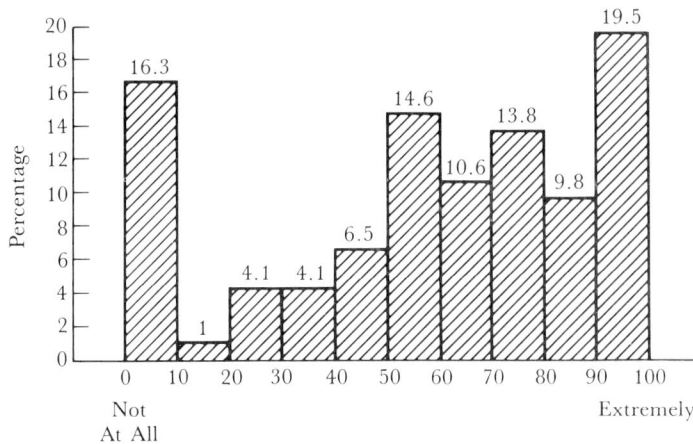

FIGURE 10.2   Distribution of diabetic subject's responses to the question "Considering all of your personal experiences watching your blood sugars flucuate, to what degree do you think stress affects your blood sugar?" The majority of subjects believed stress affected their blood sugar. From "The Relationship Between Psychological Stress and Insulin-Dependent Diabetic Blood Glucose Control: Preliminary Investigations" by D. J. Cox, A. G. Taylor, G. Nowacek, P. Holley-Wilcox, S. L. Pohl, and E. Guthrow, 1984, *Health Psychology, 3*, p. 71. Reprinted by permission.

impact on blood glucose levels. The patients were also asked to rate the effects of specific emotions on blood glucose. Worry, sadness, and frustration were the emotions most consistently associated with perceived blood glucose increases. Happiness was most consistently associated with reported blood glucose decreases. However, there was a considerable range of responses to the questions assessing the impact of different emotions. The investigators concluded that future research needs to determine the characteristics of diabetic patients who are vulnerable to specific types of psychological stress and to determine what can be done to reduce their vulnerability.

# Social Factors

FAMILY FUNCTIONING   Diabetes may be a source of stress for families as well as for patients. When a family member is diabetic, the entire family may have to alter eating patterns, daily schedules, and leisure activities. Moreover, the parents of a diabetic child are expected to assume responsibility for the child's diabetic regimen. This responsibility can be anxiety arousing; indeed, mothers of diabetic children have reported frequent concerns about diabetic control, hypoglycemic reactions, and long-term complications of diabetes (Banion, Miles, & Carter, 1983).

Several authors have suggested that diabetes has a negative impact on family functioning (Crain, Sussman, & Weil, 1966; Klusa, Habbick, & Abernathy, 1983; Zeidel, 1970). For example, Crain et al. (1966) reported more marital dysfunction in parents of diabetic children than in parents of healthy children. However, the results were significant on only one of four measures of marital functioning. A more recent study found that parents of diabetic children and parents of healthy children did not differ as to levels of marital adjustment or divorce rate (Lavigne, Traisman, Marr, & Chasnoff, 1982).

In fact, reviews of the research on the functioning of diabetic families have concluded that most families cope effectively with the stress associated with diabetes (Johnson, 1980; Pond, 1979; Turk & Speers, 1983). In addition to studying the impact of diabetes on the family, researchers have attempted to determine if specific family characteristics (e.g., cohesion) are associated with good metabolic control in diabetic children. For example, Hanson and her colleagues administered a questionnaire assessing family behavior to a sample of adolescent Type I diabetics and their parents (Hanson, Henggeler, Harris, Burghen, & Moore, 1989). Level of metabolic control in the adolescents was determined by $HbA_1$ values. Good metabolic control was associated with high family cohesion and flexibility. However, these associations were strong only for adolescents with short duration of diabetes. As duration of diabetes lengthened, the associations decreased substantially. Similar results were found in a longitudinal study of school-aged children with Type I diabetes (Kovacs, Kass, Schnell, Goldstein, & Marsh, 1989). Data collected over a six-year period failed to reveal any significant association between aspects of family life and the children's metabolic control.

Investigators have started to assess the family functioning of adult patients with diabetes. Social support from family members and friends appears to be an important variable influencing the adherence of adult patients to their diabetic regimen (Glasgow & Toobert, 1988) and also their level of metabolic control (Edelstein & Linn, 1985; Kaplan & Hartwell, 1987). The results suggest that certain types of social support may be beneficial for some patient groups but not for others (see Chapter 5 for a discussion of social support). Additional research is needed to examine the family functioning of adult diabetics.

# Psychological and Behavioral Reactions

## The "Diabetic Personality"

Early psychosomatic theorists proposed that specific personality types were associated with particular illnesses. In the case of diabetes mellitus, Dunbar (1954) hypothesized that diabetic patients were anxious, depressed, paranoid individuals with dependence-independence conflicts and poor sexual adjustment. Similarly, Menninger (1935) thought that anxiety and depression were characteristic of the "diabetic personality" pattern. It was thought that the diabetic personality might either (a) predispose individuals to the development of the disease or (b) represent a significant consequence of diabetes. The lack of evidence for the role of psychological variables in the etiology of diabetes has focused the attention of researchers on the impact of diabetes on personality. Contrary to the diabetic personality hypothesis, most diabetic adults, adolescents, and children appear to be well-adjusted individuals.

For example, Sullivan (1978) compared a large sample of adolescent female diabetics with a sample of healthy adolescent females using a self-esteem scale and the Beck Depression Inventory (BDI; Beck, 1967). No significant differences were found between diabetic and nondiabetic adolescents on self-esteem scores. Although the diabetic females reported more depression than the nondiabetic females, their elevated BDI scores were due to positive responses to items indicating physiological signs of depression such as appetite change and fatigability. As these signs may be symptoms of diabetes as well as depression, the elevated BDI scores of the diabetic adolescents probably reflected their disease status rather than depression.

Indeed, a subsequent study of adolescent girls with diabetes found that the majority of the teenagers reported adequate adjustment in the areas of dependence-independence conflicts, peer relationships, family relationships, school adjustment, body-image concerns, and attitudes toward diabetes (Sullivan, 1979).

Healthy personality characteristics have also been found in samples of pediatric (Rovet & Ehrlich, 1988; Tavormina, Kastner, Slater, & Watt, 1976) and adult diabetic patients (Murawski, Chazan, Balodimas, & Ryan, 1970). When the MMPI was administered to Type I adults who had been diabetics for at least 25 years, their average scores were within normal limits on all scales (Murawski et al., 1970). Similarly, when diabetic children were administered a large battery of personality tests, only a few of their subtest scores differed from those of healthy children or children with other chronic diseases (Tavormina et al., 1976).

In sum, the research results described above have contributed to the conclusion that the diabetic personality is a myth and that the majority of diabetic patients are well adjusted (Dunn & Turtle, 1981). Moreover, the range of personality characteristics exhibited by diabetic patients appears to be no different from that exhibited by healthy individuals or patients with other chronic diseases.

# Good Versus Poor Control

Although the majority of diabetic individuals have adjusted well to their chronic illness, certain subgroups within the diabetic population may tend to demonstrate psychological reactions such as anxiety and depression (Lustman, Harper, Griffith, & Clouse, 1986). Several investigations have found that diabetic patients in poor metabolic control demonstrated more psychological problems than patients in good control (Gath, Smith, & Baum, 1980; Simonds, 1977). For example, Mazze and his colleagues followed a large sample of Type I diabetics over a thirty-six-week period in order to determine psychological correlates of metabolic control (Mazze, Lucido, & Shamoon, 1984). Half of the patients were receiving conventional medical therapy including urine glucose testing; the other half received intensive therapy with blood glucose monitoring. For all patients, self-reports of anxiety, depression, and quality of life were significantly correlated with metabolic control, as measured by $HbA_1$ levels. Patients in poor metabolic control reported more anxiety, depression, and life problems than patients in good control. Figure 10.3 graphs the relationships between level of metabolic control and the psychological variables at the beginning of the study.

Significant correlations were also found between changes in metabolic control during the course of the study and changes in anxiety, depression, and quality of life. Patients whose metabolic control decreased tended to report increases in anxiety, depression, and number of life problems. The converse was true for patients whose metabolic control improved. The authors concluded that improved diabetic control is associated with improved quality of life as well as with decreased anxiety and depression. From the results of this study, it cannot be determined if the changes in metabolic control produced the changes in psychological functioning or vice versa. Nevertheless, the results suggest that health professionals should monitor psychological variables in patients with poor diabetic control or whose control has recently decreased.

## Psychosocial Adjustment

Psychosocial problems frequently demonstrated by diabetic patients include school problems, subtle neuropsychological deficits, and sexual dysfunction. In a study of diabetic children aged seven to fifteen, interviews with teachers and mothers revealed that the majority of the children had significant school problems (Fallstrom, 1974). Similarly, Frankel (1970) found that high-school-aged diabetics did not perform as well academically as healthy control students. However, the elementary school diabetics performed as well as their healthy peers. In another sample of students aged five to sixteen, significantly more diabetic as compared to healthy control students were delayed in reading development, as measured by standardized achievement tests (Gath et al., 1980).

The school problems of diabetic children are apparently not due to a lack of intellectual ability. Diabetic students have generally performed as well as healthy peers on standardized intelligence tests (Frankel, 1970). However, frequent absences from school due to illness can interfere with school performance. The anxiety and depression associated with poor metabolic control can also disrupt academic performance. In addition, episodes of hypoglycemia or hyperglycemia that affect the central nervous system may produce acute or long-term learning deficits.

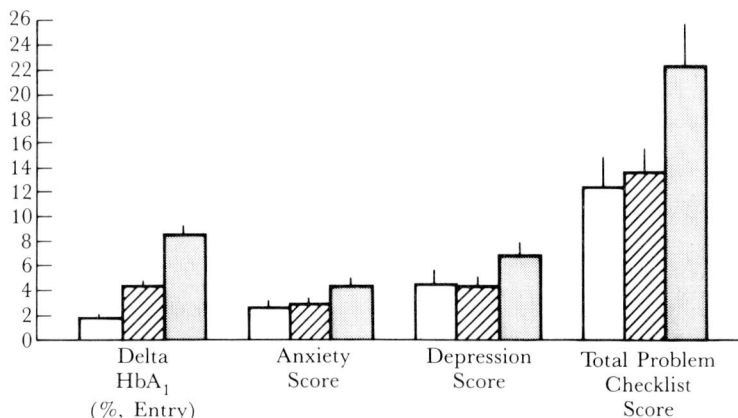

FIGURE 10.3   Mean anxiety, depression, and problem check list
scores for diabetic subjects in good, average, and poor control.
Control was measured by Hemoglobin Al levels, and had a range
of 0% to 16%. Subjects in good control (open bar) were the least
emotionally distressed and those in poor control (shaded bar) were
the most distressed. Subjects in average control were intermediate.
From "Psychological and Social Correlates of Glycemic Control" by
R. S. Mazze, D. Lucido, and H. Shamoon, 1984, *Diabetes Care, 7,*
p. 363. Reprinted by permission.

The long-term effects of variable blood glucose levels may include subtle
neuropsychological deficits in some diabetic patients. Several studies have
found significant differences between the performance of diabetic and
healthy subjects on tests assessing visual-motor coordination, memory, abstract
reasoning, and verbal skills (Bale, 1973; Franceschi, Cecchetto, Minicucci,
Smizne, Baio, & Canal, 1984; Ryan, 1988; Ryan, Vega, Longstreet, & Drash,
1984). It should be noted that most of the diabetic patients in these studies
performed within normal limits. The lower performance level of the diabetic
as compared to healthy subjects could be related to several factors, including
structural changes within the brain, abnormal blood glucose levels at the time
of testing, and psychological and behavioral reactions to diabetes.

Another psychosocial problem frequently encountered by diabetic patients
is sexual dysfunction. An increased frequency of erectile impotence in diabetic
men, as compared to healthy males, has been found in a number of studies
(Ellenberg, 1979; Schiavi & Hogan, 1979). The prevalence of impotence in
samples of diabetic men has ranged from 28% to 59%, with older diabetic
men demonstrating more dysfunction than younger diabetics. The high incidence of impotence in diabetic males is thought to be the result of autonomic
neuropathy and/or metabolic changes related to poorly controlled diabetes
(Ellenberg, 1979).

The research on the sexual functioning of diabetic women has produced inconsistent results. Several studies have found only minor differences in sexual functioning between diabetic females and healthy controls (Jensen, 1981; Tyrer, Steel, Ewing, Bancroft, Warner, & Clarke, 1983). However, other studies have found a high incidence of orgasmic dysfunction (Kolodny, 1971), inhibited sexual excitement and painful intercourse (Newman & Bertelson, 1986) reported in samples of Type I and II diabetic women. Additional research is needed to explore the possible effects of diabetes on sexual functioning in female patients.

# Treatment Interventions

The primary goal of the medical treatment of diabetes is the normalization of blood glucose levels (Seltzer, 1980). In the attempt to achieve euglycemia, diabetic patients are asked to follow the complex behavioral regimen previously described. A multidisciplinary team composed of physicians, nurses, dieticians, social workers, psychologists, psychiatrists, and other health professionals is often used to help patients follow the diabetic regimen and achieve control of blood glucose levels. Psychological interventions for diabetic patients have usually consisted of relaxation, biofeedback, or other stress management techniques and interventions designed to increase adherence to the diabetic regimen.

## Relaxation and Biofeedback Therapies

Research on the effects of stress on diabetic control has encouraged psychologists to study the possible benefits of relaxation training, biofeedback therapy, and other stress management techniques for diabetic patients. Surwit and Feinglos (1983) reported the first controlled group study of the effects of a biofeedback-assisted relaxation therapy on diabetic control. Twelve patients with Type II diabetes in poor control were chosen for participation in the study because they reported variation in diabetic control as a consequence of stressful events. The patients were hospitalized in a clinical research unit and administered glucose-tolerance and insulin-sensitivity tests. The glucose-tolerance test measured the patients' ability to metabolize orally administered glucose. The insulin-sensitivity test assessed the decline in blood glucose levels after intravenously administered insulin. Half of the patients then received instruction in progressive muscle relaxation techniques. They were given a cassette recording of the exercises and instructed to practice twice a day for five days. In addition, the patients in the relaxation group received five EMG biofeedback sessions. The six patients assigned to the control group remained in the hospital under identical conditions but did not receive relaxation or biofeedback training.

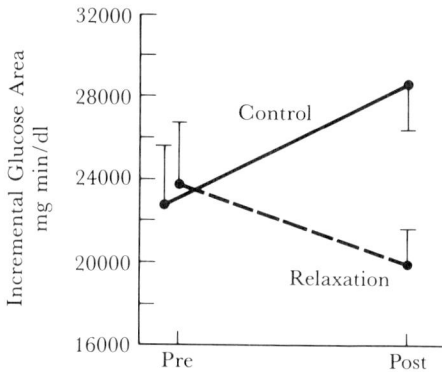

FIGURE 10.4    The effect of relaxation on incremental glucose area, a measure of diabetic control calculated from glucose tolerance tests. Values are shown before and after relaxation training, and are for hospitalized patients with non-insulin-dependent diabetes. Relaxation improved glucose tolerance. From "The effects of Relaxation on Glucose Tolerance in Non-Insulin-Dependent Diabetes" by R. S. Surwit and M. N. Feinglos, 1983, *Diabetes Care, 6*, p.177. Reprinted by permission.

At the end of one week, the glucose-tolerance and insulin-sensitivity tests were repeated on all patients. The results revealed that the biofeedback-assisted relaxation therapy affected glucose tolerance but did not change insulin sensitivity. As compared to pretreatment, the relaxation group demonstrated significantly greater glucose tolerance at posttreatment (see Figure 10.4). In contrast, the glucose tolerance of the control group deteriorated from pre- to posttreatment. The results of this study indicate that biofeedback-assisted relaxation therapy is beneficial for Type II diabetic patients who report that stress affects their metabolic control. However, it should be noted that the long-term effects of relaxation therapy were not determined in this study. Surwit and Feinglos (1983) concluded that additional studies with larger patient-samples are needed to determine if the improvement in glucose tolerance can be maintained in the home environment.

Anxiety-management training (AMT) that included relaxation therapy has been employed successfully with Type I diabetics in poor control (Rose, Firestone, Heick, & Faught, 1983). Five adolescents who reported that emotional stress affected their diabetic control were chosen to receive the AMT. A multiple-baseline design across subjects was used to evaluate treatment efficacy. Following a baseline phase that varied in length across patients, an attention-control phase consisting of psychological testing was begun in order to control for possible placebo effects. The AMT phase, initiated after each patient's attention-control phase, consisted of three stages. In the first stage, patients were taught deep muscle relaxation exercises. Next, they were asked to visualize stressful life situations and to identify their physiological responses to the stressful imaging (e.g., increased heart rate). In the third stage, the patients were stressed again using mental imaging and were taught to use a cue (e.g., a deep breath) to reduce their physiological response to stress. In addition, each patient was given a cassette recording of the relaxation instructions and was asked to practice at least three times a week and whenever stressful situations occurred. The length of the treatment phase ranged from ten to sixteen weeks.

Diabetic control during the study was assessed using the results of daily urine tests. Analysis of the test results revealed that all patients exhibited significant decreases in their mean urine glucose levels by the end of the AMT phase. The patients demonstrated nonsignificant decreases in urine glucose values during the attention-control phase. However, the differences in mean urine glucose levels between the baseline and AMT phases were significant for all the adolescents. Surprisingly, the patients' self-report of anxiety and tension did not vary during the study.

Rose and colleagues concluded that the AMT intervention effectively improved metabolic control by reducing sympathetic nervous system activity that may increase urine glucose levels and/or by encouraging patients to self-monitor their control and to adhere to their diabetic regimens. Although the results of this study indicated that AMT with relaxation therapy for Type I diabetics improved metabolic control, it should be noted that several investigations have found that relaxation therapy was not beneficial to all of the Type I diabetic patients studied (Feinglos, Hastedt, & Surwit, 1987; Landis et al., 1985; Seeburg & DeBoer, 1980). It is possible that relaxation and other anxiety management therapies are effective only for patients who report that emotional stress affects their diabetic control.

To summarize the preceding section, biofeedback therapy, and relaxation and anxiety management training appear to be effective treatments for diabetic patients who state that stress affects their blood glucose levels. The benefits of the relaxation-based treatments include improvement in metabolic control of diabetes. However, none of the controlled studies to date have examined possible long-term effects of relaxation, biofeedback, or AMT therapies.

## Strategies for Improving Adherence

As nonadherence is a major problem with diabetic patients, psychologists are beginning to develop programs to improve adherence. These programs have focused on the use of psychological techniques to increase the knowledge, skills, and motivation necessary for adherence.

Epstein and his colleagues have developed a treatment to improve the urine testing skills of diabetic children (Epstein et al., 1981). A sample of diabetic children who demonstrated frequent errors in urine testing were randomly assigned to treatment or control groups. Patients in the treatment group were asked to test ten urine solutions that contained predetermined amounts of glucose. The children were given feedback on their testing accuracy and were told the correct answers. Patients in the control group also tested the ten urine solutions but were not provided with any feedback.

Following the feedback and control training, all patients were retested using ten urine solutions under no-feedback conditions. The results indicated that patients in the treatment group had significantly fewer urine testing errors at

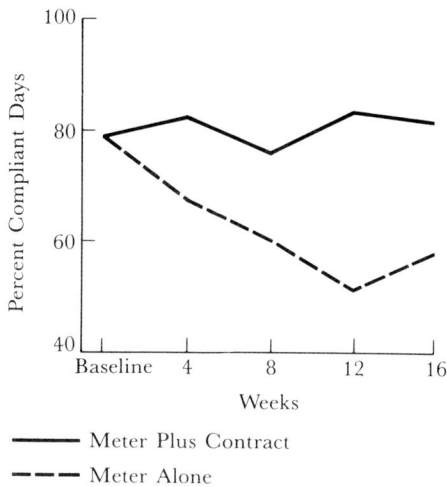

FIGURE 10.5   Mean percentage of days on which children completed prescribed blood glucose self-monitoring schedules. Children who contracted with their parents for rewards for appropriate testing were more likely to monitor glucose as prescribed. From "Blood Glucose Monitoring by Diabetic Adolescents: Compliance and Metabolic Control" by T. Wysocki, L. Green, and K. Huxtable, 1989, *Health Psychology, 8*, p. 274. Reprinted by permission.

posttreatment than at pretreatment. In contrast, the accuracy of the control group declined slightly from pre- to posttreatment. Thus, the simple procedure of providing informational feedback improved the skills of diabetic children. It has been suggested that a similar treatment program could be used to improve blood glucose testing skills of diabetic patients (Wysocki, 1989).

Once patients possess the knowledge and skills required for adherence, they may need adequate motivation (i.e., reinforcement) for performing the behaviors in the diabetic regimen. Several studies have examined the effects of positive reinforcement on the adherence of diabetic patients (Carney et al., 1983; Wysocki, Green, & Huxtable, 1989). Wysocki and his colleagues used a behavioral contract with Type I diabetic adolescents to increase adherence to blood glucose testing (Wysocki et al., 1989). Thirty adolescents were given special blood glucose meters with a computer memory that automatically recorded the results of blood glucose tests. Half of the adolescents also agreed to a behavioral contract that permitted them to earn money (i.e., positive reinforcement) for adhering to their prescribed blood glucose testing schedules. As indicated in Figure 10.5, the behavioral contract group demonstrated significantly greater compliance than the meter alone group during the course of the study. The results of this study indicate that positive reinforcement techniques can be used successfully to improve the adherence of diabetic adolescents.

Behavioral programs with multiple treatment components have also been used to increase diabetic adherence (Epstein, et al., 1979; Hartwell, Kaplan, & Wallace, 1986; Schafer, Glasgow, & McCaul, 1982). A behavioral weight-control program was developed to improve the dietary adherence of Type II obese diabetics (Wing, Epstein, Nowalk, Koeske, & Hagg, 1985). The diabetic patients were randomly assigned to behavior modification, nutrition education, or standard-care groups. Both the behavior modification and nutrition groups met weekly for sixteen weeks. The behavior modification treatment consisted of education on nutrition, exercise, and diabetes, plus behavioral strategies to help patients adhere to their dietary and exercise regimens. The behavioral strategies included self-monitoring, goal setting, contingency contracts, and positive self-statements. Patients in the nutrition group received education on exercise and the diabetic diet but did not learn behavioral strategies.

At the end of the treatment period, patients in the behavior modification group had lost significantly more weight than patients in the other two groups. However, the weight losses of the behavioral group were not maintained at a sixteen-month follow-up assessment. Self-report questionnaires were used to measure patient adherence during the study. In all three groups, the patients who reported adhering to positive exercise and eating behaviors demonstrated the greatest weight losses. Wing (1989) has suggested that weight-loss programs for obese diabetic patients should include training in diet and exercise as well as intensive, long-term treatment.

In summary, several behavioral treatments for the nonadherence of diabetic patients appear to be effective. However, the studies to date have failed to demonstrate the long-term efficacy of the behavioral approaches. Additional well-controlled group research is needed to determine the most effective strategies for improving long-term adherence to the different behaviors in the diabetic regimen.

## Prevention

As the etiology of diabetes is not understood, there have been few studies on the primary prevention of this chronic disease. It has been suggested that the prevention of Type I diabetes may eventually be based on a vaccine to prevent the viral destruction of the beta cells of the pancreas (Hawthorne & Cowie, 1984). In contrast, behavioral factors may play an important role in the prevention of Type II diabetes. Because obesity is a major risk factor for the development of Type II diabetes, psychological treatments for obesity may help to prevent the development of this chronic disease. Unfortunately, no research studies have examined the effectiveness of psychological weight control techniques for the prevention of Type II diabetes. A prospective study using obese adults with additional risk factors for the development of Type II diabetes (e.g., family history) would help to determine if a behavioral weight-control program is a successful preventive strategy (see Chapter 6 for a discussion of psychological treatments for obesity).

Secondary prevention in Type I and Type II diabetes has focused on the prevention of serious complications such as retinopathy and renal failure. Recent research has suggested that careful control of blood glucose levels may help to prevent long-term complications of diabetes (Santiago, 1984). Thus, the medical and psychological treatments that promote euglycemia can be considered strategies for secondary prevention.

Secondary prevention has also focused on the early identification of patients with diabetes. However, researchers have questioned the utility and cost-effectiveness of community programs that screen large numbers of individuals for diabetic symptoms (Hawthorne & Cowie, 1984). It has been suggested that screening programs should focus on groups that are at risk for the development of diabetes such as obese adults and pregnant women (Bennett & Knowler, 1984). Early diagnosis and effective treatment may help to prevent or ameliorate at least some of the complications of diabetes.

# Summary

Diabetes mellitus is a common chronic disease of unknown etiology that may produce significant complications and/or early mortality. As the complications of diabetes have been attributed to chronic hyperglycemia, medical treatment of diabetes attempts to normalize blood glucose levels. For most diabetics, medical treatment involves a behavioral regimen that can include diet, medication, exercise, and monitoring of urine or blood glucose levels. Because the diabetic regimen typically requires patients to perform complex behaviors with no immediate reinforcement, it is not surprising that nonadherence to the diabetic regimen is a major problem.

Psychological stress appears to play a role in the course of diabetes for a significant number of patients. The adverse effects of stress on diabetic control may be the result of stress-related physiological changes and/or nonadherence. Although most diabetic patients appear to cope well with their chronic illness, patients in poor metabolic control demonstrate more psychological problems than patients in good control. In addition, many diabetic patients have to cope with psychosocial issues such as changes in family functioning, school concerns, and/or sexual dysfunction.

As the diabetic regimen is composed of specific behaviors, it has been suggested that diabetes is a behavioral illness (Surwit et al., 1983). Indeed, psychologists are beginning to play an important role in the assessment and treatment of diabetic patients. Biofeedback and relaxation therapies have been used successfully to improve diabetic control. Behavioral treatments have also been employed to improve adherence to the diabetic regimen. Future research is expected to evaluate the long-term benefits of psychological interventions for diabetic patients.

# References

ALOGNA, M. (1980). Perception of severity of disease and health locus of control in compliant and noncompliant diabetic patients. _Diabetes Care, 3,_ 533–534.

BALE, R. N. (1973). Brain damage in diabetes mellitus. _British Journal of Psychiatry, 122,_ 337–341.

BALODIMOS, M. C. (1971). Diabetic nephropathy. In A. Marble, P. White, R. Bradley, & L. Krall (Eds.), *Joslin's diabetes mellitus* (11th ed.). Philadelphia: Lea and Febiger.

BANION, C. R., MILES, M. S., & CARTER, M. C. (1983). Problems of mothers in management of children with diabetes. *Diabetes Care, 6,* 548–551.

BECK, A. (1967). *Depression — Causes and treatment.* Philadelphia: University of Pennsylvania Press.

BENNETT, P. H., & KNOWLER, W. C. (1984). Early detection and intervention in diabetes mellitus: Is it effective? *Journal of Chronic Diseases, 37,* 653–666.

BLOOM, A., & IRELAND, J. (1980). *Color atlas of diabetes.* Chicago: Year Book Medical Publishers.

BRADLEY, C. (1979). Psychophysiological effects of stressful experiences and the management of diabetes mellitus. In D. J. Osborne, M. M. Gruneberg, & J. R. Eiser (Eds.), *Research in psychology and medicine* (Vol. 1). London: Academic Press.

BUNN, H. G. (1981). Evaluation of glycosylated hemoglobin in diabetic patients. *Diabetes, 30,* 613–617.

CARNEY, R. M., SCHECHTER, K., & DAVIS, T. (1983). Improving adherence to blood glucose testing in insulin-dependent diabetic children. *Behavior Therapy, 14,* 247–254.

CARTER, W. R., GONDER-FREDERICK, L. A., COX, D. J., CLARKE, W. L., & SCOTT, D. (1985). Effect of stress on blood glucose in IDDM. *Diabetes Care, 8,* 411–412.

CHASE, H. P., & JACKSON, G. G. (1981). Stress and sugar control in children with insulin-dependent diabetes mellitus. *Journal of Pediatrics, 98,* 1011–1013.

COHEN, A. S., VANCE, V. K., RUNYAN, J. W., & HURWITZ, D. (1960). Diabetic acidosis: An evaluation of the cause, course and therapy of 73 cases. *Annals of Internal Medicine, 52,* 55–86.

COX, D. J., TAYLOR, A. G., NOWACEK, G., HOLLEY-WILCOX, P., POHL, S. L., & GUTHROW, E. (1984). The relationship between psychological stress and insulin-dependent diabetic blood glucose control: Preliminary investigations. *Health Psychology, 3,* 63–75.

CRAIN, A. J., SUSSMAN, M. B., & WEIL, W. B. (1966). Effects of a diabetic child on marital integration and related measures of family functioning. *Journal of Health and Human Behavior, 7,* 122–127.

DAVIDSON, M. B. (1981). *Diabetes mellitus: Diagnosis and treatment.* New York: J. Wiley.

DUNBAR, H. F. (1954). *Emotions and bodily changes.* New York: Columbia University Press.

DUNN, S. M., & TURTLE, J. R. (1981). The myth of the diabetic personality. *Diabetes Care, 4,* 640–646.

EDELSTEIN, J., & LINN, M. W. (1985). The influence of the family on control of diabetes. *Social Science and Medicine, 21,* 541–544.

EFENDIC, S., CERASI, E., & LUFT, R. (1974). Trauma: Hormonal factors with special reference to diabetes mellitus. *Acta Anaesthesiologica Scandinavica, 55s,* 107–119.

ELLENBERG, M. (1979). Sex and diabetes: A comparison between men and women. *Diabetes Care, 2,* 4–8.

EPSTEIN, L. H., BECK, S., FIGUEROA, J., FARKAS, G., KAZDIN, A. E., DANEMAN, D., & BECKER, D. (1981). The effects of targeting improvements in urine glucose on metabolic control in children with insulin-dependent diabetes. *Journal of Applied Behavior Analysis, 14,* 365–375.

EPSTEIN, L. H., FIGUEROA, J., FARKAS, G. M., & BECK, S. (1981). The short-term effects of feedback on accuracy of urine glucose determinations in insulin-dependent diabetic children. *Behavior Therapy, 12,* 560–564.

ETZWILER, D. D. (1962). What the juvenile diabetic knows about his disease. *Pediatrics, 29,* 135–141.

FAERMAN, I., JADZINSKY, M., & PODOLSKY, S. (1980). Diabetic neuropathy and sexual dysfunction. In S. Podolsky (Ed.), *Clinical diabetes: Modern management.* New York: Appleton-Century-Crofts.

FALLSTROM, K. (1974). On the personality structure in diabetic schoolchildren aged 7–15 years. *Acta Paediatrica Scandinavica, 64* (Suppl. 251), 1–53.

FEINGLOS, M. N., HASTEDT, P., & SURWIT, R. S. (1987). Effects of relaxation therapy on patients with Type I diabetes mellitus. *Diabetes Care, 10,* 72–75.

FISHER, E. B., JR., DELAMATER, A. M., BERTELSON, A. D., & KIRKLEY, B. G. (1982). Psychological factors in diabetes and its treatment. *Journal of Consulting and Clinical Psychology, 50,* 993–1003.

FRANCESCHI, M., CECCHETTO, R., MINICUCCI, F., SMIZNE, S., BAIO, G., & CANAL, N. (1984). Cognitive processes in insulin-dependent diabetes. *Diabetes Care, 7,* 228–231.

FRANKEL, J. J. (1970). In Z. Laron (Ed.), *Habilitation and rehabilitation of juvenile diabetes.* Baltimore: Williams and Watkins.

GATH, A., SMITH, M. A., & BRAUM, J. D. (1980). Emotional, behavioural, and educational disorders in diabetic children. *Archives of Disease in Childhood, 55,* 371–375.

GILBERT, B. O., JOHNSON, S. B., SILVERSTEIN, J., & MALONE, J. (1989). *Journal of Pediatric Psychology, 14,* 577–591.

GLASGOW, R. E., & TOOBERT, D. J. (1988). Social environment and regimen adherence among Type II diabetic patients. *Diabetes Care, 11,* 377–386.

GOETSCH, V. L. (1989). Stress and blood glucose in diabetes mellitus: A review and methodological commentary. *Annals of Behavioral Medicine, 11,* 102–107.

GONDER-FREDERICK, L., COX, D. J., POHL, S. L., & CARTER, W. (1984). Patient blood glucose monitoring: Use, accuracy, adherence, and impact. *Behavioral Medicine Update, 6,* 12–16.

GRABER, A. L., CHRISTMAN, B. G., ALOGNA, M. T., & DAVIDSON, J. K. (1977). Evaluation of diabetes patient-education programs. *Diabetes, 26,* 61–64.

HANSON, C. L., HENGGELER, S. W., HARRIS, M. A., BURGHEN, G. A., & MOORE, M. (1989). Family system variables and the health status of adolescents with insulin-dependent diabetes mellitus. *Health Psychology, 8,* 239–253.

HARRIS, M. (1982). Classification and diagnosis of diabetes mellitus. In J. D. Schnatz (Ed.), *Diabetes mellitus: Problems in management.* Menlo Park, CA: Addison-Wesley.

HARTWELL, S. L., KAPLAN, R. M., & WALLACE, J. P. (1986). Comparison of behavioral interventions for control of Type II diabetes mellitus. *Behavior Therapy, 17,* 447–461.

HAWTHORNE, V. M., & COWIE, C. C. (1984). Some thoughts on early detection and intervention in diabetes mellitus. *Journal of Chronic Diseases, 37,* 667–669.

HINKLE, L. E., & WOLF, S. (1952). Importance of life stress in course and management of diabetes mellitus. *Journal of the American Medical Association, 148,* 513–520.

HOLMES, T. H., & RAHE, R. H. (1967). The Social Readjustment Rating Scale. *Journal of Psychosomatic Research, 11,* 213–218.

HULKA, B. S., KUPPER, L. L., CASSEL, J. C., & MAYO, F. (1975). Doctor-patient communication and outcomes among diabetic patients. *Journal of Community Health, 1,* 15–27.

JENSEN, S. B. (1981). Diabetic sexual dysfunction: A comparative study of 160 insulin-treated diabetic men and women and an age-matched control group. *Archives of Sexual Behavior, 10,* 493–504.

JOHNSON, S. B. (1980). Psychosocial factors in juvenile diabetes: A review. *Journal of Behavioral Medicine, 3,* 95–116.

JOHNSON, S. B., POLLAK, T., SILVERSTEIN, J. H., ROSENBLOOM, A. L., SPILLAR, R., McCALLUM, M., & HARKAVY, J. (1982). Cognitive and behavioral knowledge about insulin-dependent diabetes among children and parents. *Pediatrics, 69,* 708–713.

KANNER, A. D., COYNE, J. C., SCHAEFER, C., & LAZARUS, R. S. (1981). Comparison of two modes of stress measurement: Daily hassles and uplifts versus major life events. *Journal of Behavioral Medicine, 4,* 1–39.

KAPLAN, R. M., & HARTWELL, S. L. (1987). Differential effects of social support and social network on physiological and social outcomes in men and women with Type II diabetes mellitus. *Health Psychology, 6,* 387–398.

KEMMER, F. W., BISPING, R., STEINGRUBER, H. J., BAAR, H., HARDTMANN, R., SCHLAGHECKE, R., & BERGER, M. (1984). Psychological stress and metabolic control in patients with Type I diabetes. *New England Journal of Medicine, 314,* 1078–1084.

KLUSA, Y., HABBICK, B. F., & ABERNATHY, T. J. (1983). Diabetes in children: Family responses and control. *Psychosomatics, 24,* 367–372.

KOLODNY, R. C. (1971). Sexual dysfunction in diabetic females. *Diabetes, 20,* 557–559.

KOVACS, M., KASS, R. E., SCHNELL, T. M., GOLDSTEIN, D., & MARSH, J. (1989). Family functioning and metabolic control of school-aged children with IDDM. *Diabetes Care, 12,* 409–414.

LAMMERS, C. A., NALIBOFF, B. D., & STRAATMEYER, A. J. (1984). The effects of progressive relaxation on stress and diabetic control. *Behaviour Research and Therapy, 22,* 641–650.

LANDIS, B., JOVANOVIC, L., LANDIS, E., PETERSON, C. M., GROSHEN, S., JOHNSON, K., & MILLER, N. E. (1985). Effect of stress reduction on daily glucose range in previously stabilized insulin-dependent diabetic patients. *Diabetes Care, 8,* 624–626,

LAVIGNE, J. V., TRAISMAN, H. S., MARR, T. J., & CHASNOFF, I. J. (1982). Parental perceptions of the psychological adjustment of children with diabetes and their siblings. *Diabetes Care, 5,* 420–426.

LIPSETT, L. F. (1980). Overview of diabetes mellitus. *Behavioral Medicine Update, 2,* 15–17.

LUSTMAN, P. J., HARPER, G. W., GRIFFITH, L. S., & CLOUSE, R. E. (1986). Use of the Diagnostic Interview Schedule in patients with diabetes mellitus. *Journal of Nervous and Mental Disease, 174,* 743–746.

MARBLE, A. (1971). Current concepts of diabetes. In A. Marble, P. White, R. Bradley, & L. Krall (Eds.), *Joslin's diabetes mellitus* (11th ed.). Philadelphia: Lea and Febiger.

MAZZE, R. S., LUCIDO, D., & SHAMOON, H. (1984). Psychological and social correlates of glycemic control. *Diabetes Care, 7,* 360–366.

MENNINGER, W. C. (1935). Psychological factors in the etiology of diabetes. *Journal of Nervous and Mental Diseases, 81,* 1–13.

METZGER, B. E. (1980). Complications in pregnancy and fetal development. In B. A. Hamburg, L. F. Lipsett, G. E. Inoff, & A. L. Drash (Eds.), *Behavioral and psychosocial aspects of diabetes: Proceedings of a national conference* (NIH Publication No. 80–1993). Washington, D.C.: U. S. Government Printing Office.

MINUCHIN, S., ROSMAN, B. L., & BAKER, L. (1978). *Psychosomatic families.* Cambridge: Harvard University Press.

MORRIS, L. R., McGEE, J. A., & KITABCHI, A. E. (1981). Correlation between plasma and urine glucose in diabetes. *Annals of Internal Medicine, 94,* 469–471.

MURAWSKI, B. J., CHAZAN, B. I., BALODIMOS, M. C., & RYAN, J. R. (1970). Personality patterns in patients with diabetes mellitus of long duration. *Diabetes, 19,* 259–263.

NALIBOFF, B. D., COHEN, M. J., & SOWERS, J. D. (1985). Physiological and metabolic responses to brief stress in non-insulin dependent diabetic and control subjects. *Journal of Psychosomatic Research, 29,* 367–374.

NEWMAN, A. S., & BERTELSON, A. D. (1986). Sexual dysfunction in diabetic women. *Journal of Behavioral Medicine, 9,* 261–270.

O'GRADY, G. E. (1980). Diabetic retinopathy. In S. Podolsky (Ed.), *Clinical diabetes: Modern management.* New York: Appleton-Century-Crofts.

POHL, S. L., GONDER-FREDERICK, L., & COX, D. J. (1984). Diabetes mellitus: An overview. *Behavioral Medicine Update, 6,* 3–7.

POND, H. (1979). Parental attitudes toward children with a chronic medical disorder: Special reference to diabetes mellitus. *Diabetes Care, 2,* 425–431.

PYKE, D. A. (1981). Diabetes: The genetic connection. *Diabetologia, 17,* 333–343.

ROBINSON, N., & FULLER, J. H. (1985). Role of life events and difficulties in the onset of diabetes mellitus. *Journal of Psychosomatic Research, 29,* 583–591.

ROSE, M. I., FIRESTONE, P., HEICK, H. M. C., & FAUGHT, A. K. (1983). The effects of anxiety management training on the control of juvenile diabetes mellitus. *Journal of Behavioral Medicine, 6,* 381–395.

ROVET, J. F., & EHRLICH, R. M. (1988). Effect of temperament on metabolic control in children with diabetes mellitus. *Diabetes Care, 11,* 77–82.

RYAN, C. M. (1988). Neurobehavioral complications of Type I diabetes: Examination of possible risk factors. *Diabetes Care, 11,* 86–91.

RYAN, C. M., VEGA, A., LONGSTREET, C., & DRASH, A. (1984). Neuropsychological changes in adolescents with insulin-dependent diabetes. *Journal of Consulting and Clinical Psychology, 52,* 335–342.

SANTIAGO, J. V. (1984). Effect of treatment on the long-term complications of IDDM. *Behavioral Medicine Update, 6,* 26–31.

SCHAFER, L. C., GLASGOW, R. E., & McCAUL, K. D. (1982). Increasing the adherence of diabetic adolescents. *Journal of Behavioral Medicine, 5,* 353–362.

SCHIAVI, R. C., & HOGAN, B. (1979). Sexual problems in diabetes mellitus: Psychological aspects. *Diabetes Care, 2,* 9–17.

SCHLENK, E. A., & HART, L. K. (1984). Relationship between health locus of control, health values, and social support and compliance of persons with diabetes mellitus. *Diabetes Care, 7,* 566–574.

SEEBURG, K. N., & DeBOER, K. F. (1980). Effects of EMG biofeedback on diabetes. *Biofeedback and Self-Regulation, 5,* 289–293.

SELTZER, H. S. (1980). Prime consideration in diagnosis and treatment. In S.

Podolsky (Ed.), *Clinical diabetes: Modern management.* New York: Appleton-Century-Crofts.

SIMONDS, J. F. (1977). Psychiatric status of diabetic youth matched with a control group. *Diabetes, 26,* 921–925.

SKYLER, J. S. (1979). Complications of diabetes mellitus: Relationship of metabolic dysfunction. *Diabetes Care, 2,* 499–509.

SLAWSON, P., FLYNN, W., & KOLLAR, E. (1963). Psychological factors associated with the onset of diabetes mellitus. *Journal of the American Medical Association, 185,* 166–170.

SPEERS, M. A., & TURK, D. C. (1982). Diabetes self-care: Knowledge, beliefs, motivation, and action. *Patient Counselling and Health Education, 3,* 144–149.

STEIN, S., & CHARLES, E. (1971). A study of early life experiences of adolescent diabetics. *American Journal of Psychiatry, 128,* 700–704.

SULLIVAN, B. J. (1978). Self-esteem and depression in adolescent diabetic girls. *Diabetes Care, 1,* 18–22.

SULLIVAN, B. J. (1979). Adjustment in diabetic adolescent girls: I. Development of the Diabetic Adjustment Scale. *Psychosomatic Medicine, 41,* 119–126.

SURWIT, R. S., & FEINGLOS, M. N. (1983). The effects of relaxation on glucose tolerance in non-insulin-dependent diabetes. *Diabetes Care, 6,* 176–179.

SURWIT, R. S., & FEINGLOS, M. N. (1988). Stress and autonomic nervous system in Type II diabetes: A hypothesis. *Diabetes Care, 11,* 83–85.

SURWIT, R. S., & FEINGLOS, M. N., & SCOVERN, A. W. (1983). Diabetes and behavior: A paradigm for health psychology. *American Psychologist, 38,* 255–262.

TAVORMINA, J. B., KASTNER, L. S., SLATER, P. M., & WATT, S. L. (1976). Chronically ill children: A psychologically and emotionally deviant population? *Journal of Abnormal Child Psychology, 4,* 99–110.

TURK, D. C., & SPEERS, M. A. (1983). Diabetes mellitus: A cognitive-functional analysis of stress. In T. G. Burish & L. A. Bradley (Eds.), *Coping with chronic disease.* New York: Academic Press.

TYRER, G., STEEL, J. M., EWING, D. J., BANCROFT, J., WARNER, P., & CLARKE, B. F. (1983). Sexual responsiveness in diabetic women. *Diabetologia, 24,* 166–171.

U. S. DEPARTMENT OF HEALTH AND HUMAN SERVICES (1984). Summary of births, deaths, marriages, and divorces: United States—1983 (DHHS publication No. 84–1120). Washington, D.C.: U. S. Government Printing Office.

U. S. DEPARTMENT OF HEALTH AND HUMAN SERVICES (1985). Diabetes in America (DHHS publication No. 85–1468). Washington, D.C.: U. S. Government Printing Office.

WALLSTON, K. A., WALLSTON, B. S., & DeVELLIS, R. (1978). Development of the multidimensional Health Locus of Control (MHLC) scales. *Health Education Monographs, 6,* 160–170.

WATKINS, J. D., WILLIAMS, T. F., MARTIN, D. A., HOGAN, M. D., & ANDERSON, E. (1967). A study of diabetic patients at home. *American Journal of Public Health, 57,* 452–459.

WATTS, F. N. (1980). Behavioural aspects of the management of diabetes mellitus: Education, self-care and metabolic control. *Behaviour Research and Therapy, 18,* 171–180.

WILLIAMS, T. F., ANDERSON, E., WATKINS, J. D., & COYLE, V. (1967). Dietary errors made at home by patients with diabetes. *Journal of the American Dietetic Association, 51,* 19–25.

WING, R. R. (1989). Behavioral strategies for weight reduction in obese Type II diabetic patients. *Diabetes Care, 12,* 139–144.

WING, R. R., EPSTEIN, L. H., & NOWALK, M. P. (1984). Dietary adherence in patients with diabetes. *Behavioral Medicine Update, 6,* 17–21.

WING, R. R., EPSTEIN, L. H., NOWALK, M. P., KOESKE, R., & HAGG, S. (1985). Behavior change, weight loss, and physiological improvements in Type II diabetic patients. *Journal of Consulting and Clinical Psychology, 53,* 111–122.

WING, R. R., LAMPARSKI, D. M., ZASLOW, S., BETSCHART, J., SIMINERIO, L., & BECKER, D. (1985). Frequency and accuracy of self-monitoring of blood glucose in children: Relationship to glycemic control. *Diabetes Care, 8,* 214–218.

WYSOCKI, T. (1989). Impact of blood glucose monitoring on diabetic control: Obstacles and interventions. *Journal of Behavioral Medicine, 12,* 183–205.

WYSOCKI, T., GREEN, L., & HUXTABLE, K. (1989). Blood glucose monitoring by diabetic adolescents: Compliance and metabolic control. *Health Psychology, 8,* 267–284.

ZEIDEL, A. (1970). Emotional adjustment of juvenile diabetics and their families. In Z. Laron (Ed.), *Habilitation and rehabilitation of juvenile diabetics.* Baltimore: Williams and Watkins.

ZINMAN, B. (1984). Diabetes mellitus and exercise. *Behavioral Medicine Update, 6,* 22–25.

# Respiratory Disease

## Biological and Psychophysiological Components

### Biological Components

THE APPARATUS OF THE RESPIRATORY SYSTEM: HOW DO WE BREATHE? The major function of the respiratory system is to provide the blood with oxygen. At the same time it rids blood of carbon dioxide before blood circulates throughout the body. The major structures involved in respiration resemble an upside-down tree with the trunk being the *trachea*. The trachea separates into two branches, the *bronchi*. Each bronchus leads to a lung. The bronchi divide into smaller and smaller air tubes like the branches of a tree. They end in air sacs called *alveoli*.

In the process of breathing, air enters and leaves the lungs. The walls of the bronchi are elastic and expand and contract during breathing. Air passes through the bronchial tubes with the help of a smooth membrane. The glands of this membrane secrete a mucus that acts as a lubricant. It is in the alveoli that the exchange of oxygen for carbon dioxide occurs. Nests of capillaries, very small blood vessels, surround alveoli. Oxygen passes through the alveolar membrane into the blood and carbon dioxide moves in the opposite direction into the alveolus. From here, oxygen circulates to body tissues, and carbon dioxide is exhaled.

Although it is known that breathing occurs in response to voluntary and involuntary factors, the mechanisms controlling respiration have not been precisely defined. Voluntary acts of breathing, such as hyperventilation (rapid breathing) and holding one's breath are thought to be under the control of higher structures within the cerebral cortex. Involuntary breathing probably involves neurons in the pons and medulla.

RESPIRATORY DISORDERS   There are many types of respiratory disorders. As experts in this area point out, the environment of our contemporary society is constantly being poisoned with various chemicals and pollutants that result in the identification of new variants of respiratory diseases (Creer, 1979). The most common group of respiratory disorders is referred to as chronic obstructive diseases, which are characterized by chronic obstruction to airflow during the course of breathing. Asthma, chronic bronchitis, and emphysema are included in this group. Asthma differs from emphysema and chronic bronchitis in that its airflow obstruction is partially and, at times, totally reversible. Asthma is usually referred to as a reversible obstructive airway disease (ROAD), as opposed to a chronic obstructive pulmonary disease (COPD).

*Asthma*   In asthma, interference in normal breathing occurs when there is a constriction of airways in segments of the bronchial tree. Airflow to and from the alveoli is obstructed, and the body must work harder to empty and fill the lungs. An excess of mucus is produced and secreted. This excess mucus collects in the bronchial tubes and further reduces the flow of air. Air becomes trapped in the lungs. The major problem in most obstructive pulmonary disorders is getting the stale air out of the lungs, and the fresh air in. Individuals with asthma experience shortness of breath, tightness in the chest, dyspnea (air hunger), a choking sensation, and a coughing spasm that is an effort of the airways to remove the obstruction. Wheezing also occurs as a result of the bronchial constriction.

Not all asthmatics experience the same symptoms or severity of symptoms. A definition of asthma helpful in understanding this variability was suggested by Chai (1975): He defined asthma as an *intermittent, variable*, and *reversible* airway obstruction. *Intermittent* means that attacks usually occur periodically, as opposed to continuously. A patient may experience severe asthma symptoms for two weeks and then remain relatively symptom-free for several months.

*Variable* refers to the variability in the severity of the symptoms experienced by the patient. An attack may be experienced as a fairly mild obstruction in breathing, such as a slight wheeze, or it may be a *status asthmaticus condition* (steadily worsening asthma) that may be so severe as to threaten the patient's life. *Reversible* means that the asthma condition can change to a normal state with or without treatment. This reversible characteristic sets asthma apart from other respiratory diseases in which reversibility is more unlikely.

There are several triggers that produce asthma attacks. Some individuals react to specific allergens such as cigarette smoke, pollen, or dust. These asthmatics are said to experience *extrinsic* or *allergic* asthma. If such triggers cannot be specified, the patient is said to suffer from *intrinsic* asthma. Not all asthmatics fit neatly into these two categories, and more elaborate descriptive classifications have been devised (Reed and Townley, 1978).

About 5% of the adult population of the United States suffer from asthma, and at one time or another 7% of the population have suffered from asthma (Davis, 1972; McFadden, 1987). Creer (1979) points out that incidence and prevalence estimates vary because many different methods are used to identify asthmatic sufferers. A number of reports indicate that at least half of all asthmatics are under the age of fifteen (Creer, 1979). One estimate indicated that between 7% and 10% of American children are afflicted with asthma (McFadden, 1987).

*Other Common Respiratory Disorders* Chronic inflammation and swelling of the cells lining the inside of the bronchi (air tubes) is known as *chronic bronchitis*. When inflamed, these cells produce excess quantities of mucus that narrow the air tubes, making breathing more difficult. The major cause of chronic bronchitis is prolonged irritation of the bronchial lining. Heavy smoking and air pollution are two of many stimuli that cause bronchial irritation.

*Emphysema* is an abnormal and permanent enlargement of respiratory air spaces involving a reduced number of alveoli. Fewer alveoli result in a lessening of the elasticity of the lung. Thus, the patient with emphysema has difficulty squeezing air out of the lungs. Although no single cause for emphysema has been pinpointed, smoking is a major factor (Matthay, 1988).

# Psychophysiological Components of Asthma

THE ROLE OF EMOTIONS The role of emotions in respiratory disease, particularly asthma, has historically been a controversial topic. Some have viewed asthma as solely a medical disease, whereas others have contended it was purely a psychological disorder. Today, it is generally accepted that asthma is a physical disease that can be exacerbated by allergic, infectious, and/or psychological factors. Psychological factors may trigger an asthma attack or may be relevant to how successfully an individual copes with the consequences of the disease. Behavioral patterns influence both the development and the course of respiratory diseases.

That emotions play a role in precipitating and/or aggravating attacks of asthma is not a new idea. As early as the twelfth century, Maimonides, the physician to the court of Saladin, believed emotions to play a primary role in asthma. Hippocrates, also commenting on the role of emotions in asthma, allegedly said, "The asthmatic patient must guard against anger" (Knapp, Mathe, & Vachon, 1976).

The role of anxiety in triggering asthma attacks has been of particular interest to researchers. As early as 1886, Sir James McKenzie studied anxiety and its association with airway obstruction. He presented an artificial rose to an asthmatic patient who was allergic to roses. The patient not only wheezed in the presence of real roses, but also in the presence of artificial ones. The conclusion was drawn that asthmatic patients anxiously expect to respond to certain stimuli. That expectation, in and of itself, was thought to be sufficient to elicit an attack. More recent studies have confirmed the notion that expectation plays an important part in the onset of asthma attacks for some individuals (McFadden, Luparello, Lyons, & Bleecker, 1969).

In understanding the role that emotions play in asthma, it is important to emphasize that this role is unique to the individual and that generalizations are at this time impossible to make. McFadden et al. (1969), for example, studied the role of expectation in the elicitation of asthma attacks and found that when subjects were presented with neutral substances with the instructions that they would likely experience an attack, asthma attacks would result. One-third of their subjects, however, did not respond in this manner. It is important, therefore, to understand the characteristics of asthmatics who do respond to suggestion in this way, as well as the characteristics of those who do not. Horton, Suda, Kinsman, Souhrada, and Spector (1978), interested in determining which factors would predict response to suggestion, found that on a variety of pulmonary measures, asthmatics with the *least* reactive airways showed less response to suggestion than those with *hyperreactive* airways. Asthmatics with hyperreactive airways, then, were thought to be most susceptible to attacks of asthma induced by emotional arousal. Those with less activity were thought to be least susceptible to attacks. Thus, one must consider that there is likely an interplay between the pathophysiological aspects of asthma and strong emotion. The precise nature of this interplay awaits further clarification.

THE ROLE OF LEARNING   The role of learned responses in asthma has long been of interest to scientists. An early article by Turnbull (1962) addressed this question. Turnbull, in a review of some animal studies, suggested that asthma symptoms may be acquired through classical conditioning. The typical paradigm exploring the role of classical conditioning involved exposing presensitized animals to allergic inhalants that subsequently resulted in asthma attacks. Other stimuli present in the original situation in which the asthma attack occurred were then found to elicit the asthmalike response. Justeson, Braun, Garrison, and Pendleton (1970), for example, classically conditioned an asthmalike response in a group of sixteen guinea pigs. Although Turnbull suggested that such studies provide evidence for the conditioning of asthmalike behavior, he also noted these conditioned responses generally extinguished quite rapidly. The conditioned asthmalike behavior failed to appear within a few trials after the unconditioned stimulus was withdrawn. Because of this rapid extinction, the classical conditioning paradigm is thought to be inadequate in explaining how asthmalike behaviors endure (Knapp et al., 1976).

To more adequately explain the role of learning in the asthma response, Turnbull suggested that for this conditioned response to persist, it must be reinforced. Unlike the original formulations that linked learning models to asthma through a classical conditioning paradigm, Turnbull posited a two-factor theory of asthma. His theory states that although the asthmalike response may be learned through classical conditioning, it persists as a result of strong reinforcement of that response via operant conditioning. For example, a child's asthma response may be reinforced and thereby maintained by parental attention to the behavior. Turnbull further suggested that the specific asthma symptoms that result have been formed through the reinforcement of progressively closer approximations to asthmatic breathing. More recent studies have focused on the effects both of suggestion and the acquisition of specific symptoms of respiratory distress through operant conditioning procedures (Creer, Chai, & Hoffman 1977; Mumford, Reardon, Liberman, & Allen 1976). The evidence for classical conditioning as a sole cause for bronchial asthma may not be convincing, but it is plausible that operant conditioning may account for the symptoms of some asthmatics (Knapp et al., 1976).

# Behavioral, Psychological, and Social Factors

## Behavioral Factors

Behavioral patterns influence both the development and the course of respiratory diseases. Some behaviors may promote the onset or contraction of a respiratory disease and other behaviors that occur after the respiratory problem is diagnosed can affect the course of the disorder. Smoking is an example of the first type of behavioral pattern, and the underusage or overusage of medication prescribed for the respiratory disease patient is an example of the second type of behavioral pattern.

We have already seen, in Chapter 6, that smoking is a major contributor to health problems. Cigarette smoking is highly correlated to the onset of respiratory disorders (Wynder & Hoffman, 1979). One may view the habit of smoking as a behavioral excess (a behavior that has developed as a result of its reinforcing qualities), or as a behavioral deficit (a maladaptive behavior that has developed in the absence of more adaptive coping strategies for dealing with stress) (Creer, 1979). However one views the etiology and maintenance of smoking behavior, it is undeniably an important variable in the etiology of life-threatening pulmonary problems.

A behavioral pattern that can certainly influence the course of a respiratory disease is the patient's misuse of medications designed to facilitate breathing and to control the worsening of respiratory problems. Because most respiratory diseases are chronic in nature and require some form of medication in order for the individual to function optimally, the use of prescribed medications becomes particularly important in the treatment of respiratory diseases. Asthmatics, for example, are generally prescribed a medication regimen that may need to be taken indefinitely in order to control their disease. Misusing medications can lead to asthma mismanagement and to flare-ups of the disorder.

Although characteristics of asthmatics who overuse or underuse medications to control their asthma have yet to be fully defined, studies have been conducted that suggest that one's tendency to over- or underrespond to asthma symptoms relates to medication usage (Kinsman, Dirks, & Dahlem, 1980a). Some medication is taken on a regular schedule and other medication is taken on a symptomatic basis, whenever the patient feels medication is required. Kinsman et al. (1980a) described the personality patterns that may lead to over- or underuse of medications taken on a symptomatic basis. Those patients who underuse medications tend or seem to view themselves as unrealistically capable and able to deal with problems in living. They experience relatively little anxiety as signs of asthma increase and underrespond to their symptoms.

Patients prone to overuse medication have different personality characteristics. These patients see themselves as less able to cope than most people, having little control over their asthma. They are described as exceptionally anxious, worried, and prone to hyperventilation during asthma attacks. Such patients are found to use medications at times when objective information about their breathing indicates that they may not need to.

# Psychological Factors

Psychological factors may be relevant to the development and care of respiratory disease in two ways: (1) psychological factors may influence the onset or contraction of a respiratory disease, such as when a person denies that smoking may be endangering his or her general health and pulmonary status, and (2) psychological factors may influence the course of the disorder after the respiratory problem has been diagnosed.

Kinsman, Dirks, & Jones (1982) have stressed that in order to understand the psychological components influencing the course of asthma, one must take into account at least four factors: (1) patients' personality styles, (2) the attitudes held with regard to illness, (3) the asthma symptoms reported, and (4) the manner by which the first three factors interact to affect behavior associated with the management of illness.

These four factors are important determinants of how the patient regards his or her asthma, experiences asthma, and behaves during its treatment. The Battery of Asthma Illness Behavior evaluates variables such as optimism regarding prognosis, regard for medical staff, beliefs about ability to cope with and master asthma, panic and anxiety related to asthma attacks, and the degree to which asthma is regarded as a psychological flaw. Scores on the Battery of Asthma Illness Behavior have been found to predict rates of rehospitalization (Dirks, 1982; Dirks & Kinsman, 1981).

One important dimension related to illness management is the degree to which one feels in control of one's health status. Patients who tend to feel helpless emphasize their distress and give up easily in many situations, and they tend to be pessimistic about their own ability to control and cope with their asthma. They see their illness as being in the hands of medical care givers, and respond to breathing problems with extreme anxiety, exaggeration of affective distress, and helplessness. Such individuals will not take appropriate, independent action to deal with their asthma but will, rather, rely on medical assistance (Kinsman, Dirks, & Jones, 1980b).

Patients on the opposite end of this psychological continuum are described as counterdependent. They experience a strong need to be independent and capable. They thereby have their own ideas about how to manage their asthma and are unrealistically optimistic about their ability to master their asthma independently. They do not rely on medical attention when perhaps they are in need of it. They tend to be unaware of early signs of respiratory distress and respond with very little anxiety. Such individuals may be prone to delay seeking medical attention and, by doing so, may exacerbate their symptoms (Kinsman et al., 1980b).

## Social Factors

PARENTAL CHARACTERISTICS   Early studies investigating the role of parental characteristics in childhood asthma tended to focus on potential psychopathological characteristics of this group as causative factors in the disease process. Block, Harvey, Jennings, and Simpson (1966) and Block (1969) introduced the notion of the "asthmatogenic mother," whose particular personality or behavior was thought to increase the frequency and severity of asthma attacks in her children. The notion that parental characteristics are primary determinants of the course of this disorder is referred to as a *linear model* of family functioning.

That psychopathological parental characteristics reinforce or induce asthma symptoms was thought to be supported by the observation that removal of asthmatic children from their homes often resulted in marked improvement of their symptoms (Purcell, Brady, Chai, Muser, Mulk, Gordon, & Means, 1969). This led to the *parentectomy* approach to the treatment of asthma in which children were removed from their homes for treatment (Peshkin, 1960). It was hoped that they would gain psychological strength and that they might better cope with the characteristics of their parents and relationships to them.

Numerous studies have attempted to document psychopathological characteristics of parents of asthmatic children. There has been little success in doing so (Creer & Kotses, 1983). For example, there have been attempts to relate heightened maternal anxiety, overprotectiveness, and/or maternal depression to the onset and maintenance of the disease (Parker & Lipscombe, 1979; Byrne & Murrell, 1977; Davis, 1977). Consistent support for increased parental psychopathology, or even increased anxiety and overprotectiveness, has not been found. Indeed, some contend that the overprotectiveness often described in mothers of asthmatic children is likely the consequence, not the cause, of asthmatic symptoms (Parker & Lipscombe, 1979). Further, some studies have seriously questioned the theory of a pathological relationship between mother and child and have actually found these individuals to be quite well adjusted (Gauthier, Fortin, Drapeau, Briton, Gosselin, Quental, Weisnagel, & Lamarre, 1978). The varied quality of studies in this area and the general failure of such studies to employ reliable and valid instruments in assessing mother-child interactions, limit any conclusions supporting the role of parent-child interactions and/or parental psychopathology on the development and/or exacerbations of asthma (Creer & Kotses, 1983).

CHARACTERISTICS OF FAMILY FUNCTIONING  A theory that focuses on the role of *family interactions* in the initiation and maintenance of intractable asthma has been posited by Minuchin and his coworkers (1975). They have pointed out that the linear models suggesting that parental functioning has a direct effect on childhood illness have hindered advancement in this field. Instead, they have emphasized the impact that family members have on each other and how such interactions govern a family member's behavior. Such a view of asthma is termed a *psychosomatic family model*. In contrast to a *linear model*, this approach is called a *systems model* of family functioning.

In this model, four characteristics of psychosomatic families are emphasized. These characteristics are thought to lead to the presence of a physical disorder such as asthma:

1. *Enmeshment*, wherein the boundaries usually drawn between parental and child roles are blurred. This results in confusion regarding behaviors appropriate to one's role. Members tend to be overinvolved with each other. Independent action is not valued but instead punished. It is believed that such relationships thwart each member's striving for independent functioning.

2. *Overprotectiveness*, wherein a high degree of nurturance and overinvolvement is apparent between members. Such overinvolvement also limits the extent to which an individual member may grow independently.

3. *Rigidity*, wherein the family tenaciously strives to maintain its existing family patterns of interaction. Change is viewed as a threat to family members. The asthmatic symptoms are maintained in order to deflect family attention away from conflict that might challenge the status quo. Symptoms, for example, allow a couple to avoid dealing with conflicts in their marriage because they must attend to their sick child.

4. *Lack of conflict resolution*, wherein problems within the family are denied and, therefore, remain unresolved.

This perspective posits three factors that initiate and maintain childhood illness:

1. Physiological susceptibility of the child to the condition.
2. The presence of the four transactional characteristics previously described.
3. The sick child plays a major role in family conflict avoidance and is reinforced for his symptoms because of this role.

Although some evidence has been cited to support the existence of these characteristics within families with children with asthma (Liebman, Minuchin, & Baker, 1974), such evidence is hardly compelling and has generally involved too many methodological insufficiencies to warrant drawing any firm conclusions. In addition, there is some evidence to indicate that the transactional patterns described within these families may not relate to the severity of asthma (Burbeck, 1979). A review of studies of the family systems model of asthma indicates that the relationship between asthma and family variables is equivocal at best. The use of unreliable and invalid measures of family interaction poses major problems in this area of research (Creer & Kotses, 1983).

OCCUPATIONAL EXPOSURE   A factor related to the onset of some asthma in adults are substances to which one may be exposed to on the job. Asthma can be caused by substances manufactured by or used by a worker in his job setting, or such substances may aggravate a pre-existing asthmatic condition. Asthma caused by substances encountered on the job is called *occupationally induced asthma*.

A number of substances may lead to this condition. Animal dusts and secretions may lead to asthma attacks. Asthmatics exposed to such substances may be reacting to animal hairs or dander or substances associated with animals (e.g., insects or molds). Wood and vegetable dusts (oak, cotton, grain, and flour) and industrial chemicals and detergents may also induce asthma (McFadden, 1987).

From a social and psychological standpoint, occupationally induced asthma brings with it both positive and negative effects. Because the diagnosis of occupational asthma can isolate the allergen causing the disease, the asthma can be controlled by simply avoiding the substance. For many adults, however, this requires that they change jobs and, perhaps, even occupations. Psychologically, for some individuals, this would be quite difficult. It requires not only the acquisition of new skills but also may pose a financial burden for a period of time while retraining occurs. The individual may feel a sense of loss and depression when forced to give up an occupation that has been enjoyable and/or lucrative.

# Psychological, Behavioral, and Physical Reactions

## Psychological and Behavioral Reactions

A number of psychological reactions to respiratory problems have been observed by clinicians (Agle & Baum, 1977; Creer, 1979; Agle, Baum, Chester, & Wenott, 1973; Kent & Smith, 1977). Depression is a common reaction to a pulmonary disease in that the disease may dramatically affect and extensively limit one's life-style (Kent & Smith, 1977). Patients frequently experience symptoms of depression including frequent sadness, tearfulness, lack of motivation, a sense of worthlessness, suicidal ideation, loss of appetite, and sleep disturbance (Agle & Baum, 1977). The depression felt by pulmonary patients may be thought of as an experience of painful loss. This involves not only loss of one's physical vitality but may also include alteration of one's life-style and loss of livelihood.

In diagnosing depression as a psychological reaction to respiratory disease, one must be aware that changes in mood may also be the result of the pharmacological treatment often applied to this problem, namely, the use of corticosteroid therapy. Corticosteroids, discussed in more detail below, have been shown to induce mood changes. Patients become depressed as well as elated. Symptoms of depression, such as physical fatigue and sleeplessness, may also result from the pulmonary disease in and of itself. Sleep disturbance, a symptom of depression, will occur in pulmonary patients who cough frequently in the middle of the night. One must ascertain if the disturbance in sleep is due to depression, to the physical nature of the pulmonary problems, or to the medication.

Anxiety is another common psychological reaction and is often related to the experience of air hunger, or shortness of breath. The fear that one may not be able to breathe once symptoms of asthma are noticed may lead to anxiety. For some people, anxiety becomes a conditioned response to the symptoms of asthma, and extreme anxiety is elicited when asthma symptoms are noticed. Neff and Petty (1971) suggest that when this occurs, "respiratory panic" may cause a patient to struggle harder and less efficiently for breath. Anxiety may in that manner compound the pulmonary patient's fight to breathe when asthma symptoms are perceived.

Some patients respond to symptoms of respiratory distress with heightened anxiety or panic, whereas others tend to ignore such symptoms (Kinsman, Dirks, & Jones, 1982). The tendencies to react emotionally to stress and to be sensitive to changes in breathing ability appear to be related. Asthmatics who are most able to sense airway obstruction are also most sensitive to emotional arousal under stress (Steiner, Higgs, Fritz, Laszlo, & Harvey, 1987). Asthmatics prone to panic and anxiety may respond anxiously to small changes in breathing ability, and thereby increase their breathing problems. Conversely, those who do not respond anxiously also may not notice early signs of an asthma attack. They are thus at risk for delaying treatment until the attack becomes severe.

## Physical Reactions to Pharmacological Treatments

Early in the 1940s sophisticated methods for the synthesis and isolation of chemical compounds were developed. These compounds could then be used as agents in treating some disease processes. The major pharmacological agents for treatment of bronchial asthma are *corticosteroids*. These drugs resemble compounds produced by the human adrenal gland. Corticosteroids have been found to have an anti-inflammatory effect on lung structures and thus are an effective treatment for some types of pulmonary diseases.

Morris (1977), in a review of the pharmacological treatments of asthma, indicated that there are many studies confirming specific steroid-induced complications. The adverse effects of corticosteroid treatment have been found to be related to the dose and duration of the drug therapy. The most frequent physical complications associated with corticosteroid therapy include obesity, cataracts, and osteoporosis (the breakdown of calcium in the bones). Some patients become bloated, particularly in the facial and stomach areas. Many of the adverse effects of steroid therapy are eliminated when its use is discontinued. Some complications, like osteoporosis and cataracts, will persist despite discontinuance of the medication.

An important complication of steroid usage found in a sizable number of patients is memory difficulties. Specifically, patients on high doses of steroids have been found to be forgetful and inattentive (Schraa & Dirks, 1982). Although such effects are thought to be short lived and dose-dependent, the long-term effects of steroid usage on memory awaits further investigation.

## *Psychotherapeutic Interventions*

The psychotherapeutic treatment approaches to asthma fall into one of two general categories. The first category includes those treatments aimed at decreasing the anxiety-arousing effect of stimuli associated with the asthma attack. Such stimuli are thought to increase anxiety that may stimulate or exacerbate attacks. The second category includes those treatments aimed at decreasing the reinforcing stimuli that serve to maintain asthma symptoms. Associated with the former treatment aim are such techniques as relaxation training and systematic desensitization. The latter approaches are characterized by the use of biofeedback training and by programs designed to decrease the asthma-related behaviors that may be reinforcing the asthma response.

## Changing Reactions to Anxiety-Arousing Stimuli

RELAXATION TRAINING    Anxiety is a common response to symptoms of acute respiratory difficulty. Not surprisingly, anxiety may become associated with specific aspects of respiratory distress and become an aggravating factor of the disorder. That such associations may aggravate or stimulate asthma symptoms has been shown by studies that have induced asthma in patients by exposing them to a stressful situation or by suggesting that certain stimuli will elicit such symptoms (Creer & Kotses, 1983). The purpose of relaxation training is to interrupt the relationship between anxiety and bronchoconstriction by teaching the patient an alternative and competing response to the stimuli that typically elicit anxiety. This competing response is relaxation.

The method of relaxation training that is typically used with respiratory patients is the Jacobsonian relaxation training technique (see Chapter 4). Patients are taught to alternately tense and relax specific muscle groups. To this relaxation technique some have added "guided imagery." Patients are taught to create visual images of a state of comfort and relaxation, such as lying on a beach or sailing on a calm lake (Hock, Rodgers, Reddi, & Kennard, 1978).

Although the efficacy of relaxation training in the treatment of respiratory disorders remains unconfirmed, as a result of many methodologic weaknesses (Erskine-Milliss & Schonell, 1981; Richter & Dahme, 1982), it is likely that relaxation training can improve patients' pulmonary function (Knapp & Wells, 1978; Creer & Kotses, 1983). However, it is unclear whether this positive change is clinically significant (Alexander, 1981). Studies have also not adequately addressed the effect of relaxation training on measures other than pulmonary function (e.g., verbal reports of asthma discomfort, medication usage, hospitalization rates, and attack frequency). The long-range effects of the relaxation technique also await investigation.

SYSTEMATIC DESENSITIZATION    Systematic desensitization, described in detail in Chapter 4, is a technique used to provide the patient with an anxiety-competing response to anxiety generated by respiratory symptoms. Patients are taught the Jacobsonian relaxation procedure. They are then asked to describe the particular thoughts and feelings related to their experience of respiratory distress. From these descriptions emerges a series of statements that characterize the anxiety-provoking aspects of the attack. These statements are then ranked in order of the intensity of anxiety associated with them. In this way a *hierarchy* of anxiety-arousing situations related to acute respiratory distress is constructed.

The initial stage of the systematic desensitization procedure involves training in relaxation and the construction of the anxiety hierarchy. Then the patient is presented with each statement from the hierarchy while in a relaxed state. The patient is instructed to relax away any tension that is aroused when the statements are presented.

Systematic desensitization has generally been found to be superior to relaxation training in increasing pulmonary function measures (Yorkston, McHugh, Brady, Server, & Sergeant, 1974; Moore, 1965). In a review of studies assessing the effectiveness of relaxation training and systematic desensitization, Creer and Kotses (1983) conclude that it not only appears to be superior to relaxation training but it has also been found to affect parameters other than pulmonary function levels, including asthma attack frequency, the use of inhaled asthma treatments, and subjective measures of asthma severity.

# Reinforcing Positive and Punishing Negative Asthma-Related Behaviors

BIOFEEDBACK TRAINING    Biofeedback is a technique that has been used to train patients to monitor their respiratory functions and to change physiological variables related to bronchoconstriction. Feedback with regard to his or her pulmonary condition is provided for the patient. This feedback may take the form of different-colored lights, for example, that correspond to measures of pulmonary function. The patient is instructed to maintain the colored light that reflects increased pulmonary function and is rewarded for doing so (Vachon & Rich, 1976).

Although studies employing careful methodologies have shown biofeedback to be effective in helping asthmatics increase their pulmonary functions (Vachon & Rich, 1976), the long-term therapeutic effects of this expensive technique remain unknown (Richter & Dahme, 1982). Typically, studies have failed to include adequate control groups. One can question whether the effects are due to biofeedback or to other variables such as patient motivation or placebo factors (Creer & Kotses, 1983).

OPERANT CONDITIONING    Operant conditioning techniques have been used to alter the consequences of asthma attacks, and thereby change the frequency of the attacks. Hochstadt, Shepard, and Lulla (1980) decreased the number of hospitalizations of children who tended to overuse the hospital. Hochstadt and his colleagues identified a group of asthmatic children who apparently received secondary gains or reinforcers as a result of being hospitalized for asthma flare-ups. For example, one child gained the company of a friend by being hospitalized at the same time. An operant conditioning program was instituted in which hospitalization was paired with negative reinforcers. The negative reinforcers included such conditions as the removal of comic books, loss of social interactions with other patients, and limited or no use of the television while in the hospital. Results revealed a significant reduction in the amount of time children spent in the hospital when hospitalization no longer resulted in positive consequences.

Renne and Creer (1976) also used operant reinforcement techniques in teaching children to use a breathing device devised to transport medication to their lungs. Particular behaviors relevant to the successful use of the breathing machine, such as eye fixation and diaphragmatic breathing, were taught by reinforcing children for these appropriate behaviors. The training program was found to be effective. Their data suggested that proper use of the machine led to the delivery of more medication to the lungs and, hence, greater effectiveness of the medication and treatment.

# Summary

The respiratory system provides blood with oxygen and removes carbon dioxide from blood. Air travels down the trachea into the bronchi. The bronchi lead into the lungs, divide into progressively smaller air tubes, and eventually end in air sacks called alveoli. Oxygen and carbon dioxide exchange occurs in the alveoli.

Asthma is an intermittent, variable, and reversible airway obstruction. Extrinsic asthma is diagnosed when specific allergens cause asthma attacks. If no specific allergens can be identified, intrinsic asthma is diagnosed. Estimates are that 5% of adults and 7% to 10% of children are afflicted with asthma.

Chronic bronchitis is a chronic inflammation and swelling of the bronchi, leading to excess mucus production and difficult breathing. Emphysema involves a permanent reduction in the number of alveoli and reduced lung elasticity.

Asthma is a physical disease that may be exacerbated by allergic, infectious, or psychological factors. Psychological and behavioral factors may be important in both the triggering of an asthma attack and how an individual copes with the disease. In some asthmatics, the expectation of an imminent asthma attack can increase the probability that an attack will occur. Asthmatics with hyperreactive airways are most likely to be susceptible to asthma attacks induced by emotional arousal.

Asthmatics may underuse or overuse medication. Those who underuse medication may see themselves as unrealistically capable and able to deal with problems in living. They do not respond adequately to symptoms, and thus take too little medication. Asthmatics who overuse medication may feel that they have poor coping ability and little control over symptoms. They become quite anxious with minor breathing problems, and thus may take medication when it is unwarranted.

Personality style, attitude toward asthma, and asthma symptoms may all influence how people respond to the disease. Patients who feel helpless tend to react to breathing problems with anxiety and feel dependent on medical care givers. Counterdependent patients often delay seeking medical attention because they are unrealistically optimistic about their ability to cope with asthma attacks.

Some investigators have argued that parental psychopathology or family interaction patterns reinforce or induce asthma attacks. However, support for the role of parental pathology and family interactions in asthma is equivocal.

Occupationally induced asthma involves asthma attacks stimulated by exposure to substances encountered on the job. Animal dusts and secretions, wood and vegetable dusts, and industrial chemicals and detergents may induce asthma attacks. A job change necessitated by occupationally induced asthma may be quite stressful because of the need to learn new skills and the potential financial loss.

Depression and anxiety may be seen after asthma or another respiratory disease is diagnosed or when symptoms recur. Depression may be associated with a sense of loss, and anxiety is a frequent reaction to shortness of breath. Some patients experience attention and memory difficulties as a result of corticosteroids prescribed to treat asthma. Corticosteroids can also induce obesity, cataracts, and osteoporosis.

Relaxation training and systematic desensitization have been used to improve pulmonary functioning in asthmatics. Systematic desensitization appears superior to relaxation, although there is debate as to whether the improvements in pulmonary functioning with either technique are large enough to be clinically significant. Operant conditioning procedures have been successful in reducing unnecessary hospitalizations and in training asthmatics to use medication delivery devices.

# References

AGLE, D. P., & BAUM, G. L. (1977). Psychological aspects and management. In E. Middleton, Jr., C. Reed, & E. Ellis (Eds.), *Allergy: Principles and practice* (2nd ed.). St. Louis: Mosby.

AGLE, D. P., BAUM, G. L., CHESTER, E. H., & WENDT, M. (1973). Multidiscipline treatment of chronic pulmonary insufficiency. I. Psychological aspects of rehabilitation. *Psychosomatic Medicine, 35,* 41–49.

ALEXANDER, A. B. (1981). Behavioral approaches in the treatment of bronchial asthma. In C. K. Prokop & L. A. Bradley (Eds.), *Medical psychology: Contributions to behavioral medicine* (pp. 373–394). New York: Academic Press.

BLOCK, J. (1969). Parents of schizophrenic, neurotic, and asthmatic and congenitally ill children. *Archives of General Psychiatry, 20,* 659.

BLOCK, J., HARVEY, E., JENNINGS, P. H., & SIMPSON, E. (1966). Clinicians' conceptions of the asthmatogenic mother. *Archives of General Psychiatry, 15,* 610.

BURBECK, T. W. (1979). An empirical investigation of the psychosomatogenic family model. *Journal of Psychosomatic Research, 23,* 327–337.

BYRNE, D. G., & MURRELL, T. G. C. (1977). Self-descriptions of mothers of asthmatic children. *Australian and New Zealand Journal of Psychiatry, 11,* 179.

CHAI, H. (1975). Management of severe chronic perennial asthma in children. *Advances in Asthma and Allergy, 1975,* 1–12.

CREER, T. L. (1979). *Asthma therapy: A behavioral health care system for respiratory disorders.* New York: Springer.

CREER, T. L., CHAI, H., & HOFFMAN, A. (1977). A single application of an aversive stimulus to eliminate chronic cough. *Journal of Behavior Therapy and Experimental Psychiatry, 8,* 107–109.

CREER, T. L., & KOTSES, H. (1983). Asthma: Psychologic aspects and management. In E. Middleton, Jr., C. Reed, & E. Ellis (Eds.), *Allergy: Principles and practice* (2nd ed.). St. Louis: Mosby.

DAVIS, D. J. (1972). NIAID initiatives in allergy research (1972). *The Journal of Allergy and Clinical Immunology, 49,* 323–328.

DAVIS, J. B. (1977). Neurotic illness in the families of children with asthma and wheezy bronchitis: A general practice population study. *Psychological Medicine, 7*, 305–310.

DIRKS, J. F. (1982). Bayesian prediction of psychomaintenance related to rehospitalization in asthma. *Journal of Personality Assessment, 46*, 159–163.

DIRKS, J. F., & KINSMAN, R. A. (1981). Clinical prediction of medical rehospitalization: Psychological assessment with the Battery of Asthma Illness Behavior. *Journal of Personality Assessment, 45*, 608–613.

ERSKINE-MILLISS, J., & SCHONELL, M. (1981). Relaxation therapy in asthma: A critical review. *Psychosomatic Medicine, 43* (4.).

GAUTHIER, Y., FORTIN, C., DRAPEAU, P., BRETON, J., GOSSELIN, J., QUINTAL, L., WEISNAGEL, J., & LAMARRE, A. (1978). Follow-up study of 35 asthmatic preschool children. *Journal of the American Academy of Child Psychiatry, 17*, 679–694.

HOCHSTADT, N., SHEPARD, J., & LULLA, S. H. (1980). Reducing hospitalizations of children with asthma. *Journal of Pediatrics, 97*, 1012–1015.

HOCK, R. A., RODGERS, C. H., REDDI, C., & KENNARD, D. W. (1978). Medicopsychological interventions in male asthmatic children: An evaluation of physiological change. *Psychosomatic Medicine, 40*, 210–215.

HORTON, D. J., SUDA, W. L., KINSMAN, R. A., SOUHRADA, N. J., & SPECTOR, S. L. (1978). Bronchoconstrictive suggestion in asthma: A role for airways hyperreactivity and emotions. *American Review of Respiratory Disease, 117*, 1029–1038.

JUSTESON, D. R., BRAUN, E. W., GARRISON, R. G., & PENDLETON, R. B. (1970). Pharmacological differentiation of allergic and classically conditioned asthma in guinea pigs. *Science, 170*, 864–866.

KENT, D. C., & SMITH, J. K. (1977). Psychological implications of pulmonary disease. *Clinical Notes on Respiratory Disease*, Winter, 3–11.

KINSMAN, R. A., DIRKS, J. F., & DAHLEM, N. W. (1980a). Noncompliance to prescribed-as-needed (PRN) medication use in asthma: Usage patterns and patient characteristics. *Journal of Psychosomatic Research, 24*, 97–107.

KINSMAN, R. A., DIRKS, J. F., & JONES, N. F. (1982). Psychomaintenance of chronic physical illness: Clinical Assessment of Personal Styles Affecting Medical Management. In T. Millon, C. Green, & R. Meagher (Eds.), *Handbook of clinical health psychology*, NY: Plenum.

KINSMAN, R. A., DIRKS, J. F., & JONES, N. F. (1980b). Levels of psychological experience in asthma: General and illness-specific concomitants of panic-fear personality. *Journal of Clinical Psychology, 36*, 552–561.

KNAPP, P. H., MATHE, A. A., & VACHON, L. (1976). Psychosomatic aspects of bronchial asthma. In E. B. Weiss & M. S. Segal (Eds.), *Bronchial asthma: Mechanisms and therapeutics*, pp. 1055–1080. Boston: Little Brown.

KNAPP, T. J., & WELLS, L. A. (1978). Behavior therapy for asthma: A review. *Behavior Research and Therapy, 16*, 103–115.

LIEBMAN, R., MINUCHIN, S., & BAKER, L. (1974). The use of structural family therapy in the treatment of intractable asthma. *American Journal of Psychiatry, 131*, 535–540.

MATTHAY, R. A. (1988). Chronic airway disease. In J. B. Wyngaarden & L. H. Smith (Eds.), *Cecil textbook of internal medicine* (18th ed.), pp. 410–418. Philadelphia: Saunders.

MCFADDEN, E. R., Jr. (1987). Asthma. In E. Braunwald, K. J. Isselbacher, R. G. Petersdorf, J. D. Wilson, J. B. Martin, & A. S. Fauci (Eds.), *Harrison's principles of internal medicine* (11th ed.), pp. 1060–1065. New York: McGraw-Hill.

MCFADDEN, E. R., JR., LUPARELLO, T., LYONS, H. A., & BLEECKER, E. (1969). The mechanism of action of suggestion in the induction of acute asthma attacks. *Psychosomatic Medicine, 31,* 134–143.

MINUCHIN, S., BAKER, L., ROSMAN, B. L., LIEBMAN, R., MILMAN, L., & TODD, T. C. (1975). A conceptual model of psychosomatic illness in children. *Archives of General Psychiatry, 32,* 1031.

MOORE, N. (1965). Behaviour therapy in bronchial asthma: A controlled study. *Journal of Psychosomatic Research, 9,* 257.

MORRIS, H. G. (1977). Pharmacology of corticosteroids in asthma. In E. Middleton, Jr., C. E. Reed, & E. F. Ellis (Eds.), *Allergy: Principles and practice* (2nd ed.). St. Louis: Mosby.

MUMFORD, P. R., REARDON, D., LIBERMAN, R. P., & ALLEN, L. (1976). Behavioral treatment of hysterical coughing and mutism: A case study. *Journal of Consulting and Clinical Psychology, 44,* 1008–1014.

NEFF, T. A., & PETTY, T. L. (1971). Outpatient care for patients with chronic airway obstruction: Emphysema and bronchitis. *Chest* (Supplement), *60,* 11S–17S.

PARKER, G., & LIPSCOMBE, P. (1979). Parental overprotection and asthma. *Journal of Psychosomatic Research, 7,* 305–310.

PESHKIN, M. M. (1960). Management of the institutionalized child with intractable asthma. *Annals of Allergy, 18,* 75–79.

PURCELL, K., BRADY, K., CHAI, H., MUSER, J., MOLK, L., GORDON, N., & MEANS, J. (1969). The effect of asthma in children of experimental separation from the family. *Psychosomatic Medicine, 31,* 144.

REED, C. E., & TOWNELY, R. G. (1978). Asthma: Classification and pathogenesis. In E. Middleton, Jr., C. E. Reed, & E. F. Ellis (Eds.), *Allergy: Principles and practice.* St. Louis: Mosby.

RENNE, C. M., & CREER, T. L. (1976). The effects of training on the use of inhalation therapy equipment by children with asthma. *Journal of Applied Behavior Analysis, 9,* 1–11.

RICHTER, R., & DAHME, B. (1982). Bronchial asthma in adults: There is little evidence for the effectiveness of behavioral therapy and relaxation. *Journal of Psychosomatic Research, 26,* 533–540.

SCHRAA, J. C., & DIRKS, J. F. (1982). The influence of corticosteroids and theophylline on cerebral function. A review. *Chest, 82,* 181–185.

STEINER, H., HIGGS, C. M. B., FRITZ, G. K., LASZLO, G., & HARVEY, J. E. (1987). Defense style and the perception of asthma. *Psychosomatic Medicine, 49,* 35–44.

TURNBULL, J. W. (1962). Asthma conceived as a learned response. *Journal of Psychosomatic Research, 6,* 59–70.

VACHON, L., & RICH, E. S. (1976). Visceral learning in asthma. *Psychosomatic Medicine, 38,* 122–130.

WYNDER, E. L., & HOFFMAN, D. (1979). Tobacco and health. *New England Journal of Medicine, 300,* 894–903.

YORKSTON, H. J., MCHUGH, R. B., BRADY, R., SERBER, M., & SERGEANT, H. G. S. (1974). Verbal desensitization in bronchial asthma. *Journal of Psychosomatic Research, 18,* 371–376.

# Rheumatoid Arthritis

*Rheumatoid arthritis* (RA) is a chronic disease with no known cause or cure that is characterized primarily by inflammation of the joints. The disease affects approximately 1% of the general population and is most common among individuals between the ages of twenty and fifty. The ratio of female to male patients, however, is approximately 3:1 (K. O. Anderson, Bradley, Young, McDaniel, & Wise, 1985; Masi & Medsger, 1979). Although RA is rarely identified as a cause of death, the mortality rate of RA patients has been shown to be as much as three times that of persons of the same gender and age in the general population (D. M. Mitchell et al., 1986; Monson & Hall, 1976; Prior, Symmons, Scott, Brown, & Hawkins, 1984). For example, a prospective study of 112 RA patients in Great Britain revealed that 54% of the patients were dead (35%) or severely disabled (19%) 20 years after beginning treatment (Scott, Symmons, Coulton, & Popert, 1987). Significant causes of death among RA patients include circulatory, respiratory, digestive, and genitourinary disorders as well as infections (Prior et al., 1984).

Treatment of RA patients has traditionally emphasized the medical and physical consequences of the disease process. Relatively little attention was paid to the possibility of altering the psychological and behavioral effects of RA until the late 1970s. However, two factors have interacted with one another to facilitate increased collaboration between rheumatologists and health psychologists in RA treatment and research. First, during the 1960s and 1970s, the focus of psychological research concerning RA began to shift from the role of psychodynamics in the development of RA to the psychological and behavioral consequences of the disease (cf. K. O. Anderson et al., 1985; Moos, 1964). Second, during the early 1980s, a number of influential rheumatologists began to emphasize that the psychological and behavioral outcomes of RA are as important as the physical outcomes (e.g., Fries, 1983; Rogers, Liang, & Partridge, 1982). As a result of the converging interests described above, rheumatologists have encouraged psychologists to devote greater effort to rheumatology research concerning the assessment of the psychosocial consequences of RA as well as the efficacy of medical and nonmedical treatment interventions. Moreover, as psychologists have become increasingly involved in rheumatic disease research, they have begun to develop and test behaviorally oriented interventions that may allow RA patients to better cope with the psychosocial and physical effects of RA.

# Biological and Psychophysiological Components

## Biological Components

It has been suggested that a complicated sequence of biological events leads to the development of RA (Zvaifler, 1983). The sequence is thought to begin when some causative agent (e.g., a virus), that at present is unidentified, enters one or more joints, causing injury to the small blood vessels within the *synovium*, or the lining membrane of the joints (see Figure 12.1). This initial damage to the synovial blood vessels leads to inflammation within the joints and the excessive production of *antibodies* that together with *antigens* form immune complexes. The cause of this unrestrained antibody production is also currently unknown. It has been suggested, however, that due to a lack of suppressor T cells, the interaction between helper T cells and B cells that produces antibodies cannot be "turned off." At this point in the disease process, the affected joints often appear swollen and feel puffy to the touch. The joints also tend to feel warm as a result of increased blood flow caused by the inflammatory process. Furthermore, the inflammatory response causes the

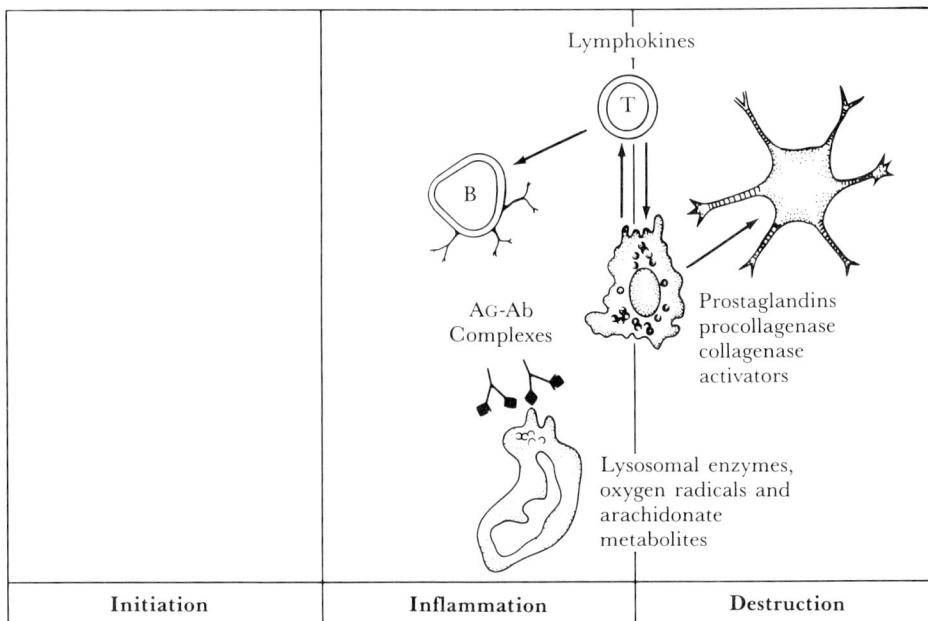

| Initiation | Inflammation | Destruction |

FIGURE 12.1  Schematic depiction of the etiology of RA and of the cellular and immune interactions responsible for joint inflammation and destruction in that condition. Reproduced from "Etiology and Pathogenesis of Rheumatoid Arthritis" by N. J. Zvaifler, 1989, D. J. McCarty (Ed) *Arthritis and Allied Conditions: A Textbook of Rheumatology* (p. 667) Philadelphia: Lea & Febiger.

number of synovial cells to increase, and slender projections of synovial tissues protrude into the joint spaces. Inflammation within the blood vessels of the synovium also occurs. Eventually, as the immune complexes are ingested by phagocytes, several substances, such as lyposomal enzymes, oxygen-free radicals, and metabolites of arachidonic acid, are released within the joint spaces. This process leads to further inflammation and damage to the synovium and connective tissues of the joints.

As the synovium becomes increasingly enlarged, a granulation tissue, termed *pannus*, accumulates within the joints, producing large amounts of fatty acids called *prostaglandins* and other substances that destroy the peripheral cartilage and bone around the joint spaces. Thus, RA appears to be an *autoimmune disease* in that an immune response to some causative agent leads to a sequence of events that results in the destruction rather than the protection of joint tissues.

If the aforementioned disease process continues without remission, deformities or dislocations of the joints eventually occur. The joints most frequently involved are the small joints of the hand and wrist. Other body areas that often are affected include the cervical spine as well as the knees, ankles, and the small joints of the feet, shoulders, and elbows. Several additional complications may result from RA such as damage to peripheral nerves, cardiovascular and lymph systems, as well as eye disease. It should be stressed, however, that the degree to which RA progresses is quite different from one person to another. It is not possible to predict with great accuracy whether an individual will experience only a mild illness involving a few joints or a highly deforming condition involving many joints and other organ systems. Furthermore, the disease is characterized by a series of improvements and exacerbations for most people. Thus, RA patients often report difficulty in coping with the unpredictable nature of the disease (Achterberg-Lawlis, 1982; Wiener, 1977).

Many bacteria and viruses have been suggested as possible causative agents that might initiate the immunologic responses leading to the development of RA. For example, a virus designated as RA-1 was isolated from the synovial tissue of an RA patient. When mice were injected with the RA-1 virus, they developed a set of symptoms that were very much like RA (Simpson et al., 1984). In addition, it is known that the Epstein-Barr virus (EBV) can trigger B cells to proliferate indefinitely and to produce antibodies. Compared to healthy people, RA patients tend to have greater amounts of EBV-related antibodies and appear to be defective in their ability to control EBV infections (Zvaifler, 1989). However, it remains to be determined whether RA-1, EBV, or some other virus or bacteria will be identified with certainty as the causative agent in RA. It may even be possible that RA actually is a set of disease conditions with several different causal agents (Littler, 1980).

Genetic factors also may play a role in the development of RA among the majority of patients. For example, those who report a slow, insidious onset of the disease represent about 80%–85% of the RA population. These people show a much higher incidence of RA among their relatives and tend to experience more severe disease than do those who report an acute onset of the disease (K. O. Anderson et al., 1985; Rimón, 1969). Indeed, Rimón (1969; Rimón, Belmaker, & Ebstein, 1977) has speculated that there may be two types of RA: one with a slow onset that is strongly influenced by genetic factors and one with an acute onset that often is preceded by high levels of psychological stress.

## Psychophysiological Components

A small amount of evidence has been accumulated regarding the psychophysiological responses of people with RA. Several studies using electromyographic (EMG) measurement techniques have consistently demonstrated that RA patients show elevated muscle tension levels at or near affected joints (e.g., Moos & Engel, 1962). In addition, RA patients tend to respond to psychological stressors with extremely large increases in muscle tension levels at affected joints that subside more slowly than normally expected (C. D. Anderson, Stoyva, & Vaughn, 1982). It has been suggested, then, that these psychophysiological responses may be related to the development of RA among the relatively small number of patients who report high levels of psychological stress prior to disease onset (cf. K. O. Anderson et al., 1985; Howath & Hollander, 1949). However, attempts to study the influence of stress on the onset and course of RA have produced both positive and negative results (Koehler, 1985). These investigations generally have required RA patients and age-matched healthy controls to recall from memory the occurrence of stressful life events prior to the onset of patients' disease. Thus, it is quite possible that the positive relationships found between stress and RA have been due to distorted patient recollections. Nevertheless, a recent longitudinal study that did not rely upon patients' memories revealed that stressful life events are associated with negative changes in cellular and humoral immune responses among RA patients (Zautra et al., 1989).

What might link the impact of negative life events on the nervous system with changes in immune system activity? It is known that hyperactivity of the sympathetic nervous system is associated with some painful neurological diseases such as causalgia and reflex sympathetic dystrophy. In fact, applying norepinephrine to the skin of a patient with causalgia greatly increases perceptions of pain (Levine, Collier, Basbaum, Moskowitz, & Helms, 1985). It also is known that a neuropeptide involved in transmission of pain signals through the nervous system, substance P, is released by sensory nerve fibers within joints when they are injured or inflamed. It also stimulates the release of cytokines and substances such as prostaglandins that increase inflammation and destruction of the joint tissues (Lotz, Carson, & Vaughan, 1987; Lotz, Vaughan, & Carson, 1988). Moreover, animal studies have revealed that the joints most severely affected by experimentally-induced arthritis have the highest concentrations of substance P (Levine et al., 1984). Injection of an antirheumatic drug, gold sodium thiomalate, in rats significantly reduces substance P levels (Levine, Moskowitz, & Basbaum, 1988). Finally, persons with paralyzing lesions in the central or peripheral nervous systems who later develop RA do not suffer from inflammation or joint damage in their paralyzed limbs (Levine et al., 1985). Thus, stress or other environmental events that increase sympathetic nervous system activity in RA patients may lead to the release of substance P within joints. Substance P, then, amplifies or prolongs the inflammatory response and stimulates the release of other substances that damage joint tissues. This hypothesis suggests that treatment interventions that reduce substance P release directly or indirectly (e.g., by reducing sympathetic nervous system effects) would be beneficial to RA patients.

# Behavioral, Psychological, and Social Factors

## The Arthritic-Personality Hypothesis

Early psychosomatic theorists believed that there might exist a specific personality type that predisposed individuals to the development of RA. Many descriptive investigations suggested that the arthritic personality was characterized by a wide variety of somewhat contradictory traits such as perfectionism, excessive interest in athletic pursuits, competitiveness, and passivity (Moos, 1964). However, more recent research efforts that have utilized appropriate control groups as well as valid and reliable assessment procedures have failed to find support for the existence of an arthritic personality (e.g., Spergel, Ehrlich, & Glass, 1978). Spergel et al., for example, reported that patients with RA and several other chronic diseases (e.g., multiple sclerosis, gastric ulcers) produced highly similar MMPI profiles (see Figure 12.2). Thus, it appears that any psychological disturbances observed among RA patients may be more likely to represent reactions to the suffering caused by exposure to chronic illness rather than symptoms of an underlying cause.

## The Learned-Helplessness Hypothesis

*Learned helplessness* refers to a phenomenon characterized by emotional, motivational, and cognitive deficits in adaptive coping with stressful situations. The deficits are produced by an individual's perception that no viable solutions are available to eliminate or reduce the source of stress (Garber & Seligman, 1980). Bradley and his colleagues (1984) have suggested that the learned helplessness phenomenon might underlie a portion of the behavioral disabilities shown by RA patients. That is, as noted in the previous section, the psychological problems and functional disabilities of RA patients may be attri-

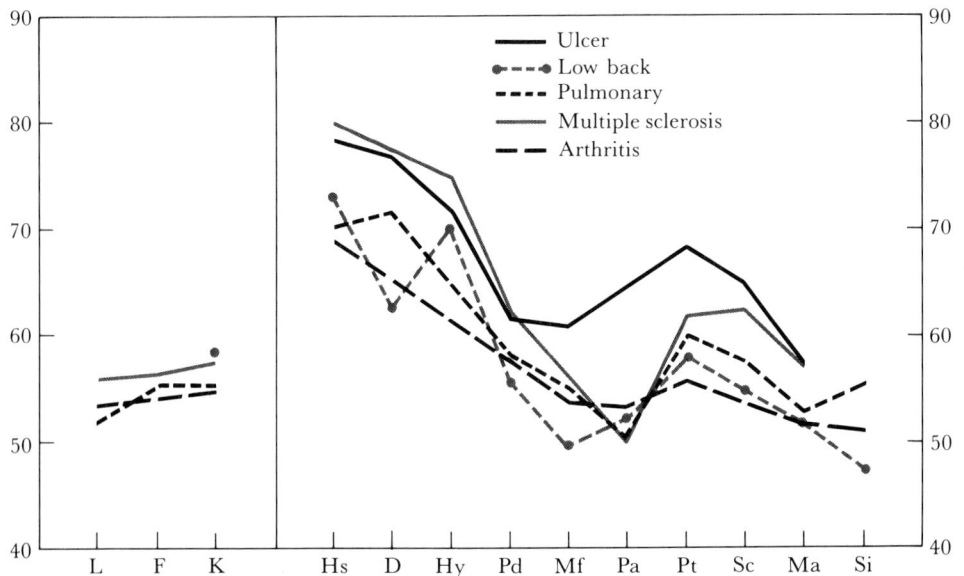

FIGURE 12.2   Mean MMPI scale scores of patients with RA or other chronic disease. Reproduced from "The Rheumatoid Arthritic Personality: A Psychodiagnostic Myth" by P. Spergel, G. E. Ehrlich and D. Glass, 1978 *Psychosomatics, 19*, pp. 79–86.

buted in part to the disease process itself. However, given that the exact cause and cure of RA are unknown and that the course of the disease is chronic and unpredictable, many RA patients may develop the belief that the disease is beyond their effective control (Achterberg-Lawlis, 1982; Bradley et al., 1984; Wiener, 1977). These patients perceive that regardless of the number or nature of the coping responses they employ, they will not be able to reduce the pain, disabilities, or other symptoms associated with RA. The perception of uncontrollability may cause these RA patients to experience anxiety and depression (i.e., emotional deficits) that, in turn, may lead to increased pain and reduced attempts to engage in activities of daily living (i.e., motivational deficits) or to develop new means of coping with their disabilities (i.e, cognitive deficits). These deficits may be particularly profound and resistant to change among some RA patients who may tend to view the consequences of RA to be (a) beyond the effective control of themselves *or* their physicians (given that the disease may be managed but not cured); (b) relatively stable over time (due to the chronicity of the disease); and (c) relatively global in nature (because numerous vocational, recreational, social, and marital-sexual activities may be affected by the disease). In short, many RA patients may suffer excessive disabilities, or disabilities that are greater than would be expected given their actual physical conditions, as a result of the learned-helplessness phenomenon.

A team of rheumatologists and behavioral scientists have developed a questionnaire designed to assess learned helplessness among RA patients and people with other rheumatic diseases. The Arthritis Helplessness Index (AHI) measures the extent to which individuals believe they can control their arthritis symptoms (Nicassio, Wallston, Callahan, Herbert, & Pincus, 1985). Figure 12.3 shows the items that are included in the AHI.

The learned helplessness hypothesis has been tested in several studies using the AHI. It has been shown that perceived lack of control over RA symptoms is associated with low levels of self-esteem (Nicassio et al., 1985), use of maladaptive pain coping strategies and high levels of pain and depression (Nicassio et al., 1985; Stein, Wallston, & Nicassio, 1988; Stein, Wallston, Nicassio, & Castner, 1988), and high levels of impairment in performing daily activities such as walking, dressing, and hygiene (Callahan, Brooks, & Pincus, 1988). Conversely, perceptions of high control over daily RA symptoms is correlated with positive mood among patients with moderate or severe pain and joint stiffness; perceived control is unrelated to mood among patients with only mild RA symptoms (Affleck, Tennen, Pfeiffer, & Fifield, 1987).

Is it desirable for RA patients to believe they can control all aspects of their disease? The answer appears to be "no." Affleck and colleagues (1987) found that patients' perceptions of control over the long-term outcomes of their disease (i.e., will it improve or at least not become worse) were correlated with negative mood in patients with moderately or severely active disease (e.g., those with greatly deformed joints or who required frequent hospitalizations). However, perceived control over disease outcome was associated with positive

Name _____

Date _____

This section is concerned with your attitudes toward how you see yourself dealing with arthritis or a related condition. Each item is a belief with which you may: (1) STRONGLY DISAGREE, (2) DISAGREE, (3) AGREE, or (4) STRONGLY AGREE. Circle the number beside each statement that best describes how you feel about the statement. Since these questions are a measure of your personal beliefs, there are no right or wrong answers.

|  | | Strongly Disagree | Disagree | Agree | Strongly Agree |
|---|---|---|---|---|---|
| 1. | Arthritis is controlling my life. | 1 | 2 | 3 | 4 |
| 2. | Managing my arthritis is largely my own responsibility. | 1 | 2 | 3 | 4 |
| 3. | I can reduce my pain by staying calm and relaxed. | 1 | 2 | 3 | 4 |
| 4. | Too often, my pain just seems to hit me from out of the blue. | 1 | 2 | 3 | 4 |
| 5. | If I do all the right things, I can successfully manage my arthritis. | 1 | 2 | 3 | 4 |
| 6. | I can do a lot of things myself to cope with my arthritis. | 1 | 2 | 3 | 4 |
| 7. | When it comes to managing my arthritis, I feel I can only do what my doctor tells me to do. | 1 | 2 | 3 | 4 |
| 8. | When I manage my personal life well, my arthritis does not flare up as much. | 1 | 2 | 3 | 4 |
| 9. | I have considerable ability to control my pain. | 1 | 2 | 3 | 4 |
| 10. | I would feel helpless if I couldn't rely on other people for help with my arthritis. | 1 | 2 | 3 | 4 |
| 11. | Usually, I can tell when my arthritis will flare up. | 1 | 2 | 3 | 4 |
| 12. | No matter what I do, or how hard I try, I just can't seem to get relief from my pain. | 1 | 2 | 3 | 4 |
| 13. | I am coping effectively with my arthritis. | 1 | 2 | 3 | 4 |
| 14. | It seems as though fate and other factors beyond my control affect my arthritis. | 1 | 2 | 3 | 4 |
| 15. | I want to learn as much as I can about arthritis. | 1 | 2 | 3 | 4 |

FIGURE 12.3   Items included in the Arthritis Helplessness Index. Patients respond a four-point scale ranging from "strongly disagree" to "strongly agree." Adapted from "The Measurement of Helplessness in Rheumatoid Arthritis: The Development of the Arthritis Helpessness Index" by P. M. Nicassio, K. A. Wallston, L. F. Callahan, M. Herbert, and T. Pincus, 1985, *Journal of Rheumatology, 12,* pp. 462–467.

mood among patients with mild disease. Why did the investigators find that perceived control over RA symptoms generally was positive whereas perceived control over disease course generally was negative? The investigators reasoned that perceptions of symptom control could be validated by experience. For instance, even people with high levels of pain could prevent even greater pain by carefully pacing their activities (e.g., scheduling rest periods during the day). However, it would be unrealistic and frustrating for patients to believe that they could lessen their disease activity in the future if they have been hospitalized frequently or if their joints have become highly deformed.

# Self-efficacy

Another psychological factor that is closely associated with perceptions of helplessness or control is *self-efficacy* (Lorig, Chastain, Ung, Shoor, & Holman, 1989). Perceptions of control or helplessness represent a tendency to believe that one generally can or cannot manage RA symptoms. Self-efficacy (SE), however, represents a belief that one can perform relatively specific behaviors or tasks in the future. For example, one may have high SE for using relaxation training to reduce RA pain; one might also have low SE for performing exercises to improve physical function. It is possible to modify perceptions of helplessness with psychological therapy (Linton, Bradley, Jensen, Spangfort, & Sundell, 1989) but it may be easier for SE to be altered by environmental events such as receiving positive feedback following task performance. Thus, SE for exercise performance might increase if learning to integrate exercise within one's daily activities is followed by improvements in strength or other physical functions.

The importance of SE for behaviors that affect health status is that it tends to predict actual health status, given that individuals believe that performing the behavior will lead to improved health and that they value improved health status (Lorig et al., 1989). For example, O'Leary, Shoor, Lorig, and Holman (1988) examined the relationship between changes in patients' perceptions of SE for behaviors intended to decrease pain and physical disability and actual changes in pain and disability as they participated in a psychological treatment program for RA (see Treatment Interventions). Significant correlations were found between increases in SE and reductions in average pain ($r = -.47$) and physical disability ($r = -.49$). Thus, nearly 25% of the variance in pain and disability reductions could be predicted by SE change.

The results just described indicate that RA patients' beliefs about their abilities to *control their symptoms* and to *perform health-related behaviors* are associated with their levels of pain, disability, and mood. These findings have encouraged health psychologists to develop treatment programs for reducing helplessness and improving SE and health status among patients. The success of these psychological treatments for RA will be described later in this chapter. It should be considered, however, that the ultimate value of measuring helplessness and SE may be judged by the degree to which it will allow psychologists and physicians to accurately identify patients who are most likely to benefit from psychological intervention. The predictive utility of helplessness and SE measures has not yet been evaluated by health psychologists.

# Psychological and Behavioral Reactions

## Depression

Many investigators have attempted to assess the emotional reactions associated with RA. The early studies that were designed to test the arthritic personality hypothesis relied on projective tests and other measures of questionable reliability and validity. However, more recent investigations often have used objective standardized tests such as the MMPI and the Beck Depression Inventory (BDI). Polley and colleagues (Polley, Swenson, & Steinhilber, 1970), for example, compared the MMPI profiles produced by a large sample of hospitalized RA patients with those produced by general medical patients and healthy control subjects. It was found that the depression scale scores of the RA patients were significantly higher than those of the other subject groups. Similar findings also have been reported in studies of outpatients with RA (Nalven & O'Brien, 1964).

Some critics have argued, however, that the MMPI Depression Scale and the BDI may be poor measures for use with RA patients because many of their items deal with symptoms that are associated with chronic disease such as RA (e.g., Smythe, 1984). For example, three MMPI Depression Scale items (e.g., "I am about as able to work as I ever was") that reliably discriminate RA patients from healthy age-matched controls also have been found to be significantly associated with high levels of impairment in performing daily activities (Pincus, Callahan, Bradley, Vaughn, & Wolfe, 1986). Similar findings have been reported with the BDI (Peck, Smith, Ward, & Milano, 1989). It has been suggested, then, that great caution be exercised when interpreting the MMPI and BDI scores produced by patients with chronic painful conditions such as RA (Smythe, 1984; Watson, 1982).

Significant levels of depression also have been reported among RA patients in studies that have used relatively uncontaminated measures such as the Center for Epidemiological Studies Depression Scale (CES–D) and the Diagnostic Interview Schedule (Blalock, DeVellis, Brown, & Wallston, 1989; Frank et al., 1988). The prevalence of depressive disorders in these studies has ranged from 30% to 42%. Thus, the consistent finding of high-depression levels among RA patients has not resulted solely from reliance upon a single and possibly contaminated instrument. However, as noted in the discussions of the arthritic personality and the learned-helplessness hypothesis, it is now generally accepted that depression among RA patients represents in most instances a reaction to suffering from a chronic and potentially disabling illness (Spergel et al., 1978).

Some investigators have examined the factors that best predict or are associated with depression among RA patients. These studies have found that pain severity and factors such as age, lack of satisfaction with current lifestyle, and degree of impairment in daily activities are better predictors of depression than measures of disease activity such as number of swollen joints (Frank et al., 1988; Hawley & Wolfe, 1988). The low correlation between disease activity and depression may seem surprising. However, it should be remembered that the potential effects of disease activity upon patients' psychological reactions are modified by patients' strategies for coping with their illnesses (Hawley & Wolfe, 1988). These strategies are discussed in the next section.

## Coping Strategies

Coping is defined as efforts "to manage (i.e., to master, tolerate, reduce, minimize) environmental and internal demands, and conflicts among them, which tax or exceed a person's resources" (Lazarus & Launier, 1978). Numerous methods have been used to assess coping (Burish & Bradley, 1983). However, studies of RA patients' coping strategies primarily have relied on two measures, the Ways of Coping Scale (Folkman & Lazarus, 1980) and the Coping Strategies Questionnaire (Rosenstiel & Keefe, 1983). The former measure was designed to evaluate the strategies people use to cope with a wide variety of situations whereas the latter was developed to assess the strategies people employ to cope with chronic, painful conditions. Despite the differences in these coping measures, it has been found consistently that the use of poor coping strategies such as catastrophizing and escapist fantasies are correlated with high levels of depression on measures such as the CES-D and BDI (Keefe, Brown, Wallston, & Caldwell, 1989; Parker, McRae et al., 1988; Revenson & Felton, 1989). Catastrophizing is defined as anticipating or misinterpreting the outcome of an event to be a catastrophe (e.g., "I don't think this pain will ever let up"). Escapist fantasies represent an attempt to reduce emotional distress by using fantasies (e.g., "I wish I didn't have this disease; I wish a miracle would happen so that I wouldn't have to hurt so badly"). Conversely, psychological adjustment has been found to be associated with strategies such as attempts to derive personal meaning from the illness experience (e.g., "This is an opportunity to discover what is really important in life") and information-seeking (e.g., "I want to learn as much as I can about this illness") (Manne & Zautra, 1989; Revenson & Felton, 1989).

Patients' coping strategies are especially important in modifying the potential effects of disease activity on patients' emotional states. As a result, it is quite common to see RA patients who suffer from severe RA but who maintain relatively positive outlooks and who find ways to enjoy their lives within the limits imposed on them by their disease. Also common are patients who appear to have "given up" on life and who are highly depressed despite suffering from comparatively mild forms of RA. Similar to the findings concerning learned helplessness and self-efficacy, research on depression and coping strategies has encouraged health psychologists to devise treatments for improving the coping repertoires of RA patients. Before describing these treatments, however, additional psychological and behavioral reactions to RA will be described.

## Impairment in Activities of Daily Living

The majority of RA patients experience some difficulty in performing activities of daily living such as walking, dressing and grooming, or gripping objects. These difficulties often are referred to as *functional impairments*. The American Rheumatism Association (ARA) has developed a system of four classes with which the functional impairments of RA patients may be classified. Class 1 patients are considered to have the ability to perform all of their usual activities; only about 15% of RA patients are found in this category. Class 2 patients, or about 40% of the patient population, are moderately impaired but are able to perform their normal activities. Approximately 30% of the population is represented in class 3; these patients are unable to perform most of their occupational or self-care tasks. Finally, class 4 patients, or about 15% of the population, are confined to bed or wheelchair (K. O. Anderson et al., 1985).

The ARA classification system is useful for general assessment of RA patients in the clinic or physician's office but it is not sufficiently sensitive to detect small changes in patient status that might result from therapeutic interventions or from disease progression (Liang & Jette, 1981). Thus, a number of instruments have been developed for the purpose of assessment of functional impairments. These instruments primarily utilize patients' self-reports, although a few include direct observations of patient behavior. The two best constructed and validated self-report instruments probably are the Arthritis Impact Measurement Scales or AIMS (Meenan, Gertman, & Mason, 1980) and the Health Assessment Questionnaire, or HAQ (Fries, Spitz, Kraines, & Holman, 1980). Several representative HAQ items are shown in Figure 12.4.

The importance of careful evaluation of functional impairment has been highlighted in a series of reports by Pincus and his colleagues. These investigators first evaluated the predictive validity of several behavioral and demographic variables with respect to mortality among seventy-five RA patients who were followed over a nine-year period (Pincus et al., 1984). Two major findings emerged from the investigation. First, there were substantial increases in functional impairment across the study period. Of the fifty patients who survived and provided data regarding functional impairment at the initial and final assessments, forty-six reported increased functional impairment. These self-reports were corroborated by large decreases in measures of grip strength and fine motor dexterity (measured by the time required to unbutton five buttons on a standard cloth and then rebutton them). The second important finding was that three measures of functional impairment served as better predictors of mortality than did age. These measures were fine motor dexterity, self-report ratings, and the time required to rise from a

| | Without Difficulty | With Difficulty | With Some Help from Another Person | Unable to Do |
|---|---|---|---|---|
| **1. *Dressing and Grooming*** Are you able to: | | | | |
| a. get your clothes out of the closet and drawers | — | — | — | — |
| b. dress yourself including handling of closures (buttons, zippers, snaps) | — | — | — | — |
| c. shampoo your hair | — | — | — | — |
| **2. *Arising*** Are you able to: | | | | |
| a. stand up from a straight chair without using your arms for support | — | — | — | — |
| **3. *Eating*** Are you able to: | | | | |
| a. cut your meat | — | — | — | — |
| b. lift a full cup or glass to your mouth | — | — | — | — |
| **4. *Walking*** Are you able to: | | | | |
| a. walk outdoors on flat ground | — | — | — | — |
| **5. *Hygiene*** Are you able to: | | | | |
| a. wash and dry your entire body | — | — | — | — |
| b. use the bathtub | — | — | — | — |
| c. turn faucets on and off | — | — | — | — |
| d. get on and off the toilet | — | — | — | — |
| **6. *Reach*** Are you able to: | | | | |
| a. comb your hair | — | — | — | — |
| b. reach and get down a 5 lb. bag of sugar which is above your head | — | — | — | — |
| **7. *Grip*** Are you able to: | | | | |
| a. open push-button car doors | — | — | — | — |
| b. open jars which have been previously opened | — | — | — | — |
| c. use a pen or pencil | — | — | — | — |
| **8. *Activity*** Are you able to: | | | | |
| a. drive a car (For reasons other than arthritis, I do not drive._____ ) | — | — | — | — |
| b. run errands and shop | — | — | — | — |

| | Without Any Difficulty | Somewhat Uncomfortable | Limited to Certain Positions or Very Uncomfortable | Impossible Because of Arthritis |
|---|---|---|---|---|
| **9. *Sex*** Are you able to: | | | | |
| a. have sex (I am not involved in a sexual relationship. _____ ) | — | — | — | — |

FIGURE 12.4 Functional impairment items included in the Health Assessment Questionnaire. Patients respond on a four-point scale ranging from "without difficulty" to "unable to do." Reproduced from "Measurement of Patient Outcome in Arthritis" by J. F. Fries, P. Spitz, R. G. Kraines, and H. R. Holman, 1980, *Arthritis and Rheumatism, 23*, pp. 137–145.

chair, walk twenty-five feet, and sit in a chair at the twenty-five-foot mark. More than 75% of the patients with severe impairment on at least one of the three measures died during the study period. A second analysis of these data showed that the increased risk of mortality associated with functional impairment could not be explained by factors such as gender, disease duration, smoking, effects of other diseases, or type of medical treatment (Pincus, Callahan, & Vaughn, 1987).

Is functional impairment associated with other variables that might explain its predictive relationship with mortality? Psychological factors such as learned helplessness, coping strategies, anxiety, and depression are not highly correlated with impairment when education and other socioeconomic variables are controlled statistically (K. O. Anderson et al., 1988; Hagglund, Haley, Reveille, & Alacón, 1989; Parker et al., 1989). However, low education level does predict functional impairment (Callahan & Pincus, 1988) and mortality (Pincus & Callahan, 1985) independently of the influence of age, gender, and duration of disease. It has been suggested, then, that people who are poorly educated may engage in maladaptive health behaviors such as maintaining poor diets, failing to follow physicians' prescriptions for medication and physical therapy, and poor problem-solving or coping strategies (Pincus, 1988). These negative behaviors, in turn, may lead to relatively rapid declines in functional ability and relatively early death. Regardless of the exact causal sequence, however, the data suggest that even people with moderate levels of functional impairment or low levels of education require increased attention from health care professionals given their increased risk of mortality. It is possible that medical, surgical, or behavioral interventions that reduce functional impairment also may have a secondary, positive effect on patient survival.

Pincus and his colleagues have suggested that it may not be sufficient to only identify specific functional impairments that require intervention (Pincus, Summey, Soraci, Wallston, & Hummon, 1983). They have noted that it may also be worthwhile to assess the degree to which RA patients are satisfied with their functional abilities. Indeed, these investigators recently modified the HAQ in order to allow evaluation of patients' (a) levels of satisfaction with their performance of daily activities; (b) perceptions of change in difficulty of performing daily activities; and (c) need for help in performing these activities. It was found that the best predictors of RA patients' reports of satisfaction in performing daily activities were their reports of present difficulty and change in difficulty of activity performance. However, more than 40% of responses indicating that an activity was performed "with some difficulty" and nearly 20% of responses indicating "with much difficulty" were associated with responses of satisfaction with performance of that activity. In addition, 7% of responses signifying "without any difficulty" were accompanied by "dissatisfied" responses. Thus, reports of patient satisfaction were not always associated with reports of low levels of difficulty in performing activities of daily living. It was concluded that assessment of patient satisfaction was necessary for appropriate choices concerning which activities of daily living among individual patients require professional aid and the degree of aggressiveness with which these interventions should be undertaken. "Treatment goals and programs may be quite different in the 60% of patients responding 'with some difficulty' and indicating dissatisfaction than in the 40% with similar difficulty who express satisfaction" (Pincus et al., 1983, p. 1352).

# Pain

Patients with RA suffer pain from a number of sources. These sources include joint pain due to inflammation or chronic injuries to the joint tissues, depression or anxiety, medication side effects, and the complications that may occur in various organ systems due to RA (Hart, 1974). Physicians and others involved in the treatment of RA have become increasingly aware of the importance of pain in the health status of RA patients. Kazis, Meenan, and Anderson (1983), for example, reported that patients' pain-intensity ratings represented a stronger predictor of their medication usage than either their physical or psychological disabilities. These investigators also found that patients' pain ratings were significant determinants of physicians' and patients' assessments of the patients' general health. Moreover, these pain ratings were significant predictors of subsequent physical disability among the patients.

Although physicians and basic scientists have developed a wide variety of medications for the reduction of RA pain (cf. K. O. Anderson et al., 1985), psychologists did not attempt to produce interventions for the reduction of pain among RA patients until the late 1970s. The pharmacological and psychological interventions for RA pain will be examined later in this chapter. The remainder of this discussion will be devoted to the measurement of RA pain and the factors that best predict patients' pain levels.

RA PAIN MEASUREMENT   It is very difficult to accurately measure patients' pain levels because pain is a subjective and multidimensional experience (Bradley, Prokop, Gentry, Van der Heide, & Prieto, 1981). The term *subjective* as it applies here means that it is impossible for any person to understand precisely the internal pain perceptions of another individual. The description of pain as multidimensional indicates that the pain experience is not composed merely of perceptions of sensory phenomena such as tearing, burning, cutting, or aching. Rather, pain also entails various emotions such as anxiety or depression.

The majority of investigations in the rheumatology literature have used patients' reports of pain intensity on various types of rating scales as measures of the pain experience. It is clear, however, that although pain intensity ratings may allow one to better understand one aspect of patients' subjective experiences, they do not reflect the multidimensional nature of pain and may be affected by numerous extraneous factors. For example, patients who receive a placebo medication during a controlled clinical trial of an anti-inflammatory drug may reduce their pain ratings due to high expectations of pain relief. Given the difficulties associated with pain rating scales, one team of psychologists and rheumatologists has attempted to evaluate RA pain by measuring the frequencies with which RA patients display specific behaviors that are indicative of pain (McDaniel et al., 1986).

Eight potential pain behaviors were identified by the investigators while viewing a large number of ten-minute video tape recordings of RA patients as they performed a standardized sequence of sitting, walking, standing, and reclining maneuvers. Additional observers were then trained to identify the behaviors and to record how frequently they were emitted by the patients during each 10-minute sequence of maneuvers. It was found that seven of the eight behaviors could be reliably recorded by trained observers and were significantly associated with patients' pain intensity ratings and HAQ ratings of functional impairment. Moreover, although the patients' pain intensity ratings were significantly associated with their scores on a measure of depression, their pain behavior frequencies were not correlated with their depression scores. Thus, pain behavior represented a more objective measure than pain intensity ratings. Two subsequent studies demonstrated that the measurement of patients' pain behaviors show good test-retest reliability over periods ranging from 6 to 28 days and that pain behavior is significantly associated with measures of disease activity such as grip strength and number of painful joints (K. O. Anderson et al., 1987a, 1987b). Thus, it now is accepted that the seven behaviors represent reliable, objective, and valid indicators of RA pain. The operational definitions of the pain behaviors are shown in Figure 12.5.

FACTORS ASSOCIATED WITH RA PAIN    Most studies that have examined the determinants of RA pain have focused on rating scale measures of pain. It has been found that disease activity and other variables of medical status do not correlate highly with RA patients' pain ratings (Hagglund et al., 1989; Parker, Frank, Beck, Finan, et al., 1988); however, psychological variables such as depression, anxiety, daily stresses, maladaptive coping strategies (e.g., catastrophization), and helplessness are significantly associated with patients' reports of pain (Brown & Nicassio, 1987; Hagglund et al., 1989; Parker, Frank, Beck, Smarr, et al., 1988; Parker et al., 1989).

Only one study has examined the relationships among pain behavior, medical status, and psychological factors (K. O. Anderson et al., 1988). In contrast to pain ratings, pain behavior was predicted best by measures of disease activity and duration of disease; depression, anxiety, and helplessness were not associated with pain behavior once the medical status factors were controlled statistically.

Why are pain ratings and pain behavior associated with such different variables? It seems that when patients are asked to rate their subjective pain experiences, their responses invariably are influenced by other subjective experiences such as anxiety and depression. When patients are asked to perform physical maneuvers in a relatively neutral situation, such as the videorecording laboratory, the recorded behaviors reflect disease activity,

## Operational Definitions of the Pain Behaviors

| | |
|---|---|
| Guarding | Abnormally stiff, interrupted or rigid movement during shifting or pacing. |
| Bracing | Position in which an almost fully extended limb supports and maintains an abnormal distribution of weight. |
| Grimacing | An obvious facial expression of pain which may include a furrowed brow, narrowed eyes, tightened lips, corners of mouth pulled back, and clenched teeth. |
| Sighing | An obvious exaggerated exhalation of air usually accompanied by a rise and fall of the shoulders. |
| Rigidity | *Excessive* stiffness of an affected joint or body part (with the exception of fingers and toes) that is not directly involved in locomotion. |
| Passive rubbing | Touching, resting, or holding an affected joint or body part on another body part for at least three consecutive seconds. |
| Active rubbing | Massaging an affected joint or body part for at least three consecutive seconds. |

FIGURE 12.5 Operational definitions of the RA pain behaviors identified by McDaniel and her colleagues. Reproduced from "Development of an Observation Method for Assessing Pain Behavior in Rheumatoid Arthritis Patients" by L. K. McDaniel, K. O. Anderson, L. A. Bradley, L. D. Young, R. A. Turner, C. A. Agudelo, and F. J. Keefe, 1986, *Pain, 24,* pp. 165–184.

functional impairment, and subjective pain experience, but they are relatively independent of emotional distress. In contrast, when the same patients are observed by technicians as they are examined by their physicians, patients' pain behaviors are associated with their ratings of anxiety and depression (K. O. Anderson et al., 1989). Therefore, although pain behavior is not equivalent to pain ratings, the *context* in which pain behavior is observed can alter the degree to which that behavior also signifies emotional distress.

## Psychosocial Functioning

Many RA patients experience problems in their vocational activities, self-esteem, and social relationships. A survey of RA patients, for example, revealed that 59% of the sample who had been employed when their disease began eventually had to give up their jobs (Meenan, Yelin, Nevitt, & Epstein, 1981).

Furthermore, the patients who were still working at the time of the survey earned on the average only 50% of their expected income. These findings are particularly striking given that 70% of the patient sample consisted of individuals in ARA functional classes 1 and 2. Indeed, the annual income losses due to RA have been estimated to be 6.5 billion dollars (J. M. Mitchell, Burkhauser, & Pincus, 1988).

The financial hardships of RA patients are compounded by the costs of medical care for the disease. A survey of the medical costs of RA showed that the costs were three times the national average; only 50% of these medical costs were covered by insurance (Meenan, Yelin, Henke, Curtis, & Epstein, 1978). An independent survey of RA patients corroborated these findings (Liang, Larson et al., 1984). The Liang et al. survey revealed that RA patients paid an average of $36.33 each month on medications, assistive devices, and outpatient services. In addition, the patients reported an average of 6.8 days each month during which their activities were limited as a result of arthritis symptoms. Patients who required hospitalization reported an average expenditure of $3,296 in hospital charges and $1,134 in physician fees. The economic costs of RA might best be appreciated by the fact that the per capita lifetime costs of RA have been estimated to be $20,142 in *1977 dollars* (Stone, 1984). These costs are nearly equivalent to those for coronary heart disease ($24,742) and stroke ($29,832).

Several recent studies have examined the impact of RA upon patients' levels of self-esteem and life satisfaction. Earle and colleagues (1979), for example, used several attitude scales in order to assess psychosocial adjustment among RA patients and healthy control individuals. It was found that RA patients produced significantly lower ratings of self-esteem and work satisfaction as well as significantly higher ratings of sense of meaninglessness than did the controls. Other investigators using standardized assessment instruments or structured interviews have reported that substantial numbers of patients (43%–70%) reported difficulties in social interaction, communication, emotional behavior or independent functioning (Deyo, Inui, Leininger, & Overman, 1982; Liang, Rogers et al., 1984).

Given the serious effects of RA on a person's ability to function effectively at home and in the workplace as well as the pain and medical costs produced by the disease, it is not surprising that the families of RA patients often suffer. Two studies have found that approximately 60% of the patients reported experiencing at least one major change in family functioning (Liang, Rogers et al., 1984; Yelin, Feshbach, Meenan, & Epstein, 1979). Studies of the marital status of RA patients have produced conflicting results; some studies have reported greater incidence of divorce among RA patients relative to normal control subjects (e.g., Cobb, Miller, & Wieland, 1959), whereas others have not (e.g., Hellgren, 1969). However, Medsger and Robinson (1972) have found a higher incidence of divorce and a lower rate of remarriage among female RA patients than among a control sample of individuals with other chronic rheumatic diseases.

Despite the inconsistent evidence regarding the effects of RA on the marital status of RA patients, several investigators have reported similar findings regarding the impact of RA on patients' sexual functioning. Each of these investigators found that a majority of patients in their samples reported negative changes in sexual activity or satisfaction since disease onset (Baldursson & Brattström, 1979; Blake, Maisiak, Alarcón, Holley, & Brown, 1987; Elst et al., 1984; Yoshino & Uchida, 1981). These findings are not surprising given that RA produces pain and fatigue, as well as reduced mobility and self-esteem—each of these factors may hinder optimal sexual performance and enjoyment (K. O. Anderson et al., 1985; Ehrlich, 1981). In addition, some arthritis medications, such as methotrexate, appear to cause erectile difficulty among male RA patients (Blake, Maisiak, Koplan, Alarcón, & Brown, 1988).

# Treatment Interventions

## Medical Treatment

The goals of medical treatment are to minimize tissue injury and loss of function, provide appropriate medication for pain relief or suppression of disease activity with few side effects, and repair the tissue damage that cannot be prevented (K. O. Anderson et al., 1985; Hunder & Bunch, 1982). The treatment of RA patients, however, must be tailored to meet the needs of individual patients who differ from one another with regard to response to medication, disease course, life-styles, and occupations, Thus, a team approach to treatment often is employed. Treatment-team members include nurses, physical and occupational therapists, psychologists, psychiatrists, and orthopedic surgeons; these members work under the direction of a rheumatologist, internist, or a family physician. This coordinated team approach has been found to be superior to uncoordinated efforts among physician and non-physician specialists (Ahlmen, Sullivan, & Bjelle, 1988).

In addition to managing the treatment team's efforts, physicians prescribe various types of drugs for RA patients to limit the disease process. A "pyramid approach" is employed in which the initial drugs usually consist of high dosages of aspirin or other nonsteroidal anti-inflammatory drugs (NSAIDs; Weinblatt & Maier, 1989). Many NSAIDs are available but patients' tolerance of the medications' side effects vary greatly, with the most common side effect being gastrointestinal discomfort and ulcerations. Thus, physicians must try various NSAIDs with their patients to determine which drugs work best and with the fewest side effects for each person.

If patients do not tolerate or respond to the NSAIDs, the next step in the treatment pyramid is to prescribe one or more disease-modifying antirheumatic drugs (DMARDs). Most of these medications were developed originally for other diseases. Thus, DMARDs include antimalarial agents such as hydroxychloroquine; drugs that slow the growth of tubercule bacilli, such as gold salts; and a drug originally developed for cancer patients, methotrexate. All of these medications are capable of producing serious side effects such as retinal damage (antimalarials), blood disorders or kidney damage (gold salts), and liver disease (methotrexate). Thus, patients who receive DMARD therapy must be monitored carefully for these potential side effects. Nevertheless, currently there is a great deal of enthusiasm among physicians for methotrexate because it often is effective among patients who do not respond to other DMARDs and most patients can continue to take the drug and benefit from it for years (Weisman, 1989).

Finally, if patients do not tolerate or respond to the DMARDs, corticosteroids or experimental medications may be prescribed. These experimental drugs include sulfasalazine, cyclosporin A, and other agents that modify various aspects of the immune response among RA patients. Moreover, some rheumatologists have demonstrated that adding fish oil to the diets of RA patients as a supplement to NSAIDs and DMARDs produces modest but significant reductions in disease activity (Cleland, French, Betts, Murphy, & Elliott, 1988; Magaro et al., 1988; Sperling et al., 1987).

## Psychological Treatment

Psychologists have begun to play important roles on treatment teams for RA. Indeed, during the 1980s there was a rapid expansion in our knowledge of effective psychological treatments for RA patients. These interventions have been classified as either educational or cognitive-behavioral and biofeedback therapies.

EDUCATIONAL INTERVENTIONS   Many of the early educational interventions for RA patients produced modest results (e.g., Kaye & Hammond, 1978; Parker et al., 1984; Potts & Brandt, 1983). However, the Arthritis Self-Management Program (ASMP), developed by Lorig, Lubeck, Kraines, Seleznick, and Holman (1985) has been shown to be an especially effective intervention. The ASMP consists of 6 two-hour sessions that provide information and home practice instructions on topics such as range of motion and isometric exercise, relaxation techniques, nutrition, and joint protection. Information is also provided regarding the causes of various types of arthritis, appropriate use of medication, and interaction with physicians. The ASMP sessions are highly experiential in nature. Thus, patients are helped to design exercise and relaxation programs tailored to their individual needs as well as to produce behavioral contracts for coping better with their illness. The most recent evaluation of the ASMP involved 543 patients with various types of arthritis (103 with RA) who were monitored for 20 months after completing the intervention (Lorig & Holman, 1989). These patients produced and maintained significant reductions in ratings of pain (20% change) and depression (13% change). Functional impairment was reduced by only 3%; thus, although the ASMP did not improve function, it may have slowed the declines in functional ability that are associated with RA and other forms of arthritis.

The ASMP was developed and tested at the Stanford University Multipurpose Arthritis Center, which is characterized by a relatively well-educated and sophisticated patient population. Thus, a similar education program, termed Bone Up on Arthritis (BUOA) was developed for use with people with reading levels as low as the sixth grade (Goeppinger, Arthur, Baglioni, Brunk, & Brunner, 1989). A home study and a small-group meeting version of the BUOA program was tested with 374 patients, 60 of whom suffered from RA. Relative to control patients who received no treatment, both the home study and small group meeting patients produced significant improvements in arthritis knowledge, self-care behavior (e.g., exercise, joint protection), and perceived helplessness that were maintained 12 months after the intervention was completed. There were no differences in improvement among the RA patients and those with other forms of arthritis. However, similar to the ASMP, the BUOA intervention did not influence functional impairment.

COGNITIVE-BEHAVIORAL AND BIOFEEDBACK THERAPIES   Research regarding learned helplessness and self-efficacy discussed earlier in this chapter has led psychologists to study the effects of cognitive-behavioral and biofeedback treatment interventions with RA patients. The assumption underlying cognitive-behavioral therapy is that patients' expectations and other evaluations of the events that occur in their life influence their emotional and behavioral reactions to those events (Tan, 1982). Therefore, in order to help patients learn that they are not helpless in their efforts to cope with RA, it is necessary to help them believe that they have the skills necessary to control their pain and other forms of disability (K. O. Anderson, Bradley, Young, & McDaniel, 1986). The cognitive-behavioral and biofeedback therapies include components, such as education, coping skill training, and rewards for displays of appropriate coping behavior, that are designed to accomplish these ends.

Three investigations have examined the effects of relaxation training and thermal biofeedback on a small number of RA patients' reports of pain and electromyographic (EMG) recordings of muscle tension levels (Burke, Hickling, Alfonso, & Blanchard, 1985; Denver et al., 1979; K. R. Mitchell, 1986). The thermal biofeedback training was designed to help patients increase skin-temperature levels. All of the studies reported decreased pain ratings among the patients during treatment. However, due to the absence of adequate control procedures, it could not be determined whether the beneficial outcomes were due directly to relaxation and biofeedback training.

Achterberg, McGraw, and Lawlis (1981) have produced one of the best investigations of the use of cognitive-behavioral and biofeedback therapies with RA patients. These researchers assigned the patients to one of two groups. The first group received training in proper body mechanics (e.g., ways to lie down or manipulate objects), relaxation skills, finger-temperature biofeedback with instructions to either increase or decrease skin-temperature levels, and exercises to be performed at home. The other group also received instruction in proper body mechanics and home exercise; however, they received physical therapy rather than the relaxation and biofeedback training provided to the first group of patients. It was found that both patient groups showed significant and positive improvement in several areas such as the time required to walk a fifty-foot course and performance of activities of daily living. Nevertheless, only the patients who received the relaxation and biofeedback training produced significant and positive changes in the number of painful joints, disability-related work changes, pain severity, physical activity, and number of nighttime awakenings due to pain.

Bradley and his colleagues recently reported the results of an investigation similar to that of Achterberg et al. (Bradley et al., 1987). The fifty-three RA patients were assigned to one of three treatment conditions. The first condition required the patients to meet in small groups with family members or close friends for ten sessions of cognitive-behavioral therapy (CBT). This CBT intervention focused on education, relaxation, and coping skills training. In addition, the patients received five sessions of thermal biofeedback training with instructions to warm the joints that were most severely affected. These patients were also provided with small portable biofeedback units for practice at home.

The second condition required patients to meet in small groups with family members or close friends for a 15-session social support program. These patients received the same educational instruction as did the CBT patients; however, they did not receive training in biofeedback, relaxation, or coping methods. Instead, the patients were encouraged to help one another to develop effective methods for coping with the problems associated with RA. The third treatment condition consisted only of standard medical treatment and did not require patients to receive any additional interventions.

The results of the study showed that, relative to social support and the no treatment control conditions, CBT and biofeedback produced significant reductions in pain behavior and disease activity at post-treatment (see Figure 12.6). These effects were not maintained at a one-year follow-up assessment but the CBT and biofeedback patients reported significantly lower levels of pain intensity and depression than the no-treatment patients at the one-year follow-up (Bradley et al., 1988). Similar to the results produced by the ASMP and BUOA programs, CBT and biofeedback did not improve patients' functional abilities.

Results similar to those of the Achterberg et al. (1981) and Bradley et al. (1987) studies have been reported by three other groups of investigators (Applebaum, Blanchard, Hickling, & Alfonso, 1988; O'Leary et al., 1988; Parker, Frank, Beck, Smarr et al., 1988). Two of these investigations have also produced important new findings. Parker and his colleagues found that CBT produced improvements at a 12-month follow-up assessment on pain ratings, the Arthritis Helplessness Index, and the Coping Strategies Questionnaire only among patients who continued to regularly practice their newly-learned

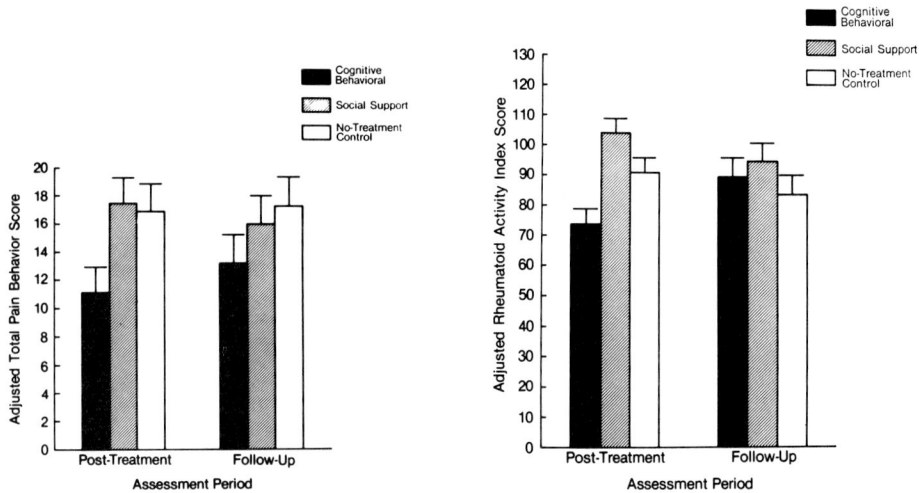

FIGURE 12.6   Mean pain behavior and rheumatoid activity index scores of RA patients. □ = group that received cognitive-behavioral group therapy and biofeedback; ▨ = group that received social support; ■ = no treatment control group. Adapted from "Effects of Psychological Therapy on Pain Behavior of Rheumatoid Arthritis Patients: Treatment Outcome and Six-Month Follow-up" by L. A. Bradley, L. D. Young, K. O. Anderson, R. A. Turner, C. A. Agudelo, L. K. McDaniel, E. J. Pisko, E. L. Semble, and T. M. Morgan, 1987, *Arthritis and Rheumatism, 30,* pp. 1105–114.

relaxation and coping skills during follow-up. O'Leary's research team reported that CBT improved patients' self-efficacy for pain and functional abilities and reduced their pain ratings and number of painful joints. Several measures of immune system activity (e.g., ratio of helper to suppressor T cells) were monitored during the study, but they were not altered by CBT. However, it was found that among the CBT patients, high levels of SE for managing pain were correlated with increases in suppressor T cells and decreases in the ratio of helper to suppressor cells. These correlations do not demonstrate that CBT had a direct effect on immune system activity, but they do indicate that potential influences of CBT on immune responses should be evaluated in future studies.

To summarize, psychological interventions for RA patients have been shown to produce improvements in patients' ratings of pain and depression that persist for 12 to 20 months after treatment. Several studies have also shown that CBT reduces disease activity or painful joints (e.g., Achterberg et al., 1981; Bradley et al., 1987; O'Leary et al., 1988), although these changes have not been maintained during follow-up periods. Nevertheless, it is intriguing to speculate that the relaxation training component of CBT may have reduced sympathetic nervous system activity and release of substance P or other immune responses. Finally, there is some evidence that psychological interventions produce improvements in helplessness, self-efficacy, and coping strategies. It will be important to determine in future studies whether the beneficial effects of the interventions are due in part to changes in these cognitive factors.

Three additional matters should be addressed by future research efforts. First, it is important to determine if patients may be helped to better maintain their improvements in pain behavior and disease activity. Second, attention should be devoted to determining what components of various psychological interventions are truly responsible for patient improvement. And third, it is necessary to determine if psychological treatment may have some direct positive effects on immune system responses.

## Summary

Rheumatoid arthritis is a chronic inflammatory disease with no known cause or cure. It is known, however, that RA is initiated by an immune response to some causative agent that cannot be suppressed. The immune response eventually results in the destruction of joint tissues. The course of the disease is unpredictable and is marked by a series of exacerbations and improvements in symptoms. Patients with RA, therefore, may experience only a mild illness with little joint involvement or a highly deforming condition that may also leave secondary effects on the cardiovascular, digestive, or other organ systems.

The unpredictable course of the disease as well as the dearth of knowledge regarding its etiology and cure may cause many patients to perceive that they are unable to control or reduce the pain or other symptoms associated with RA. This perception of uncontrollability, or helplessness, might account in part for the psychological and behavioral disabilities shown by a large number of RA patients. These disabilities include depression, functional impairment, pain, decreased self-esteem, and negative changes in family functioning. Other psychological factors that are associated with helplessness are low self-efficacy and poor coping strategies such as catastrophization. The increased functional impairment that may be partially attributed to these psychological variables seems to be particularly important given the predictive relationship between functional impairment and mortality in RA patients. Psychologists have played important roles in the development of instruments designed to measure learned helplessness (i.e., the AHI), self-efficacy, coping strategies, and functional impairment (e.g., the HAQ and the AIMS) among RA patients.

The appropriate medical treatment of RA consists of a team effort to manage or minimize patients' pain, tissue damage, and disease activity.

Rheumatologists direct these teams and also use a pyramid approach in pre-scribing medications, ranging from NSAIDs (e.g., aspirin) to DMARDs (e.g., methotrexate) to experimental drugs. Psychologists have developed important roles on treatment teams, particularly in the areas of patient education and cognitive-behavioral therapy. Several investigations (e.g., Bradley et al., 1987; Lorig & Holman, 1989) have produced improvements in pain and depression that have been maintained for 12 to 20 months after treatment.

# References

ACHTERBERG, J., McGRAW, P., & LAWLIS, G. F. (1981). Rheumatoid arthritis: A study of relaxation and temperature biofeedback training as an adjunctive therapy. *Biofeedback and Self-Regulation, 6,* 207–223.

ACHTERBERG-LAWLIS, J. (1982). The psychological dimensions of arthritis. *Journal of Consulting and Clinical Psychology, 50,* 984–992.

AFFLECK, G. A., TENNEN, H., PFEIFFER, C., & FIFIELD, J. (1987). Appraisals of control and predictability in adapting to a chronic disease. *Journal of Personality and Social Psychology, 53,* 273–279.

AHLMEN, M., SULLIVAN, M., & BJELLE, A. (1988). Team versus non-team out-patient care in rheumatoid arthritis: A comprehensive outcome evaluation including an overall health measure. *Arthritis and Rheumatism, 31,* 471–479.

ANDERSON, C. D., STOYVA, J. M., & VAUGHN, L. J. (1982). A test of delayed re-covery following stressful stimulation in four psychosomatic disorders. *Journal of Psychosomatic Research, 26,* 571–580.

ANDERSON, K. O., BRADLEY, L. A., McDANIEL, L. K., YOUNG, L. D., TURNER, R. A., AGUDELO, C. A., GABY, N. S., KEEFE, F. J., PISKO, E. J., SNYDER, R. M., & SEMBLE, E. L. (1987a). The assessment of pain in rheumatoid arthritis: Dis-ease differentiation and temporal stability of a behavioral observation method. *Journal of Rheumatology, 14,* 700–704.

ANDERSON, K. O., BRADLEY, L. A., McDANIEL, L. K., YOUNG, L. D., TURNER, R. A., AGUDELO, C. A., KEEFE, F. J., PISKO, E. J., SNYDER, R. M., & SEMBLE, E. L. (1987b). The assessment of pain in rheumatoid arthritis: Validity of a behavioral observation method. *Arthritis and Rheumatism, 30,* 36–43.

ANDERSON, K. O., BRADLEY, L. A., TURNER, R. A., AGUDELO, C. A., PISKO, E. J., & SALLEY, A. N. (1989). *Observation of pain behavior in rheumatoid arthritis pa-tients during physical examination: Relationship to disease activity and psychological variables.* Manuscript submitted for publication.

ANDERSON, K. O., BRADLEY, L. A., YOUNG, L. D., & McDANIEL, L. K. (1986). Psychological aspects of arthritis. In R. A. Turner & C. Wise (Eds.), *Concise textbook of rheumatology.* New Hyde Park, NY: Medical Examination Publishing.

ANDERSON, K. O., BRADLEY, L. A., YOUNG, L. D., McDANIEL, L. K. & WISE, C. (1985). Rheumatoid arthritis: Review of psychological factors related to etiol-ogy, effects, and treatment. *Psychological Bulletin, 98,* 358–387.

ANDERSON, K. O., KEEFE, F. J., BRADLEY, L. A., McDANIEL, L. K., YOUNG, L. D., TURNER, R. A., AGUDELO, C. A., SEMBLE, E. L., & PISKO, E. J. (1988). Pre-diction of pain behavior and functional status of rheumatoid arthritis patients using medical status and psychological variables. *Pain, 33,* 25–32.

APPLEBAUM, K. A., BLANCHARD, E. B., HICKLING, E. J., & ALFONSO, M. (1988). Cognitive-behavioral treatment of a veteran population with moderate to severe rheumatoid arthritis. *Behavior Therapy, 19,* 489–502.

BALDURSSON, H., & BRATTSTRÖM, H. (1979). Sexual difficulties and total hip replacement in rheumatoid arthritis. *Scandinavian Journal of Rheumatology, 8,* 214–216.

BLAKE, D. J., MAISIAK, R., ALARCÓN, G., HOLLEY, H. L., & BROWN, S. (1987). Sexual quality-of-life of patients with arthritis compared to arthritis-free controls. *Journal of Rheumatology, 14,* 570–576.

BLAKE, D. J., MAISIAK, R., KAPLAN, A., ALARCÓN, G. S., & BROWN, S. (1988). Sexual dysfunction among patients with arthritis. *Clinical Rheumatology, 7,* 50–60.

BLALOCK, S. J., DeVELLIS, R. F., BROWN, G. K., & WALLSTON, K. A. (1989). Validity of the Center for Epidemiological Studies Depression Scale in arthritis populations. *Arthritis and Rheumatism, 32,* 991–997.

BRADLEY, L. A., PROKOP, C. K., GENTRY, W. D., VAN DER HEIDE, L. H., & PRIETO, E. J. (1981). Assessment of chronic pain. In C. K. Prokop & L. A. Bradley (Eds.), *Medical psychology: Contributions to behavioral medicine.* New York: Academic Press.

BRADLEY, L. A., YOUNG, L. D., ANDERSON, K. O., McDANIEL, L. K., TURNER, R. A., & AGUDELO, C. A. (1984). Psychological approaches to the management of arthritis pain. *Social Science and Medicine, 19,* 1353–1360.

BRADLEY, L. A., YOUNG, L. D., ANDERSON, K. O., TURNER, R. A., AGUDELO, C. A., McDANIEL, L. K., PISKO, E. J., SEMBLE, E. L., & MORGAN, T. M. (1987). Effects of psychological therapy on pain behavior of rheumatoid arthritis patients: Treatment outcome and six-month follow-up. *Arthritis and Rheumatism, 30,* 1105–1114.

BRADLEY, L. A., YOUNG, L. D., ANDERSON, K. O., TURNER, R. A., AGUDELO, C. A., McDANIEL, L. K., & SEMBLE, E. L. (1988). Effects of cognitive-behavioral therapy on rheumatoid arthritis pain behavior: One year follow-up. In R. Dubner, G. F. Gebhart, & M. R. Bond (Eds.), *Proceedings of the Vth World Congress on Pain.* Amsterdam, Netherlands: Elsevier.

BROWN, G. K., & NICASSIO, P. M. (1987). Development of a questionnaire for the assessment of active and passive coping strategies in chronic pain patients. *Pain, 31,* 53–64.

BURISH, T. G., & BRADLEY, L. A. (1983). Coping with chronic disease: Definitions and issues. In T. G. Burish & L. A. Bradley (Eds.), *Coping with chronic disease: Research and applications.* New York: Academic Press.

BURKE, E. J., HICKLING, E. J., ALFONSO, M.-P., & BLANCHARD, E. B. (1985). The adjunctive use of biofeedback and relaxation in the treatment of severe rheumatoid arthritis: A preliminary investigation. *Clinical Biofeedback and Health, 8,* 28–36.

CALLAHAN, L. F., BROOKS, R. H., & PINCUS, T. (1988). Further analysis of learned helplessness in rheumatoid arthritis using a "Rheumatology Attitudes Index." *Journal of Rheumatology, 15,* 418–426.

CALLAHAN, L. F., & PINCUS, T. (1988). Formal education as a significant marker of clinical status in rheumatoid arthritis. *Arthritis and Rheumatism, 31,* 1346–1357.

CLELAND, L. G., FRENCH, J. K., BETTS, W. H., MURPHY, G. A., & ELLIOTT, M. J. (1988). Clinical and biochemical effects of dietary fish oil supplements in rheumatoid arthritis. *Journal of Rheumatology, 15,* 1471–1475.

COBB, S., MILLER, M., & WIELAND, M. (1959). On the relationship between divorce and rheumatoid arthritis. *Arthritis and Rheumatism, 2,* 414–418.

DENVER, D. R., LAVEAULT, D., GIRARD, F., LACOURCIERE, Y., LATULIPPE, L., GROVE, R. N., PREVE, M., & DOIRON, N. (1979). Behavioral medicine: Biobehavioral effects of short-term thermal biofeedback and relaxation in rheumatoid arthritis patients. *Biofeedback and Self-Regulation, 4,* 245–246 (Abstract).

DEYO, R. A., INUI, T. S., LEININGER, J., & OVERMAN, S. (1982). Physical and psychosocial function in rheumatoid arthritis: Clinical use of a self-administered health status instrument. *Archives of Internal Medicine, 142,* 879–882.

EARLE, J. R., PERRICONE, P. J., MAULTSBY, D. M., PERRICONE, N., TURNER, R. A., & DAVIS, J. (1979). Psychosocial adjustment of rheumatoid arthritis patients from two alternative treatment settings. *Journal of Rheumatology, 6,* 80–87.

EHRLICH, G. E. (1981). Arthritis and its problems. *Clinics in Rheumatic Disease, 1,* 305–320.

ELST, P, SYBESMA, T., VAN DER STADT, R. J., PRINS, A. P. A., MULLER, W. N., & DEN BUTTER, A. (1984). Sexual problems in rheumatoid arthritis and ankylosing spondylitis. *Arthritis and Rheumatism, 27,* 217–220.

FOLKMAN, S., & LAZARUS, R. S. (1980). An analysis of coping in a middle-aged community sample. *Journal of Health and Social Behavior, 21,* 219–239.

FRANK, R. G., BECK, N. C., PARKER, J. C., KASHANI, J. H., ELLIOTT, T. R., HAUT, A. E., SMITH, E., ATWOOD, C., BROWNLEE-DUFFECK, M., & KAY, D. R. (1988). Depression in rheumatoid arthritis. *Journal of Rheumatology, 15,* 920–925.

FRIES, J. F. (1983). Toward an understanding of patient outcome measurement. *Arthritis and Rheumatism, 26,* 679–704.

FRIES, J. F., SPITZ, P., KRAINES, R. G., & HOLMAN, H. R. (1980). Measurement of patient outcome in arthritis. *Arthritis and Rheumatism, 23,* 137–145.

GARBER, J., & SELIGMAN, M. E. P. (Eds.). (1980). *Human helplessness: Theory and applications.* New York: Academic Press.

GOEPPINGER, J., ARTHUR, M. W., BAGLIONI, A. J., BRUNK, S. E., & BRUNNER, C. M. (1989). A reexamination of the effectiveness of self-care education for persons with arthritis. *Arthritis and Rheumatism, 32,* 706–716.

HAGGLUND, K. J., HALEY, W. E., REVEILLE, J. D., & ALARCÓN, G. S. (1989). Predicting individual differences in pain and functional impairment among patients with rheumatoid arthritis. *Arthritis and Rheumatism, 32,* 851–858.

HART, F. D. (1974). The control of pain in the rheumatic disorders. In F. D. Hart (Ed.), *The treatment of chronic pain.* Philadelphia: Davis.

HAWLEY, D. J., & WOLFE, F. (1988). Anxiety and depression in patients with rheumatoid arthritis: A prospective study of 400 patients. *Journal of Rheumatology, 15,* 932–941.

HELLGREN, L. (1969). Marital status in rheumatoid arthritis. *Acta Rheumatologica Scandinavica, 15,* 271–276.

HOWATH, S. M., & HOLLANDER, J. L. (1949). Intra-articular temperature as a measure of joint reaction. *Journal of Clinical Investigation, 28,* 469–473.

HUNDER, G. G., & BUNCH, T. W. (1982). Treatment of rheumatoid arthritis. *Bulletin on the Rheumatic Diseases, 32,* 1–6.

KAYE, R. L., & HAMMOND, A. H. (1978). Understanding rheumatoid arthritis: Evaluation of a patient education program. *Journal of the American Medical Association, 239,* 2466–2467.

KAZIS, L. E., MEENAN, R. F., & ANDERSON, J. J. (1983). Pain in the rheumatic diseases. *Arthritis and Rheumatism, 26,* 1017–1022.

KEEFE, F. J., BROWN, G. K., WALLSTON, K. A., & CALDWELL, D. S. (1989). Coping with rheumatoid arthritis pain: Catastrophizing as a maladaptive strategy. *Pain, 37,* 51–56.

KOEHLER, T. (1985). Stress and rheumatoid arthritis: A survey of empirical evidence in human and animal studies. *Journal of Psychosomatic Research, 29,* 655–663.

LAZARUS, R. S., & LAUNIER, R. (1978). Stress-related transactions between person and environment. In L. A. Pervin & M. Lewis (Eds.), *Perspectives in interactional psychology.* New York: Plenum.

LEVINE, J. D., CLARK, R., DEVOR, M., HELMS, C., MOSKOWITZ, M. A., & BASBAUM, A. I. (1984). Intraneuronal substance P contributes to the severity of experimental arthritis. *Science, 226,* 547–549.

LEVINE, J. D., COLLIER, D. H., BASBAUM, A. I., MOSKOWITZ, M. A., & HELMS, C. (1985). Hypothesis: The nervous system may contribute to the pathophysiology of rheumatoid arthritis. *Journal of Rheumatology, 12,* 406–411.

LEVINE, J. D., MOSKOWITZ, M. A., & BASBAUM, A. I. (1988). The effect of gold, an antirheumatic therapy, on substance P levels in rat peripheral nerve. *Neuroscience Letters, 87,* 200–202.

LIANG, M. H., & JETTE, A. M. (1981). Measuring functional ability in chronic arthritis: A critical review. *Arthritis and Rheumatism, 24,* 80–86.

LIANG, M. H., LARSON, M., THOMPSON, M., EATON, H., McNAMARA, E., KATZ, R., & TAYLOR, J. (1984). Costs and outcomes in rheumatoid arthritis and osteoarthritis. *Arthritis and Rheumatism, 27,* 522–529.

LIANG, M. H., ROGERS, M., LARSON, M., EATON, H. M., MURAWSKI, B. J., TAYLOR, J. E., SWAFFORD, J., & SCHUR, P. H. (1984). The psychosocial impact of systemic lupus erythematosus and rheumatoid arthritis. *Arthritis and Rheumatism, 27,* 13–19.

LINTON, S. J., BRADLEY, L. A., JENSEN, I., SPANGFORT, E., & SUNDELL, L. (1989). The secondary prevention of low back pain: A controlled study with follow-up. *Pain, 36,* 197–207.

LITTLER, T. R. (1980). Pain in rheumatic conditions: Part 2. In S. Lipton (Ed.), *Persistent pain: Modern methods of treatment.* London: Academic Press.

LORIG, K., CHASTAIN, R. L., UNG, E., SHOOR, S., & HOLMAN, H. (1989). Development and evaluation of a scale to measure perceived self-efficacy in people with arthritis. *Arthritis and Rheumatism, 32,* 37–44.

LORIG, K., & HOLMAN, H. R. (1989). Long-term outcomes of an arthritis self-management study: Effects of reinforcement efforts. *Social Science and Medicine, 29,* 221–224.

LORIG, K., LUBECK, D., KRAINES, R. G., SELEZNICK, M., & HOLMAN, H. R. (1985). Outcomes of self-help education for patients with arthritis. *Arthritis and Rheumatism, 28,* 680–685.

LOTZ, M., CARSON, D. A., & VAUGHAN, J. H. (1987). Substance P activation of rheumatoid synoviocytes: Neural pathway in pathogenesis of arthritis. *Science, 235,* 893–895.

LOTZ, M., VAUGHAN, J. H., & CARSON, D. A. (1988). Effect of neuropeptides on production of inflammatory cytokines by human monocytes. *Science, 241,* 1218–1221.

MAGARO, M., ALTOMONTE, L., ZOLI, A., MIRONE, L., DESOLE, P., DiMARIO, G., LIPPA, S., & OPADEI, A. (1988). Influence of diet with different lipid compositions, on neutrophil chemiluminescence and disease activity in patients with rheumatoid arthritis. *Annals of the Rheumatic Diseases, 47,* 793–796.

MANNE, S. L., & ZAUTRA, A. J. (1989). Spouse criticism and support: Their association with coping and psychological adjustment among women with rheumatoid arthritis. *Journal of Personality and Social Psychology, 56,* 608–617.

MASI, A. T., & MEDSGER, T. A. (1979). Epidemiology of the rheumatic diseases. In D. J. McCarty (Ed.), *Arthritis and allied conditions* (9th ed.). Philadelphia: Lea & Febiger.

McDANIEL, L. K., ANDERSON, K. O., BRADLEY, L. A., YOUNG, L. D., TURNER, R. A., AGUDELO, C. A., & KEEFE, F. J. (1986). Development of an observation method for assessing pain behavior in rheumatoid arthritis patients. *Pain, 24,* 165–184.

MEDSGER, A. R., & ROBINSON, H. (1972). A comparative study of divorce in rheumatoid arthritis and other rheumatic diseases. *Journal of Chronic Diseases, 25,* 269–275.

MEENAN, R. F., GERTMAN, P. M., & MASON, J. H. (1980). Measuring health status in arthritis: The Arthritis Impact Measurement Scales. *Arthritis and Rheumatism, 23,* 146–152.

MEENAN, R. F., YELIN, E. H., HENKE, C. J., CURTIS, D. L., & EPSTEIN, W. V. (1978). The costs of rheumatoid arthritis: A patient-oriented study of chronic disease costs. *Arthritis and Rheumatism, 21,* 827–833.

MEENAN, R. F., YELIN, E. H., NEVITT, M., & EPSTEIN, W. (1981). The impact of chronic disease: A sociomedical profile of rheumatoid arthritis. *Arthritis and Rheumatism, 24,* 544–549.

MITCHELL, D. M., SPITZ, P. W., YOUNG, D. Y., BLOCH, D. A., McSHANE, D. J., & FRIES, J. F. (1986). Survival, prognosis, and causes of death in rheumatoid arthritis. *Arthritis and Rheumatism, 29,* 706–714.

MITCHELL, J. M., BURKHAUSER, R. V., & PINCUS, T. (1988). The importance of age, education, and comorbidity in the substantial earnings losses of individuals with symmetric polyarthritis. *Arthritis and Rheumatism, 31,* 348–357.

MITCHELL, K. R. (1986). Peripheral temperature autoregulation and its effect on the symptoms of rheumatoid arthritis. *Scandinavian Journal of Behavior Therapy, 15,* 55–64.

MONSON, R. R., & HALL, A. P. (1976). Mortality among arthritics. *Journal of Chronic Diseases, 29,* 459–467.

MOOS, R. H. (1964). Personality factors associated with rheumatoid arthritis: A review. *Journal of Chronic Diseases, 17,* 41–55.

MOOS, R. H., & ENGEL, B. T. (1962). Psychophysiological reactions in hypertensive and arthritic patients. *Journal of Psychosomatic Research, 6,* 227–241.

NALVEN, F., & O'BRIEN, J. (1964). On the use of the MMPI with rheumatoid arthritis patients. *Arthritis and Rheumatism, 7,* 18–29.

NICASSIO, P. M., WALLSTON, K. A., CALLAHAN, L. F., HERBERT, M., & PINCUS, T. (1985). The measurement of helplessness in rheumatoid arthritis: The development of the Arthritis Helplessness Index. *Journal of Rheumatology, 12,* 462–467.

O'LEARY, A., SHOOR, S., LORIG, K., & HOLMAN, H. R. (1988). A cognitive-behavioral treatment for rheumatoid arthritis. *Health Psychology, 1,* 527–544.

PARKER, J., FRANK, R., BECK, N., FINAN, M., WALKER, S., HEWETT, J. E., BROSTER, C., SMARR, K., SMITH, E., & KAY, D. (1988). Pain in rheumatoid arthritis: Relationship to demographic, medical, and psychological factors. *Journal of Rheumatology, 15,* 433–437.

PARKER, J., FRANK, R. G., BECK, N. C., SMARR, K. L., BUESCHER, K. L., PHILLIPS, L. R., SMITH, E. I., ANDERSON, S. K., & WALKER, S. E. (1988). Pain management in rheumatoid arthritis: A cognitive-behavioral approach. *Arthritis and Rheumatism, 31,* 593–601.

PARKER, J., MCRAE, C., SMARR, K., BECK, N., FRANK, R., ANDERSON, S., & WALKER, S. (1988). Coping strategies in rheumatoid arthritis. *Journal of Rheumatology, 15,* 1376–1383.

PARKER, J., SINGSEN, B., HEWETT, J., WALKER, S., HAZELWOOD, S., HALL, P., HOLSTEN, D., & RODON, C. (1984). Educating patients with rheumatoid arthritis: A prospective analysis. *Archives of Physical Medicine and Rehabilitation, 65,* 771–774.

PARKER, J., SMARR, K. L., BUESCHER, K. L., PHILLIPS, L. R., FRANK, R. G., BECK, N. C., ANDERSON, S. K., & WALKER, S. E. (1989). Pain control and rational thinking: Implications for rheumatoid arthritis. *Arthritis and Rheumatism, 32,* 984–990.

PECK, J., SMITH, T. W., WARD, J. R., & MILANO, R. (1989). Disability and depression in rheumatoid arthritis: A multi-trait, multi-method investigation. *Arthritis and Rheumatism, 32,* 1100–1106.

PINCUS, T. (1988). Formal education level—A marker for the importance of behavioral variables in the pathogenesis, morbidity, and mortality of most diseases? *Journal of Rheumatology, 15,* 1457–1460.

PINCUS, T., & CALLAHAN, L. F. (1985). Formal education as a marker for increased mortality and morbidity in rheumatoid arthritis. *Journal of Chronic Diseases, 38,* 973–984.

PINCUS, T., CALLAHAN, L. F., BRADLEY, L. A., VAUGHN, W. K., & WOLFE, F. (1986). Elevated MMPI scores for hypochondriasis, depression, and hysteria in patients with rheumatoid arthritis reflect disease rather than psychological status. *Arthritis and Rheumatism, 29,* 1456–1466.

PINCUS, T., CALLAHAN, L. F., SALE, W. G., BROOKS, A. L., PAYNE, L. E., & VAUGHN, W. K. (1984). Severe functional declines, work disability, and increased mortality in seventy-five rheumatoid arthritis patients studied over nine years. *Arthritis and Rheumatism, 27,* 864–872.

PINCUS, T., CALLAHAN, L. F., & VAUGHN, W. K. (1987). Questionnaire, walking time and button test measures of functional capacity as predictive markers for mortality in rheumatoid arthritis. *Journal of Rheumatology, 14,* 240–251.

PINCUS, T., SUMMEY, J. A., SORACI, S. A., WALLSTON, K. A., & HUMMON, N. P. (1983). Assessment of patient satisfaction in activities of daily living using a modified Stanford Health Assessment Questionnaire. *Arthritis and Rheumatism, 26,* 1346–1353.

POLLEY, H. F., SWENSON, W. M., & STEINHILBER, R. M. (1970). Personality characteristics of patients with rheumatoid arthritis. *Psychosomatics, 11,* 45–49.

POTTS, M., & BRANDT, K. D. (1983). Analysis of education-support groups for patients with rheumatoid arthritis. *Patient Counseling and Health Education, 4,* 161–166.

PRIOR, P., SYMMONS, D. P. M., SCOTT, D. L., BROWN, R., & HAWKINS, C. F. (1984). Cause of death in rheumatoid arthritis. *British Journal of Rheumatology, 23,* 92–99.

REVENSON, T. A., & FELTON, B. J. (1989). Disability and coping as predictors of psychological adjustment to rheumatoid arthritis. *Journal of Consulting and Clinical Psychology, 57,* 344–348.

RIMÓN, R. (1969). A psychosomatic approach to rheumatoid arthritis: A clinical study of 100 patients. *Acta Rheumatologica Scandinavica, Supplementum, 13,* 11–154.

RIMÓN, R., BELMAKER, R. H., & EBSTEIN, R. (1977). Psychosomatic aspects of juvenile rheumatoid arthritis. *Scandinavian Journal of Rheumatology, 6,* 1–10.

ROGERS, M. P., LIANG, M. H., & PARTRIDGE, A. J. (1982). Psychological care of adults with rheumatoid arthritis. *Annals of Internal Medicine, 96,* 344–348.

ROSENSTIEL, A. K., & KEEFE, F. J. (1983). The use of coping strategies in chronic low back pain patients: Relationship to patient characteristics and current adjustment. *Pain, 17,* 33–44.

SCOTT, D. L., SYMMONS, D. P. M., COULTON, B. L., & POPERT, A. J. (1987). Long-term outcome of treating rheumatoid arthritis: Results after 20 years. *Lancet, 2,* 1108–1111.

SIMPSON, R. W., McGINTY, L., SIMON, L., SMITH, C., GODZESKI, C. W., & BOYD, R. J. (1984). Association of parvoviruses with rheumatoid arthritis of humans. *Science, 223,* 1425–1428.

SMYTHE, H. A. (1984). Problems with the MMPI [Editorial]. *Journal of Rheumatology, 11,* 417–418.

SPERGEL, P., EHRLICH, G. E., & GLASS, D. (1978). The rheumatoid arthritic personality: A psychodiagnostic myth. *Psychosomatics, 19,* 79–86.

SPERLING, R. I., WEINBLATT, M., ROBIN, J-L., RAVALESE, J., HOOVER, R. L., HOUSE, F., COBLYN, J. S., FRASER, P. A., SPUR, B. W., ROBINSON, D. R., LEWIS, R. A., & AUSTEN, K. F. (1987). Effects of dietary supplementation with marine fish oil on leukocyte lipid mediator generation and function in rheumatoid arthritis. *Arthritis and Rheumatism, 30,* 988–997.

STEIN, M. J., WALLSTON, K. A., & NICASSIO, P. M. (1988). Factor structure of the Arthritis Helplessness Index. *Journal of Rheumatology, 15,* 427–432.

STEIN, M. J., WALLSTON, K. A., NICASSIO, P. M., & CASTNER, N. M. (1988). Correlates of a clinical classification schema for the arthritis helplessness subscale. *Arthritis and Rheumatism, 31,* 876–881.

STONE, C. E. (1984). The lifetime economic costs of rheumatoid arthritis. *Journal of Rheumatology, 11,* 819–827.

TAN, S-Y. (1982). Cognitive and cognitive-behavioral methods for pain control: A selective review. *Pain, 12,* 201–228.

WATSON, D. (1982). Neurotic tendencies among chronic pain patients: An MMPI item analysis. *Pain, 14,* 365–385.

WEINBLATT, M. E., & MAIER, A. L. (1989). Treatment of rheumatoid arthritis. *Arthritis Care and Research, 2,* S23–S32.

WEISMAN, M. H. (1989). Natural history and treatment decisions in rheumatoid arthritis revisited. *Arthritis Care and Research, 2,* S75–S83.

WIENER, C. (1977). Living with rheumatoid arthritis. In S. T. Fayerhaugh & A. Strauss (Eds.), *Politics of pain management: Staff-patient interaction.* Menlo Park, CA: Addison-Wesley.

YELIN, E., FESHBACH, D. M., MEENAN, R. F., & EPSTEIN, W. V. (1979). Social problems, services and policy for persons with chronic disease: The case of rheumatoid arthritis. *Social Science and Medicine, 13,* 13–20.

YOSHINO, S., & UCHIDA, S. (1981). Sexual problems of women with rheumatoid arthritis. *Archives of Physical Medicine and Rehabilitation, 62,* 122–123.

ZAUTRA, A. J., OKUN, M. A., ROBINSON, S. E., LEE, D., ROTH, S. H., & EMMANUAL J. (1989). Life stress and lymphocyte alterations among patients with rheumatoid arthritis. *Health Psychology, 8,* 1–14.

ZVAIFLER, N. J. (1983). Pathogenesis of the joint disease in rheumatoid arthritis. *American Journal of Medicine, 75* (6A), 3–8.

ZVAIFLER, N. J. (1989). Etiology and pathogenesis of rheumatoid arthritis. In D. J. McCarty (Ed.), *Arthritis and allied conditions: A textbook of rheumatology* (11th ed.). Philadelphia: Lea & Febiger.

# Gastrointestinal Disorders

This chapter will examine several gastrointestinal disorders that appear to be related both to psychological and somatic factors. Two of these disorders, *irritable bowel syndrome* and *noncardiac chest pain* are often termed *functional gastrointestinal disorders*. It has been estimated that 40%–70% of all consultations to gastroenterologists involve functional disorders (Switz, 1976; Whitehead & Bosmajian, 1982). Functional gastrointestinal disorders may also be present in a large number of people who do not seek health care for their symptoms. For example, Thompson and Heaton (1980) reported that one-fifth of a sample drawn from a general population in England had experienced abdominal pain more than six times during the previous year. This pain appeared to be related to symptoms of irritable bowel syndrome in nearly 14% of the sample. Similar findings have also been reported by American investigators (Drossman, Sandler, McKee, & Lovitz, 1982).

It should be noted that the term *functional gastrointestinal disorder* does not imply that the associated symptoms are due solely to psychological causes or that they symbolize unconscious psychological events. Rather, gastroenterologists use the term *functional* to describe any gastrointestinal disorder for which a specific, underlying disease cannot be identified. For example, a patient with recurrent abdominal pain and diarrhea may be classified after physical examination as suffering from irritable bowel syndrome, a functional disorder. Further laboratory investigation may reveal a parasitic cause for the symptoms. The patient's symptoms, then, no longer would be regarded as functional. However, it is well known that the gastrointestinal tract is highly responsive to environmental events and emotional experiences (Latimer, 1983a). It is not surprising, therefore, that emotional or other psychological disturbances are often associated with gastrointestinal disturbances that are functional in nature as well as those that are associated with disease processes (e.g., achalasia or the loss of smooth muscle ganglion cells accompanied by an absence of peristaltic activity in the lower esophagus).

There currently exists a great need for psychological services to be delivered to patients with gastrointestinal disorders. A few physicians have attempted to provide guidelines that gastroenterologists may follow in treating the psychological problems of their patients (e.g., Almy, 1977; Lennard-Jones, 1983). However, most gastroenterologists have little psychological training and feel that their efforts to effectively treat patients with functional disorders are inadequate (Whitehead & Bosmajian, 1982).

Given the complexity of the gastrointestinal system (see Chapter 3), the disorders that are reviewed in this chapter have been organized according to the anatomical divisions with which they are associated—that is, esophagus, stomach and small intestine, colon and rectum.

## The Esophagus

The *esophagus* is a narrow tube that is guarded by an *upper* and a *lower* sphincter. These sphincters must maintain high pressures relative to the pharynx and the stomach to prevent abnormal movements of air or food into the esophagus (see Figure 13.1). When a swallow is initiated, food is pushed by contraction of the tongue and pharyngeal muscles through a relaxed upper esophageal sphincter (UES) into the esophagus. The food is then transported by a peristaltic contraction wave downward through the esophagus. The lower esophageal sphincter (LES) relaxes, and the food is delivered into the stomach (cf. Stacher, 1983). This peristaltic contractile activity of the esophagus appears to be controlled by a "swallowing center" located in the reticular formation of the brain and the brainstem (Jean, 1972).

Some individuals suffer from disturbances of esophageal peristalsis or abnormalities of sphincter function, which can produce unpleasant symptoms such as difficulty in swallowing, heartburn, or food regurgitation (Castell, 1980). Gastroesophageal reflux is the most common of these esophageal disorders (Cohen & Snape, 1977).

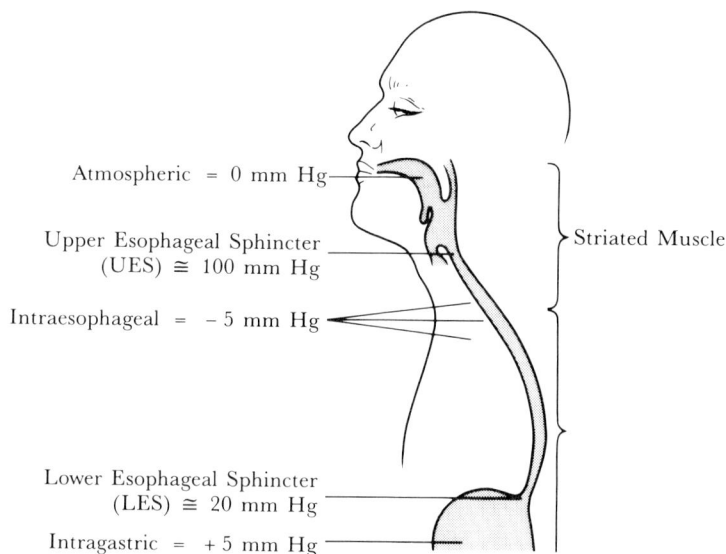

Atmospheric = 0 mm Hg

Upper Esophageal Sphincter
(UES) ≅ 100 mm Hg

Striated Muscle

Intraesophageal = – 5 mm Hg

Lower Esophageal Sphincter
(LES) ≅ 20 mm Hg

Intragastric = + 5 mm Hg

FIGURE 13.1 Schematic drawing of the esophagus showing the pressure relationships in the pharynx, esophagus, esophageal sphincters, and the stomach. Reprinted from *Esophageal Motility Testing* (p. 21) by D. O. Castell, J. E. Richter, and C. B. Dalton, 1987, New York: Elsevier.

## Gastroesophageal Reflux

BIOLOGICAL AND PSYCHOPHYSIOLOGICAL COMPONENTS Gastroesophageal reflux (GER) is characterized by the passage of acidic gastric juices upward through the LES into the esophagus. As the esophagus is repeatedly exposed to gastric acid, it becomes inflamed, and the burning pain of heartburn is usually experienced.

The physiology of GER is not completely understood. It is known, however, that persons with GER show weaker LES resting pressures than do normal individuals. In addition, unlike so-called normals, GER patients do not show increased pressures within the LES in response to elevations in intragastric pressures (e.g., due to bending or leg raising). Furthermore, these patients tend to produce lower levels of the hormone gastrin in response to meals than do normals (cf. Cohen & Snape, 1977; Schuster, 1983). It appears, then, that GER is associated both with abnormal LES functioning and abnormal hormonal response of the stomach.

If individuals experience GER over extended periods of time, they are likely to report *dysphagia*, or the sensation that their food is hindered in its normal passage from the mouth to the stomach. These individuals frequently report that solid food "sticks" or "gets caught" in the esophagus. The dysphagia tends to become progressively severe and may be associated with the development of *strictures*, or partial obstructions, within the esophagus due to ulceration or scarring of the esophageal tissue (this condition is called *reflux esophagitis*). When food becomes impacted within the esophagus, transport to the stomach may be aided by repeated swallowing, raising the arms over the head, or quickly throwing the shoulders backward. Some patients, however, report that they must force regurgitation for relief (e.g., placing a finger against the back of the throat to induce vomiting).

BEHAVIORAL, PSYCHOLOGICAL, AND SOCIAL FACTORS   Several behavioral, psychological, and social factors have been associated with decreased LES competence and GER symptoms. For example, it has been established that tobacco smoking and alcohol consumption decreases LES pressure (Cohen & Snape, 1977; Dennish & Castell, 1971). The ingestion of substances such as chocolate (Wright & Castell, 1975), coffee (Cohen, 1980), citrus juice (Price, Smithson, & Castell, 1978), as well as many fried and spicy foods (Nebel, Fornes & Castell, 1976) have also been shown to elicit GER symptoms. Pregnancy is another factor that is closely associated with reflux. Indeed, 15% of pregnant women suffer heartburn on a daily basis. The relationship between pregnancy and GER is probably mediated both by increased abdominal pressure as well as by the reductions in LES pressure produced by estrogens and progesterone (Schuster, 1983). Finally, the clinical experience of many gastroenterologists suggests that psychological stress may increase the likelihood of GER among persons with compromised LES functioning.

Several of the factors noted above may actually interact with one another. Consider, for example, an individual who suffers from chronic anxiety. This person may be especially likely to perceive environmental events as threatening and possess a relatively sparse repertoire of strategies for coping with anxiety. This individual, then, is prone to experience a large number of situations as stressful (Burish, 1981). An examination of this individual's coping strategies may reveal several behaviors that are correlated with GER symptoms. These behaviors might include smoking and drinking alcohol or coffee in a variety of situations. Furthermore, similar to many anxious persons, this individual may involuntarily swallow air under periods of high stress. Swallowed air in the esophagus tends to elicit a peristaltic wave for the purpose of clearing the esophagus; however, this wave also may relax the LES and further increase the probability of gastric acid reflux. In addition, some anxious persons will perceive increases in their reflux symptoms during stressful events even without corresponding increases in gastric acid within the esophagus (Pulliam et al., 1989).

Let us suppose that the chronically anxious individual eventually begins to experience chest pain and is diagnosed as suffering from GER. A well-intentioned physician may prescribe an antispasmodic drug in order to reduce gastric acid production. Unfortunately, this medical treatment might actually have a paradoxical effect in that the antispasmodic activity of the drug may also reduce the resting pressure of the LES. The anxious patient, therefore, may have to endure increased pain until he or she refuses to adhere to the treatment regimen or the physician changes the treatment.

PSYCHOLOGICAL AND BEHAVIORAL REACTIONS    There have been no systematic studies of the psychological reactions of GER patients. However, gastroenterologists tend to describe these patients as anxious. The patients are often concerned that the intensity of their symptoms may suddenly increase in social situations and cause them embarrassment. A small number of patients show unusual concern that their chest pain or dysphagia is caused by heart disease despite careful diagnostic evaluation and reassurance from their physicians. It is important to note that, given the absence of psychological studies, it is impossible to determine what percentage of patients may experience anxiety disorders prior to the manifestation of GER versus what percentage show high anxiety levels as a response to reflux symptoms.

TREATMENT INTERVENTIONS    The medical treatment of GER usually consists of frequent doses of antacids or histamine $H_2$ blocking drugs (e.g., cimetidine, ranitidine, famotidine). A new drug, omeprazole, has recently been made available in the United States; this drug reduces acid secretion far more effectively than the aforementioned pharmacologic agents. In addition, several behavioral changes are often recommended by physicians. These include elevating the head of the bed 6 inches to decrease reflux episodes during sleep; reducing the amount of food consumed during meals; and abstaining from eating for two or three hours before going to bed (Young, Richter, Bradley, & Anderson, 1987). These treatments are useful for symptom reduction but they do not affect the functioning of the LES. However, various drugs such as *urecholine* and *metoclopramide* have been administered to patients because they tend to increase the resting pressure of the LES.

There has been only one study of the use of a behavioral therapy for the treatment of GER. Schuster, Nikoomanesh, and Wells (1973) described the effectiveness of a biofeedback procedure for increasing resting LES pressures. The subjects in this study consisted of three healthy individuals and six patients with GER. The investigators passed a small polyethylene tube into the esophagus and stomach of each subject. The tube, called an *esophageal motility catheter*, was lined with pressure sensors, located at 5-cm intervals. It was positioned in such a manner that changes in LES pressure would be transmitted to amplifiers, registered on a meter that subjects could observe, and printed out on a strip chart recorder. This method of measuring changes in esophageal pressure is termed *esophageal manometry*.

Each control subject and patient was instructed to look at the meter and to make the needle on the meter go up (i.e., increase LES pressure) by any method available except changing respiration or contracting abdominal or other voluntary muscles. It was found that all of the subjects and patients learned to double their resting LES pressures for at least brief time periods after approximately ninety minutes of practice. These increases in resting pressures were accomplished without changes in intragastric or intra-esophageal pressures. Figure 13.2 shows a graph depicting one subject's changes in peak LES, esophagus, and stomach pressures across seven trials in a single biofeedback training session.

Schuster and his colleagues (1973) did not report any data regarding the effects of the biofeedback training procedure on the patients' clinical symptoms. However, ten years following the publication of the original report, Schuster (1983) stated that seven of ten patients who had been administered biofeedback training had learned to double their LES pressures. Moreover, two of the patients with severe GER who had not responded to conventional medical treatment had shown "excellent" (Schuster, 1983; p. 41) symptom reductions.

There is a clear need for systematic study of the effectiveness of the biofeedback training procedure developed by Schuster and his colleagues. It may be, however, that controlled investigations will reveal that the procedure is clinically effective for only a subset of patients with mildly impaired LES function. For example, Schuster (1983) has stated that resting LES pressures of normal individuals tend to vary between 14 and 16 mm Hg. Reflux esophagitis patients with resting LES pressures of 6–9 mm Hg might be expected to benefit from biofeedback training; those with resting LES pressures of 2–5 mm Hg would probably not show positive clinical responses even after learning to double their resting pressures (cf. Schuster, 1983).

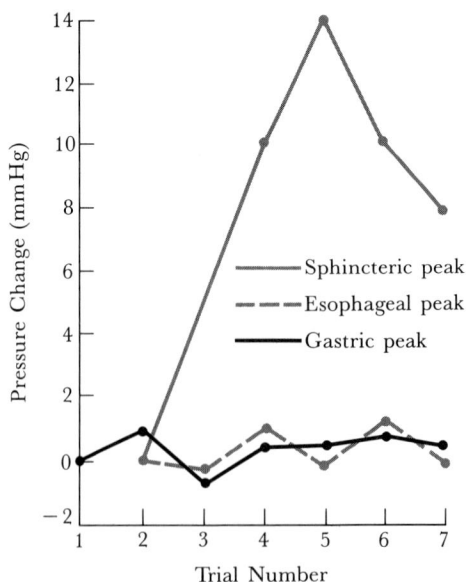

FIGURE 13.2   Graphic depiction of pressure changes in the lower esophageal sphincter, esophagus, and stomach over seven trials of a single training session for one subject. Reprinted from "Disorders of the Esophagus: Applications of Psychophysiological Methods to Treatment" by M. M. Schuster, 1983, R. Hölzl and W. E. Whitehead (Eds.) *Psychophysiology of the Gastrointestinal Tract: Experimental and Clinical Applications* (p. 42) New York: Plenum.

# Noncardiac Chest Pain

BIOLOGICAL AND PSYCHOPHYSIOLOGICAL COMPONENTS   As many as 30% of patients who seek medical care for chest pain and other symptoms of heart disease are found to have normal coronary arteries and heart function (Richter, Bradley, & Castell, 1989). Nevertheless, despite the reassuring finding that their symptoms are not due to coronary artery disease, a large number of these persons do not return to work, continue to live restricted lifestyles, and maintain the belief that they may suffer from heart disease (Lantinga et al., 1988; Ockene, Shay, Alpert, Weiner, & Dalen, 1980; Wielgosz & Earp, 1986). Moreover, it is estimated that medical costs of noncardiac chest pain, or NCCP (e.g., medication, emergency room visits), exceed 315 million dollars per year (Richter et al., 1989).

A recent review has found that esophageal disorders are involved in the etiology of NCCP in 18% to 58% of patients (Richter et al., 1989). Approximately one-half of the patients with esophageal disorders suffer from GER. The other half of the patients experience a variety of esophageal motility disorders. The most common of these is the *nutcracker esophagus* or peristaltic contractions of extremely high amplitudes ($\geq$180 mm Hg). Other motility problems include *achalasia*, *diffuse esophageal spasm* (multiple simultaneous contractions in the lower esophagus), *hypertensive lower esophageal sphincter*, and a broad spectrum of abnormalities classified as *nonspecific esophageal motility disorders*. However, approximately one-half of NCCP patients have both normal coronary arteries and normal esophageal functioning.

The confusion regarding the etiology of NCCP has led cardiologists to suggest that some of these patients may have abnormalities in coronary blood vessels that are too small to be detected by current imaging techniques (Cannon et al., 1985). However, most of the patients who have been identified as suffering from "microvascular angina" also have been shown to have esophageal motility disorders, especially the nutcracker esophagus (Ducrotte et al., 1985). For these patients, then, it is difficult to differentiate between possible coronary and esophageal causes of chest pain.

BEHAVIORAL, PSYCHOLOGICAL, AND SOCIAL FACTORS   Little is known regarding the behavioral, psychological, and social factors that underlie the development of NCCP. This is rather surprising given that it was first observed in 1883 that "psychic upset" elicited esophageal contractions (Kronecker & Meltzer, 1883). During the first half of the twentieth century, several observational studies of patients using X-ray technology also produced evidence that psychological stress may produce esophageal spasm (Faulkner, 1940; Jacobson, 1927; Wolf & Almy, 1949).

More recently, several investigators have attempted to systematically expose people to various types of psychological stressors under controlled conditions in order to examine the relationship between stress and esophageal functioning. Anderson and colleagues (Anderson, Dalton, Bradley, & Richter, 1989; Young et al., 1987) exposed normal individuals and NCCP patients to two stressors: uncontrollable bursts of white noise of 100-db intensity that were delivered via headphones and unsolvable cognitive tasks. Esophageal manometry was performed during each of the ten-minute stress exposure periods as well as during the ten-minute baselines that preceded exposure to each stressor. Of particular interest to the experimenters were the amplitudes of the subjects' peristaltic contractions as they periodically swallowed 5 ml of water during the baseline and stress exposure periods. It was found that, relative to baseline conditions, each stressor produced significant increases in the amplitudes of subjects' peristaltic contractions and measures of their anxiety levels. Moreover, after controlling for initial differences, it was found that NCCP patients with the nutcracker esophagus had significantly greater increases in contraction amplitudes during stress than the healthy controls. Similar findings have been reported by Stacher and his colleagues using normal Austrian subjects (Stacher, Schmierer, & Landgraf, 1979; Stacher, Steinringer, Blau, & Landgraf, 1979).

The results just described provide evidence that stress-related increases in the amplitudes of peristaltic contractions may be found among normal individuals and NCCP patients, especially those with the nutcracker esophagus. It may be, then, that stressors encountered in the natural environment may induce exceptionally high amplitude contractions and pain among persons who are predisposed to excessive esophageal responsivity. However, when patients' esophageal pressures have been monitored for 24 hours in their environments (rather than the laboratory), it has been found that abnormal contractions occur as frequently *after* as they do before the onset of chest pain (Peters et al., 1988). Thus, abnormal contractile activity may be a byproduct, rather than a cause, of chest pain. If so, NCCP would resemble other stress-related, chronic pain syndromes (e.g., tension headache) in which increases in the psychophysiologic markers for the syndromes (e.g., electromyographic activity) are not consistently associated with the experience of pain (Burish, 1981).

In addition to studying the effects of stress on NCCP patients, some investigators have begun to examine patients' responses to distention pressure within the esophagus. Richter and his coworkers (Barish, Castell, & Richter, 1986; Richter, Barish, & Castell, 1986) have modified the esophageal manometry probe by placing a soft, inflatable balloon 10 cm from its lower end. This balloon may be safely inflated within the esophagus with volumes of air ranging from 1 to 20 ml in order to produce perceptions of pain similar to patients' spontaneous pain experiences. It has been found consistently that NCCP patients begin to perceive pain (i.e., reach *pain threshold*) at significantly lower air volumes than healthy control individuals. It may be, then, that NCCP patients are especially sensitive to distentions of the esophagus that are nonpainful to healthy people. However, further research is needed to determine to what extent the low pain threshold levels of NCCP patients may be caused by biological factors affecting the esophagus, disordered central nervous system processing of esophageal stimulation, or psychological reactions that may influence patients' verbal reports of pain. Several of these psychological reactions are described in the section that follows.

BEHAVIORAL AND PSYCHOLOGICAL REACTIONS  For many years, the clinical experience of gastroenterologists and psychologists has been that NCCP patients are frequently anxious and depressed (Richter et al., 1986). These clinical impressions have led several groups of investigators to examine the psychological attributes of these patients. The similarities of the findings produced by these investigators are quite striking given that they were performed using different psychological measurement procedures or subject samples of different nationalities.

Clouse and Lustman (1983) administered a structured interview to fifty patients who were referred for esophageal manometry. The structured interview was the Diagnostic Interview Schedule—Version Three (DIS-III; Robins, Helzer, Croughan, & Ratcliff, 1981), which was designed to provide a reliable and valid identification of fifteen psychiatric disorders based on the criteria outlined in the *Diagnostic and Statistical Manual* (DSM-III) of the American Psychiatric Association (Committee on Nomenclature and Statistics, 1980). The DIS-III interviews were administered by professionals who had no knowledge of the patients' manometric evaluations. It was found that four of the thirteen patients (31%) with normal esophageal motility patterns fulfilled the DSM-III criteria for a psychiatric diagnosis, whereas twenty-one of the twenty-five patients (84%) with abnormal esophageal contractions (e.g., nutcracker esophagus) received psychiatric diagnoses. The most common diagnoses were depression, somatization (i.e., hypochondriasis) disorder, and anxiety disorder. These results, then, suggest that the abnormal motility patterns that often are found among NCCP patients are associated frequently with psychiatric disorders.

Richter and his colleagues (1986) compared the responses of twenty nutcracker-esophagus patients to a psychological inventory with those of four subject samples. These four samples consisted of twenty patients with the irritable bowel syndrome, a functional gastrointestinal disorder of the colon; twenty patients with painful symptoms (e.g., dysphagia) due to structural abnormalities of the esophagus; twenty healthy individuals with normal esophageal motility patterns who previously had undergone manometry several times; and twenty healthy people with little manometry experience. The psychological inventory used in this study, the Millon Behavioral Health Inventory (MBHI; Millon, Green, & Meagher, 1982), was designed specifically to aid in the psychological understanding of medical patients.

The results showed that the nutcracker esophagus and irritable bowel syndrome groups produced significantly higher scores on the Gastrointestinal Susceptibility Scale of the MBHI than did the other subject groups. Thus, both the nutcracker esophagus and irritable bowel syndrome patients produced MBHI responses very similar to those of medical patients who are likely to react to psychological stress with frequent and severe gastrointestinal symptoms. A nearly identical pattern of results was found on the Somatic Anxiety Scale. This indicated that the MBHI responses of the two patient groups with functional gastrointestinal disorders were much like those of persons with hypochondriacal tendencies, unusual amounts of fear regarding bodily functions, and depression. Figure 13.3 shows a graphic representation of these findings.

The consistency of the findings independently reported by Clouse and Lustman (1983) and Richter et al. (1986) are quite striking given that they employed very different methods of assessment. That is, regardless of whether a psychiatric interview or a self-report inventory were employed, patients with abnormal esophageal motility were characterized as hypochondriacal, anxious, and depressed. Moreover, the nutcracker-esophagus patients' high scores on the Gastrointestinal Susceptibility Scale were consistent with clinical impressions and laboratory data regarding the effects of stress on the esophagus (cf. Anderson et al., 1989; Stacher et al., 1979).

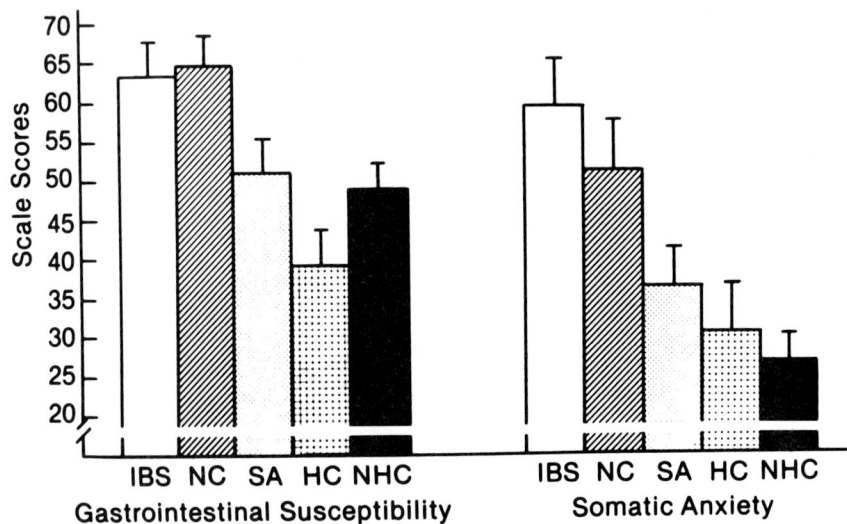

FIGURE 13.3   Mean Millon Behavioral Health Inventory scores of patients with irritable bowel syndrome (IBS), nutcracker esophagus (NC), structural abnormalities of the esophagus (SA), and healthy controls with manometry experience (HC) or with no manometry experience (NHC). Reprinted from "Psychological Comparison of Patients with Nutcracker Esophagus and Irritable Bowel Syndrome" by J. E. Richter, W. F. Obrecht, L. A. Bradley, L. D. Young, and K. O. Anderson, 1986, *Digestive Diseases and Sciences, 31*, pp. 131–138.

The results described have been given some additional support by a study that was performed in Great Britain. Bass and Wade (1984) administered a psychiatric interview to ninety-nine patients with complaints of chest pain after the patients underwent coronary angiography for the assessment of coronary artery disease. Neither the interviewers nor the patients were aware of the angiography results before the interviews were completed. It was found that a significantly higher proportion of individuals with normal coronary arteries (NCCP patients) were assigned psychiatric diagnoses on the basis of the interviews relative to persons with significant coronary vessel obstruction. Similar results have been reported among a sample of Swedish NCCP patients (Roll & Theorell, 1987).

Psychiatrists recently have become interested in patients with NCCP and have begun to evaluate these patients for a specific anxiety disorder, panic disorder, that usually responds well to psychotropic medication. Panic disorder is characterized by episodes of intense fear or discomfort accompanied by at least four of the following symptoms: shortness of breath or smothering sensations, choking, palpitations or accelerated heart rate, sweating, faintness, dizziness, lightheadedness, nausea or abdominal distress, depersonalization, numbness or tingling sensations, hot flashes or chills, trembling, fear of dying, and fear of going crazy or doing something uncontrolled. Several investigations have reported that between 30% and 47% of NCCP patients meet the criteria for panic disorder (Beitman et al., 1989; Cormier et al., 1988; Katon et al., 1988). It also has been found that NCCP patients with psychiatric disturbances such as panic disorder use different strategies for coping with their pain than do patients without such disturbances. The former are more likely to use strategies such as *avoidance* ("tried to forget the whole thing") and *wishful thinking* ("wished you could change the situation"), whereas the latter are more likely to use relatively positive strategies such as *seek social support* ("talked to others and accepted their sympathy") and *problem-focused coping* ("made a plan of action and followed it") (Vitaliano, Katon, Maiuro, & Russo, 1989).

How may the psychological factors and reactions just reviewed interact with the biological and psychophysiological components described earlier in this discussion to cause or exacerbate chest pain in the absence of coronary artery disease? Mayou (1989) recently suggested three possible interactions.

1. The autonomic and hormonal responses to anxiety and panic disorder may affect esophageal or cardiac function and thus produce chest pain.
2. Psychological distress may produce altered perceptions of cardiac function, chest pain, or other somatic symptoms.
3. The biological causes of minor chest pain may produce high levels of psychological distress in some predisposed individuals (e.g., those with abnormal esophageal contractions), which, in turn, may increase the severity of the chest pain or prolong its duration.

TREATMENT INTERVENTIONS   A variety of medical and pharmacological interventions have been tested with NCCP patients. These have included the use of antidepressant and antianxiety drugs, dilation or surgery of the esophagus, and medications designed to relax smooth muscles such as those found in the lower esophagus (cf. Richter, Spurling, Cordova, & Castell, 1984). Unfortunately, controlled experimental trials have shown that medical and pharmacological interventions can reduce esophageal contraction amplitudes but they do not reliably alter patients' reports of pain or other symptoms (Richter, Dalton, Bradley, & Castell, 1987; Richter et al., 1984).

A good example of the problems found with medical interventions for NCCP may be found in a controlled study of the antidepressant medication trazodone for patients with esophageal contraction abnormalities (Clouse, Lustman, Eckert, Ferney, & Griffith, 1987). This investigation found that trazodone, relative to a placebo, produced significant improvements in patients' ratings of overall improvement. However, trazodone was not superior to placebo in reducing esophageal symptoms, chest pain, or contraction abnormalities. Thus, trazodone helped patients to "feel better" but was no better than placebo in reducing more specific aspects of NCCP.

There are currently no controlled trials of psychological or behavioral interventions for NCCP. However, two case studies have appeared regarding the use of relaxation training or forehead EMG training to reduce the symptoms of two esophageal motility disorders related to NCCP, diffuse esophageal spasm (Latimer, 1981) and constriction of the throat and upper esophagus (Haynes, 1976).

Levenkron, Goldstein, Adamides, and Greenland (1985) have reported the successful use of a behavior therapy intervention with an NCCP patient. This treatment required 6½ weeks of hospitalization in a behavior therapy unit and included reinforcement of physical activity and other healthy behaviors, relaxation and assertiveness training, family therapy, and antidepressant (desimipramine) medication. A great deal of expense and professional time was devoted to this patient, but the one-year follow-up results were quite striking. The patient returned to work and experienced only two episodes of chest pain (producing only six days of work absences) during this period. A similar case study of outpatient treatment of NCCP with relaxation and stress management training as well as antidepressant medication also has been reported (Schwartz, Large, DeGood, Wegener, & Rowlingson, 1984).

It is clear that psychological therapies must become the focus of controlled outcome studies with NCCP patients in the near future. That is, the powerful and consistent evidence (e.g., Clouse & Lustman, 1983; Richter et al., 1986) that these patients suffer anxiety and depression suggests that it may well be necessary to improve their psychological status before any medical therapies may be effective. Indeed, this proposition recently received some indirect empirical support. A controlled, double-blind study of the effects of nifedipine, a smooth-muscle relaxant, showed that the drug produced significant reductions in the amplitudes of nutcracker-esophagus patients' peristaltic contractions. The drug failed, however, to reduce patients' reports of esophageal pain (Richter et al., 1987). Effective treatment of emotional disturbance or learned pain behaviors (see Chapter 14) as well as disordered esophageal motility may both be necessary for optimal control of NCCP.

# *The Stomach and Small Intestine*

The stomach is a stretchable sack that is bounded at one end by the lower esophageal sphincter and at the other end by the *pyloric sphincter* (see Chapter 3). The pyloric sphincter controls the rate at which the contents of the stomach are released into the small intestine and prevents reflux from the intestine into the stomach. The small intestine is composed of the *duodenum*, the *jejunum*, and the *ileum*. It is separated from the colon by the *ileocecal sphincter*. The duodenum, however, is most important for this discussion. It is the area in which the bile ducts and pancreatic ducts join the intestine and in which most *peptic ulcers* develop.

## Peptic Ulcers

*Peptic ulcer* is a term that is used to describe ulcerating lesions in either the stomach (gastric ulcer) or the duodenum (duodenal ulcer). Peptic ulcers occur in about 10% of the population at some point in their life (Whitehead & Bosmajian, 1982), the majority (about 75%) of which are duodenal ulcers. Ulcers present a hazard to health because of the significant blood loss they may produce and the possibility that they may become malignant. In addition, some ulcers will actually perforate the wall of the gastrointestinal tract, allowing the tract's contents to enter the peritoneal cavity, thus causing widespread infection (Weiss, 1984). Indeed, peptic ulcers account for approximately 10,000 deaths annually in the United States (Whitehead & Bosmajian, 1982).

BIOLOGICAL AND PSYCHOPHYSIOLOGICAL COMPONENTS  The biological mechanism involved in the development of peptic ulcers is believed to involve increased secretion of gastric acid and pepsin (a digestive enzyme), impaired functioning of the gastric mucosa (the outer lining of the stomach wall), or both. However, the biological mechanisms of gastric and duodenal ulcers appear to differ somewhat from one another. High levels of gastric acid production are typically associated with duodenal rather than gastric ulcers. Nevertheless, there is evidence based on animal studies that both gastric and duodenal ulcers increase in severity following high levels of gastric acid secretion (Weiss, 1984).

Impaired functioning of the gastric mucosa appears to be more important than gastric acid secretion in the development of gastric ulcers. The function of the mucosa is to protect the lining of the stomach from the corrosive substances (e.g., pepsin) that allow for food digestion. Many persons secrete large quantities of acid but do not develop ulcers, presumably due to the integrity of the gastric mucosa. The evidence from several animal studies (e.g., Hase & Moss, 1973) suggests that restriction of normal blood flow to the mucosa (ischemia) leads to gastrointestinal erosions that may eventually develop into ulcers. However, the exact process that leads from mucosal ischemia to impaired mucosal functioning remains unclear. It has been suggested that extreme mucosal ischemia leads to rupturing of the small blood vessels within the mucosa. The hemorrhaging of blood into the mucosa impedes normal cell metabolism that eventually results in mucosal tissue death or lesion development (Ivey, Grossman, & Bachrach, 1950; Kristt & Freimark, 1973; Weiss, 1984). However, it is also possible that the mucosal hemorrhaging observed in animals and humans follows rather than precedes lesion development.

Little is known regarding the psychophysiology of ulcer development. Most psychophysiological studies with humans have involved direct measurement of gastric acid secretion before and after exposure to environmental stressors by insertion of a pH monitor or aspiration of stomach contents (Whitehead & Bosmajian, 1982). These recording methods, however, are quite intrusive and disturbing to some subjects. In addition, the data recorded by these devices may be confounded by the normal digestive functions of the stomach and spontaneous stomach activity (Stern, 1983). Most investigators attempt to control for the effects of normal digestive functions by asking subjects to fast for several hours before testing. However, fasting reduces the external validity of the laboratory situation (Stern, 1983).

Noninvasive recording devices, such as the *electrogastrogram* (Hölzl, 1983) have been developed to measure stomach motility. The electrogastrogram records electrical activity from the abdomen's surface that reflects stomach movement. Nevertheless, the relationships among stomach motility, gastric acid secretion, and ulcer development are unclear. In short, there are few meaningful data regarding the psychophysiological components of ulcer development.

BEHAVIORAL, PSYCHOLOGICAL AND SOCIAL FACTORS   Despite the difficulties that have been encountered in psychophysiological studies, correlational studies with humans have provided consistent evidence that the experience of chronic stress is involved in the etiology of peptic ulcer disease (Gilligan, Furig, Piper, & Tennant, 1987; Wolf et al., 1979). For example, Cobb and Rose (1973) found that peptic ulcers were nearly twice as prevalent among air-traffic controllers relative to second-class airmen. There was also a significantly greater prevalence of peptic ulcer disease among controllers at air-traffic centers characterized by high stress compared to those at low-stress centers.

Moreover, the assumption has been made that the relationship between chronic stress and ulcer development is mediated either by high levels of gastric acid secretion or deficient mucous secretion because medications that reduce acid secretion effectively promote ulcer healing (Whitehead & Bosmajian, 1982).

This assumption was supported by a series of studies performed by Feldman and his associates (Feldman, Walker, Green, & Weingarden, 1986; Walker, Luther, Samloff, & Feldman, 1988). These investigators examined the relationships among several physiological, environmental, behavioral, and psychological factors found in patients with gastric or duodenal ulcers, control patients with kidney stones or gallstones, and healthy controls. The factors that best discriminated the peptic ulcer patients from the two control groups were high levels of depression, highly stressful negative life events, family history of peptic ulcer disease, and high blood serum levels of pepsinogen (this was especially true for the duodenal ulcer patients). In addition, high levels of serum pepsinogen ( which is a measure of gastric acid secretion) were correlated across all subject groups with general psychological distress, poor coping abilities, and hostility. It was proposed, then, that an individual with a family history of peptic ulcer disease, poor coping skills, and who is exposed to severe stressors would be more likely to develop peptic ulcers than an equally stressed individual without a genetic predisposition to the disease. Moreover, it was suggested that serum pepsinogen is the physiological factor that mediates the relationship between stress and peptic ulcer disease. That is, genetically predisposed individuals who cannot cope well with high levels of stress (i.e., describe themselves as depressed) may secrete relatively high levels of gastric acid and thus be at high risk for peptic ulcer disease development.

A number of investigators have attempted to use primates or other animals to assess more directly the relationship between stress and the development of peptic ulcers. There is some controversy regarding the degree to which the results of animal studies may teach us about the development of peptic ulcers in humans (Weiss, 1984; Whitehead & Bosmajian, 1982). Nevertheless, the animal studies have produced some intriguing results.

The first animal study that examined the relationship between coping with stress and peptic ulcer disease has become known as the "executive monkey" study (Brady, Porter, Conrad, & Mason, 1958; Porter et al., 1958). This study examined four pairs of monkeys; in each pair, one monkey was chosen as the "executive" whereas the other served as the "yoked" control. Both monkeys were restrained during experimental trials. However, the executive monkey could press a lever in order to avoid a strong, electrical shock that was presented on a fixed-interval schedule. The yoked monkey, however, received the shock whenever the executive failed to prevent its presentation. Thus, both monkeys received the same number of shocks but only the executive could exert control over the shocks. It was found that each of the four executive monkeys developed duodenal ulcers and died, whereas the yoked controls showed no ulcer development.

The executive monkey study generated a great deal of excitement. It appeared that Brady and his colleagues had demonstrated that the stress induced by the avoidance learning procedure resulted in the development of severe gastrointestinal pathology. Unfortunately, several subsequent attempts to replicate the original investigation failed to reproduce the dramatic results.

Some investigations, in fact, demonstrated that "executive rats" that could avoid shock following the presentation of a warning signal by performing a selected response showed significantly less severe gastric lesions than yoked-control rats (Weiss, 1968, 1971a).

Weiss has attempted to reconcile his findings and those of Brady and colleagues in a series of papers (1971b, 1977, 1984). He has suggested that the development of gastric lesions in the laboratory testing situation is related to two factors: the number of avoidance responses made by the animal and the amount of relevant feedback received by the animal immediately following its responses. Thus, gastric lesions are most likely to occur when an animal shows a large number of avoidance responses but receives little feedback following those responses.

Careful examination of the original executive-monkey study has revealed that the executive and the yoked-control monkeys were not randomly assigned to the experimental conditions. That is, those monkeys that eventually were assigned to the executive condition had shown a higher rate of avoidance responses on an initial pretest than did those that were placed in the yoked-control condition. Moreover, the avoidance-learning task used in the original investigation did not include a warning signal prior to the presentation of shock. Thus, the executive monkeys received very little relevant feedback concerning the effectiveness of their numerous avoidance responses.

In contrast to the executive-monkey study, Weiss did randomly allocate his animal subjects to experimental and control conditions. Weiss also provided the executive rats with relevant feedback in the form of a warning signal that could be terminated with the emission of the correct avoidance response. Thus, the executive rats were tested under conditions that were vastly different from those in which the executive monkeys were tested. It is not surprising, then, that the executive role produced different degrees of gastrointestinal pathology in the original and subsequent investigations.

The experiments described above provide a fascinating demonstration of the process of scientific inquiry. However, the implications of these experiments for our understanding of the cause of gastrointestinal pathology are not entirely clear. That is, the investigations did not attempt to determine what physiological factors may mediate the relationships among stress, behavior, and gastrointestinal pathology. Nevertheless, it is interesting to speculate that the executive monkeys' high levels of avoidance responses and lack of relevant feedback may be analogous to the poor coping responses to stress displayed by Feldman's human subjects with peptic ulcer disease. Consider Weiss's (1984) description of the poorly organized coping behaviors he observed during his first psychotherapeutic interview with an ulcer patient.

> This patient, a man in his late 30's, had recently undergone surgery to extirpate an ulcer. In the interview, the patient responded to my rather nondescript opening statement ("Tell me about what brings you to see me") by talking nonstop

for 1 hour, precluding any verbal intervention on my part. If verbal output can be considered a measure of response rate or activity, it is hard to imagine how anyone could have scored higher than this man.

This patient was also one of my most salient treatment failures. I was only able to maintain contact with him for a few months, during which he missed the majority of his therapy appointments and finally terminated after missing six consecutive sessions. It is with considerable sadness and frustration that I must report that this young man died 3 years later of a heart attack. (p. 211)

PSYCHOLOGICAL AND BEHAVIORAL REACTIONS    Relatively little research has been conducted regarding the psychological and behavioral reactions of peptic ulcer patients. This may be because until recently, many psychosomatic investigators continued to accept Franz Alexander's (1950) hypothesis that certain unique psychological attributes of peptic ulcer patients served as causes rather than consequences of their disease. Alexander (1950) had postulated that the common psychological attribute underlying peptic ulcer disease was an unconscious desire to be dependent upon others much as an infant is dependent upon its parents. In order to avoid awareness of these infantile dependency needs, many ulcer patients tend to use reaction formation and overcompensation as defense mechanisms. Thus the patients attempt to present themselves as highly independent, self-reliant, and highly competitive and aggressive.

Some ulcer patients, however, may partially express their dependency needs by behaving in an ingratiating manner in order to please others. Furthermore, a third category of ulcer patients may attempt to satisfy their dependency needs by insistently making demands on others in the environment (Engel, 1975).

As you might imagine, the behavior of many different ulcer patients may be viewed as consistent with the psychosomatic model of Alexander given that dependency needs may be expressed in numerous ways. A prospective study, however, showed that psychiatrists found it difficult to correctly differentiate duodenal ulcer patients from those with other "psychosomatic" diseases (e.g., asthma, rheumatoid arthritis, essential hypertension) on the basis of clinical interview data alone (Alexander, French, & Pollack, 1968). Although the psychiatrists classified patients more accurately than would be expected by chance alone, the percentage of correctly classified patients in each disease category was generally less than 50%. Moreover, recent studies have shown a great deal of variability among peptic ulcer patients with respect to psychological factors such as emotional stability, dependency, anxiety, and hostility (Langeluddecke, Goulston, & Tennant, 1987; Magni, DiMario, Rizzardo, Pulin, & Naccarato, 1986). It is clear, therefore, that studies of ulcer patients have provided little meaningful information regarding the psychological consequences of peptic ulcer disease.

# Treatment Interventions

The three major medical treatments for peptic ulcers consist of surgery, diet, and pharmacological agents. Although 20% of all ulcer patients undergo some form of surgery, surgical interventions are highly expensive (Sonnenberg, 1989), do not represent a "cure" for peptic ulcers, and often produce discomforting side effects. For example, one common surgical intervention is *vagotomy*, or the severing of the two large vagal nerve trunks that innervate the stomach. This procedure decreases the secretion of gastric acid but also inhibits the emptying of the stomach contents into the duodenum. Thus, an additional surgical procedure may be required to widen the pylorus and promote gastric emptying. Regardless of the technical skill with which these procedures are employed, there are often side effects such as weight and strength loss, gastric pain, diarrhea, or constipation (Walker, 1983).

The pharmacological alternatives to surgery have traditionally consisted of antacids and drugs that inhibit gastric acid secretion. However, controlled studies that have compared the effectiveness of these pharmacological agents to that of placebos have not produced consistent evidence. The current drugs of choice for duodenal and gastric ulcers are those that inhibit gastric secretion by blocking histamine receptors such as *cimetidine* and *ranitidine*. However, side effects, such as mental confusion and breast changes among males, may occur. In addition, these medications tend to be more effective with duodenal than gastric ulcers.

Dietary treatments for peptic ulcers have traditionally included bland diets featuring milk, cottage cheese, and white meat. There is evidence, nevertheless, that milk or cream actually may increase rather than inhibit gastric acid secretion (Lennard-Jones & Babouris, 1965).

Given the inconsistent evidence regarding the efficacy of some of the traditional medical treatments for peptic ulcer as well as the negative side effects of these treatments, a few investigators have attempted to use behavioral or cognitive-behavioral therapies with ulcer patients. For example, biofeedback studies with both patients (e.g., Welgan 1974, 1977) and healthy people (e.g., Whitehead, Renault, & Goldiamond, 1975) have shown that it is possible for humans to learn to control gastric acid secretion. Extensive training is required, however, and there are many technical difficulties associated with the measurement procedures. Thus, biofeedback training is currently not a cost-effective treatment for ulcer patients (Whitehead & Bosmajian, 1982).

Cognitive-behavioral therapy and other short-term forms of psychological treatment appear to be more promising interventions than biofeedback training. Brooks and Richardson (1980) demonstrated the long-term effectiveness of an anxiety management and assertiveness training program for duodenal ulcer patients. The training program included education, relaxation training, cognitive restructuring of irrational beliefs related to anxiety and assertiveness, and coping skills training. It was found that, compared to patients who received short-term supportive psychotherapy, patients who received the anxiety-management and assertiveness training reported significantly lower levels of anxiety, pain, emotional constriction, and antacid consumption as well as significantly higher levels of assertiveness following treatment. Moreover, during a three-and-a-half year follow-up period, significantly fewer patients in the anxiety-management and assertiveness-training condition, relative to patients in the supportive psychotherapy condition, experienced a recurrence of ulcers or required surgery for ulcers.

Results similar to those of Brooks and Richardson have been produced in a controlled investigation performed in Sweden of the efficacy of a coping-skills training program (Sjödin, 1983). Peptic ulcer patients in the experimental treatment condition reported significantly lower levels of pain and social maladjustment at posttreatment than did control patients. A fifteen-month follow-up showed that the experimental patients, relative to the controls, reported significantly fewer symptoms of ulcers as well as significantly greater levels of self-confidence, coping ability, and belief in their abilities to resolve their life problems.

Some interest recently has been generated in the use of hypnosis with peptic ulcer patients. Klein and Spiegel (1989) have demonstrated that hypnotic instructions to imagine eating a series of delicious meals increased gastric acid output by 89% among healthy subjects. Conversely, instructions to remove all thoughts of hunger and to experience deep relaxation reduced acid production by 39%. In Great Britain, Colgan, Faragher, and Whorwell (1988) added either hypnotic instructions to control gastric acid secretions or nonspecific professional attention (placebo) to a regimen of ranitidine among 30 patients with frequently relapsing duodenal ulcers. It was reported at a one-year follow-up assessment that hypnotherapy was associated with a significantly lower relapse rate (53%) than the attention-placebo (100%).

The aforementioned results suggest that cognitive-behavioral therapy or hypnotherapy may be highly useful adjuncts to the medical management of peptic ulcer disease. However, given that only a small number of controlled studies have appeared since 1980, it will be necessary to perform additional research to determine if psychological therapies may be used successfully with large numbers of peptic ulcer patients.

# The Colon and Rectum

The colon, or large intestine, is comprised of four segments: the ascending, transverse, descending, and sigmoid colons (see Chapter 3). The lower end of the colon is guarded by an internal and external anal sphincter and terminates on the rectum. Pelvic floor muscles loop around the rectum to form an additional sphincter.

## Irritable Bowel Syndrome

The irritable bowel syndrome (IBS) is the most common disorder among patients who are referred to gastrointestinal clinics, accounting for 40% to 50% of these referrals (Sammons & Karoly, 1987). Symptoms of IBS are reported by 8% to 19% of adults in any given year (Thompson, Dotevale, Drossman, Heaton, & Kruis, 1989) and result in approximately 115,000 hospital admissions per year (Mendeloff, 1979). Following many years of disagreement among gastroenterologists, there now is a consensus that the diagnostic criteria for IBS consist of (1) abdominal pain, relieved with defecation or associated with a change in frequency or consistency of stool; and/or (2) disturbed defecation (e.g., changes in stool frequency, form, or passage, or evacuation of mucus); usually with (3) bloating or feelings of abdominal distention; and (4) no evidence of organic disease (Thompson et al., 1989). People with IBS typically experience periods in which they are free of symptoms as well as periods during which they suffer symptoms of varying severity (Latimer, 1983a). Most IBS sufferers can adequately cope with their symptoms, although a substantial minority do suffer disruptions of their life activities. It is currently not clear whether IBS represents a precursor of any other, more threatening gastrointestinal diseases.

BIOLOGICAL AND PSYCHOPHYSIOLOGICAL COMPONENTS    The biological and psychophysiological components of IBS have been examined by inserting polyethylene tubes within the first 25 cm of the rectum and sigmoid colon to measure pressure changes indicative of colonic motor activity (i.e., contractions) or electrical control activity of the smooth muscle of the bowel wall. Early investigators reported that the total amount of colonic motor activity was greater among IBS patients relative to normal control individuals (e.g., Champion, 1973; Wangel & Deller, 1965). At first, it was suggested that this increased contractile activity might account for the bowel symptoms and pain of IBS. However, Latimer and his colleagues (Latimer, Sarna, Campbell, Latimer, Waterfall, & Daniel, 1981) later demonstrated that the colonic motor activity of IBS patients was greater than that of normal individuals but was equivalent to that of patients with neurotic disorders (e.g., anxiety, depression) who had no IBS bowel symptoms. This is a particularly important finding given that IBS patients tend to report a wide variety of psychological disturbances, especially anxiety and depression (see section on Psychological and Behavioral Reactions). That is, the findings of Latimer et al. indicate that increased contractile activity of the colon may be associated with psychological distress but it is not sufficient to account for the pain and disturbed defecation that characterize IBS.

Other investigators have attempted to determine if there may be specific types of physiological activity that distinguish IBS patients from normal or neurotic-control subjects. Several investigators have independently found differences between IBS patients and healthy control persons in electrical control activity (Snape, Carlson, Matarazzo, & Cohen, 1970; Taylor, Duthie, Hammond, & Basu, 1978; Whitehead, Engel, & Schuster, 1980). However, Latimer and his colleagues (1981) failed to find any differences in electrical control activity between IBS patients and either neurotic or normal control subjects. Latimer (1983a, 1983b) has noted that there were important differences between his investigation and those of the other investigators with respect to bowel preparation (e.g., use of a pretreatment enema), recording site, and methods of data analysis that might account for the discrepant results. Thus, until the methodological differences among the various investigators are resolved, it is not possible to determine with certainty whether electrical control activity plays a role in IBS symptoms.

It should be noted that one additional factor may complicate attempts to identify a specific biological abnormality unique to IBS. Several British investigators have found that esophageal symptoms or motility abnormalities similar to those observed with noncardiac chest pain are found among substantial numbers of IBS patients (Moriarty & Dawson, 1982; Watson, Sullivan, Corke, & Rush, 1976; Whorwell, Clouter, & Smith, 1981). In addition, Richter et al. (1986) have reported some psychological similarities between IBS and NCCP patients with the nutcracker esophagus. Thus, IBS and NCCP may actually be subtypes of a more inclusive disorder such as an "irritable gut syndrome" (Latimer, 1983a; Richter et al., 1986).

BEHAVIORAL, PSYCHOLOGICAL, AND SOCIAL FACTORS  Four behaviorally or psychologically oriented hypotheses have been advanced regarding the etiology of IBS. The first has been described as the *abnormal stimulation hypothesis* (Latimer, 1983a, 1983b). This hypothesis suggests that both IBS patients and normals show increased colonic motility following exposure to stressful situations (cf. Narducci, Snape, Battle, London, & Cohen, 1985). However, IBS patients develop bowel symptoms and psychological disturbances because they more frequently experience stress relative to normals. It has been found that IBS patients tend to report that stress exacerbates their symptoms (Hislop, 1971) and that they experience more stressful life events than patients with other gastrointestinal diseases (Mendeloff, Monk, Siegel, & Lilienfield, 1970). Nevertheless, IBS patients' psychological characteristics are similar to those of patients with other stress-related disorders (West, 1970). Thus, exposure to stress is not uniquely associated with the development of IBS. Other factors must be involved.

The *abnormal interoception hypothesis* posits that IBS patients experience normal colonic responses as abnormal and thus behave in an abnormal fashion (Latimer, 1983a, 1983b). Indeed, several investigators have reported that IBS patients are more likely than normal controls to report pain in response to distension of the sigmoid colon produced by the inflation of an inserted balloon (Ritchie, 1973, 1977; Whitehead et al., 1980). Latimer and his colleagues, however, reported that IBS patients were no more likely than neurotic patients or normals to report pain at various levels of colonic distension (Latimer et al., 1979). Similar to the studies of colonic electrical activity described earlier, there were important differences in the colonic distension procedure used by Latimer's group and that used by the other investigators. Latimer and his colleagues successively inflated and deflated the balloon every sixty seconds; there was a standard increase in the colonic distension with each inflation. The previous investigators either used a standard distension (Ritchie, 1973) or cumulative distensions that were not alternated with periods of balloon deflation (Whitehead et al., 1980). It may well be, then, that the inconsistencies in the evidence may be due to methodological differences among the studies performed to date. However, the findings of Ritchie and Whitehead are similar to the relatively low pain thresholds found among NCCP patients. These data, then, provide additional support to the concept that IBS and NCCP are subtypes of an irritable gut syndrome.

The *learning hypothesis* suggests that disturbed defecation is an unlearned response to stress. However, some people who have a genetic predisposition to neuroticism (i.e., anxiety and depression) and who receive positive reinforcement for complaints of pain, diarrhea, or constipation following stress, are likely to develop the psychological and physical symptoms of IBS (Latimer, 1983a, 1983b). Some evidence for this hypothesis was provided by the following two research groups. Whitehead and colleagues demonstrated that a significantly greater number of IBS patients, compared to peptic ulcer patients and healthy controls, reported that they had received gifts (i.e., positive reinforcement) when they were ill during childhood (Whitehead, Winget, Fedoravicious, Wooley, & Blackwell, 1982). Drossman's group found that IBS patients, relative to healthy people, reported more stomach pain, school absences, doctor visits, and family stresses during childhood (Lowman, Drossman, Cramer, & McKee, 1987)

Despite the positive evidence for the learning hypothesis, it should be remembered that genetic studies of neuroticism among IBS patients have never been performed. Furthermore, the leaning hypothesis cannot account for the prevalence of IBS symptoms among large numbers of individuals (about 17% of the population) who are not psychologically distressed and who do not seek medical care (Drossman et al., 1982; Thompson & Heaton, 1980). Some work, however, has been directed toward defining why some persons with IBS seek medical care whereas others cope with their symptoms without medical assistance. This work will be discussed in the Psychological and Behavioral Reactions section that follows.

The final hypothesis represents an attempt to reconcile the conflicting evidence reviewed above. This *heterogeneity hypothesis* emphasizes that IBS patients may be quite different from one another with respect to etiology of their disorder and the three behavioral dimensions of IBS—abnormal colonic motility or electrical activity, verbal complaints of pain, and such motor behavior as frequent defecation. These dimensions may independently vary along a continuum from normal to abnormal in any person with IBS (Latimer, 1983a). In addition, the hypothesis suggests that these dimensions show a great deal of variability among different individuals with IBS. Put another way, there are many variations among IBS patients in the causes of their disorder and the type and severity of symptoms they experience; these symptoms also vary over time in individual IBS patients. The utility of the heterogeneity hypothesis lies in its implications for treatment. That is, the hypothesis implies that treatments should be tailored for individual IBS patients on the basis of a careful assessment of the role of each behavioral dimension in their symptoms. For example, patients with relatively normal colonic motility but who frequently report abdominal pain when exposed to stressful situations might benefit more from stress management training than from a dietary regimen designed to reregulate colonic motor activity patterns. However, patients who are characterized primarily by unusual colonic motor activity might best respond to a bowel sound biofeedback training regimen (see Treatment Interventions section).

To summarize, a variety of hypotheses have been advanced concerning the etiology of IBS. All of these hypotheses have received some support from research studies but none can sufficiently account for all aspects of IBS. Although a unifying theory of the cause of IBS does not currently exist, Sammons and Karoly (1987) have suggested that several features drawn from the aforementioned hypotheses should be evaluated in future studies of the origins of IBS. These are: (1) potential hereditary and physiological factors; (2) learning factors (e.g., operant conditioning of behavior associated with IBS); (3) critical positive or negative (e.g., stresses) life events; and (4) cognitive factors (e.g., perceptions of internal bodily events, attitudes toward seeking health care). Progress in understanding and developing treatments for IBS will depend on the ability of future investigators to link these features together in a meaningful way.

PSYCHOLOGICAL AND BEHAVIORAL REACTIONS   A large number of controlled and uncontrolled investigations have examined the psychological characteristics of IBS patients. The four most rigorous studies have shown that the prevalence of psychological disturbance ranges between 72% and 100% of the IBS patient population that seeks medical care (Hislop, 1971; Liss, Alpers, & Woodruff, 1973; Young, Alpers, Norlund, & Woodruff, 1976; Latimer et al., 1981). The most common psychiatric diagnoses assigned to the IBS patients have been hysteria, depression, and anxiety disorder. Other psychological characteristics associated with IBS include fatigue, anorexia, insomnia, and weeping.

Given the exceptionally high prevalence and severity of psychological disturbance among IBS patients, it is tempting to assume that nearly all persons with IBS suffer from psychological disorders. This assumption has been evaluated by two independent groups of investigators, who compared the psychological profiles of IBS patients sampled from medical clinics, healthy individuals drawn from the community, and people from the same community who meet the diagnostic criteria for IBS but who have not obtained medical care (IBS nonpatients). Drossman and colleagues (1988) reported that IBS patients, relative to IBS nonpatients, reported more severe symptoms of pain and diarrhea. However, even after statistically controlling for these differences, the IBS patients reported greater psychological distress, fewer positive life experiences, and poorer coping abilities than the IBS nonpatients and healthy controls (Drossman et al., 1988). Similar results, obtained using somewhat different psychological assessment instruments, were reported by Whitehead's group (Whitehead, Bosmajian, Zonderman, Costa, & Schuster, 1988). Thus, although the bowel symptoms underlying IBS are common within the general population (about 17%), people who are most likely to seek medical care experience relatively severe pain, diarrhea, and psychological distress. This means that it is the "interaction of psychological factors and the degree of altered bowel physiology that determine the illness experience and behaviors such as health care utilization" (Drossman et al., 1988, p. 707).

TREATMENT INTERVENTIONS   The traditional medical treatment of IBS has consisted of the use of high-fiber diets and antispasmodic pharmacological agents to reduce the frequency, duration, and magnitudes of bowel contractions (Latimer, 1983a). It should be noted, however, that only a few controlled clinical trials have been performed regarding the efficacy of high-fiber diets or antispasmodic agents in managing IBS. The evidence that has been accumulated thus far does not suggest that either of these interventions is clearly superior to placebo (Klein, 1988; Latimer, 1983a).

A few medical investigators have attempted to pharmacologically treat the psychological difficulties of IBS patients and have also recorded the effects of treatment on the IBS symptoms (e.g., Greenbaum et al., 1987; Steinhart, Wong, & Zarr, 1981). Unfortunately, these investigators' efforts have not produced convincing evidence of the superiority of antidepressant or antianxiety agents to placebo in IBS symptom reduction. This does not suggest, however, that these medical treatments are not effective with any IBS patients. Rather, the difficulties involved in producing valid outcome studies in this area have prevented investigators from generating compelling evidence that current medical treatments are effective with large numbers of IBS patients (Klein, 1988).

As a result of the difficulties encountered in the medical treatment of IBS, a few individuals have produced case studies of the efficacy of biofeedback (Bueno-Miranda, Cerulli, & Schuster, 1976; Furman, 1973) among IBS patients. Both of these investigations have produced positive results. However, the results of the Bueno-Miranda et al. study were limited to the learned control of colonic contractions; the critical clinical effects (control of pain or diarrhea) of the biofeedback treatment were not reported. Furman (1973) taught five IBS patients to increase and decrease bowel sounds using biofeedback from an electronic stethoscope placed on the abdomen. Recently, Radnitz and Blanchard (1988) employed a multiple baseline design to study the clinical effectiveness of this biofeedback procedure with five patients. Two of the patients learned to reliably control their bowel sounds and showed pretreatment to post-treatment reductions in their IBS symptoms (e.g., pain, diarrhea, constipation) that were greater than 50%. These improvements were maintained at a one-year follow-up assessment.

Three groups of investigators have performed controlled studies of the efficacy of psychotherapy in treating IBS. Svedlund and his associates (Svelund, Sjödin, Ottosson, & Dotevall, 1983) compared the effects of ten sessions of psychological therapy and conventional medical treatment (high-fiber agents, antispasmodic and antianxiety drugs, and antacids) to those of conventional medical treatment alone. Figure 13.4 shows that patients who received the psychological therapy reported significant improvements in total somatic symptoms, abdominal pain, and bowel dysfunction relative to the patients who received only conventional medical treatment. These improvements were maintained for twelve months following the end of treatment. Thus, it appeared that the addition of psychotherapy to medical treatment resulted in long-term improvements in IBS symptoms that reduced patients' needs for extended periods of medical care.

Whorwell, Prior, and Faragher (1984) performed a study that compared the effects of hypnotherapy that focused on control of gut functioning to those of supportive psychotherapy on IBS symptoms. The purpose of this hypnotherapy technique, then, was similar to that of Furman's biofeedback procedure, although Whorwell and his colleagues did not attempt to measure

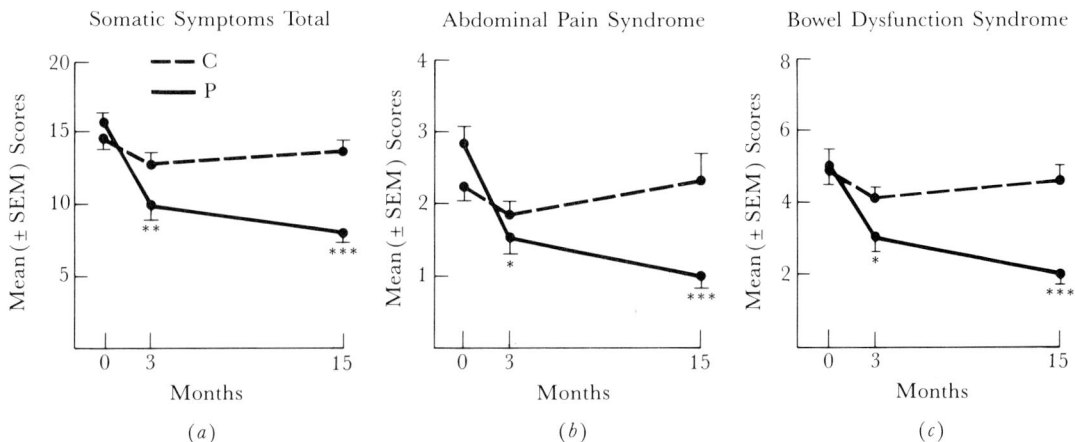

FIGURE 13.4   Mean IBS patient ratings at pretreatment (0 months), after 3 months' treatment, and at 15 months for total (a) somatic symptoms, (b) abdominal pain, and (c) bowel dysfunction. P = psychotherapy group and C = conventional medical treatment group. Reprinted from "Controlled Study of Psychotherapy in Irritable Bowel Syndrome" by J. Svedlund, I. Sjödin, J-O Ottosson, and G. Dotevall, 1983, *Lancet, 2*, pp. 589–592.

patients' control of gut functioning. During the three-month course of treatment, hypnotherapy produced significantly greater improvements than did supportive psychotherapy upon patients' reports of abdominal pain, bowel habit, abdominal distension, and general well-being. The hypnotherapy patients were followed for an average of eighteen months after treatment and all maintained their initial improvements (Whorwell, Prior, & Colgan, 1987). As noted by the investigators, however, it is not known how the hypnosis actually produced the beneficial effects reported by the patients (Whorwell et al., 1987).

Blanchard and his colleagues have performed the most comprehensive series of studies of the effects of psychological therapy on IBS patients. Neff and Blanchard (1987) developed a psychological intervention consisting of educational information, relaxation training, thermal biofeedback for increasing hand temperature (to promote general relaxation), and stress-management training. The intervention originally was designed for use with individual patients. Six of ten IBS patients treated with this intervention achieved pre-treatment to post-treatment reductions in their IBS symptoms that met criteria for clinical success (greater than 50% reduction). None of nine IBS control patients showed this level of clinical success. However, of the seven controls who later received the intervention, three achieved clinical success. Fourteen of the total of seventeen treated patients participated in a two-year follow-up assessment (Blanchard, Schwarz, & Neff, 1988). Eight of these patients were still clinically improved two years after treatment. Similarly, nine of fourteen IBS patients who received the psychological intervention in a group format, rather than an individual one, met the criteria for clinical success at a six-week follow-up assessment (Blanchard & Schwarz, 1987).

To conclude, several psychological treatments (bowel sound biofeedback, hypnotherapy, individual or group psychotherapy) appear to produce sustained improvements in IBS symptoms. These improvements have been shown to be greater than those produced by medical treatment alone, because all of the patients were receiving medical care while they participated in the psychological treatment studies. However, it is not clear why all of the psychological interventions, which have varied greatly in treatment technique, have produced such similar results. It may be that any psychological intervention that promotes distraction from pain (e.g., hypnotherapy, bowel sound biofeedback, relaxation training) and reduces anxiety and depression will have a secondary positive effect on disturbed defecation and other IBS symptoms. However, additional research is necessary to test this hypothesis or determine what other factors account for the successful psychological treatment of IBS.

# *Summary*

This chapter examined four gastrointestinal disorders. *Gastroesophageal reflux* (GER) is characterized by the passage of acidic stomach contents through the lower esophageal sphincter into the esophagus. *Noncardiac chest pain*

(NCCP) is the perception of chest pain in the absence of coronary heart disease. It is considered to be a *functional* disorder because a specific disease underlying the pain has not been identified. *Peptic ulcer* disease is a term that describes ulcerating lesions in either the stomach (gastric ulcer) or the duodenum (duodenal ulcer). *Irritable bowel syndrome* (IBS) is another functional disorder that is characterized by abdominal pain, disturbed defecation, bloating or feelings of abdominal distention, and no evidence of organic disease.

One factor that is common to all of the disorders reviewed in this chapter is the exacerbating effect of stress. Patients with these disorders report that their symptoms are increased when they are exposed to stressful situations. Another factor that is often associated with these disorders is anxiety. This is especially true for patients with GER, NCCP, and IBS. Indeed, anxiety and other psychological disturbances appear to be particularly important in deciding to seek medical attention for IBS symptoms. Although IBS symptoms are common within the general population, people who are most likely to seek medical care are those with relatively severe levels of pain, diarrhea, and psychological distress.

Studies of the psychophysiological components and psychological factors associated with NCCP and IBS suggests that these functional disorders actually may be subtypes of a single disorder, the "irritable gut." For example, the psychological profiles of NCCP and IBS patients are very similar to one another. Furthermore, both NCCP and IBS patients show relatively low pain thresholds in response to balloon distention of the esophagus and colon, respectively. Abnormal motor activity often is found in both the esophagus and colon of NCCP and IBS patients. Indeed, substantial numbers of IBS patients display esophageal symptoms or motility disturbances similar to those associated with NCCP. However, the pain symptoms of these gastrointestinal disorders cannot be caused only by altered contractile activity of the esophagus or colon.

Effective psychological treatments have been developed for peptic ulcers and IBS. Hypnosis and psychotherapy both have been shown to produce sustained improvements among patients with ulcers and IBS. In addition, bowel sound biofeedback has been documented as an effective treatment for some IBS patients. Little work has been devoted to the psychological treatment of GER and NCCP patients. Nevertheless, studies of NCCP patients suggest that it may be necessary to improve the psychological status of these patients before any medical therapies can be effective.

# References

ALEXANDER, F. (1950). *Psychosomatic medicine: Its principles and applications*. New York: Norton.

ALEXANDER, F., FRENCH, T. M., & POLLACK, G. H. (Eds.) (1968). *Psychosomatic specificity* (Vol. 1). Chicago: University of Chicago Press.

ALMY, T. P. (1977). Therapeutic strategy in stress-related digestive disorders. *Clinics in Gastroenterology, 6*, 709–722.

ANDERSON, K. O., DALTON, C. B., BRADLEY, L. A., & RICHTER, J. E. (1989). Stress induces alteration of esophageal pressures in healthy volunteers and non-cardiac chest pain patients. *Digestive Diseases and Sciences, 34*, 83–91.

BARISH, C. F., CASTELL, D. O., & RICHTER, J. E. (1986). Graded esophageal balloon distention: A new provocative test for noncardiac chest pain. *Digestive Diseases and Sciences, 31*, 1292–1298.

BASS, C., & WADE, C. (1984). Chest pain with normal coronary arteries: A comparative study of psychiatric and social morbidity. *Psychological Medicine, 14*, 51–61.

BEITMAN, B. D., MUKERJI, V., LAMBERTI, J. W., SCHMID, L., DEROSEAR, L., KUSHNER, M., FLAKER, G., & BASHA, I. (1989). Panic disorder in patients with chest pain and angiographically normal coronary arteries. *American Journal of Cardiology, 63*, 1399–1403.

BENJAMIN, S. B., & CASTELL, D. O. (1983). Chest pain of esophageal origin: Where are we, and where should we go? *Archives of Internal Medicine, 143*, 772–776.

BENJAMIN, S. B., GERHARDT, D. C., & CASTELL, D. O. (1979). High amplitude, peristaltic esophageal contractions associated with chest pain and/or dysphagia. *Gastroenterology, 77*, 478–483.

BLANCHARD, E. B., & SCHWARZ, S. P. (1987). Adaptation of a multicomponent treatment for irritable bowel syndrome to a small group format. *Biofeedback and Self-Regulation, 12*, 63–69.

BLANCHARD, E. B., SCHWARZ, S. P., & NEFF, D. F. (1988). Two-year follow-up of behavioral treatment of irritable bowel syndrome. *Behavior Therapy, 19*, 67–73.

BRADY, J. V., PORTER, R. W., CONRAD, D. G., & MASON, J. W. (1958). Avoidance behavior and the development of gastroduodenal ulcers. *Journal of the Experimental Analysis of Behavior, 1*, 69–72.

BRAND, D. L., MARTIN, D. & POPE, C. E. (1977). Esophageal manometrics in patients with angina-like chest pain. *American Journal of Digestive Diseases, 22*, 300–304.

BROOKS, G. R., & RICHARDSON, F. C. (1980). Emotional skills training: A treatment program for duodenal ulcer. *Behavior Therapy, 11*, 198–207.

BUENO-MIRANDA, F., CERULLI, M., & SCHUSTER, M. M. (1976). Operant conditioning of colonic motility in irritable bowel syndrome (IBS). *Gastroenterology, 70*, 867.

BURISH, T. G. (1981). EMG biofeedback in the treatment of stress-related disorders. In C. K. Prokop & L. A. Bradley (Eds.), *Medical psychology: Contributions to behavioral medicine*. New York: Academic Press.

CANNON, R. O., BONOW, R. O., BACHARACH, S. L., GREEN, M. V., ROSING, D. R., LEON, M. B., WATSON, R. M., & EPSTEIN, S. E. (1985). Left ventricular dysfunction in patients with angina pectoris, normal epicardial coronary arteries, and abnormal vasodilator reserve. *Circulation, 71*, 218–226.

CASTELL, D. O. (1980). Esophageal manometric studies: A perspective of their physiologic and clinical relevance. *Journal of Clinical Gastroenterology, 2*, 191–196.

CHAMPION, P. (1973). Some cases of the irritable bowel syndrome studied by intraluminal pressure recordings. *Digestion, 9*, 21–29.

CLOUSE, R. E., & LUSTMAN, P. J. (1983). Psychiatric illness and contraction abnormalities of the esophagus. *New England Journal of Medicine, 309*, 1337–1342.

CLOUSE, R. E., LUSTMAN, P. J., ECKERT, T. C., FERNEY, D. M., & GRIFFITH, L. S. (1987). Low-dose trazodone for symptomatic patients with esophageal contraction abnormalities. *Gastroenterology, 92,* 1027–1036.

COBB, S., & ROSE, R. M. (1973). Hypertension, peptic ulcer, and diabetes in air traffic controllers. *Journal of the American Medical Association, 224,* 489–492.

COHEN, S. (1980). Pathogenesis of coffee-induced gastrointestinal symptoms. *New England Journal of Medicine, 303,* 122–124.

COHEN, S. I., & REED, J. L. (1968). The treatment of "nervous diarrhea" and other conditioned autonomic disorders by desensitization. *British Journal of Psychiatry, 114,* 1275–1280.

COHEN, S., & SNAPE, W. J. (1977). The role of psychophysiological factors in disorders of aesophageal function. *Clinics in Gastroenterology, 6,* 569–579.

COLGAN, S. M., FARAGHER, E. B., & WHORWELL, P. J. (1988). Controlled trial of hypnotherapy in relapse prevention of duodenal ulceration. *Lancet, 2,* 1299–1300.

COMMITTEE ON NOMENCLATURE AND STATISTICS, AMERICAN PSYCHIATRIC ASSOCIATION (1980). *Diagnostic and statistical manual of mental disorders. 3rd ed.* Washington, D.C. : American Psychiatric Association.

CORMIER, L. E., KATON, W., RUSSO, J., HOLLIFIELD, M., HALL, M. L., & VITALIANO, P. P. (1988). Chest pain with negative cardiac diagnostic studies: Relationship to psychiatric illness. *Journal of Nervous and Mental Disease, 176,* 351–358.

DENNISH, G., & CASTELL, D. O. (1971). Effect of smoking on lower esophageal sphincter pressure. *New England Journal of Medicine, 289,* 1136–1137.

DIAMANT, N. E. (1977). How now esophageal peristalsis? *Gastroenterology, 73,* 1353–1354.

DROSSMAN, D. A., McKEE, D. C., SANDLER, R. S., MITCHELL, C. M., CRAMER, E. M., LOWMAN, B. C., & BURGER, A. L. (1988). Psychosocial factors in irritable bowel syndrome: A multivariate study of patients with irritable bowel syndrome. *Gastroenterology, 95,* 701–708.

DROSSMAN, D. A., SANDLER, R. S., McKEE, D. C., & LOVITZ, A. J. (1982). Bowel patterns among subjects not seeking health care: Use of a questionnaire to identify a population with bowel dysfunction. *Gastroenterology, 83,* 529–534.

DUCROTTE, P. H., BERLAND, M. J., DENIS, P. H., GALMICHE, J. P., CRIBIER, A., LETAC, B., & PASQUIS, P. (1985). Coronary sinus lactate estimation and esophageal motor anomalies in angina with normal coronary angiograms. *Digestive Diseases and Sciences, 29,* 305–310.

ENGEL, G. L. (1975). Psychophysiological gastrointestinal disorders. I. Peptic ulcer. In A. M. Freedman, H. I. Kaplan, & B. J. Sadock (Eds.), *Comprehensive textbook of psychiatry II* (Vol. 2). Baltimore: Williams & Wilkins.

FAULKNER, W. B. (1940). Severe esophageal spasm: An evaluation of suggestion-therapy as determined by means of the esophagoscope. *Psychosomatic Medicine, 2,* 139–140.

FELDMAN, M., WALKER, P., GREEN, J. L., & WEINGARDEN, K. (1986). Life events stress and psychosocial factors in men with peptic ulcer disease: A multidimensional case-controlled study. *Gastroenterology, 91,* 1370–1379.

FURMAN, S. (1973). Intestinal biofeedback in functional diarrhea: A preliminary report. *Journal of Behavior Therapy and Experimental Psychiatry, 4,* 317–321.

GILLIGAN, I., FURIG, L., PIPER, D. W., & TENNANT, C. (1987). Life event stress and chronic difficulties in duodenal ulcer: A case control study. *Journal of Psychosomatic Research, 31,* 117–123.

GREENBAUM, D. S., MAYLE, J. E., VANEGREN, L. E., JEROME, J. A., MAYOR, J. W., GREENBAUM, R. B., MATSON, R. W., STEIN, G. E., DEAN, H. O., HALVORSEN, N. A., & ROSEN, L. W. (1987). Effects of desimipramine on irritable bowel syndrome compared with atropine and placebo. *Digestive Diseases and Sciences, 32,* 257–266.

HASE, T., & MOSS, B. (1973). Microvascular changes of gastric mucosa in the development of stress ulcer in rats. *Gastroenterology, 65,* 224–234.

HAYNES, S. N. (1976). Electromyographic biofeedback treatment of a woman with chronic dysphagia. *Biofeedback and Self-Regulation, 1,* 121–126.

HISLOP, I. G. (1971). Psychological significance of the irritable colon syndrome. *Gut, 12,* 452–457.

HÖLZL, R. (1983). Stomach, In R. Hölzl & W. E. Whitehead (Eds.), *Psychophysiology of the gastrointestinal tract: Experimental and clinical applications.* New York: Plenum.

IVY, A. C., GROSSMAN, M. I., & BACHRACH, W. H. (1950). *Peptic ulcer.* Philadelphia: Blakiston.

JACOBSON, E. D. (1927). Spastic esophagus and mucus colitis: Etiology and treatment by progressive relaxation. *Archives of Internal Medicine, 39,* 433–445.

JEAN, A. (1972). Localization and activity of medullary swallowing neurones. *Journal de Physiologie, 64,* 227–268.

KATON, W., HALL, M. L., RUSSO, J., CORMIER, L., HOLLIFIELD, M., VITALIANO, P. P., & BEITMAN, B. D. (1988). Chest pain: Relationship of psychiatric illness to coronary arteriographic results. *American Journal of Medicine, 84,* 1–9.

KLEIN, K. B. (1988). Controlled treatment trials in the irritable bowel syndrome: A critique. *Gastroenterology, 95,* 232–241.

KLEIN, K. B. & SPIEGEL, D. (1989). Modulation of gastric secretion by hypnosis. *Gastroenterology, 96,* 1383–1387.

KRISTT, D. A., & FREIMARK, J. J. (1973). Histopathology and pathogenesis of behaviorally induced gastric lesions in rats. *American Journal of Pathology, 73,* 411–420.

KRONECKER, H., & MELTZER, J. (1883). Der Schluckmechanismus, seine Erregung und seine Hemmung. *Archives für Anatomic und Physiologie, Physiologische Abteilung, 7,* 328–362.

LANGELUDDECKE, P., GOULSTON, K., & TENNANT, C. (1987). Type A behavior and other psychological factors in peptic ulcer disease. *Journal of Psychosomatic Research, 31,* 335–340.

LANTINGA, L. J., SPRAFKIN, R. P., McCROSKERY, J. H., BAKER, M. T., WARNER, R. A., & HILL, N. E (1988). One year psychosocial follow-up of patients with chest pain and angiographically normal coronary arteries. *American Journal of Cardiology, 62,* 209–213.

LATIMER, P. R. (1981). Biofeedback and self-regulation in the treatment of diffuse esophageal spasm: A single case report. *Biofeedback and Self-Regulation, 6,* 181–189.

LATIMER, P. R. (1983a). *Functional gastrointestinal disorders: A behavioral medicine approach.* New York: Springer.

LATIMER, P. R. (1983b). Colonic psychophysiology: Implications for functional bowel disorders. In R. Hölzl & W. E. Whitehead (Eds.), *Psychophysiology of the gastrointestinal tract: Experimental and clinical applications*. New York: Plenum.

LATIMER, P., CAMPBELL, D., LATIMER, M., SARNA, S., DANIEL, E., & WATERFALL, W. (1979). Irritable bowel syndrome: A test of the colonic hyperalgesia hypothesis. *Journal of Behavioral Medicine, 2*, 285–295.

LATIMER, P., SARNA, S., CAMPBELL, D., LATIMER, M., WATERFALL, W. & DANIEL, E. E. (1981). Colonic motor and myoelectrical activity: A comparative study of normal subjects, psychoneurotic patients, and patients with irritable bowel syndrome. *Gastroenterology, 80*, 893–901.

LENNARD-JONES, J. E. (1983). Current concepts: Functional gastrointestinal disorders. *New England Journal of Medicine, 308*, 431–435.

LENNARD-JONES, J. E., & BABOURIS, N. (1965). Effect of different foods on the acidity of the gastric contents in patients with duodenal ulcer. *Gut, 6*, 113–117.

LEVENKRON, J. C., GOLDSTEIN, M. G., ADAMIDES, O. & GREENLAND, P. (1985). Chronic chest pain with normal coronary arteries: A behavioral approach to rehabilitation. *Journal of Cardiopulmonary Rehabilitation, 5*, 475–479.

LISS, J. L., ALPERS, D., & WOODRUFF, R. A. (1973). The irritable colon syndrome and psychiatric illness. *Diseases of the Nervous System, 34*, 151–157.

LOWMAN, B. C., DROSSMAN, D. A., CRAMER, E. M., & MCKEE, D. C. (1987). Recollection of childhood events in adults with irritable bowel syndrome. *Journal of Clinical Gastroenterology, 9*, 324–330.

MAGNI, G., DIMARIO, F., RIZZARDO, R., PULIN, S., & NACCARATO, R. (1986). Personality profiles of patients with duodenal ulcer. *American Journal of Psychiatry, 143*, 1297–1300.

MAYOU, R. (1989). Invited review: Atypical chest pain. *Journal of Psychosomatic Research, 33*, 393–406.

MENDELOFF, A. I. (1979). Epidemiology of the irritable bowel syndrome. *Practical Gastroenterology, 3*, 12–18.

MENDELOFF, A. I., MONK, M., SIEGEL, C. I., & LILLIENFELD, A. (1970). Illness experience and life stresses in patients with irritable colon and with ulcerative colitis. *New England Journal of Medicine, 282*, 14–17.

MILLON, T., GREEN, C. J., & MEAGHER, R. B. (1982). *Millon behavioral health inventory manual* (3rd ed.). Minneapolis: National Computer Systems.

MORIARTY, K. J., & DAWSON, S. M. (1982). Functional abdominal pain: Further evidence that whole gut is affected. *British Medical Journal, 284*, 1670–1672.

NARDUCCI, F., SNAPE, W. J., BATTLE, W. M., LONDON, R. L., & COHEN, S. (1985). Increased colonic motility during exposure to a stressful situation. *Digestive Diseases and Sciences, 30*, 40–44.

NEBEL, O. T., FORNES, M. F., & CASTELL, D. O. (1976). Symptomatic gastroesophageal reflux: Incidence and precipitating factors. *American Journal of Digestive Diseases, 21*, 953–956.

NEFF, D, F., & BLANCHARD, E. B. (1987). A multi-component treatment for irritable bowel syndrome. *Behavior Therapy, 18*, 70–83.

OCKENE, I. S., SHAY, M. J., ALPERT, J. S., WEINER, B. H., & DALEN, J. E. (1980). Unexplained chest pain in patients with normal coronary arteriograms. *New England Journal of Medicine, 303*, 1249–1252.

PETERS, L. J., MAAS, L. C., PETTY, D., DALTON, C., PENNER, D., WU, W. P., CASTELL, D., & RICHTER, J. (1988). Spontaneous non-cardiac chest pain: Evaluation by 24-hour ambulatory esophageal motility and pH monitoring. *Gastroenterology, 94*, 878–886.

PORTER, R. W., BRADY, J. V., CONRAD, D., MASON, J. W., GALAMBOS, R., & RIOCH, D. (1958). Some experimental observations on gastrointestinal lesions in behaviorally conditioned monkeys. *Psychosomatic Medicine, 20*, 379–394.

PRICE, S. F., SMITHSON, K. W., & CASTELL, D. O. (1978). Food sensitivity in reflux esophagitis. *Gastroenterology, 75*, 240–243.

PULLIAM, T. J., BRADLEY, L. A., DALTON, C. B., SALLEY, A. N., CASE, L. D., & RICHTER, J. E. (1989). Psychological factors influence the relationship between stress and reports of gastroesophageal reflux symptoms. Manuscript submitted for publication.

RADNITZ, C. L., & BLANCHARD, E. B. (1988). Bowel sound biofeedback as a treatment for irritable bowel syndrome.. *Biofeedback and Self-Regulation, 13*, 169–179.

RICHTER, J. E., BARISH, C. F., & CASTELL, D. O. (1986). Abnormal sensory perception in patients with esophageal chest pain. *Gastroenterology, 91*, 845–852.

RICHTER, J. E., BRADLEY, L. A., & CASTELL, D. O. (1989). Esophageal chest pain: Current controversies in pathogenesis, diagnosis, and therapy. *Annals of Internal Medicine, 110*, 66–78.

RICHTER, J. E., & CASTELL, D. O. (1984). Diffuse esophageal spasms: A reappraisal. *Annals of Internal Medicine, 100*, 242–245.

RICHTER, J. E., DALTON, C. B., BRADLEY, L. A., & CASTELL, D. O. (1987). Oral nifedipine in the treatment of noncardiac chest pain in patients with the nutcracker esophagus. *Gastroenterology, 93*, 21–28.

RICHTER, J. E., OBRECHT, W. F., BRADLEY, L. A., YOUNG, L. D., & ANDERSON, K. O. (1986). Psychological comparison of patients with the nutcracker esophagus and irritable bowel syndrome. *Digestive Diseases and Sciences, 31*, 131–138.

RICHTER, J. E., SPURLING, T. J., CORDOVA, C. M., & CASTELL, D. O. (1984). Effects of oral calcium blocker, diltiazem, on esophageal contractions: Studies in volunteers and patients with nutcracker esophagus. *Digestive Diseases and Sciences, 29*, 649–656.

RITCHIE, J. A. (1973). Pain from distension of the pelvic colon by inflating a balloon in the irritable colon syndrome. *Gut, 14*, 125–132.

RITCHIE, J. A. (1977). The irritable bowel syndrome. Part II. Manometric and cineradiographic studies. *Clinics in Gastroenterology, 6*, 622–631.

ROLL, M., & THEORELL, T. (1987). Acute chest pain without obvious organic cause before age 40: Personality and recent life events. *Journal of Psychosomatic Research, 31*, 215–221.

ROBINS, L. N., HELZER, J. E., CROUGHAN, J., & RATCLIFF, K. S. (1981). National Institute of Mental Health Diagnostic Interview Schedule: Its history, characteristics, and validity. *Archives of General Psychiatry, 38*, 381–389.

SAMMONS, M. T., & KAROLY, P. (1987). Psychosocial variables in irritable bowel syndrome: A review and proposal. *Clinical Psychology Review, 7*, 187–204.

SCHUSTER, M. M. (1983). Irritable bowel syndrome: Applications of psychophysiological methods to treatment. In R. Hölzl & W. E. Whitehead (Eds.), *Psychophysiology of the gastrointestinal tract: Experimental and clinical applications*. New York: Plenum.

SCHUSTER, M. M., NIKOOMANESH, P., & WELLS, D. (1973). Biofeedback control of lower esophageal sphincter contraction. *Rendiconti di Gastroenterologica, 5*, 14–18.

SCHWARTZ, D. P., LARGE, H. S., DEGOOD, D. E., WEGENER, S. T., & ROWLINGSON, J. C. (1984). A chronic emergency room visitor with chest pain: Successful treatment by stress management training and biofeedback. *Pain, 18*, 315–319.

SJÖDIN, I. (1983). Psychotherapy in peptic ulcer disease: A controlled outcome study. *Acta Psychiatrica Scandinavica, 67*, (Supplement 307), 1–90.

SNAPE, W. J., CARLSON, G. M., MATARAZZO, S. A., & COHEN, S. (1977). Evidence that abnormal myoelectrical activity produces colonic motor dysfunction in the irritable bowel syndrome. *Gastroenterology, 72*, 383–387.

SONNENBERG, A. (1989). Costs of medical and surgical treatment of duodenal ulcer. *Gastroenterology, 96*, 1445–1452.

STACHER, G. (1983). The responsiveness of the esophagus to environmental stimuli. In R. Hölzl & W. E. Whitehead (Eds.), *Psychophysiology of the gastrointestinal tract: Experimental and clinical applications.* New York: Plenum.

STACHER, G., SCHMIERER, G., & LANDGRAF, M. (1979). Tertiary esophageal contractions evoked by acoustical stimuli. *Gastroenterology, 77*, 49–54.

STACHER, G., STEINRINGER, H., BLAU, A., & LANDGRAF, M. (1979). Acoustically evoked esophageal contractions and defense reaction. *Psychophysiology, 16*, 234–241.

STEINHART, M. J., WONG, P. Y., & ZARR, M. L. (1981). Therapeutic usefulness of amitriptyline in spastic colon syndrome. *International Journal of Psychiatry in Medicine, 11*, 45–57.

STERN, R. M. (1983). Responsiveness of the stomach to environmental events. In R. Hölzl & W. E. Whitehead (Eds.), *Psychophysiology of the gastrointestinal tract: Experimental and clinical applications.* New York: Plenum.

SVEDLUND, J., SJÖDIN, I., OTTOSSON, J-O., & DOTEVALL, G. (1983). Controlled study of psychotherapy in irritable bowel syndrome. *Lancet, 2*, 589–592.

SWITZ, D. M. (1976). What the gastroenterologist does all day: A survey of a state society's practice. *Gastroenterology, 70*, 1048–1050.

TAYLOR, I., DUTHIE, C., HAMMOND, P., & BASU, P. (1978). Is there a myoelectric abnormality in the irritable colon syndrome? *Gut, 19*, 391–395.

THOMPSON, W. G., DOTEVALL, G., DROSSMAN, D. A., HEATON, K. W., & KRUIS, W. (1989). Irritable bowel syndrome: Guidelines for the diagnosis. *Gastroenterology International, 2*, 92–95.

THOMPSON, W. G., & HEATON, K. W. (1980). Functional bowel disorder in apparently healthy people. *Gastroenterology, 79*, 283–288.

VITALIANO, P. P., KATON, W., MAIURO, R. D., & RUSSO, J. (1989). Coping in chest pain patients with and without psychiatric disorders. *Journal of Consulting and Clinical Psychology, 57*, 338–343.

WALKER, B. B. (1983). Treating stomach disorders: Can we reinstate regulatory processes? In R. Hölzl & W. E. Whitehead (Eds.), *Psychophysiology of the gastrointestinal tract: Experimental and clinical applications.* New York: Plenum.

WALKER, P., LUTHER, J., SAMLOFF,. I. M., & FELDMAN, M. (1988). Life events stress and psychosocial factors in men with peptic ulcer disease. II. Relationships with serum pepsinogen concentrations and behavioral risk factors. *Gastroenterology, 94*, 323–330.

WANGEL, A, G., & DELLER, D. J. (1965). Intestinal motility in man. III. Mechanisms of constipation and diarrhea with particular reference to the irritable colon syndrome. *Gastroenterology, 48,* 69–84.

WATSON, W. C., SULLIVAN, S. N., CORKE, M., & RUSH, D. (1976). Incidence of oesophageal symptoms in patients with irritable bowel syndromes. *Gut, 17,* 827.

WEILGOSZ, A. J., & EARP, J. (1986). Perceived vulnerability to serious heart disease and persistent pain in patients with minimal or no coronary disease. *Psychosomatic Medicine, 48,* 118–124.

WEISS, J. M. (1968). Effects of coping responses on stress. *Journal of Comparative and Physiological Psychology, 65,* 251–260.

WEISS, J. M. (1971a). Effects of coping behavior in different warning-signal conditions on stress pathology in rats. *Journal of Comparative and Physiological Psychology, 77,* 1–13.

WEISS, J. M. (1971b). Effects of coping behavior with and without a feedback signal on stress pathology in rats. *Journal of Comparative and Physiological Psychology, 77,* 22–30.

WEISS, J. M (1977). Ulcers. In J. D. Maser & M. E. P. Seligman (Eds.). *Psychopathology: Experimental models.* San Francisco: Freeman.

WEISS, J. M. (1984). Behavioral and psychological influences on gastrointestinal pathology: Experimental techniques and findings. In W. D. Gentry (Ed.), *Handbook of behavioral medicine.* New York: Guilford Press.

WELGAN, P. R. (1974). Learned control of gastric acid secretions in peptic ulcer patients. *Psychosomatic Medicine, 36,* 411–419.

WELGAN, P. R. (1977). Biofeedback control of stomach acid secretions and gastrointestinal reactions. In J. Beaty & H. Legewie (Eds.), *Biofeedback and behavior.* New York: Plenum.

WEST, K. L. (1970). MMPI correlates of ulcerative colitis. *Journal of Clinical Psychology, 26,* 214–219.

WHITEHEAD, W. E., & BOSMAJIAN, L. S. (1982). Behavioral medicine approaches to gastrointestinal disorders. *Journal of Consulting and Clinical Psychology, 50,* 972–983.

WHITEHEAD, W. E., BOSMAJIAN, L., ZONDERMAN, A. B., COSTA, P. T., & SCHUSTER, M. M. (1988). Symptoms of psychologic distress associated with irritable bowel syndrome: Comparison of community and medical clinic samples. *Gastroenterology, 95,* 709–714.

WHITEHEAD, W. E., ENGEL, B. T., & SCHUSTER, M. M. (1980). Irritable bowel syndrome: Physiological and psychological differences between diarrhea-predominant and constipation-predominant patients. *Digestive Diseases and Sciences, 25,* 404–413.

WHITEHEAD, W. E., RENAULT, P. F., & GOLDIAMOND, I. (1975). Modification of human gastric acid secretion with operant-conditioning procedures. *Journal of Applied Behavior Analysis, 8,* 147–156.

WHITEHEAD, W. E., WINGET, C., FEDORAVICIUS, A. S., WOOLEY, S., & BLACKWELL, B. (1982). Learned illness behavior in patients with irritable bowel syndrome and peptic ulcer. *Digestive Diseases and Sciences, 27,* 202–208.

WHORWELL, P. J., CLOUTER, C., & SMITH, C. L. (1981). Oesophageal motility in the irritable bowel syndrome. *British Medical Journal, 282,* 1101–1102.

WHORWELL, P. J., PRIOR, A., & COLGAN, S. M. (1987). Hypnotherapy in severe irritable bowel syndrome: Further experience. *Gut, 28,* 423–425.

WHORWELL, P. J., PRIOR, A., & FARAGHER, E. B. (1984). Controlled trial of hypnotherapy in the treatment of severe refractory irritable-bowel syndrome. *Lancet, 3,* 1232–1234.

WOLF, S., & ALMY. T. P. (1949). Experimental observations on cardiospasm in man. *Gastroenterology, 13,* 401–421.

WOLF, S., ALMY, T. P., BACHRACH, W. H., SPIRO, H. M., STURDEVANT, R. A. L., & WEINER, H. (1979). The role of stress in peptic ulcer disease. *Journal of Human Stress, 5,* 27–37.

WRIGHT, L. E., & CASTELL, D. O. (1975). The adverse effect of chocolate in lower esophageal sphincter pressure. *American Journal of Digestive Diseases, 20,* 703–707.

YOUELL, K. J., & MCCOLLOUGH, J. P. (1975). Behavioral treatment of mucous colitis. *Journal of Consulting and Clinical Psychology, 43,* 740–745.

YOUNG, L. D., RICHTER, J. E., ANDERSON, K. O., BRADLEY, L. A., KATZ, P. O., MCELVEEN, L., OBRECHT, W. F., DALTON, C., & SNYDER, R. M. (1987). The effects of psychological and environmental stress on peristaltic esophageal contractions in healthy volunteers. *Psychophysiology, 24,* 132–141.

YOUNG, L. D., RICHTER, J. E., BRADLEY, L. A., & ANDERSON, K. O. (1987). Disorders of the upper gastrointestinal system: An overview. *Annals of Behavioral Medicine, 9,* 7–12.

YOUNG, S. J., ALPERS, D. H., NORLAND, C. C., & WOODRUFF, R. A. (1976). Psychiatric illness and the irritable bowel syndrome: Practical implications for the primary physician. *Gastroenterology, 70,* 162–166.

# Chronic Pain Syndromes

Everyone has experienced pain, and at first glance pain would seem to be one of the most easily understood aspects of health and illness. We all quickly make the association between injury and pain, and few people would argue immediately with the proposition that pain is due to tissue damage and provides a signal of illness or injury. However, a little reflection suggests that pain is not as simple a phenomenon as it first appears to be. For example, what about situations when an injury occurs but the injured person does not experience pain? It is doubtful that any readers of this book have not been engaged in some strenuous activity and later found that they cut, bruised, or otherwise injured themselves without noticing it at the time. Similarly, soldiers in combat or accident victims are sometimes able to function during a crisis without noticing the extent of their injury or feeling its pain. How do psychological events, such as involvement in activities and attention to external stimuli, interfere with the experience of pain?

At the opposite end of the spectrum, consider those situations in which a person complains of the presence of pain, yet no physical cause may be found. It is common to hear it said that a person's pain is "all in his head" in such situations, but what does this really mean? Even if no physical damage or illness is present, the person reporting the pain experiences discomfort just as if a clearly identifiable cause were present, and it is not likely to be helpful to dismiss the pain as "imaginary." After all, pain is an experience ultimately verifiable only by the sufferer, and if an individual reports the presence of pain, it is very difficult to deny the possibility that it may indeed exist. The situation may become even more complicated if an injury or illness once existed but has since healed or been cured. A man may physically recover from a back injury suffered in an automobile accident yet continue to experience pain in the formerly injured, but now healed, back. What is causing the continuing subjective experience of pain in this case, and if physical recovery has not stopped the pain, what alternative treatments may exist? As an extreme example of pain without a clear physical explanation, consider *phantom limb pain*. In this disorder a person who has lost a leg or arm reports the presence of pain in the now absent limb. It is clear that pain in a missing limb is in reality impossible, yet the sufferer experiences pain nonetheless. And what of those who have experienced a psychological trauma, such as a divorce, and express their feelings by saying that they "feel hurt"? Is this pain the same as the pain of a injured arm? Might the man who has recovered from back surgery still feel pain because of the loss of his job as a construction worker and the consequent psychological trauma of a deteriorating financial situation?

In an effort to deal with the difficulties involved in the study of such an elusive phenomenon as pain, the International Association for the Study of Pain has suggested that pain be defined as "an unpleasant sensory and emotional experience associated with actual or potential tissue damage, or described in terms of such damage" (Brena, 1983, p. 15). Note that this definition avoids the pitfall of insisting on a direct relationship between physical damage and pain but instead focuses on the experience of the individual. The pain experience may be understood and treated differently dependent on the physical status of the sufferer, but there is no argument concerning the presence or absence of pain based on physical findings. The sufferer's experience determines the presence of pain.

Acute pain, or pain of a few days to a few weeks duration, seldom presents a major problem in treatment or results in serious psychological and social problems. However, chronic pain, commonly defined as pain lasting more than six months, represents a much larger problem. It has been estimated that 75 million Americans suffer from some type of chronic pain; about 23 million suffer from backaches and 24 million from severe headaches. These numbers suggest that the total economic cost of chronic pain is about $57 billion per year, although it may be as high as $80 billion per year (Brena, 1983). Thus, chronic pain not only poses a difficult set of scientific questions but also represents an issue of major economic and social importance. The balance of this chapter is devoted to an overview of the two most prevalent types of chronic pain: headache and back pain.

# *Headache*

Headache is one of the most common health complaints. It has been estimated that 80% of the U.S. population suffers from at least one headache each year and 10%–15% of the population of the U.S. and Northern Europe suffer from severe, recurrent headaches (Ziegler, 1984). Headache was the chief complaint in 8,684,000 visits to physicians in 1985, making it the seventeenth most common reason for visits to the doctor in the United States (National Center for Health Statistics, 1987). In a review synthesizing the statistics regarding headaches of various types, Kurtz (1982) estimated that about 10% of the population suffer from migraine headache, and 15% of the population suffer from tension headache or some other type of headache. The differences in tension and migraine headache are discussed in more detail below.

Treatment for headache may involve both medical and psychological procedures and varies dependent on the nature of the headache. Medication may be used to relax muscles and/or reduce vascular dilation. Relaxation training and biofeedback may be employed to increase an individual's control over and awareness of psychophysiological responses. Additionally, psychotherapy may be suggested as a means of dealing with conflicts related to continuing stress in the headache sufferer's life. All of the above treatment strategies have been shown to be effective in some cases, but there is considerable debate as to the reasons for the success of most treatment approaches. The physical and psychological phenomena associated with headache are also less clearly understood than might be expected in so common a disorder. The following pages review the current state of the art in the understanding and treatment of migraine and tension headache.

## Biological and Psychophysiological Components

The biological events associated with a headache differ dependent on the variety of headache involved. In *tension headache*, also referred to as *muscle contraction headache*, the sufferer typically reports pain over the entire head. The pain is often described as a dull and steady ache, and some individuals report feeling pressure, as if there is a tight band around their head. Often the headache begins in the occipital (rear) region of the skull or in the neck and shoulders and then moves up to involve the rest of the skull.

As the name implies, tension headache has typically been explained as due to sustained contraction of the muscles of the head, neck, and/or shoulders. However, the role of elevated muscle tension is not as clear as might be expected, particularly tension in the muscles of the forehead. Philips (1977) found that frontal (forehead) EMG levels were higher in tension headache patients than in people without tension headache, but frontal EMG levels were not higher when the patients were experiencing a headache than when they were headache free. In contrast, Haynes et al. (1983) reported that neck, but not frontal, EMG levels were higher during headache periods than during headache-free periods. Tension headache sufferers trained to *increase* frontal muscle tension have shown reductions in headache activity similar to that shown in patients trained to decrease their levels of frontal muscle tension (Andrasik & Holroyd, 1980). Similarly, Onorato and Tsushima (1983) found no relationship between reductions in frontal EMG activity with biofeedback training and reductions in pain behaviors associated with tension headache. It thus appears that factors other than elevated muscle tension in the forehead must be related to the pain experienced in muscle contraction headache, but the exact nature of these additional factors remains unclear. One possibility involves abnormalities in blood flow. Tension headache sufferers have been reported not only to experience elevated neck muscle EMG levels but also to experience dilation of the temporal artery during a headache (Haynes et al., 1983). Vasodilation is characteristic of migraine headaches, so there is some evidence that tension and migraine headache share some elements.

The pain of *migraine headache* is often unilateral; that is, it is experienced on only one side of the head. Migraine sufferers describe the pain as a throbbing sensation and often experience nausea, vomiting, and extreme sensitivity to light and sound during the headache. Many migraine sufferers experience a tension headache after the most painful portion of the migraine has passed. This usually viewed as a result of tension in the muscles of the neck and shoulders induced by the individual's attempts to cope with the migraine pain.

A migraine is composed of two stages, with distinct physiological events occurring in each stage. Initially, cranial and cerebral arteries constrict, thus reducing the supply of blood and oxygen to the brain. During this first phase, the sufferer may experience prodromal, or preheadache, symptoms, also referred to as an *aura*. Symptoms during the aura may include visual irregularities, such as blind spots or flashes of light, and muscle weakness or other motor or sensory problems. The aura typically lasts for a few minutes to an hour. The alert reader will note that these symptoms are similar to those associated with a transient ischemic attack, described previously in Chapter 8. The symptoms in both disorders are associated with a temporarily reduced supply of blood and oxygen to the brain. Migraine headache with prodromal symptoms is referred to as classic migraine. If no aura is present the headache is referred to as common migraine. About 15% of migraineurs report experiencing an aura (Friedman, 1979).

It is in the second stage of the migraine that the sufferer is likely to experience pain. During this phase the cerebral arteries, which were previously constricted, dilate, or expand. It is this sudden overexpansion of the blood vessels that leads to the throbbing and pulsing pain of the migraine headache itself; the walls of arteries become inflamed and *vascular edema*, or an oversupply of blood, occurs. As the vasculature returns to normal, the pain of the migraine gradually subsides.

Although the pattern of physiological events that occur in a migraine is well established, the psychophysiological characteristics that make migraineurs prone to such vascular events are less certain. It has been suggested that the vasculature of migraine sufferers is less stable than the vasculature of persons free of migraine (Dalessio, 1980), and this instability increases the risk of the sudden contractions and dilations that result in a migraine headache. There is also evidence that migraine headache may be related to increased vascular response to stress. Rojahn and Gerhards (1986) subjected migraine sufferers and headache-free controls to an aversive noise. Migraine sufferers showed a significantly greater increase in the volume of blood pulsing through the temporal artery during the stressful noise than did the controls. Other evidence suggests that there is no difference in the stability of the vasculature of migraineurs and normals but instead that migraineurs show consistently warmer head and hand temperatures than normals. This increased temperature is presumably associated with increased blood flow in migraine sufferers (Cohen, Rickles, & McArthur, 1978). Although migraine does appear to be associated with some irregularity in blood flow, the exact nature of this irregularity is unclear.

## Behavioral and Psychosocial Factors

Behavioral and psychosocial factors have long been suspected of playing important causative roles in both tension and migraine headache. Migraine headache sufferers have been described as perfectionistic, rigid, preoccupied with success, resentful, and unconsciously hostile. Tension headache has been characterized as related to dependence, depression, worry, and sexual conflicts (Blanchard, Andrasik, & Arena, 1984). However, the great majority of these descriptors have been derived from uncontrolled case studies and may be questioned based on the weaknesses of the case study approach discussed in Chapter 2. The headache sufferers described in these case studies are unlikely to be representative of all headache sufferers. Instead, the unusual nature of their cases probably play a large part in why they were selected for detailed study and publication. Thus, it may be that only individuals experiencing headaches resistant to the standard treatment approaches possess these personality characteristics. Perhaps more importantly, the question arises as to whether the behavioral and psychological factors noted were really causes of the headaches or if instead they were results of experiencing chronic pain and its associated problems in living.

Potential psychological causes of headache have been investigated in more tightly controlled studies as well, usually using standardized psychological tests and/or interviews. In general, the results of these studies indicate that persons experiencing difficulties with headaches do appear more psychologically distressed than headache-free individuals. A powerful determinant of the degree of disturbance present is the *pain density* of the headache symptom picture

(Sternbach, Dalessio, Kunzel, & Bowman, 1980). Pain density is a summary indicator of the severity of pain and is derived by multiplying headache frequency by headache intensity. Migraineurs would be likely to score lower on pain density than tension headache sufferers because migraine headaches tend to occur less frequently than tension headaches and are not always more painful than tension headaches.

Migraine sufferers usually appear less disturbed than tension headache patients (Blanchard et al., 1984), perhaps as a result of the lower pain density of migraine. The nature of their disturbance might best be characterized as generalized psychological distress rather than a specific "headache personality." In fact, Hundleby and Loucks (1985) compared 91 migraineurs to 126 nonmigraineurs and concluded that there was insufficient evidence to support the contention that there was any real usefulness to the construct of a "migraine personality." Migraine headaches have been reported to be associated with the presence of the Type A Behavior Pattern (Hicks & Campbell, 1983; Rappaport, McAnulty, & Brantley, 1988). Type A behavior may thus be a risk factor for vascular disorders other than heart disease (Rappaport et al., 1988). However, chronic migraine headaches might also contribute to the development of Type A behavior. The risk of frequent headaches that interfere with the ability to attend to daily tasks may easily be imagined to promote a sense of a need to accomplish more and more in less and less time, as suggested by the Type A findings.

The current view of psychological and behavioral contributions to headache may be described as one of an interaction between a physiological predisposition, psychological factors, and perceived environmental stresses. Levor, Cohen, Naliboff, McArthur, and Heuser (1986) examined the daily activities, stresses, emotions, and headache symptoms of 33 migraine headache sufferers. Their data suggested that a headache was the culmination of a multiday cycle of increasing perceived stress and declining physical activity. As stresses increased and physical activity declined, a headache became more likely. The authors suggested that physiological arousal in migraineurs occurs at lower stress levels than in nonmigraineurs, but it is not possible to say whether heightened physiological arousal leads the headache sufferer to be more sensitive to stress or whether migraineurs are less tolerant of stress than headache-free individuals. In tension headaches, stressful events may prevent a person from relaxing and returning to a normal arousal level. When someone's attention is directed toward stressful events, he or she may not notice the warning signs of an impending headache, such as increased muscle tension. This continuing unnoticed arousal may eventually result in a tension headache (Hovanitz, Chin, & Warm, 1989). The position is thus one of interaction between psychosocial and physiological factors. It is uncertain, and perhaps not crucial, whether psychological or physiological events are primary. Indeed, it may be that the most important causative factor in some headache sufferers is physiological, whereas in others the most important factors may be psychological. From a practical point of view, psychological, behavioral, and physiological phenomena are likely to need attention in treatment.

## Treatment Programs

The treatment programs most commonly used for migraine and tension headaches share many features. Differences that exist are related to the physiological characteristics of the two types of headaches. The most common treatments include several modalities of biofeedback and relaxation training.

ELECTROMYOGRAPHIC BIOFEEDBACK   The most frequently used form of biofeedback treatment for headaches is electromyographic biofeedback, also referred to as *EMG biofeedback*. All forms of biofeedback use instrumentation to allow the subject to become aware of physiological responses usually below the threshold of awareness. In the case of EMG feedback, the subject is provided with information concerning levels of muscle tension. This information, usually provided by an auditory or visual signal such as a tone or a light display, can then be used by the subject to learn how to control muscle tension. The learning processes underlying biofeedback are those of operant conditioning, discussed in Chapter 4. As the subject experiments with his or her behavior, the biofeedback signal acts as a reinforcer of responses that alter the signal in the desired fashion. Thus, a headache patient participating in EMG biofeedback treatment may learn what he or she can do to lower the pitch of the biofeedback signal, reflecting a decrease in muscle tension.

This treatment program would appear at first glance to be an excellent intervention for tension headache sufferers. For this reason, EMG biofeedback has been the focus of considerable research and has been used in the clinic in the treatment of many patients experiencing tension headaches. The biofeedback subject usually sits quietly with eyes closed and uses the biofeedback signal as an aid to relaxation. Electrodes are attached by a tapelike adhesive to the surface of the subject's skin over the tense muscles, usually the forehead or neck. The electrodes measure the level of electrical activity in the subject's muscles. No electrical current flows through the electrodes to the subject. The more tense the muscles are, the higher the level of electrical activity measured by the biofeedback equipment.

One of the earliest studies of the use of EMG biofeedback in tension headache was conducted by Budzynski, Stoyva, and Adler (1970). These three investigators reported that after four to eight weeks of EMG biofeedback training five tension headache patients experienced a significant reduction in their levels of frontal (forehead) muscle tension and headache activity. Since this early report, numerous other studies have appeared suggesting that EMG biofeedback is an effective treatment for tension headache.

Despite this general agreement, there is considerable controversy about the relative efficiency of EMG biofeedback and other treatment approaches and the active elements in EMG biofeedback. Much of this debate has been stimulated by the findings mentioned earlier regarding the lack of evidence that tension headache is reliably associated with increased muscle tension. If increased muscle tension is not a consistent problem in tension headache patients, why does learning to reduce muscle tension help many tension headache sufferers? And furthermore, how could it be that training to increase muscle tension may also lead to a reduction in headaches, as demonstrated by the studies of Andrasik, Holroyd, and colleagues discussed in Chapter 2 (Andrasik & Holroyd, 1980; Holroyd et al., 1984)?

The most likely explanation of this apparent paradox is that EMG biofeedback, like the other treatment strategies to be discussed, provides the subject with two primary benefits: (1) education in a relaxation strategy and (2) an experience of success in controlling physiological reactivity. The experiences of success may alter the expectations of the subject, so stressful situations previously seen as inevitably leading to a headache are dealt with adaptively. Successful coping leads to a reduction in the subject's stress responses, and thus to a reduction in headache activity (Holroyd et al., 1984).

TEMPERATURE BIOFEEDBACK  If EMG biofeedback initially appears to be a program tailor-made for tension headache, then temperature biofeedback seems to be correspondingly appropriate for migraine. A person participating in this form of biofeedback training learns to increase surface skin temperature, usually on a finger. Skin temperature increases are due to an increase in blood flow, so the subject is really learning to control the blood flow to the region of the body to which the temperature sensor is attached. Because migraine headaches are related to irregularities in blood flow, this type of biofeedback may provide a way to teach a migraineur to control the underlying cause of her or his headache.

The use of finger-temperature biofeedback for migraine headache was first reported by Sargent, Green, and Walters (1972). In this initial study, migraine patients received finger-temperature biofeedback and autogenic training, a form of relaxation training in which subjects attempt to induce physiological changes by repeating phrases such as "My hands are heavy and warm, my whole body is relaxed and warm." Biofeedback was used during the early phases of the treatment program. A majority of the migraine patients were rated as being improved as a result of this treatment program.

This early investigation suffered from several weaknesses, most notably the lack of a control group, the combination of biofeedback with autogenic training, and the impressionistic nature of the outcome data. However, the encouraging results lead to a series of investigations of the effectiveness of temperature biofeedback for migraine headache. The results of many such studies suggest that temperature biofeedback may be an effective treatment for migraine headache and is superior to medication-placebo treatments, but it is generally no more effective than other treatment approaches such as relaxation training and autogenic training. In fact, it is likely that most of the successful behavioral treatments for migraine headache work by training in relaxation procedures (Blanchard, Andrasik, Ahles, & Teders, 1980). Relaxation training is discussed in more detail below.

The use of temperature biofeedback as a treatment for migraine headache hinges on the assumption that peripheral blood flow and blood flow in the arteries in the head where the headache occurs are related. In the typical temperature biofeedback program, a migraine sufferer learns to alter the temperature of a finger. If the effectiveness of the training program is directly related to the biofeedback, and resultant control over peripheral blood flow, there should be a demonstrable relationship between blood flow in the fingers and in the head. There is reason to question the existence of this relationship.

Largen, Mathew, Dobbins, Meyer, and Claghorn (1978) trained different subjects to increase or decrease finger temperature and later measured cerebral blood flow. Although the subjects were documented to have learned to alter finger temperature in the desired direction, no relationship between finger temperature changes and cerebral blood flow were found. Those suffering from migraine and those without migraine have also been reported to show increases, not decreases, in temporal artery blood flow when finger temperature increased (Price & Tursky, 1976). It may therefore be more reasonable to train migraine sufferers to control cerebral blood flow by providing feedback directly from the temporal artery.

*Temporal cooling* has been suggested as one means of directly altering cerebral blood flow. In this form of biofeedback, a subject is provided with information concerning the temperature of the temporal artery and attempts to learn to lower the temperature of the blood vessel. A reduction in temperature should be a reflection of reduced blood flow. Gauthier, Bois, Allaire, and Drolet (1981) reported that finger-warming, finger-cooling, temporal-warming, and temporal-cooling feedback were all equally effective in reducing migraine symptoms, and Gamble and Elder (1983) reported that temporal cooling was associated with a reduction in hours per week of migraine pain. These results suggest that learned control of the temperature of the temporal artery may result in headache improvement, but the pattern of the results indicates that the reason for the improvement is unlikely to be as simple as might be hoped. If a reduction in blood flow was the reason for the success of the treatment, why would training in warming the temporal artery, which should increase blood flow, also result in improvement? If blood flow in the fingers and the head is unrelated, why should finger and temporal biofeedback be equally effective? Gauthier et al. (1981) speculated that it may be that the important ingredient is learned *stabilization* of blood flow rather than learned increases or decreases in blood flow. If a migraine sufferer learns to control blood flow, and thus stabilize her or his vascular responses, this might result in the avoidance of the vasoconstriction followed by vasodilation involved in the migraine headache.

CEPHALIC VASOMOTOR RESPONSE BIOFEEDBACK    Cephalic vasomotor response (CVMR) biofeedback is a technique that avoids the problem of the presence or absence of a relationship between skin temperature and blood flow by providing feedback based directly on blood flow. In order to do this, a tiny light is focused on the temporal artery. Reflection from this light provides an indication of the diameter of the artery, and thus blood flow in the artery itself. Information from this apparatus, called a *photoplethysmograph*, is then fed to a computer, and, information regarding the artery's dilation is provided to the migraine sufferer by means of a tone, a light, or some other signal.

Perhaps the most influential study of CVMR feedback was conducted by Bild and Adams (1980). In this study, seven migraine sufferers receiving CVMR feedback were compared to six receiving EMG feedback and six waiting-list control patients. CVMR feedback patients reported significantly fewer headaches per week than the other two groups, a significant reduction in headache duration in comparison to the control group, and showed decreases in medication use, although the pattern of medication changes was not statistically analyzed. However, as with temperature feedback, the mechanisms underlying the potential effectiveness of CVMR feedback in the treatment of migraine headache may not be as simple as it initially appears.

This lack of simplicity is illustrated in a more recent study by Gauthier, Doyon, Lacroix, and Drolet (1983). In this project, some migraineurs received the typical form of CVMR feedback and were trained to constrict the temporal artery. However, other migraine sufferers were taught to *dilate* the temporal artery through the use of CVMR feedback. Both types of feedback resulted in equal improvement in headache activity, and the amount of learned dilation or constriction was unrelated to the amount of headache improvement. However, headache improvement was associated with a reduction in variability of the blood flow in the temporal artery. As with temperature feedback, Gauthier et al. (1983) suggested that the effectiveness of CVMR feedback may be related to reduced variability (or increased stability) in the vascular system. It may not be important whether one learns to expand or contract the temporal artery, for either type of learning results in control leading to stability.

RELAXATION TRAINING    Relaxation training is often used in the treatment of tension and headaches. The rationale for using relaxation training is essentially the same as that for EMG biofeedback, as patients are given direct instructions regarding how to relax their muscles with the hope that reduced levels of muscle tension will lead to reduced headache activity.

A variety of relaxation methods exist. However, most encourage subjects to concentrate on the sensations in their muscles and then provide specific instructions for how to begin to let those muscles relax. One of the most common techniques is Progressive Muscle Relaxation (Jacobson, 1938). In this procedure, subjects are asked to physically tense various muscle groups, hold this tension for a few seconds, and then to release the tension and allow the muscles to relax. A patient is thus asked to first tense the muscles in the hands, hold the tension, and then let it go. Next the subject tenses the muscles in the forearms, holds it, and lets it go. This procedure then continues until all the muscle groups in the body have been relaxed. By first tensing and then relaxing the muscles, subjects are able to feel the contrast between tense and relaxed muscles and learn procedures for controlling muscle tension as they release the tension they have induced. Other relaxation procedures do not include an initial tensing period but instead give suggestions for letting tension go. Subjects may be encouraged to visualize their muscles becoming longer and looser, and to feel warmth and relaxation spreading over their body. Some of these procedures may have a meditative or hypnotic quality, as subjects are encouraged to focus inwardly and ignore outward distractions as they concentrate on the sensations in their body.

There is some evidence that relaxation training may be as effective as biofeedback in the treatment of tension headache. Haynes, Griffin, Mooney, and Parise (1975) reported equal headache improvement in persons receiving EMG biofeedback and relaxation training. Holmes and Burish (1983) reviewed the tension headache treatment literature and concluded that EMG biofeedback had no advantages over relaxation training. In fact, they suggested that EMG biofeedback might be viewed as less advantageous as a result of the cost of the biofeedback equipment.

However, relaxation training and biofeedback have not always been found to yield equivalent results. Daley, Donn, Galliher, and Zimmerman (1983) found that tension and migraine headache patients who received biofeedback reported fewer headaches per month than those who received only relaxation training. It is not uncommon for biofeedback and relaxation training to be combined. Janssen (1983) found no differences in headache improvement between tension headache sufferers who received EMG biofeedback and those who received EMG biofeedback and relaxation training, although those receiving the combined treatment reported fewer days of sick leave and fewer days of incapacitating pain than those receiving only biofeedback.

Whether biofeedback, relaxation, or a combination of the two is used, it is important that the patients practice the skills that they are learning and try to apply them outside the treatment setting. Patients are often given a tape recording of a relaxation procedure to use as they practice. In some cases, home practice with a relaxation tape in combination with relatively few contacts with the therapist may be a cost-effective treatment (Blanchard et al., 1988; Teders et al., 1984). It is important to remember that these home-based treatment programs were preceded by a careful professional diagnosis. All patients met with the therapist to be instructed in the relaxation procedure, were given manuals to follow for home practice, and met personally with the therapist a total of three times over an eight-week program. Phone contacts were also made during two of the appointment-free weeks. A case in which biofeedback and relaxation training with home practice were combined is presented in Boxed Highlight 14.1.

BOXED HIGHLIGHT 14.1

# Treatment of a Case of Tension Headache

Mrs. P. G. was a forty-two-year-old female with a five-year history of tension headaches. Her headaches had gradually worsened to the point that she was unable to remember more than two consecutive days without a headache during the last year before she came for treatment. She had been treating her headaches with aspirin and rest.

The first session was devoted to taking a history of Mrs. P. G.'s headache symptoms and a description of her current social and marital situation. Her marriage and family life was described as "fine," although her three children had been moving out of the house and going to college during the last four years. She now spent her headache-free days doing housework and getting together with her friends. Except for the interference with her activities caused by the headaches and some mild depression she attributed to this interference, she felt satisfied with her daily life.

The patient was introduced to the biofeedback equipment at the end of the first session. Her forehead and neck muscle EMG levels were found to be moderately elevated, although she did not report a headache at that time. EMG biofeedback was used for the first half of the second session, and the patient was able to see that her muscles began to relax as she calmed and became habituated to the treatment room. She was then introduced to relaxation training; she expressed a preference for the relaxation training over the biofeed-

back because she found the biofeedback signal to be distracting as she tried to relax. She was given a tape recording of the procedure and instructed to use it at home twice a day.

At the third session, the patient was connected to the biofeedback equipment, but the signal was not turned on. Instead, the equipment was used to monitor her muscle tension levels as she relaxed. A similar procedure was followed during sessions four through eight, and Mrs. P. G.'s muscle tension levels gradually decreased. She also reported fewer and less-severe headaches. After a total of eight weekly sessions she reported having gone for a week without a headache, and she felt much encouraged about her ability to control her headaches in the future.

She was seen every other week for four more sessions. During this time her headaches continued to be mild and infrequent, and her EMG levels continued to be in the normal range. She also reported that she had begun to look for a job outside the house. She started a job at a local community service organization just before the final regular session. At this last session she commented that because her headaches were under control she felt able to become involved in the activities she had not had time for while her children were at home, and she was looking forward to her outside work. She was given an appointment for a follow-up session a month later.

(continued)

*BOXED HIGHLIGHT 14.1 (continued)*

At the follow-up meeting she reported that she had not had a headache for three weeks, and she was enjoying her job and the friends she had made at work. Her EMG levels continued to be normal.

---

On the average, it appears that biofeedback and relaxation training are equally effective for most tension headache patients. However, there may be some patients who benefit more from one treatment as opposed to the other or from a combination of the two treatments. Using biofeedback as a follow-up treatment to relaxation training in persons who continue to experience headache problems may offer a cost-efficient and reasonable alternative in some cases (Masters, Burish, Hollon, & Rimm, 1987). People also differ in their preferences for relaxation versus biofeedback, and the individual's perception that a reliable tool for relaxation is available may be more important in inducing relaxation than the actual use of the relaxation procedure (Prokop, Pratt, & Rhodes, 1987). The data of Holroyd et al. (1984) strongly suggest that it is the sense of competence and control over previously uncontrollable symptoms that is responsible for much of the improvement seen with biofeedback. It is thus important that the headache-treatment program be selected to fit the patient in order to increase the probability of success experiences. As the case of Mrs. P. G. suggests, it is not uncommon to see patients begin to make other changes in their life as their headaches improve and they begin to feel more confident in their abilities.

# Chronic Benign Pain

As was noted earlier in this chapter, chronic pain is typically defined as pain lasting for more than six months. However, many types of conditions may lead to chronic pain, ranging from muscle spasms to disease processes such as cancer, and the underlying physical or psychological reason for the chronic pain may have important implications for the most appropriate treatment. The term *chronic benign pain* refers to chronic pain that is *not* due to a malignant disease process, such as cancer. Low back pain is the prototypical example of chronic benign pain, and the following material concentrates on problems associated with low back pain.

Although slightly fewer people suffer from back pain as compared to headache, it has been estimated that about 5% of the U.S. population suffer from lower-back pain (Kurtzke, 1982). Back symptoms are the ninth most common reason for visits to physicians and accounted for 11,311,000 visits in 1985 (National Center for Health Statistics, 1987). The costs of low back pain to society are immense. A sense of the economic impact of chronic low back pain may be gained from considering the following figures. As noted earlier in this chapter, it has been estimated that 23 million persons in the United States suffer from back pain (Brena, 1983), and Brena, Chapman, and Decker (1981) estimated that the total costs to society of 1 million pain-disabled persons is $20 billion per year. The social costs of low back pain extend well beyond medical care directly related to pain relief but also include factors such as time lost from work, disability and compensation payments, and psychological treatment for distress related to continuing pain and the loss of normal interpersonal, vocational, and recreational activities that often accompanies pain and disability. Consider how your life would change if you began to experience severe pain whenever you exerted yourself or even stayed on your feet for more than a few minutes, and you may begin to appreciate the degree of life change and psychological distress that often exists coincident with low back pain. Not only does low back pain affect psychological and social functioning, but there is also substantial evidence that psychological and social factors may have a significant impact on low back pain itself.

## Biological and Psychophysiological Components

The most definitive causes of low back pain are *herniated disk* and arthritis. In cases of disk herniation, a vertebral disk in the spinal cord pushes out of place and exerts pressure on nerve roots. (Arthritis was discussed in detail in Chapter 12.) In other cases, low back pain appears to be related to chronic musculoskeletal stress. Chronic muscle stresses and strains may lead to the development of sensitive *trigger points* in the muscle tissue and *fascia*, or the fibrous membrane that covers the muscles. Pressure on the trigger points will lead to pain. Pain of this nature is referred to as *myofascial pain* (Melzack & Wall, 1983). As noted below, in many cases no clear physical reason for the pain may be found.

One of the most intriguing and perplexing problems concerning low back pain (as well as many other types of pain) involves the mechanisms underlying the interaction between psychological and physiological factors in pain perception. People differ in how they experience the pain of similar injuries or diseases. The pain experienced by any given individual fluctuates, even without any changes in physical condition. Thus, it is clear that pain may not be explained as simply a direct result of tissue injury. Low back pain provides a particularly graphic example of this problem, as it is often difficult to specify the exact nature of the physiological dysfunction underlying the pain, and discomfort of chronic low back pain waxes and wanes in many patients, often without obvious physical causes. In fact, it has been estimated that about 70% of low back pain patients have no demonstrable physical pathology underlying their pain (Loeser, 1980), and it appears that about 52.5% of patients treated for chronic low back pain are diagnosed as suffering from *functional* pain

(Prokop, 1988). The term *functional* is commonly applied to cases of low back pain where no physical reason for the pain can be found or where the pain is out of proportion to physical pathology.

The *gate-control theory* of pain (Melzack & Wall, 1983) has been proposed as a model for understanding how factors other than tissue damage may exert powerful influences on pain perception. According to the gate-control theory, activity in the spinal cord and the brain influence pain perception. (The gate-control model is illustrated in Figures 14.1a and 14.1b. Refer frequently to the figures to best understand the following discussion of gate-control theory.)

Sensory signals from the skin and viscera enter the spinal cord through the *dorsal horns*; the dorsal horns are the terminals on the dorsal, or back, side of the spinal cord where sensory neurons enter. Incoming sensory signals may be modulated, or changed, in the spinal cord, and they may be affected by signals traveling down the spinal cord from the brain. This interaction between incoming sensory signals from the skin and viscera and information from the brain occurs primarily in the *substantia gelatinosa*, located in the spinal cord. This name comes from its gelatinous, or gelatinlike, texture. (See Figure 14.1a for the location of this region.) The hypothesized "gate" is located in the substantia gelatinosa.

Three types of neural fibers are particularly important in the experience of pain, and all three types of fibers activate cells in the substantia gelatinosa. These include two types of small fibers, called *A-delta fibers* and *C fibers*, and one type of large fiber, called *A-beta fibers*. A-delta fibers transmit fast, sharp, and well-localized pain, while C fibers transmit pain experienced as slow, aching, and poorly localized (Mountcastle, 1980). The large A-beta fibers are sensitive to light pressure, and they activate cognitive processes that may influence activity in the gate by means of neural fibers descending from the brain (Melzack & Wall, 1983). The balance of activity in these large and small fibers determines whether or not pain will be experienced. Activity in the small fibers potentiates (increases) the experience of pain, and activity in the large fibers may potentiate or inhibit pain, dependent on circumstances to be discussed.

Large- and small-fiber stimulation results not only in activation of the substantia gelatinosa, but also in activation of transmission cells. The transmission cells sense the input from the gate in the substantia gelatinosa and transmit this information to the brain stem. Brain stem activity may inhibit pain by sending information down the spinal cord to the gate.

The gating mechanism is also affected by cognitive processes acting as a central control trigger in the brain. Large-fiber activity has direct and indirect effects on the gate. In addition to sending sensory information directly to the gate, large-fiber activity also stimulates cognitive processes in the brain; the resulting cognitive activity then affects the gate. Stimulation traveling up the spinal cord through the large fibers provides information that is interpreted

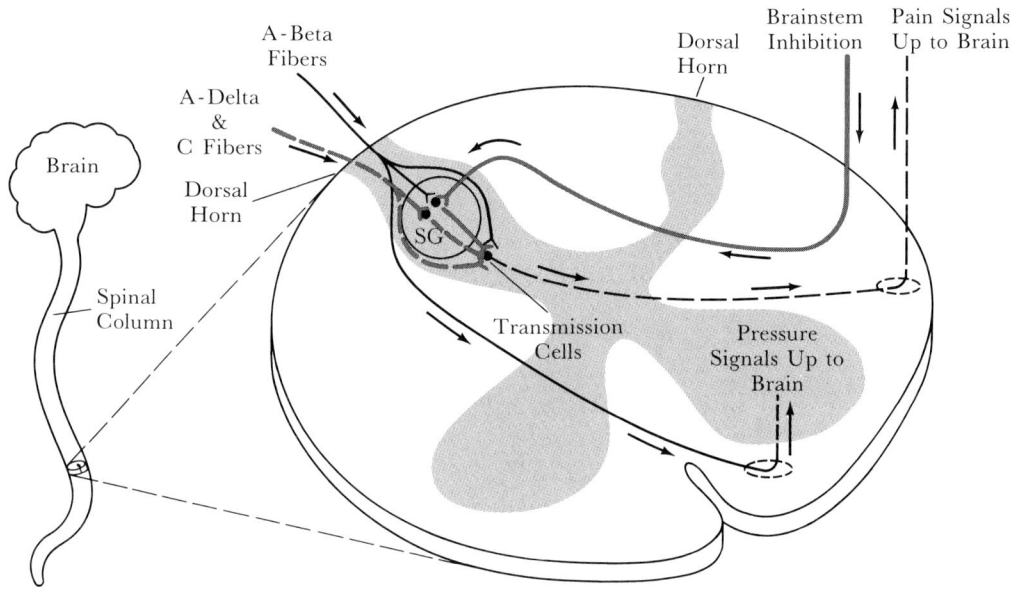

A

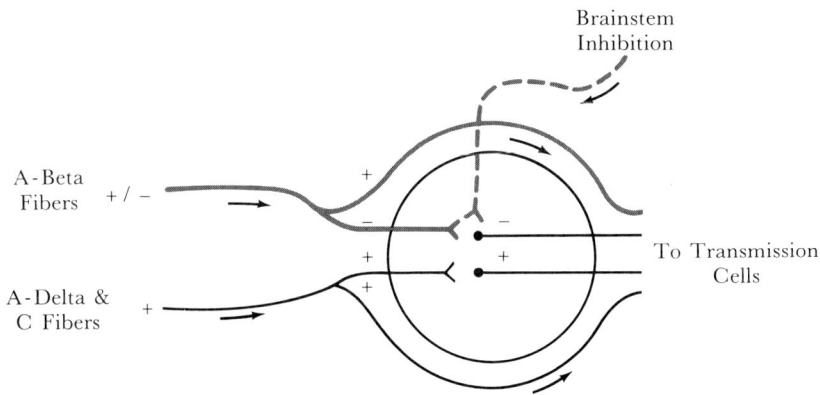

B

FIGURE 14.1   (a) Stylized cross-section of the spinal cord. The gate control theory of pain hypothesizes the existence of a "gate" in the spinal cord. The diagram shows the location of the gate and the nerve fibers leading into and out of the gate. The arrows indicate the direction of information flow in the nervous system. (b) Detail of gate in the substantia gelatinosa. Neural stimulation increasing pain is indicated by a plus (+) sign, and stimulation decreasing pain is indicated by a minus (−) sign. The "±" shows that stimulation of the A-beta fibers may increase or decrease pain.

in the brain, and information then travels back down the spinal cord to modify the sensory experience. In this way, personality factors and emotional reactions may have an impact on pain as activity in the brain will act to open or close the gate by means of this central control triggering mechanism. Anxiety, depression, and other negative emotions may act to open the gate and thus intensify the experience of pain, whereas pleasant experiences such as relaxation or distraction by involvement in other activities may close the gate and thereby reduce pain.

According to gate-control theory, pain is a complex process dependent on the relative activity in the large- and small-diameter fibers, the influence of central control processes from the cerebral cortex, and the presence of inhibitory controls from the brain stem. The transmission cells send information directly to the brain, while the substantia gelatinosa regulates, or "gates" the amount of information transmitted to the brain (Melzack & Wall, 1983). Stimulation of the small fibers (A-delta and C) activates the transmission cells and tends to open the gate. Activity in the large fibers (A-beta) activates the transmission cells but also tends to close the gate by calling central control processes into play and by direct action upon cells in the substantia gelatinosa. Inhibitory controls from the brainstem may also act to close the gate.

Gate-control theory provides a means of explaining many of the otherwise puzzling ways in which we experience pain. Gentle pressure, such as massage, may at times relieve pain and at other times increase pain. This is because in some cases the activity in the small fibers is so intense that the gate is open too much for the stimulation of large-diameter fibers by pressure to close the gate. Instead the stimulation of the large fibers only increases activity in the transmission cells, resulting in more extreme pain. At other times the small-fiber activity may be less extreme, the pressure may close the gate by means of the large-diameter fibers, and pain is reduced.

Gate-control theory also provides a mechanism to begin to understand how psychological or attentional factors may influence pain. For example, soldiers in combat or athletes engaged in strenuous competition may not notice injuries when they occur because the distraction of the activity acted to close the gate through the central control trigger. When the competition or battle ends, the gate opens as stimulation through the central control trigger lessens. We may also be more sensitive to pain when anxious or depressed because these negative emotions also act to open the gate. Similarly, the chronic low back pain patient's discomfort may wax and wane as a function of emotional and attentional factors and be independent or nearly independent of physiological status. If a person becomes sufficiently vigilant for the experience of pain, and anticipates pain to occur, this may actually make pain more likely as central control mechanisms are not acting to close the gate, and very small amounts of stimulation may lead to pain perception. As will be seen when psychological factors in pain and pain treatment procedures are discussed, gate-control theory also provides a useful model for understanding how psychological factors may be capitalized upon to influence pain perception.

# Behavioral and Psychological Factors

Chronic benign pain has been found to be associated with behavioral and psychological factors in a variety of ways. Chronic pain may be maintained through operant conditioning procedures, and chronic pain may also be associated with specific psychological conditions as documented by psychological assessment procedures.

CHRONIC PAIN AND OPERANT CONDITIONING   Behavioral and psychosocial factors may play a large part in low back pain and other types of pain and have their most notable impact on *pain behaviors*. It is important to remember that pain is a completely private experience; no one but the person in pain can actually document the existence of pain because only the sufferer may observe the pain itself. All others must observe the verbal or nonverbal pain-related communications of the sufferer. Pain behaviors are "the things people do when they suffer or are in pain" (Fordyce, 1988, p. 278), such as verbal reports of pain, crying, grimacing, medication requests, and withdrawal from normal activities. As with all behaviors, pain behaviors may be powerfully affected by environmental circumstances and by the reactions of other individuals.

Fordyce (1976) has emphasized the role of behavioral and psychosocial factors in chronic pain and its treatment. He has particularly stressed that many treatment procedures and people in the pain patient's environment may actually act to reward pain behavior rather than reduce it by concentrating attention on patients when they are complaining of pain or otherwise exhibiting pain behavior and ignoring patients when they are exhibiting well behavior. For example, consider when a patient receives emotional support from family, friends, or the health care system; it is most commonly when the patient is reporting the presence of pain, crying, or staying in bed and withdrawing from normal activities. Similarly, a patient is also most likely to receive medication at these same times, so the receipt of potentially addictive pain medication may very well act to reinforce the presence of pain complaints. Pain complaints may therefore be maintained by an operant conditioning process, as a patient is rewarded for displaying pain behaviors and is thus more likely to display these same behaviors in the future.

As Keefe and Gil (1986) have pointed out, there is evidence to support the assumption that pain may be subject to operant conditioning procedures. Normal subjects will give increased ratings of the pain of electrical shocks when social reinforcement is associated with increased pain complaints (Linton & G'otestam, 1985), and pain patients with a supportive spouse have been found to rate their pain as more severe when in the presence of their spouse (Block, Kremer, & Gaylor, 1980).

PSYCHOLOGICAL ASSESSMENT OF CHRONIC PAIN   The Minnesota Multiphasic Personality Inventory (MMPI) and the McGill Pain Questionnaire

(Melzack, 1975; MPQ) are used frequently in psychological assessment of chronic-pain patients. These two techniques provide very different types of information about the psychological status of the pain patient. The MMPI gives an overview of the psychological functioning of the patient and is particularly useful as an indicator of the presence or absence of any psychological disturbance that may need attention during the patient's treatment. The MPQ does not directly assess psychopathology. Instead, it allows the pain patient to described the pain experience by choosing the words that most accurately match her or his pain sensations and to rate the intensity of the pain.

The use of the MMPI with chronic pain was briefly mentioned in Chapter 2 in the discussion of descriptive group studies. An early study by Hanvik (1951) reported that functional-back-pain patients could be differentiated from organic-back-pain patients by their MMPI profiles. Functional-back-pain patients produced significantly more elevated MMPI profiles, particularly on the Hypochondriasis (*Hs*) and Hysteria (*Hy*) scales. This profile came to be referred to as the "Conversion V" profile, and was interpreted as meaning that the patient producing this profile was concentrating on physical symptoms in order to avoid psychologically distressing issues. This interpretation draws on the psychoanalytic defense mechanism of conversion, in which a psychological conflict is converted into a physical symptom because many people find it less threatening to experience and seek help for a physical disorder than to acknowledge the presence of a psychological problem. Physical illness typically carries much less social stigma than psychological illness.

A "Conversion V" MMPI profile from a chronic-pain patient is presented in Figure 14.2. As you can see, the *Hs* and *Hy* scales are the highest scales in the profile. The patient producing this profile was complaining of low back pain, and there appeared to be no physical reason for the pain. It was later learned that the pain had begun just after the patient began to experience marital problems, and she felt unable to cope with the life changes that a divorce might lead to. Rather than acknowledging her fears of being alone, which she probably viewed as suggesting psychological weakness, she was instead focusing on physical pain and thus deflecting attention away from the actual source of her distress. In fact, her focus on the pain complaints was also mobilizing a significant amount of social support as her family and friends were spending a great deal of time caring for her and expressing sympathy. This illustrates *secondary gain*, another psychological factor that may serve to maintain chronic pain in such a case. Whereas the primary gain of the pain complaints was to allow for the avoidance of psychologically threatening thoughts and feelings, the secondary gain may be seen in the care and sympathy the physical symptoms elicited from others. The secondary gain concept thus acknowledges the role that operant conditioning processes may play in chronic pain.

It is important to remember that although recent attempts to understand the psychology of chronic pain have emphasized behavioral and operant conditioning concepts rather than personality theory, the two ways of under-

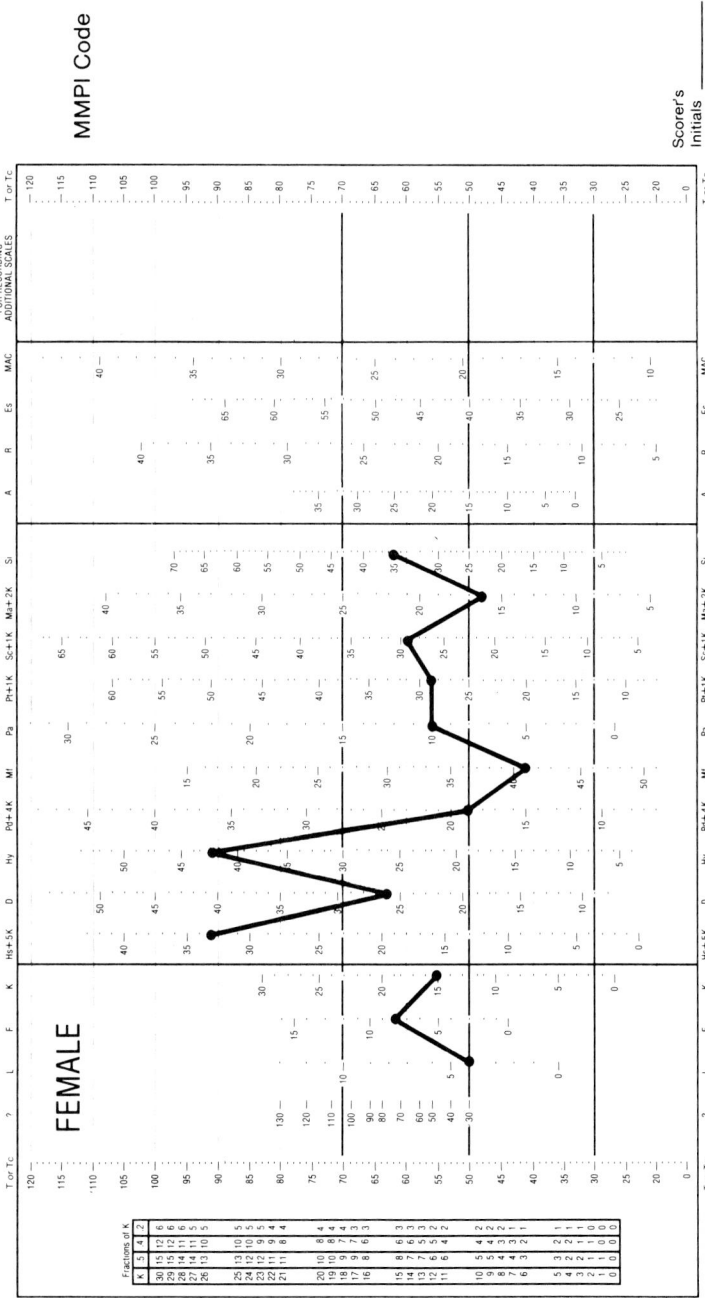

FIGURE 14.2  A "Conversion V" MMPI Profile from a low back pain patient. Minnesota Multiphasic Personality Inventory. Copyright The University of Minnesota, 1943, renewed 1970. This form 1982. Reprinted by permission.

standing pain are not incompatible. Personality may predispose someone to view certain types of experiences, such as sympathy and dependence on others, as very rewarding. Some people see the acknowledgment of psychological problems as unacceptable or threatening whereas others do not. Personality structure may thus increase the risk of developing chronic pain, given the appropriate circumstances. Personality assessment may thus be useful, even in cases where there are clear operant conditioning processes underlying the patient's pain problem.

The use of the MMPI with chronic pain patients has received a great deal of research attention since Hanvik's initial report. Although many studies, such as that of Gentry, Shows, and Thomas (1974), mentioned in Chapter 2, have confirmed that the average MMPI profile of chronic pain patients is the Conversion V, the existence of other profiles has been noted and the interpretation of the Conversion V as always indicating the presence of repressed psychological disturbance has been questioned. Perhaps most important, it has become clear that the MMPI is not a reliable instrument for the differentiation of pain without an organic basis from pain with an organic basis (Prokop, 1988). Bradley, Prokop, Margolis, and Gentry (1978) studied the MMPI profiles of chronic pain patients using cluster analysis, a statistical technique in which profiles are sorted into groups sharing common features. These investigators reported the presence of several other MMPI profile subgroups in addition to the Conversion V. In fact, the Conversion-V profile subgroup was found only in female patients and accounted for only about 34% of the female MMPI profiles. About 42% of the pain patient MMPI profiles were sorted into a normal subgroup. Thus, a substantial number of patients did not appear to be psychologically disturbed. Other investigators have reported similar results using cluster analysis (Hart, 1984; McCreary, 1985), and it is now generally recognized that many MMPI profiles reflecting a wide variety of psychological distress are seen in chronic-pain patients.

A more recent study by Prokop (1986) questioned the assumption that the Conversion-V MMPI profile always indicates a tendency to deny psychological distress by focusing on physical symptoms. The MMPI *Hy* scale contains items pertaining to physical complaints and to psychological features such as needs for affection and tendencies to deny social anxiety; Harris and Lingoes developed subscales of the *Hy* scale reflecting these different categories of items (described in Greene, 1980). Prokop reported that differences between chronic-back-pain patients and people without any psychological or physical disorders occurred primarily on the subscales of the *Hy* scale relating to physical symptoms. Similar findings were also reported by Ornduff, Brennan, and Barrett (1988). It is therefore important to determine in a specific pain patient whether or not a *Hy* scale elevation is reflecting only physical distress or whether other psychological factors, such as need for affection, are also leading to the *Hy* elevation. For example, the patient whose profile was presented in Figure 14.2 elevated both the physical symptom subscales and the subscales with a more purely psychological content. In that patient's case, it was appropriate to consider the possibility that the pain was a reflection of a need to deny psychological conflict and to solicit affection through pain complaints. The patient's history and current situation was then examined for signs confirming or disconfirming that interpretation.

The MMPI plays a valuable part in assessing the psychological status of chronic-pain patients. However, it is important to remember that no single MMPI profile is characteristic of pain patients, and it is necessary to account for the possibility that the patient's physical complaints may require the profile to be interpreted differently than it would be in a patient not suffering from chronic pain. It has also been recognized that the most important information to be derived from the MMPI profiles of chronic pain patients is not the probability that the patient's pain is actually caused by psychological factors but is instead related to the current psychological status of the patient and the resulting implications for treatment selection. The psychological needs of a pain patient are important, whether or not medical treatment for a physical disorder is indicated.

The McGill Pain Questionnaire (Melzack, 1975) was developed to provide a way to gain insight into the personal experience of pain. The MPQ assesses the pain experience by compartmentalizing it into three categories of descriptive adjectives representing the sensory, affective, and evaluative components of pain. The patient is asked to select the word from each adjective group that best describes his or her pain at the time the MPQ is administered. Sensory adjectives apply to the actual sensations characterizing the pain, such as pulsing, gnawing, or itching. Affective adjectives apply to the emotional reaction of the patient to the pain, such as tiring, cruel, or frightful. Evaluative adjectives allow the pain sufferer to rate the degree of interference the pain causes, from annoying to unbearable. A Pain Rating Index is computed by totaling the values of the adjectives chosen, and the patient also rates his or her Present Pain Intensity on a six-point scale ranging from no pain to excruciating pain. By reviewing the MPQ the evaluator is able to get a picture of the internal experience of the pain patient.

Dubisson and Melzack (1976) reported that specific constellations of pain descriptors were chosen by patients experiencing pain resulting from different disorders. For example, arthritis was commonly described as gnawing, aching, exhausting, and annoying, whereas cancer pain was more likely to be described as shooting, sharp, gnawing, and unbearable. Leavitt and Garron (1980) found that patients with functional pain were more likely to consistently choose specific affective words to described their pain, whereas those with pain of organic origin were more likely to choose specific sensory adjectives. Bradley and Van der Heide (1984) reported that patients with more elevated MMPI profiles also produced higher scores on several of the MPQ measures. Data from the MPQ thus suggest that even though pain is a private experience, there may be some commonalities in how different people experience pain of similar origin, and these descriptions may be useful in gaining an understanding of the nature of the individual patient's disorder.

# Treatment Program

Treatment programs for chronic pain are similar to those for headache and include such techniques as relaxation training and biofeedback. However, chronic pain treatment is often conducted while a person is an inpatient in a hospital or pain-treatment program, whereas headache treatment is more likely to be completed on an outpatient basis. This difference is due to the operant conditioning influences that frequently play an important role in the maintenance of the patient's pain. The controlled environment of an inpatient program provides a better opportunity for the modification of the reinforcers that are contributing to the patient's pain problem. Comprehensive pain treatment programs commonly include a variety of treatment approaches in combination with an education program covering the nature of chronic pain and the rationale for the treatments.

OPERANT TREATMENT PROGRAMS   It was noted earlier in this chapter that pain behavior may be reinforced by a variety of environmental influences. A pain sufferer is often inadvertently reinforced for pain behavior rather than healthy behavior. For example, it is common to exercise or work until pain becomes too intense and then to rest. Although this initially appears reasonable, in the case of chronic benign pain the pain is not serving a useful warning function, and by resting when pain intensifies the pain patient is actually reinforcing the experience of pain by resting. Pain becomes the signal for the opportunity to relax, and thus pain may become more likely to occur. In the same way, taking pain medication when pain intensifies may reinforce the pain. Medication is particularly likely to act as a reinforcer because the muscle relaxant and/or tranquilizing properties of many pain medications may be pleasant experiences for many people. Operant pain treatment programs work to counteract these reinforcing behavioral patterns.

Fordyce (1976) has developed several techniques to begin to break the association between pain behavior and rewarding consequences. When first admitted to a pain treatment program, a patient is asked to exercise in her or his normal fashion, stopping when the pain becomes too intense to continue. After it is determined where the patient's personal pain threshold is, a target number of exercise repetitions, or *movement cycles*, is chosen. This target number is below the pain threshold. During treatment, the patient exercises until the target is reached, and then the patient rests. In this way, the reward of rest becomes contingent upon completion of an appropriate amount of exercise rather than upon pain. The target number is then gradually increased over a period of weeks, allowing the endurance of the patient to increase. Medication is given on a regular schedule, such as every six hours, rather than when pain becomes intense, thus breaking the association between pain and the potentially reinforcing effects of the medication. The patient may also be gradually withdrawn from medication by mixing the drug with flavored syrup that masks the taste of the medication. The amount of drug in this *pain cocktail* is gradually reduced during the treatment program. Perhaps most important, staff attention and privileges are contingent upon the display of healthy, nonpain behavior rather than illness behavior. Pain complaints evoke little or no response from the staff, but reaching exercise goals leads to positive comments and encouragement.

Operant treatment programs are often useful for increasing activity levels and decreasing medication usage. Increased activity is particularly important in recovery. Excessive inactivity makes movement painful, and pain due to disuse may be misinterpreted by the patient as pain due to a lack of healing (Fordyce, 1988). Cairns and Pasino (1977) found that social reinforcement, such as compliments and encouragement, caused patients to increase their activity levels if the social reinforcement was contingent upon healthy behavior such as reaching exercise goals. White and Sanders (1985) studied chronic pain patients undergoing medication withdrawal. They reported that administering medication on a regular schedule led to lower pain ratings and better mood ratings than when medication was administered based on pain complaints. Fordyce, Brockway, Bergman, and Spengler (1986) compared an operant treatment program to a traditional let-pain-be-your-guide exercise program. Nine to twelve months after treatment the patients in the operant program reported less impairment and less use of health care resources than patients in the traditional management program. The Fordyce et al. (1986) study is especially noteworthy because the subjects had all been injured just before the program began, and the results therefore suggest that operant programs may actually help prevent the development of a chronic-pain problem.

Operant programs may be criticized for focusing too heavily on pain behavior at the expense of the pain itself (Keefe & Gil, 1986). Although pain is sometimes reported to be lower following operant treatment (White & Sanders, 1985), this is not always the case. Kincey and Benjamin (1984) reported that although activity level increased after operant treatment and the relationship between pain and daily activity also decreased, pain was not significantly lower after treatment than before. Similarly, Linton and G'otestam (1985) found that relaxation training led to greater pain relief than operant treatment, although the operant program led to greater reductions in medication and increases in activity. Relaxation and biofeedback are therefore often included in comprehensive pain treatment programs.

RELAXATION TRAINING AND BIOFEEDBACK   Many chronic pain patients, especially those suffering from low back pain, report the presence of muscle spasms associated with pain. However, the evidence for an association between increased muscle tension and pain is far from clear. Dolce and Raczynski (1985) reviewed the literature regarding muscle tension levels and back pain and concluded that it is unclear that the resting muscle tension levels of most back pain patients are unusually high, and there is even evidence that EMG levels during movement are abnormally *low* in some back pain patients. In cases where muscle tension is abnormally low, it may be that the low muscle tension levels cause spinal instability, which leads to irritation of spinal nerves. It is therefore important for any muscle relaxation or biofeedback treatment program to be carefully matched to the individual patient's condition.

In patients with high levels of muscle tension, EMG biofeedback from the painful, tense muscles may reduce tension and pain (Flor, Haag, Turk, & Koehler, 1983; Large & Lamb, 1983). However, it is not always true that lowered EMG levels correlate perfectly with reduced pain. Nouwen and Solinger (1979) reported that although pain and tension reduced during biofeedback treatment, three months after treatment some of the patients maintained or increased their pain reduction even though their muscle tension levels had returned to the pretreatment levels. Patients with larger decreases in EMG levels during treatment were most likely to show continued pain relief. Successful biofeedback treatment may have led those patients to be more confident in their self-control abilities, and this increased confidence may have led to decreases in pain. This interpretation is similar to Holroyd et al.'s (1984) suggestions regarding the reasons for the effectiveness of biofeedback for tension headaches. It is also possible that the lowering of muscle tension levels during treatment allowed inflamed muscles to heal, and thus allowed pain to be reduced (Dolce & Raczynski, 1985).

In pain patients with abnormal EMG levels during movement, biofeedback may be used to help the patient relearn correct muscle tension patterns and thus reduce the risk of abnormal and pain-inducing postures. This use of biofeedback is quite new, but successful retraining of muscle tension habits and consequent reduction in pain have been reported in two single-subject studies (Jones & Wolf, 1980; Wolf, Nacht, & Kelly, 1982). In both of these cases, biofeedback was delivered while the patients were in motion, and the feedback allowed the patients to observe muscle tension patterns and learn ways to tense specific muscles at the appropriate times during movement.

# Summary

Headaches and low back pain are serious health problems that result in high costs to society as well as to the individual sufferer. It has been estimated that 75 million Americans suffer from some type of chronic pain. Chronic pain is usually defined as pain lasting more than six months.

The pain of tension headache is dull and steady. Elevated muscle tension is not always present in tension headache patients. Migraine headaches are characterized by throbbing pain that is often unilateral. Nausea and sensitivity to light and sound are other symptoms often present. Migraines are related to irregularities in blood flow.

No specific personality style is characteristic of headache sufferers, although psychological distress may accompany headaches. The degree of psychological distress is related to the pain density of the headaches. Headache onset may be related to continuing stressful events and physiological arousal that may go unnoticed.

Biofeedback and relaxation training are often used to treat headaches. EMG biofeedback may train patients in relaxation and provide an experience of success in controlling physiological reactivity. Temperature and CVMR biofeedback may help migraine sufferers learn to stabilize blood flow. Relaxation training is generally as effective as biofeedback in the treatment of tension headaches, although some patients may benefit from a combination of the two treatments.

Low back pain may be caused by herniated disk, arthritis, or chronic muscle stresses and strains. In many cases low back pain is present in the absence of demonstrable physical pathology. The gate-control theory attempts to explain how physical and psychological events interact in the pain experience. Psychological factors such as attention and emotion may act to either open or close the gate and make the experience of pain more or less likely.

Environmental circumstances and the reactions of other individuals influence pain behaviors. Unfortunately, many common treatment procedures may reward pain behavior rather than well behavior. Psychological tests such as the MMPI and McGill Pain Questionnaire are often used with chronic pain patients. No single MMPI profile is characteristic of chronic pain patients. The most important information to be gained from psychological assessment concerns the pain patient's current psychological condition and the implications of this condition for treatment selection. Operant treatment programs attempt to break the association between pain behavior and reinforcing consequences by rewarding well behaviors such as increased activity and decreased medication usage. Operant programs are often combined with biofeedback and relaxation training.

# References

ANDRASIK, F., & HOLROYD, K. A. (1980). A test of specific and nonspecific effects in the biofeedback treatment of tension headache. *Journal of Consulting and Clinical Psychology, 48*, 575–586.

BILD, R., & ADAMS, H. E. (1980). Modification of migraine headaches by cephalic blood volume pulse and EMG biofeedback. *Journal of Consulting and Clinical Psychology, 48*, 51–57.

BLANCHARD, E. B., ANDRASIK, F., AHLES, T. A., & TEDERS, S. J. (1980). Migraine and tension headache: A meta-analytic review. *Behavior Therapy, 11*, 613–631.

BLANCHARD, E. B., ANDRASIK, F., & ARENA, J. G. (1984). Personality and chronic headache. In B. A. Maher & W. B. Maher (Eds.), *Progress in experimental personality research: Vol. 13: Normal personality processes* (pp. 303–364). New York: Academic Press.

BLANCHARD, E. B., APPELBAUM, K. A., GUARNIERI, P., NEFF, D. B., ANDRASIK, F., JACCARD, J., & BARRON, K. D. (1988). Two studies of long-term follow-up of minimal therapist contact treatments of vascular and tension headache. *Journal of Consulting and Clinical Psychology, 56*, 427–432.

BLOCK, A., KREMER, E., & GAYLOR, M. (1980). Behavioral treatment of chronic pain: The spouse as a discriminative cue for pain behavior. *Pain, 9*, 243–252.

BRADLEY, L. A., PROKOP, C. K., MARGOLIS, R. D., & GENTRY, W. D. (1978). Multivariate analyses of the MMPI profiles of low back pain patients. *Journal of Behavioral Medicine, 1,* 253–272.

BRADLEY, L. A., & VAN DER HEIDE, L. H. (1984). Pain-related correlates of MMPI profile subgroups among back pain patients. *Health Psychology, 3,* 157–174.

BRENA, S. F. (1983). Pain control facilities: Roots, organization and function. In S. F. Brena & S. C. Chapman (Eds.), *Management of patients with chronic pain* (pp. 11–20). Jamaica, NY: Spectrum.

BRENA, S. F., CHAPMAN, S. L., & DECKER, R. (1981). Chronic pain as a learned experience. In L. K. Y. Ng (Ed.), *New approaches to treatment of chronic pain* (pp. 76–83). Washington, D.C.: U. S. Department of Health and Human Services.

BUDZYNSKI, T., STOYVA, J., & ADLER, C. (1970). Feedback-induced muscle relaxation: Application to tension headache. *Journal of Behaviour Therapy and Experimental Psychiatry, 1,* 205–211.

CAIRNS, D., & PASINO, J. (1977). Comparison of verbal reinforcement and feedback in the operant treatment of disability due to chronic low back pain. *Behavior Therapy, 8,* 621–630.

COHEN, M. J., RICKLES, W. H., & MCARTHUR, D. L. (1978). Evidence for physiological response stereotypy in migraine headache. *Psychosomatic Medicine, 40,* 344–354.

DALESSIO, D. J. (1980). *Wolff's headache and other head pain.* New York: Oxford University Press.

DALEY, E. J., DONN, P. A., GALLIHER, M. J., & ZIMMERMAN, J. S. (1983). Biofeedback applications to migraine and tension headache. *Biofeedback and Self-Regulation, 8,* 135–152.

DOLCE, J. J., & RACZYNSKI, J. M. (1985). Neuromuscular activity and electromyography in painful backs: Psychological and biomechanical models in assessment and treatment. *Psychological Bulletin, 97,* 502–520.

DUBISSON, D., & MELZACK, R. (1976). Classification of clinical pain by multiple group discriminant analysis. *Experimental Neurology, 51,* 480–487.

FLOR, H., HAAG, G., TURK, D. C., & KOEHLER, H. (1983). Efficacy of EMG biofeedback, pseudotherapy, and rheumatic medical treatment for chronic rheumatic back pain. *Pain, 17,* 21–31.

FORDYCE, W. E. (1976). *Behavioral methods for chronic pain and illness.* St. Louis: Mosby.

FORDYCE, W. E. (1988). Pain and suffering: A reappraisal. *American Psychologist, 43,* 276–283.

FORDYCE, W. E., BROCKWAY, J. A., BERGMAN, J. A., & SPENGLER, D. (1986). Acute back pain: A control-group comparison of behavioral vs. traditional management methods. *Journal of Behavioral Medicine, 9,* 127–140.

GAMBLE, E. H., & ELDER, S. T. (1983). Multimodal biofeedback in the treatment of migraine. *Biofeedback and Self-Regulation, 8,* 383–392.

GAUTHIER, J., BOIS, R., ALLAIRE, D., & DROLET, M. (1981). Evaluation of skin temperature training at two different sites for migraine. *Journal of Behavioral Medicine, 4,* 407–420.

GAUTHIER, J., DOYON, J., LACROIX, R., & DROLET, M. (1983). Blood volume pulse biofeedback in the treatment of migraine headache: A controlled evaluation. *Biofeedback and Self-Regulation, 8,* 427–442.

GENTRY, W. D., SHOWS, W. D., & THOMAS, M. (1974). Chronic low back pain: A psychological profile. *Psychosomatics, 15,* 174–177.

GREENE, R. L. (1980). *The MMPI: An interpretive manual.* New York: Grune & Stratton.

HANVIK, L. J. (1951). MMPI profiles in patients with low back pain. *Journal of Consulting Psychology, 15,* 350–353.

HART, R. (1984). Chronic pain: Replicated multivariate clustering of personality profiles. *Journal of Clinical Psychology, 40,* 129–133.

HAYNES, S. N., GANNON, L. R., CUEVAS, J., HEISER, P., HAMILTON, J., & KATRANIDES, M. (1983). The psychophysiological assessment of muscle-contraction headache subjects during headache and nonheadache conditions. *Psychophysiology, 20,* 393–399.

HAYNES, S. N., GRIFFIN, P., MOONEY, D., & PARISE, M. (1975). Electromyographic feedback and relaxation instructions in the treatment of muscle contraction headaches. *Behavior Therapy, 6,* 672–678.

HICKS, R. A., & CAMPBELL, J. (1983). Type A-B behavior and self-estimates of the frequency of headaches in college students. *Psychological Reports, 52,* 912.

HOLMES, D. S., & BURISH, T. G. (1983). Effectiveness of biofeedback for treating migraine and tension headaches: A review of the evidence. *Journal of Psychosomatic Research, 27,* 515–532.

HOLROYD, K. A., PENZIEN, D. B., HURSEY, K. G., TOBIN, D. L., ROGERS, L., HOLM, J. E., MARCILLE, P. J., HALL, J. R., & CHILA, A. G. (1984). Change mechanisms in EMG biofeedback training: Cognitive changes underlying improvements in tension headache. *Journal of Consulting and Clinical Psychology, 52,* 1039–1053.

HOVANITZ, C. A., CHIN, K., & WARM, J. S. (1989). Complexities in life stress-dysfunction relationships: A case in point—tension headache. *Journal of Behavioral Medicine, 12,* 55–76.

HUNDLEBY, J. D., & LOUCKS, A. D. (1985). Personality characteristics of young adult migraineurs. *Journal of Personality Assessment, 49,* 497–500.

JACOBSON, E. (1938). *Progressive relaxation.* Chicago: University of Chicago Press.

JANSSEN, K. (1983). Differential effectiveness of EMG-feedback versus combined EMG-feedback and relaxation instructions in the treatment of tension headache. *Journal of Psychosomatic Research, 27,* 243–253.

JONES, A. L., & WOLF, S. L. (1980). Treating chronic low back pain: EMG biofeedback training during movement. *Physical Therapy, 60,* 58–63.

KEEFE, F. J., & GIL, K. M. (1986). Behavioral concepts in the analysis of chronic pain syndromes. *Journal of Consulting and Clinical Psychology, 54,* 776–783.

KINCEY, J., & BENJAMIN, S. (1984). Desynchrony following the treatment of pain behaviour. *Behaviour Research and Therapy, 22,* 85–86.

KURTZKE, J. F. (1982). The current neurologic burden of illness and injury in the United States. *Neurology, 32,* 1207–1214.

LARGE, R. G., & LAMB, A. M. (1983). Electromyographic (EMG) feedback in chronic musculoskeletal pain: A controlled trial. *Pain, 17,* 167–177.

LARGEN, J. W., MATHEW, R. J., DOBBINS, K., MEYERS, J. S., & CLAGHORN, J. L. (1978). Skin temperature self-regulation and non-invasive regional cerebral blood flow. *Headache, 18,* 197–202.

LEAVITT, F., & GARRON, D. C. (1980). Validity of a back-pain classification scale for detecting psychological disturbance as measured by the MMPI. *Journal of Clinical Psychology, 36,* 186–189.

LEVOR, R. M., COHEN, M. J., NALIBOFF, B. D., McARTHUR, D., & HEUSER, G. (1986). Psychosocial precursors and correlates of migraine headache. *Journal of Consulting and Clinical Psychology, 54,* 347–353.

LINTON, S. J., & G'OTESTAM, K. G. (1985). Controlling pain reports through operant conditioning. *Perceptual and Motor Skills, 60,* 427–437.

LOESER, J. D. (1980). Low back pain. In J. J. Bonica (Ed.), *Pain* (pp. 363–377). New York: Raven.

McCREARY, C. (1985). Empirically derived MMPI profile clusters and characteristics of low back pain patients. *Journal of Consulting and Clinical Psychology, 53,* 558–560.

MASTERS, J. C., BURISH, T. G., HOLLON, S. D., & RIMM, D. C. (1987, 1989). *Behavior therapy* (3rd ed.). Orlando, FL: Harcourt Brace Jovanovich.

MELZACK, R. (1975). The McGill Pain Questionnaire: Major properties and scoring methods. *Pain, 1,* 277–299.

MELZACK, R., WALL, P. D. (1983). *The challenge of pain.* New York: Basic Books.

MOUNTCASTLE, V. B. (1980). *Medical physiology.* St. Louis: Mosby.

NATIONAL CENTER FOR HEALTH STATISTICS. (1987). *Advance data from vital and health statistics, No. 128* (DHHS Publication No. PHS 87–1250). Hyattsville, MD: U.S. Public Health Service.

NOUWEN, A., & SOLINGER, J. W. (1979). The effectiveness of EMG biofeedback training in low back pain. *Biofeedback and Self-Regulation, 4,* 103–111.

ONORATO, V. A., & TSUSHIMA, W. T. (1983). EMG, MMPI, & treatment outcome in the biofeedback therapy of tension headache and posttraumatic pain. *American Journal of Clinical Biofeedback, 6,* 71–81.

ORNDUFF, S. R., BRENNAN, A. F., & BARRETT, C. L. (1988). The Minnesota Multiphasic Personality Inventory (MMPI) Hysteria (Hy) scale: Scoring bodily concern and psychological denial subscales in chronic back pain patients. *Journal of Behavioral Medicine, 11,* 131–146.

PHILIPS, C. (1977). A psychological analysis of tension headache. In S. Rachman (Ed.), *Contributions to medical psychology: Vol. 1* (pp. 91–114). New York: Pergamon.

PRICE, K. P., & TURSKY, B. (1976). Vascular reactivity of migraineurs and nonmigraineurs: A comparison of responses to self-control procedures. *Headache, 16,* 210–217.

PROKOP, C. K. (1986). Hysteria scale elevations in low back pain patients: A risk factor for misdiagnosis? *Journal of Consulting and Clinical Psychology, 54,* 558–562.

PROKOP, C. K. (1988). Chronic pain. In R. L. Greene (Ed.), *The MMPI: Use with specific populations* (pp. 22–49). Philadelphia: Grune & Stratton.

PROKOP, C. K., PRATT, D. L., & RHODES, L. A. (1987). Relaxation depth and perceived utility of biofeedback. Paper presented at the meeting of the Southeastern Psychological Association, Atlanta, Georgia.

RAPPAPORT, N. B., McANULTY, D. P., & BRANTLEY, P. J. (1988). Exploration of the Type A Behavior Pattern in chronic headache sufferers. *Journal of Consulting and Clinical Psychology, 56,* 621–623.

ROJAHN, J., & GERHARDS, F. (1986). Subjective stress sensitivity and physiological responses to an aversive auditory stimulus in migraine and control subjects. *Journal of Behavioral Medicine, 99,* 203–212.

SARGENT, J. D., GREEN, E. E., & WALTERS, E. D. (1972). The use of autogenic feedback training in a pilot study of migraine and tension headaches. *Headache, 12,* 120–125.

STERNBACH, R. A., DALESSIO, D. J., KUNZEL, M., & BOWMAN, G. E. (1980). MMPI patterns in common headache disorders. *Headache, 20,* 311–315.

TEDERS, S. J., BLANCHARD, E. B., ANDRASIK, F., JURISH, S. E., NEFF, D. F., & ARENA, J. G. (1984). Relaxation training for tension headache: Comparative efficiency and cost-effectiveness of a minimal therapist contact versus a therapist-delivered procedure. *Behavior Therapy, 15*, 59–70.

WHITE, B., & SANDERS, S. H. (1985). Differential effects on pain and mood in chronic pain patients with time versus pain-contingent medication delivery. *Behavior Therapy, 16*, 28–38.

WOLF, S. L., NACHT, M., & KELLY, J. L. (1982). EMG feedback training during dynamic movement for low back pain patients. *Behavior Therapy, 13*, 395–406.

ZIEGLER, D. K. (1984). An overview of the classification, causes, and treatment of headache. *Hospital and Community Psychiatry, 35*, 263–267.

# Child Health Psychology

Children pose a particular challenge to health psychologists. Childhood is a period of rapid change, and a child's developmental level influences the nature of the health risks to which he or she is exposed and the illnesses from which he or she is likely to suffer. Cognitive development particularly affects how a child reacts to and understands the causes and treatments of illness. A child's health is also profoundly affected by the prenatal environment, and the behaviors of expectant mothers are crucial to healthy growth and development. Adolescence provides opportunities for the adoption of a healthy lifestyle or the initiation of health-endangering behaviors such as smoking. Childhood chronic illness can exert stress on children and families, leading to developmental delays and poor compliance with medical regimens. Alternatively, family interactions can help an ill child cope and improve his or her adaptation to illness. This chapter surveys issues of current importance in child health psychology, with particular attention to the impact of cognitive development on understanding of illness and the problems of adolescent smoking and childhood chronic illness.

# Developmental Issues in Child Health Psychology

An understanding of child development is necessary when considering important issues in child health care and childhood illness. The term *development* refers to a normal process of orderly change over time in physical, emotional, and intellectual status. Just as children's motor, cognitive, and emotional abilities change, so do their health beliefs, attitudes, and behaviors. These health-related changes reflect an underlying maturational process that is predictable, understandable, and measurable.

The development of motor, cognitive, and emotional abilities of children affect the nature of their exposure to health hazards and illnesses, their understanding of the interaction between behavior and health, their assumptions concerning their personal responsibility for health, and their emotional responses to illness and injury. Progressive changes in a child's ability to think, reason, relate, understand, and perform motor tasks are the foundation for an increasing ability to make reasoned decisions about health. Such changes also allow for the performance of progressively complex health behaviors. Because the understanding of personal responsibility for health behaviors and outcomes and the emotional capacity for managing this personal responsibility increase with age, children become increasingly able to take personal responsibility for health care. Thinking about the physical and emotional capacities of an infant in comparison to those of an adolescent graphically underscores obvious developmental differences in abilities to understand behavior–health connections and to perform appropriate health-related actions.

## Exposure to Health Hazards

One of the most noticeable manifestations of a child's motor development is increased mobility. As a child becomes more mobile and begins to explore his or her environment, the nature of the child's interaction with the physical environment changes. Increased possibilities for interactions with the environment lead to an increase in the number of potential environmental hazards to which children will be exposed (Maddux, Roberts, Sledden, & Wright, 1986). Infants, for example, whose limited mobility decreases their contact with a great number of potential hazards, are less likely to encounter the types of hazards that a curious, mobile toddler might. It is also true, however, that infants' less developed physical capacities render them more susceptible to certain other environmental hazards. They may be more susceptible to brain injury, for example, because of their softer brain consistency and skull construction (Alcoff, 1982). Dependent on their care givers for protection, they may further be more susceptible to careless and potentially hazardous caretaking behavior on the part of their parents.

Accidents are the leading cause of death among children, and the nature of the accidents for which children are at risk varies with age (Califano, 1979). Injuries in the home, such as accidental poisonings and falls, account for the majority of deaths in preschoolers, whereas vehicular accidents are the leading cause of death in adolescents. Injuries account for nearly 80% of deaths of adolescents between the ages of fifteen and nineteen (National Center for Health Statistics, 1988).

Information concerning the risks for accidental injury at different ages has been provided in "anticipatory guidance" sessions (Roberts & Wright, 1982). In these sessions, health care providers meet with parents and provide information about accident risk and prevention strategies. For example, very young children are at risk for injury from hot water scalds. Christophersen, Williams, and Barone (cited in Christophersen, 1989) educated expectant parents and parents of two year olds about the effect that lower hot water heater temperatures could have on the rate of injury from hot water scalds. Expectant parents who received the educational message had lowered hot water heater settings than expectant parents who did not receive the message. However, the message had no significant effect on the parents of two year olds. Christophersen (1989) noted that the parents of older children reported that they had not had previous problems with hot water scalds, so they did not see any need to reduce water temperature. However, the expectant parents reported an eagerness to do anything possible to protect their children. It is thus important to time anticipatory guidance sessions appropriately so parents are most likely to believe that the information is applicable to their child's health.

## Children's Understanding of Health and Illness

Children's cognitive and intellectual capacities are crucial to their understanding of health and illness. These capacities are the foundation for the ability to assume responsibility for one's own health behavior, and affect psychological and behavioral reactions to illness, injury, and treatment programs. Perhaps most importantly, a child's level of cognitive development influences how he or she understands the nature of illness and how an illness may be related to behavior (Maddux et al., 1986).

At any point during development, children's cognitive capacities influence their understanding of and their perceptions about health. Based on Piaget's theory of development of cognitive ability, Bibace and Walsh (1980) described a six-stage theory where each stage of development represents an increased level of sophistication in thinking regarding the causes of specific health outcomes. According to Bibace and Walsh, a child's understanding of illness reflects the child's understanding of cause and effect relationships, and is consistent with Piaget's (1930) and Werner's (1948) theories about the development of cause and effect reasoning. One of the main features of this development is the child's increasing ability to differentiate, or see differences, between self and other. This differentiation allows for an increasing appreciation for what may be inside, such as an illness inside one's body, and what may be outside, such as the cause of an illness. Bibace and Walsh's (1980) six stages are discussed in the following paragraphs. Illustrative explanations of illness characteristic of each stage are presented in Table 15.1.

1. *Phenomenism*: Explanations at this stage are the most developmentally immature. Illness is attributed to an external concrete phenomenon. The phenomenon may coincide temporally with the illness, but be spatially remote. Children are unable to explain how the presumed causative events lead to the illness.

2. *Contagion*: During this stage, illness is attributed to proximity to a person, place, or object. The ill person need not actually contact another person or object to contract the illness, but only be near the causative agent. The connection between the illness and the cause is understood in "magical" terms.

3. *Contamination*: The child at this stage perceives the cause of illness as a person, object, or action external to the child. The cause is viewed as something that is bad for or harmful to the body. Children at this stage understand that illness is contracted by contact with the harmful agent or by engaging in an action that allows for contact with the harmful agent. Thus, the child sees a distinction between the cause of an illness (the harmful agent itself) and how the cause becomes effective (behavior leading to exposure to the harmful agent).

4. *Internalization*: In this stage, the cause of illness is an external agent that has an internal effect on the body. The external cause is thus internalized, or taken in, and illness results. Internalization is usually explained as occurring through swallowing or inhalation. Although internalized, the illness itself is still described in vague and nonspecific terms.

5. *Physiologic*: In this stage, children believe that the cause of illness is external, but the cause acts as a trigger for internal events. In contrast to children at the internalization stage, children at this stage understand illness as existing in specific internal physiologic structures and functions. Illness is thus seen as an internal process set in motion by some external stimulus, such as an infectious agent.

6. *Psychophysiologic*: As during the physiologic stage, children at the psychophysiologic stage understand illness as an internal physiologic process. However, they also see that psychological events such as thoughts and emotions can affect physical functioning.

Bibace and Walsh (1980) contended that these six stages were consistent with the cognitive development process outlined by Piaget (1930). They argued that phenomenism and contagion reflected preoperational thinking, contamination and internalization were manifestations of concrete operational thinking, and the physiologic and psychophysiologic stages reflected formal

TABLE 15.1  Explanations of illness characteristic of children at various stages of cognitive development. Experimenters' questions are followed by children's responses, in quotes.

| |
|---|
| *Phenomenism* |
| How do people get colds? "From the sun." |
| How does the sun give you a cold? "It just does, that's all." |
| *Contagion* |
| How do people get colds? "From the outside." |
| How do they get colds from the outside? "They just do, that's all. They come when someone gets near you." |
| How? "I don't know—by magic, I think." |
| *Contamination* |
| What is a cold? "It's like in the wintertime." |
| How do people get them? "You're outside without a hat and you start sneezing. Your head would get cold—the cold would touch it—and then it would go all over your body." |
| *Internalization* |
| What is a cold? "You sneeze a lot, you talk funny, and your nose is clogged up." |
| How do people get colds? "In winter, they breathe in too much air into their nose and it blocks up the nose." |
| How does this cause colds? "The bacteria gets in by breathing . . . ." |
| *Physiologic* |
| What is a cold? "It's when you get all stuffed up inside, your sinuses get filled up with mucus. Sometimes your lungs do, too, and you get a cough." |
| How do people get colds? "They come from viruses, I guess. Other people have the virus and it gets into your bloodstream and it causes a cold." |
| *Psychophysiologic* |
| What is a heart attack? "It's when your heart stops working right. Sometimes it's pumping too slow or too fast." |
| How do people get a heart attack? "It can come from being all nerve wracked. You worry too much. The tension can affect your heart." |

SOURCE:  Bibace, R., & Walsh, M. E. (1980). Development of children's concepts of illness. *Pediatrics, 66*, 912–917.

and operational thinking. Bibace and Walsh (1980) provided no statistical analysis to support their conclusions. However, the results of other studies suggest that children's conceptions of illness do develop systematically and predictably in a sequence compatible with Piaget's theories of cognitive development (Burbach & Peterson, 1986). Children's understanding of illness moves from vague and global ideas to more sophisticated concepts that recognize that illness is an internal process that may be affected by both external phenomena and internal events.

Educational approaches to the promotion of positive health behaviors, such as nutrition or dental care, must consider children's cognitive capacity. The ability to understand cause and effect determines how the link between behavior and health is perceived and thereby influences children's capacity and motivation to understand and comply with health regimens. However, it is important to avoid underestimating the ability of children to understand the connections between behavior and illness. It is also necessary to take into account the nature of the illness and health-care instructions being communicated to children. Siegal (1988) presented evidence that although 93% of preschoolers knew that children could catch a cold by playing with a friend who had a cold, 47% of these same children believed that a toothache could be transmitted in the same way. However, 90% of third grade children correctly rejected contagion as a cause of toothaches. These data suggest that dental-care information might need to be presented differently to preschoolers and third graders, even if information about contagious diseases such as colds could be presented similarly.

Level of cognitive development also may influence the capacity to cope emotionally with information about health. Medical information may increase rather than decrease emotional distress if children are unable to comprehend it and its implications for their health status and functioning (Willis, Elliot, & Jay, 1982). This suggests that cognitive capacity is important in determining the nature of the information that would be most effective to present to a child regarding his or her health-related problem and/or behavior. For example, since younger children may be more impressed with immediacy than with long-term consequences of behavior, emphasizing immediate consequences may elicit more compliance than would emphasizing future consequences of behavior. In their antismoking work with children, for example, Evans et al. (1978) emphasize knowledge of the immediate physiological effects of smoking rather than the long-term consequences, which seem more obscure and abstract to children.

# Emotional Development and Health and Illness

In discussing the child's emotional development, the term *psychosocial* has been used to refer to changes in the child's relationships with other people, particularly in the ability to function as an autonomous individual, separate from others (Maddux et al., 1986). This realm of functioning has significant implications for the question of who may be viewed as responsible for health-related behaviors, the child or the parents. It bears on the issue of the child's increasing ability to engage in *health self-regulation*, a term coined to describe the cognitive and emotional skills involved in the child's ability to autonomously regulate his or her own health behavior (Karoly, 1982).

The child's level of emotional development affects reactions to the onset of physical illness and/or occurrence of physical injury (Willis et al., 1982). Separations from parents because of hospitalization for illness, for example, will impact the child differently depending on his or her developmental capacity for coping with such an event. The factors relevant to children's emotional response to illness will be discussed in detail later in this chapter.

In summary, the motor, cognitive, and emotional development of children influences the nature of the health risks they encounter, their understanding of health–behavior–illness connections, their ability to take responsibility for health care, and their emotional responses to illness and/or injury. Intervention programs designed to promote child health care must therefore consider the following factors in their program development:

1. The health-care issue of importance for the particular age of the child
2. The target of the prescribed health program; that is, whether the locus of responsibility and education about child health should rest with the parent, the child, or with both of them
3. The content and nature of the health program or intervention; that is, the manner in which it is imparted and its level of complexity

# The Prenatal Period

The integrity of the prenatal environment critically affects the developing fetus. Placental membranes, which filter substances that pass between mother and fetus, are resistant to substances of a potentially harmful nature. However, the protection the uterine environment provides the fetus is far from perfect. This barrier has been found to be vulnerable to penetration by a large number of substances that are destructive to the developing fetus. These substances are referred to as *teratogens*: "environmental agents that produce structural and functional abnormalities in prenatal organisms" (LaBarba, 1984, p. 42). The timing of the exposure to teratogens and the dosage of the teratogens encountered are critical factors in determining whether an abnormality in development will occur. Avoidance of risk from exposure to teratogens rests not only on the expectant mother's awareness of them but also on her health-related behavior. Counseling programs to educate expectant parents, and counsel those with identifiable genetic risk factors, have attempted to affect the parents' knowledge and health behavior (Wright, Schaefer, & Solomons, 1979). As the list of potential risk factors grows, so does the amount of information about them made available to expectant parents.

Disease, ionizing radiations, and drugs and chemicals all have known teratogenic effects. The health behavior of the mother largely affects the degree to which such factors play a role in fetal development.

Rubella (German measles), cytomegalovirus, and herpes simplex are three infectious viral diseases that have been found to exert damaging prenatal effects (Langman, 1975). Rubella, for example, has been found to produce cardiovascular defects, blindness, deafness, and/or mental retardation in 50% of newborns when the mother has contracted it during the first month of pregnancy. Herpes simplex, or syphilis, may also exert damaging prenatal effects resulting in mild intellectual impairment, hearing loss, or skin lesions. Furthermore, about 50% of newborns whose mothers have genital herpes contract the disease, with only half of these infants surviving it (Babson, Pernol, Benda, & Simpson, 1980). One can easily see how health education programs for those at high risk for such maternal complications would be useful. Wright et al. (1979) have reported such an effort where maternal counseling programs were provided to adolescents at risk for such problems.

An increasing number of children are contracting Acquired Immune Deficiency Syndrome (AIDS) during the prenatal period. It has been estimated that by 1991 3,000 children in the United States will have been diagnosed as suffering from AIDS, and an additional 10,000 children will carry the human immunodeficiency virus (HIV), but not be diagnosed with AIDS (National Academy of Sciences, 1986). Seventy-eight percent of children with AIDS contracted the disease prenatally or during birth: prenatal infection occurs when HIV in the blood of an infected mother crosses the placental barrier. The symptoms of pediatric AIDS often appear during the first year of life, and include recurring infections, swollen lymph glands, failure to thrive, and developmental delays. Neurological symptoms such as abnormal reflexes, cognitive deficits, brain diseases, and abnormally small skulls may be present in 60% to 70% of pediatric AIDS cases (Task Force on Pediatric AIDS, 1989).

Pediatric AIDS can best be prevented by reducing the incidence of AIDS in pregnant women. Education encouraging monogamy, condom use, the avoidance of needle sharing, and drug rehabilitation must be provided. Information about AIDS prevention should be provided in language that is unambiguous and matched to the cultural and language background of the clients. Prevention efforts should also go beyond education and provide free condoms to high-risk women of childbearing age and their partners. Drug rehabilitation programs should also be expanded and made available to drug users interested in behavioral change (Task Force on Pediatric AIDS, 1989).

Exposure to diagnostic or therapeutic radiation during pregnancy is generally inadvisable. This is particularly true for radiation procedures involving the pelvic region, but even low-level exposure, such as from dental X rays, should be avoided. Prenatal exposure to radiation has been reported to have a variety of harmful effects, including intellectual and growth retardation, cancer, and spontaneous abortion (LaBarba, 1984). Numerous drugs and chemicals have been found to affect the fetus negatively and most pregnant women are advised by their physicians to take as few drugs as possible. Nevertheless, 90% of expectant mothers have been found to take one or more drugs during the course of their pregnancy, with 65% of these women taking self-administered drugs without medical advice (Howard & Hill, 1979).

Heavy smoking also affects fetal development negatively. Smoking is the most preventable cause of prematurity and low birth weight; spontaneous abortion, growth retardation, and behavioral abnormalities have been associated with maternal smoking during pregnancy (LaBarba, 1984). Nicotine and reduced fetal oxygenation may be responsible for these effects. The need for continued work on smoking cessation programs for pregnant women is clear, although the most effective programs may be those designed to prevent school-aged children from beginning to smoke.

Danaher, Shisslak, Thompson, and Ford (1978) reported on an exploratory study of a smoking cessation program for pregnant women. Eleven women participated in this study and met in a group for six two-hour sessions over seven weeks. They received an intensive program of risk education and behavioral skills training to help them stop smoking, including self-monitoring of cigarette usage and smoking urges, deep muscle relaxation techniques, and other methods of coping with smoking urges. Although the program was generally found to assist women in stopping smoking, the small number of participants in this study limits the confidence one may place in its findings. Nevertheless, further attempts of this nature are needed.

The use of alcohol during pregnancy also is a serious risk factor. Pregnant women who are heavy drinkers or even moderate drinkers may be at risk for the appearance of fetal alcohol syndrome (FAS) in their newborns. FAS is characterized by the presence of growth deficiencies and physical abnormalities, including a small head, a wide space between the margins of the eyelids, and malformed cheekbones and jaws. Central nervous system defects such as mental retardation, irritability, hyperactivity, and poor coordination may also be present. Some infants may show signs of alcohol withdrawal soon after birth (Clarren & Smith, 1978).

FAS is present in between one and two of every 1,000 live births in the United States, or in between 4,000 and 5,000 children born each year (LaBarba, 1984). The risk for FAS grows with increasing alcohol consumption. One or two drinks (one-half to one ounce of alcohol) per day may increase the risk of growth retardation (Mills, Graubard, Harley, Rhoads, & Berendes, 1984). The four-year-old children of mothers who had three drinks (one and one-half ounces of alcohol) per day during pregnancy have been reported to be at risk for an average decrement of five IQ points in comparison to children of mothers who drank less than this (Streissguth, Barr, Sampson, Darby, & Martin, 1989). Because the evidence is mixed as to whether or not there is a "safe" level of alcohol consumption during pregnancy, expectant mothers are advised to avoid alcohol completely (National Institute on Alcohol Abuse and Alcoholism, 1986). However, it has been reported that 2% of middle-class pregnant women consume two drinks or more per day. Drinking rates are higher among expectant mothers in lower socioeconomic classes (Abel, 1980). Programs designed to reduce the alcohol consumption of expectant mothers are clearly needed.

Although not a teratogen in itself, maternal age also has an effect on fetal health. Biochemical changes associated with aging or exposure to environmental hazards over many years may adversely affect ova stored in the potential mother's body. Women over thirty-five years of age are therefore at somewhat greater risk for problems during pregnancy and in fetal development. The incidence of Down's syndrome is positively related to maternal age with some studies showing that the risk of a Down's syndrome child is only about 1 in 2,500 for mothers less than twenty, 1 in 1,900 for mothers thirty to thirty-five years old, but 1 in 50 for mothers forty-five years old (Frias, 1975). The symptoms of Down's syndrome involve severe mental retardation, flattened facial features, and a variety of other birth defects. Recently it has been discovered that maternal age (and faulty cell division due to age) is not the only cause of Down's syndrome; it may also be related to paternal age, with fathers aged fifty years or older having an increased risk (LaBarba, 1984).

Although it has traditionally been thought that adolescent childbearing presents a risk to fetal development because of the physiological state of development of the mother, LaBarba (1984) notes that more recent studies that controlled for such factors as socioeconomic status, nutrition, age, prenatal care, and race reveal good obstetric outcomes among adolescents if they receive adequate prenatal care. He finds that the exception is the very young adolescent, under fourteen to fifteen years of age, especially when pregnancy occurs within twenty-four months of menarche.

Although the biological variables associated with adolescent pregnancy may present little risk, the psychosocial and economic problems common to teenage mothers may produce dismal outcomes. In comparison to children of older mothers, children of teenage mothers tend to have lower levels of school achievement, less self-control, and higher levels of aggression. These differences are probably related to the social and economic difficulties associated with early parenthood (Furstenberg, Brooks-Gunn, & Chase-Lansdale, 1989). Primary prevention programs aimed at reducing the rates of adolescent pregnancy are just beginning to be developed. These programs provide sex and contraception education, attempt to change attitudes about sexuality, and provide contraceptives and family planning services. Although all these programs are relatively new and therefore difficult to evaluate, it appears that contraceptive and family planning services are most likely to reduce rates of adolescent pregnancy. Secondary prevention programs that attempt to reduce the negative impact of adolescent pregnancy by providing education, counseling, and medical care also exist. Adolescent mothers who received educational assistance and family planning counseling after birth have been found to have better prospects for economic self-sufficiency and avoiding large families. However, many adolescents do not take advantage of such services even when they are available (Furstenberg et al., 1989).

Badger (1981) described the effectiveness of one parent education program for teenage mothers and their offspring: the Infant Stimulation–Mother Training Project. The project was based on the assumption that infancy is a critical period of development that is likely to affect future cognitive and emotional functioning. Mother–infant pairs were viewed as at risk if the mother was sixteen years of age or younger. The pairs either attended weekly classes in infant development and parenting skills or received monthly home visits where such problems as nutrition or health were discussed but no group instruction was given.

Results of the study showed that infants of high risk mothers who attended the classes performed significantly better on infant development tests than did infants of high risk mothers who received only monthly home visits. Infants of lower risk mothers did not perform differently, no matter whether these pairs attended the classes or received monthly home visits. Overall, mothers who attended weekly classes seemed to have greater awareness of their babies' physical welfare and to rely more on a health facility when they sensed a problem.

## Behavior Problems in Childhood

Between 5% and 15% of pediatric patients are identified by physicians as having mental health problems (Goldberg, Roghmann, McInerny, & Burke, 1984; Starfield et al., 1980). These estimates rely on the ability of pediatricians to recognize psychological problems in their patients and are not based on an objective formal assessment of the psychological status of pediatric patients. These figures also do not include relatively minor problems such as temper tantrums or eating problems; if minor problems were included, the incidence of psychological problems probably would be significantly higher (Christophersen, 1986). Studies also have suggested that when parents are asked who they consult when they want more information about their child's behavior and development, it is relatively unlikely that they would say they would discuss these issues with their pediatrician (Christophersen, 1986). This also may contribute to the detection of psychological problems in only a small percentage of the pediatric population. The incidence of behavior problems in children may, therefore, be higher than these estimates suggest.

Two relatively common health-related behavior problems of childhood are urinary incontinence (*enuresis*) and fecal incontinence (*encopresis*). Enuresis is much more common than encopresis; about 5% of ten-year-old children still wet the bed, but by the age of seven only 1.5% of children still lack bowel control to the degree that they soil their clothing (Campbell, 1970; Pierce, 1985b). Beyond the age of three years, problems in bladder and bowel control may result in significant psychosocial problems. Children with such difficulties are often alienated from their peer group as these problems are frequently a source of humiliation and low self-esteem. The psychosocial problems and family disruption caused by these two disorders has stimulated the development of a variety of treatment and research programs.

# Enuresis

Enuresis is generally defined as the occurrence of frequent urination in inappropriate settings after the age of three (Parker & Whitehead, 1982). Enuresis is typically thought of as urinary incontinence where psychosocial factors, as opposed to physiological abnormalities, are found to be primary in etiology (Campbell, 1970). Two types of enuresis have been identified: (1) primary enuresis, where the child has never developed bladder control, and (2) secondary enuresis, where the child has at one time attained continence but, for some reason, has suffered a relapse. Enuresis may occur during the day (diurnal enuresis) or at night (nocturnal enuresis). About 80% of enuretics are primary enuretics and 80% experience only nocturnal enuresis (Pierce, 1985b).

Nocturnal enuresis has been reported to be present in approximately 15% to 20% of all four and five year olds, and 1% to 2% of fifteen year olds (Campbell, 1970). Its occurrence appears to be significantly higher for boys than for girls (Pierce, 1985b). Although the physiology of this problem is not well understood and is quite complex, it is clear that some aspects of retention and expulsion are under voluntary control (Parker & Whitehead, 1982). The attainment of this control results from an interplay of physiological maturation and learning processes.

In a review of the problem of nocturnal enuresis, Friman and Christophersen (1986) suggested that its prominent correlates are a history of enuresis in the child's parents, small functional bladder capacity, and socioeconomic status (SES). They noted that a study of the genetics of enuresis revealed that enuresis was more common in children who had a parent who was enuretic than in children without such a parent (Bakwin, 1973), suggesting that enuresis may be a predictable phenomenon if one knows the history of enuresis in the child's parents. Reduced functional bladder size or capacity has also been found to be related to nocturnal enuresis (Zaleski, Gerrard, & Shokier, 1973). Dysfunction in the ability to experience or respond to sensory stimulation from the bladder is another organic variable of significance (Yeates, 1973). An increased number of enuretics come from families of lower SES (Gross & Dornbush, 1983), although it is not clear what is responsible for this relationship.

TREATMENT APPROACHES   The major medical intervention for enuresis, aside from surgery for organic cases in which physiological causes are responsible for symptoms, has been the use of drugs. Tricyclic antidepressants, stimulants, and tranquilizers all have been studied in the treatment of this disorder, but the most common medication used has been imipramine, an antidepressant (Pierce, 1985b). Although imipramine has been reported to result in an almost immediate cure for 40% to 50% of enuretic children, there is a very high relapse rate after the drug is withdrawn (Perlmutter, 1976). Common side effects of imipramine include sleep disturbances, headaches, weight loss, and constipation; anxiety, restlessness, and loss of concentration are less common side effects. Accidental poisonings can also occur. Drug treatment for enuresis is usually used only when other methods have been unsuccessful, and it is most effective in combination with other forms of treatment. It is sometimes used as a substitute for another treatment, such as when a child is on vacation and a temporary expedient is required (Pierce, 1985b).

Enuresis is frequently treated with one or more behavioral treatment programs. The urine alarm method was originally developed in 1938 by Mowrer and Mowrer, and is still in use today. Other behavioral approaches are based in operant theory and use a variety of reinforcement and punishment techniques. A third behavioral approach, retention control training, attempts to expand bladder capacity by asking the child to drink liquids and retain them for increasing periods of time.

*Urine Alarm Method*  The urine alarm method, also called the bell-and-pad method, was one of the first behavioral treatments for enuresis (Mowrer & Mowrer, 1938). The urine alarm consists of a multilayered pad on which the child sleeps. When urine contacts the pad, a bell or buzzer is activated. The alarm then awakens the child, and his or her parents, so that urination can be interrupted and then completed in the appropriate place. The notion underlying the development of the bell-and-pad method was that the sensation of a full bladder would eventually be paired with awakening and would thereby allow the child to engage in a more appropriate response than bedwetting. Although Mowrer and Mowrer originally described this as a classical conditional procedure, other authors have suggested that it is an operant procedure in which the child learns to avoid the buzzer (punishment) by waking up in time (Lovibond, 1964).

The bell-and-pad method has been successfully used alone in the treatment of enuresis as well as in combination with other behavioral techniques. The method has an overall success rate of 75% (Doleys, 1977), although early work that included follow-up procedures suggested a relapse rate as high as 30% (Parker & Whitehead, 1982). When the method involves an intermittent signal procedure, the effectiveness has been found to be more enduring (Turner, Young, & Rachman, 1970). Overlearning, which involves having the child drink water to increase bladder fullness while at the same time using the bell-and-pad procedure, has also been found to decrease the rate of relapse (Young & Morgan, 1972).

In summary, the bell-and-pad method has been found to be a successful approach in the treatment of enuresis, particularly when refinements in the original technique are applied. The single most common factor limiting the treatment effectiveness is lack of parental cooperation (Doleys, 1977); close supervision by the parents produces the highest success rates.

*Operant Approaches*  Several operant approaches to the treatment of enuresis have been used based upon the principles of reinforcement, punishment, shaping, and extinction. The "dry-bed program" initially described by Azrin, Sneed, and Foxx (1974) is one of the most comprehensive packages. In this procedure a urine alarm is used, as in the bell-and-pad method, but, behavioral rehearsal of the appropriate urination response is also involved, as is awakening on the first night of the procedure. If bedwetting occurs, the parents reprimand the child and the child cleans up after himself or herself. The parents use verbal reinforcement when the child remains dry. After the child remains dry for seven consecutive days, the urine alarm is removed and the rest of the procedures continued. Researchers have found the dry-bed program to be quite successful.

Daytime enuresis has also been treated by a number of operant approaches. Foxx and Azrin (1973) have developed a package involving behavioral rehearsal, such as training in lowering and raising clothes, sitting on the toilet, and urinating, and reinforcement for these appropriate behaviors. The program was initially developed to treat enuresis in retarded individuals but since has been applied to children of normal intelligence. The procedures have been found to be quite effective when applied by trained staff as well as by parents.

*Retention Control Training* Nocturnal enuresis also has been treated with retention control training, a procedure first introduced by Kimmel and Kimmel in 1970. This technique is based upon the premise that an increase is required in the functional capacity of the enuretic child's bladder. Retention control training involves increasing the child's fluid intake over a period of time while at the same time reinforcing longer and longer periods of urine retention. The hope is that training in inhibiting the urine response with larger amounts of fluid will lead to longer urine delay times and, eventually, the child's ability to sleep through the night without urination. When used alone, retention control training is effective with less than 50% of enuretic children (Doleys, Ciminero, Tollison, Williams, & Wells, 1977). However, this technique may be understandably most helpful for children whose primary problem involves an unusually small bladder capacity. Geffken, Johnson, and Walker (1986) treated enuretic children with the urine alarm method alone or with the urine alarm method combined with retention control training. Children with small bladder capacity had fewer bed-wetting episodes with the combined treatment, whereas children with larger bladder capacity had fewer bed-wetting episodes with the urine alarm method alone. An impressive 92.5% of children who completed treatment reached the treatment goal of fourteen consecutive dry nights, and all children who relapsed and returned for more treatment were subsequently cured.

# Encopresis

Encopresis is defined as voluntary or involuntary passage of feces in inappropriate places after the age toilet training should have been completed, which is generally by the age of three years (Pierce, 1985a). As in enuresis, two types of encopresis have been described: primary encopresis, where toilet training has never been achieved, and secondary encopresis, where control had been established at one time but is no longer present. Although these types have been described as resulting from toilet training that is excessively harsh or lax, the literature on encopresis has not borne this out. Additionally, research has not supported an association between encopresis and such personality characteristics as stubbornness or laziness (Friman & Christophersen, 1986).

Levine (1975) has reported the incidence of encopresis in pediatric populations to be as high as 3%. Schaefer (1979) reports the incidence to be 1.5% in seven to eight year old children. Boys have this difficulty more often than girls, with the ratio reportedly 6 to 1 (Levine, 1975). Remission of encopresis typically occurs by adolescence. About one-third of encopretic children are also enuretic (Pierce, 1985a).

TREATMENT APPROACHES    Encopresis has not been as widely studied as enuresis, probably because it is less common than enuresis. Most of the literature describing treatment of this disorder consists of case studies. Regardless of the approach used, most authors agree that a careful physical examination is the appropriate first step, and that enemas and laxatives be applied before other treatments are instituted (Christophersen & Rapoff, 1979). Enemas are thought to be the safest and most effective means of bowel evacuation (Parker & Whitehead, 1982). Although medication regimens have been reported in case studies in the literature (e.g., Musicco, 1977), the use of pharmacological interventions has not been systematically evaluated (Parker & Whitehead, 1982). Other medical procedures have involved surgical interventions to repair structural abnormalities leading to fecal incontinence, such as surgical repair of the sphincter.

As mentioned, the majority of reports in the literature describing behavioral approaches to encopresis are case studies. Behavioral approaches typically have involved the use of positive contingencies, negative contingencies, or a combination of treatment techniques. Several kinds of positive reinforcers have been applied. Parental attention has been used successfully as a positive reinforcer for continence (Balsom, 1973; Conger, 1970). Praise in conjunction with such reinforcers as pennies, stars, and candy also have been successful (Neale, 1963). In addition, punishment procedures have been employed in which consequences such as time-out and having the child clean both himself and his clothes are used (Freinden & Van Handel, 1970; Edelman, 1971).

Comprehensive treatment programs involving a number of behavioral interventions have been reported. Christophersen and Rainey (1976), for example, describe an approach involving positive reinforcement, glycerin suppositories and enemas, pants-checks with appropriate consequences, and aversive contingencies consisting of the child's cleaning himself and his soiled clothing. Using this approach, three out of three subjects maintained continence at follow-up periods ranging from two to ten months. Other programs of this nature have added a technique described as positive practice (Foxx

& Azrin, 1973). In positive practice the child performs an entire chain of behaviors involved in appropriate toileting, thereby practicing the appropriate response.

## Prevention of Enuresis and Encopresis

As with other medically related disorders, preventing enuresis and encopresis is certainly preferable to having to intervene to eliminate them. If prevented, the psychological consequences of developing these problems, such as feelings of humiliation and low self-esteem, can be circumvented. Unfortunately, little research has investigated methods to prevent either disorder.

The identification of children who are at risk for developing enuresis and/ or encopresis would be a useful place to begin when thinking of preventive measures. Children who are identified as having small functional bladder capacity, or who have family members with histories of enuresis or encopresis, may be at risk for developing such problems. The use of preventive measures would be critical for these children. It has been suggested that the best prevention strategy for all children, regardless of risk status, may be to toilet train them as soon as they are developmentally ready (Friman & Christophersen, 1986).

# *Adolescence*

Adolescence is a time of rapid physiological, cognitive, emotional, and psychosocial changes. With increasing autonomy and independence come significant changes in family and peer relationships. The adolescent is faced with the task of growing from a position of relative dependence to one in which self-direction, self-management, and self-reliance are necessary and prized abilities. This transition is not easy and may be fraught with stress and turmoil. The self-consciousness and growing self-awareness that occur in adolescence often heighten the stresses associated with this stage of life. Adolescence has come to be widely viewed as a period in the life span that is of key significance for health. Behaviors that jeopardize health, such as smoking and drug use, may be initiated during adolescence, and behavior in adolescence may have long-range consequences for health in later years (Jessor, 1984).

Jessor (1984) identified several health implications of adolescent development. First, adolescence is a time when new behaviors relevant to health status are learned and attempted. Some of these behaviors may be health endangering, such as precocious sexual activity and risk-taking behaviors, while others may be health enhancing, such as regular exercise and nutritional self-consciousness stemming from increased concern and awareness of one's body image. Second, many attributes that influence eventual health-related behavior, such as values, beliefs, and self-control, are formed during adolescence. Third, adolescence is marked by increased exposure to people and potentially more hazardous materials. Thus, the influence of peers and their health-related behaviors, as well as increased access to such materials as drugs, alcohol, and cigarettes, present the adolescent with heightened exposure to a variety of health-enhancing and health-endangering options. Fourth, adolescents typically are faced with an intense pressure to adapt, given that the changes they experience physically and socially are so rapid and dramatic. Such rapid change is accompanied by increased stress and the potential need to deal with the difficult feelings that result. Fifth, the asynchrony of changes during adolescence also may present increased stress. For example, the adolescent matures reproductively and his or her sexual interest increases while society relaxes the rules prohibiting sexual activity.

Accidents are the leading cause of death in adolescence, followed by suicide and death from homicide or legal interventions, such as a death occurring during an arrest (National Center for Health Statistics, 1988). Death rates attributable to these causes among children from ten to fourteen and fifteen to nineteen years of age are presented in Table 15.2. Accidents and violence account for 78.5% of deaths among people fifteen to nineteen years old; motor vehicle accidents alone account for 43.1% of deaths in this age group. As can be seen in Table 15.2, death rates for males are higher during adolescence. Substance use is an important contributor to the risk for accidents and violence (Halperin, Bass, Mehta, & Betts, 1983).

Adolescence is also a time that health-endangering habits such as the use of alcohol, tobacco, and other drugs may be initiated. Most initial experiences with cigarette smoking occur before the tenth grade (Severson & Lichtenstein,

TABLE 15.2   Deaths per 100,000 for (a) children ten to fourteen years old and (b) adolescents fifteen to nineteen years old.

| | *All Causes* | *Motor Vehicle Accidents* | *Other Accidents* | *Suicide* | *Homicide and Legal Interventions* |
|---|---|---|---|---|---|
| *Children Ages Ten to Fourteen Causes of Death* | | | | | |
| Total | 28.4 | 7.7 | 5.8 | 1.5 | 1.5 |
| Males | 36.1 | 10.0 | 8.9 | 2.3 | 1.7 |
| Females | 20.3 | 5.3 | 2.5 | 0.7 | 1.2 |
| *Adolescents Ages Fifteen to Nineteen Causes of Death* | | | | | |
| Total | 87.2 | 37.6 | 10.7 | 10.2 | 10.0 |
| Males | 124.3 | 52.8 | 17.7 | 16.4 | 15.1 |
| Females | 48.6 | 21.8 | 3.5 | 3.8 | 4.7 |

SOURCE:   National Center for Health Statistics. (1988). *Vital statistics of the United States, 1986* (Vol. 2, Mortality, Part A). (DHHS Publication No. PHS 88-1122). Washington, DC: U.S. Government Printing Office.

1986); in 1985 15% of adolescents between twelve and seventeen years old said that they had smoked cigarettes during the past month. About one-third of these same adolescents reported using alcohol in the past month, and 12% reported marijuana use. Figures for the use of alcohol, marijuana, and cocaine during adolescence for 1974, 1979, and 1985 are presented in Table 15.3, and Figure 15.1 illustrates changes in cigarette smoking from 1974 to 1985. The data suggest that cigarette use is declining, alcohol use is staying stable, and marijuana use is declining after increasing during the late 1970s. Cocaine use is infrequent, but has increased slightly (Schoenborn & Boyd, 1989).

Sexual behavior in adolescence also may present significant health risks, such as pregnancy in a very young woman or the contraction of sexually transmitted diseases. In 1982, 46% of 15- to 19-year-old unmarried women reported having had intercourse; in 1971, this figure was only 28% (Hofferth & Hayes, 1987; Zelnick & Kantner, 1980). Only about one-half of teenagers use contraceptives the first time they have intercourse (Zelnick & Shah, 1983). Over 25% of sexually active fifteen to nineteen year old women never use contraception, and over 16% of women in this age group become pregnant

TABLE 15.3   Percent of adolescents who reported using alcohol, marijuana, and cocaine in the past month in 1974, 1979, and 1985.

| | Alcohol | | |
| --- | --- | --- | --- |
| | *1974* | *1979* | *1985* |
| Both sexes | 34 | 37 | 31 |
| Males | 39 | 39 | 34 |
| Females | 29 | 36 | 28 |

| | Marijuana | | |
| --- | --- | --- | --- |
| | *1974* | *1979* | *1985* |
| Both sexes | 12 | 17 | 12 |
| Males | 12 | 19 | 13 |
| Females | 11 | 14 | 11 |

| | Cocaine | | |
| --- | --- | --- | --- |
| | *1974* | *1979* | *1985* |
| Both sexes | 1.0 | 1.4 | 1.5 |
| Males | — | — | 2.0 |
| Females | — | — | 1.0 |

NOTE:   Dashes indicate figures too small to reliably report.
SOURCE:   Schoenborn, C. A., & Boyd, G. (1989). *Smoking and other tobacco use: United States, 1987*. (DHHS Publication No. PHS 89-1597). Washington DC: U.S. Government Printing Office.

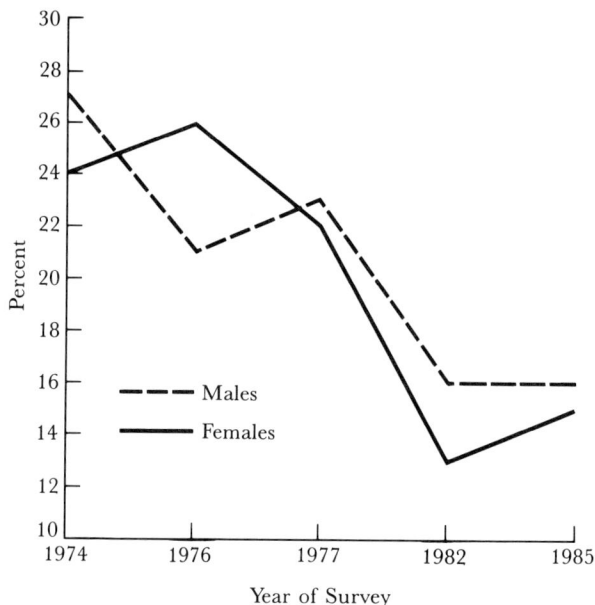

FIGURE 15.1   Percentages of male and female adolescents (between twelve and seventeen years old) who reported smoking cigarettes during the past month. Between 1974 and 1985, male smoking rates dropped from 27% to 16% and female rates dropped from 24% to 15%. The data were gathered in household interviews with a sample of the United States population. The solid line represents male respondents, and the dotted line represents female respondents. From "Smoking and Other Tobacco Use: United States, 1987", by C. A. Schoenborn and G. Boyd, 1989, DHHS Publication No. PHS 89–1597, Washington D.C.: U.S. Government Printing Office.

(Zelnick & Kantner, 1980). About half of the pregnancies among women under the age of twenty are terminated by abortion or miscarriage (Brunswick & Merzel, 1986), thereby increasing the health risk of pregnancy in this age group. Psychosocial and economic problems associated with adolescent pregnancies were discussed earlier in this chapter.

Although these figures indicate that adolescence is a time when many health-endangering habits may develop, it is important to note that not all adolescents adopt these behaviors. Relatively few adolescents smoke and smoking rates are declining, possibly because of an increase in beliefs that smoking has negative social consequences. Social concerns are strong determinants of adolescent behavior: beliefs in the negative physiological consequences of smoking may be declining and beliefs in smoking's positive psychological consequences may be increasing at the same time smoking rates are declining. It will thus be important to continue to emphasize the negative health effects of smoking in the future (Chassin, Presson, Sherman, & McGrew, 1987). Many adolescents also exercise regularly. Brown and Siegel (1988) found that seventh through eleventh graders reported about an hour or more per week of aerobics, calisthenics, running, swimming, and tennis. More importantly, exercise served as a buffer against the development of illness under stress. Adolescents who exercised were significantly less likely to become ill during periods of stress than were adolescents who did not exercise (Brown & Siegel, 1988).

## Adolescent Smoking: Initiation and Prevention

Everyone has the option of becoming a smoker or remaining a nonsmoker, and most people try cigarettes at least once. However, some people quit soon or immediately after that first trial cigarette, whereas others go on to further experimentation and eventually become smokers (Flay, d'Avernas, Best, Kersell & Ryan, 1983). The factors that influence adolescents to begin smoking, drinking alcohol, and using marijuana appear to be similar (Hansen et al., 1987). Peers have a major influence on whether or not smoking, or other substance use, is initiated. Peers may model smoking behavior, provide cigarettes or other forms of tobacco, and encourage their use (Newcomb & Bentler, 1989). Peer influence seems to be stronger than parental influence (Severson & Lichtenstein, 1986), but the family does have an impact on the development of smoking behavior. An older sibling who smokes increases the probability that other children in the family will smoke (Evans & Raines, 1982).

Socioeconomic status (SES) and gender also influence the acquisition of smoking behavior. Smoking is more common among males, and lower levels of education and SES are associated with higher smoking rates (National Center for Health Statistics, 1989). Self-esteem and self-image may also affect smoking acquisition. Smoking may reflect a desire for accelerated maturity in response to blows to self-esteem, such as academic failure, or it may be perceived as a way to look more mature and competent (Evans, Hendersen, Hill, & Raines, 1979; Flay et al., 1983).

The importance of potential influences on smoking behavior varies depending on how well developed the habit is. Family influences appear to be most important before a person first experiments with smoking, as the family affects attitudes that play a role in the selection of important peers. SES has an indirect influence at this stage, because it is associated with the child's environment, and thus the potential peer-group to which he or she may be exposed. SES is also important through its relationship to parental smoking behavior. As an adolescent confronts the opportunity to smoke the first cigarette, peer pressure and problems with self-image or social competence may become more important. Peer pressure remains important as opportunities for further experimentation arise, but social motives and the physiological effects of smoking become more dominant influences. The physiological response to nicotine becomes more and more influential as the adolescent becomes a regular smoker (Flay et al., 1983).

THE PREVENTION OF ADOLESCENT SMOKING   Because multiple factors are involved in adolescent smoking behavior, most recent programs for smoking prevention use multicomponent interventions addressing a range of potential antecedents. Prevention efforts are often targeted at sixth and seventh graders because many adolescents start smoking during these years. Most are classroom-based, and involve five to seven intervention sessions with booster sessions several months later. Many programs take a social psychological approach; they increase participants' awareness of the social pressures to smoke, include training in stress-reduction techniques and decision-making skills, and teach ways to resist the social pressure. Because information about the immediate aversive physiological consequences of smoking may provide a more effective deterrent than facts about future consequences such as heart disease and lung cancer, programs emphasize effects such as increased heart rate and blood pressure. (Evans et al., 1978; Severson & Lichtenstein, 1986).

The Houston Project of Evans and his colleagues (1978) has had a large influence on the design and strategy of smoking prevention programs. Children in the Houston Project viewed videotapes about the dangers of smoking, the advantages of not smoking, the effects of smoking on other people, and the effects of peer pressure on smoking behavior. The videotapes also discussed advertising and mass media pressures encouraging smoking, including how advertising attempts to make smoking appealing and how it hides the Surgeon General's warning about cigarette smoking. Parental influences were also covered, and the videotapes showed children modeling their parents' smoking behavior despite parental injunctions against smoking. The videotape presentations were followed by small group discussions focusing on methods to cope with the pressures to smoke. Finally, posters showing scenes from the videotapes were displayed in the participants' classrooms as reminders. Exposure to this program resulted in a 50% reduction in the onset of smoking two and one half months after the program ended.

A similar smoking prevention program was conducted with Minnesota seventh graders (Arkin, Roemhild, Johnson, Luepker, & Murray, 1981; Murray, Pirie, Luepker, & Pallonen, 1989; Murray, Richards, Luepker, & Johnson, 1987). Students in these programs were exposed to several different interventions. Some listened to lectures and watched videotapes about the long-term health consequences of smoking and others received information about social forces encouraging smoking, negative social and physiological consequences of smoking, and techniques to resist the social pressure to smoke. A final group of students received no instruction about smoking over and above the regular school curriculum. Smoking behavior was assessed repeatedly for five or six years after participation. The length of follow-up varied according to the date of participation.

The results of the prevention programs were most noticeable during the first and second years after the programs. By the time of the final follow-up, between 11.4% and 16.0% of the students were daily smokers; there were no differences in smoking behavior between groups who had participated in the different programs or had been exposed only to the regular curriculum. Despite the lack of long-term effects, Murray and his colleagues were optimistic because the early differences in smoking initiation suggested that the programs could have an effect. Even if the effect faded with time, a delay in when a person begins smoking can have significant health benefits and those who begin smoking later are more successful at quitting. Additionally, the programs included no booster sessions, and these reminders might have helped to maintain the good results of the first few years (Murray et al., 1989).

Overall, the results of the adolescent smoking prevention programs are encouraging, but much more research needs to be conducted. In a review of twenty-seven programs, Flay (1985) found that most programs seem to reduce smoking onset by about 50%. However, follow-up past two years is rare and effectiveness may decline if more than two years have passed since involvement in the program. Booster sessions appear to be important if the results of the programs are to be maintained. Most programs involve many components, and more efficient programs could be designed if research determined which components are most effective and which might be expendable.

# Chronic Illness in Childhood

From 10% to 15% of children in the United States have some chronic health problem (Gortmaker, 1985; Pless & Roghmann, 1971). Chronic illness is typically defined as illness that lasts for more than three months a year or leads to continuous hospitalization for at least one month in a year (Pless & Pinkerton, 1975). Childhood chronic illnesses include juvenile-onset diabetes, asthma, spina bifida, congenital heart disease, hemophilia, end-stage renal disease, sickle cell anemia, cystic fibrosis, and muscular dystrophy (Hobbs, Perrin, & Ireys, 1985). Although many of these disorders afflict relatively few children, the societal impact of chronic illness is much greater than their low incidence would suggest. The causes of many chronic illnesses are not well understood, and treatment focuses on illness management and symptom reduction rather than cure. Chronic illness therefore presents an ongoing, enduring threat to the child's life and developmental integrity as well as to the family's equilibrium.

# Emotional Reactions of Children to Chronic Illness

Children's emotional reactions to chronic illness are largely determined by their level of emotional and cognitive development. As noted earlier in this chapter, what children know about illness and its consequences varies depending on their developmental level. Their understanding of their illness and treatment may bear directly on their emotional responses to them. For example, children at a low level of cognitive maturity sometimes believe in immanent justice, or that people become ill because they deserve it (Kister & Patterson, 1980). A chronically ill child with this belief could easily feel guilty for being ill. In this way, chronic illness can lead to low self-esteem. Preschool children with diabetes, for example, may think that their illness was caused by eating too much candy (Perrin & Gerrity, 1981).

The prolonged hospitalization required by some chronic illnesses can inhibit the development of a strong sense of attachment between infants and parents. Medical equipment, such as tubes and machines, along with parents' fears of touching or cuddling fragile, ill infants may disrupt normal bonding and attachment. If a child is older, prolonged hospitalizations may interfere with the development of a sense of autonomy and separateness from parents. Illness and hospitalization may restrict a toddler's normal environmental exploration, and parents may fear that the ill child will suffer an injury or exacerbate his or her illness. (Hobbs et al., 1985; Magrab, 1978). Some chronic illnesses also involve impairments in sensory abilities such as sight and hearing. This sensory impairment combined with the restricted mobility imposed in the hospital may delay cognitive development in young children because it depends partly on physical exploration of the environment (Steinbauer, Mushin, & Rae-Grant, 1974).

Preschool children typically deal with developmental tasks of increasing mastery over obstacles and problems. However, chronically ill children often require higher levels of parental support than do healthy children. This may interfere with normal strivings toward independence and mastery as ill children are often less able than healthy children to take over caretaking functions. Illness may thus impose restraints that make mastery difficult, and thereby contribute to feelings of failure and low self-esteem (Hobbs et al., 1985; Steinbauer et al., 1974).

Chronically ill school-age children are unlikely to feel that illness is a punishment for wrongdoing. However they are likely to perceive differences between themselves and others. They may feel inferior or angry because they are not like others. If a chronic illness involves a physical deformity, adolescents may feel anxious or depressed because they appear different from others their own age. Ill children also may miss a great deal of school. This can lead to academic problems and may cause difficulties with interpersonal relationships. Peers are likely to be seen inconsistently and they probably do not understand or have distorted ideas about the ill child's health problems (Steinbauer et al., 1974).

Not all children with chronic illness experience psychological difficulties. Coping ability may increase as a child learns to deal with an illness, and adults who suffered from childhood chronic illness cope surprisingly well despite a higher than average incidence of problems in social adaptation (Drotar, 1981; Drotar, Owens, & Gotthold, 1980). Children who believe that their own actions can lead to a desired outcome may be better able to cope with chronic illness than are those who do not hold this belief. In a study of children with cystic fibrosis, self-efficacy was positively correlated with compliance with medical instructions (Czajkowski & Koocher, 1986).

## Effects of Chronic Illness on the Family

The families of chronically ill children deal with stresses that are unknown to many families, with every member of the family being affected. Hobbs et al. (1985) described several stresses that occur as a result of an ill child, including: (1) the shock of the initial diagnosis and the need to deal with painful feelings that occur at this time; (2) the exhausting and relentless need to provide ongoing and sometimes twenty-four-hour care for a child; (3) the unpredictable crises that sometimes occur in the child's medical condition that require emergency mobilization of psychological and often financial resources of the family; (4) the persistent financial concerns; (5) the continual witnessing of a child's pain and suffering; and (6) the stresses involved in answering the multitude of questions that arise about the fair distribution within the family of time, money, and concern.

Families may pass through several stages after a child's chronic illness is diagnosed. An initial period of shock and bewilderment is often followed by a sense that the situation is not really happening and attempts to deny its presence. Sadness, anger, and anxiety occur as the problem persists and attention to it continues. Finally, some adaptation occurs and the intensity of feelings diminishes (Hobbs et al., 1985).

Families with a recently diagnosed diabetic child have been found to differ from families with a child suffering an acute illness. Hauser et al. (1986) reported that mothers and their diabetic children engaged in more enabling interactions (interactions involving problem solving and attempting to make the other person's point of view more clear) than did mothers and their acutely ill children. Fathers of diabetic children, however, were prone to be judgmental and indifferent in their interactions with their ill children. The experimenters hypothesized that the fathers' behavior was a reaction to feelings such as anger, guilt, and sadness in reaction to learning of the child's illness (Hauser et al., 1986).

Family members are certainly affected by the demands for care of a chronically ill child. Such factors as the need for complicated special diets, as in diabetes or advanced kidney disease, or the need for physical acts, as lifting, diapering, dressing, or giving physical treatments, affect the degree of stress and nature of demands on the family. The need to adapt certain aspects of the household environment, such as extra housecleaning to eliminate dust for an asthmatic child or constructing ramps and lifts to make things more accessible for a disabled child, may occur. Sleep interruption of parents as they care for children in the middle of the night may be required, depending upon the illness. Clearly, the character of the chronic illness affects the nature of the stresses and demands upon the family (Travis, 1976).

Financial worries are reported to be a major, constant burden in families with a chronically ill child (Pearson, Stranova, & Thompson, 1976). Expenditures for such things as hospitalizations, physician visits, special medical procedures and equipment, medications, time missed from work and nursing care may be required. Typically, the insurance coverage families have for such crises is inadequate in eliminating such financial burdens.

The processes of adjusting to the realization that a child has a chronic illness and of coping with the financial and practical burdens the illness imposes can result in a variety of family problems. Parents may find themselves feeling disappointed or ashamed that their child is ill, and may simultaneously feel angry about the burden the illness imposes. They may be overprotective, overindulgent, or excessively restrictive, and may concentrate attention on the ill child and neglect other children in the family. Siblings may resent the favored attention the ill child receives, and may feel ashamed about having an abnormal brother or sister (Talbot & Howell, 1971). However, it is important to realize that although these negative effects may be present for some families, not all families with a chronically ill child experience serious problems (Kazak, 1989). The individuals involved, the nature of the illness, and the quality of family interaction all play a prominent role in the family's eventual adaptation. Further work is needed to understand what may serve to make a family resistant to dysfunction, and what factors in family functioning best promote a positive adaptation to the stress of chronic illness.

## Adjustment of Children and Their Families to Chronic Illness

Early evaluations of the effects of chronic illness on the child and family were based on the assumption that some psychopathology was necessarily intertwined with the adaptation to an illness and in some cases, the etiology of an illness. The maladaptive behavior patterns in families with chronically ill children were seen as stemming from psychological problems within the individuals in the family. The treatment focus was, therefore, aimed at curing underlying psychopathology. More recently, however, it has been argued that the behavioral patterns and coping styles of children with chronic illness and their families are best understood as the result of the psychological impact of the disease and the burdens stemming from it (Russo, 1986). When one examines the literature on the psychological adjustment of children with chronic illness, this perspective is supported.

The available literature on the effect of chronic illness on adjustment of children and their families shows inconsistent findings. Some researchers have found that divorce rates are higher among these families (Zimmerman, 1980), whereas others have found they are lower (Kazak, 1989; Lansky, Cairns, Hassanein, Wehr, & Lowman, 1978), suggesting that chronic illness may sometimes have a cohesive effect on a marriage. Some studies (Donofrio, 1979) have shown chronic illness to negatively affect family interactions, but other studies have found no difference in the quality of family interaction between families with a child who has chronic illness and with those who do not (Saur, 1980). Conflicting findings also have been apparent in studies investigating the effect of chronic illness on the siblings of these children. Although some studies have shown siblings to have greater problems, as evidenced by such qualities as greater irritability and social withdrawal (Lavigne & Ryan, 1979), other studies have found them to have an increased sense of compassion and sensitivity to the needs of others (Burton, 1975).

Family interaction patterns may either facilitate adaptive coping or hinder the child and family's ability to deal with a chronic illness. Interactions contributing to poor illness control include enmeshment, overprotection, rigidity, and lack of conflict resolution (Minuchin, Rosman, & Baker, 1978); these patterns were discussed with regard to asthmna in Chapter 11. Cohesive families have been found to be associated with adaptive coping in diabetic children. Hanson et al. (1989) reported that diabetic children in families where the individual members were relatively disengaged from one another (low cohesion) were prone to cope by avoiding and ventilating. Avoidance coping includes behaviors such as using drugs or alcohol to escape or avoiding problematic people or issues; ventilation involves reducing tension by yelling, complaining, or blaming others. The ability of the family to adapt flexibly to change was also important. The longer the child had suffered from diabetes, the more important family adaptability became in helping the child cope constructively. Avoidance and ventilation were associated with poor compliance with the demands of diabetes treatment, so family cohesion and adaptability were important to the health of the ill child as well as to his or her coping style (Hanson et al., 1989).

Parental attitudes have a significant impact on how ill children and their families cope with chronic illness. Overprotective or rejecting attitudes promote children to rebel and fail to follow medical instructions. However, parents who restrict the ill child only to the degree that is necessary and encourage self-care, school attendance, and reasonable levels of physical activity facilitate the child's ability to cope with chronic illness. Parents who remain calm in a crisis and lessen their own anxiety by familiarizing themselves with the child's illness also help the child to cope. Because children typically are affected by, and take their cues from, parental attitudes and actions, their ability to manage and cope with illness is closely related to their parents' coping abilities. The more parents are able to cope with their own feelings and help the child manage and cope, the greater the likelihood he or she will cope adequately (Mattson, 1977).

Future research should attempt to identify factors associated with good and poor adjustment to chronic illness. It is not correct to assume that the presence of illness necessarily makes for poor psychological adjustment or that psychological problems are, a priori, tied to illness. The development of psychological problems is more likely related to many factors that include the particulars of the illness itself, the burdens it places on the child and family, the way the family functions, and the quality of interactions with society at large (such as school and health care systems).

# Summary

Development is the normal process of orderly change over time in physical, emotional, and intellectual status. A child's motoric, cognitive, and psychosocial developmental levels affect health in a variety of ways. The increased mobility accompanying motor development increases the risk of accidents; anticipatory guidance sessions may reduce this risk.

Cognitive development influences how children understand illness. As children mature they develop progressively more sophisticated understanding of how illness is transmitted and are less likely to see illness as punishment for wrongdoing. They also begin to understand that illness is an internal event influenced by both external agents and psychological processes. Psychosocial developmental level determines responsibility for health self-regulation and influences a child's emotional response to separation.

Teratogens are environmental agents producing abnormalities in prenatal organisms. Diseases such as rubella and herpes simplex in pregnant women can impair fetal development. AIDS is an increasing health problem, and about 80% of pediatric AIDS cases result from exposure during the prenatal period or during birth. Exposure to diagnostic or therapeutic radiation, such as X rays, can also be harmful to the fetus. Maternal smoking is the most preventable cause of prematurity and low birth weight. Maternal drinking may also be harmful. Fetal alcohol syndrome includes physical and intellectual abnormalities, and one or two drinks per day by pregnant women may increase the risk of growth retardation. Women over thirty-five are at increased risk for problems in pregnancy and fetal development, as are women under the age of fourteen or fifteen. The major risks of adolescent pregnancy are psychosocial and economic, and children of adolescent mothers are at risk for social and behavioral problems.

Enuresis is more common than encopresis, but both present psychosocial and family problems. Enuresis may be successfully treated with behavioral techniques, including the urine alarm method, operant programs, and retention control training. Encopresis has been treated by contingency management and practice of appropriate toilet behaviors.

Life changes during adolescence provide opportunities for the adoption of many health-enhancing or health-endangering behaviors. Accidents and violence are the leading causes of death in adolescence. About 15 % of adolescents smoke at least once a month, and about one-third drink alcohol. Cigarette smoking rates are declining, and marijuana usage is decreasing now after an increase in the 1970s. A lack of contraception during sexual activity is a serious problem for adolescents today. Adolescents who exercise regularly are less susceptible to illness when under stress.

Adolescent smoking is affected by family members and peers, socioeconomic status, self-image, and social competence. Smoking prevention programs emphasize the immediate negative physiological consequences of smoking. They also stress the social pressures to smoke and provide training in ways to resist this pressure. Prevention programs appear effective initially, but may need booster sessions to maintain effects.

A child's cognitive and emotional development levels affect how he or she reacts to chronic illnesses. Chronic illness may promote low self-esteem, impair attachment between children and parents, delay the development of independence, and interfere with normal social contacts. Families of chronically ill children may be disturbed, and family interaction may help or hinder the child's adjustment to illness. Cohesive and adaptable families that encourage self-care and reasonable activity levels facilitate the child's adaptation.

# *References*

ABEL, E. L. (1980). Fetal alcohol syndrome: Behavioral teratology. *Psychological Bulletin, 87,* 29–50.

ALCOFF, J. M. (1982). Car seats for children. *American Family Physician, 25,* 167–171.

ARKIN, R. M., ROEMHILD, H. F., JOHNSON, C. A., LUEPKER, R. V., & MURRAY, D. M. (1981). The Minnesota smoking prevention program: A seventh grade health curriculum supplement. *Journal of School Health, 51,* 611–616.

AZRIN, N. H., SNEED, T. J., & FOXX, R. M. (1974). Dry-bed training: Rapid elimination of childhood enuresis. *Behaviour Research and Therapy, 12,* 147–156.

BABSON, S. G., PERNOLL, M. L., BENDA, G. I., & SIMPSON, K. (1980). *Diagnosis and management of the fetus and neonate at risk: A guide for team care (4th edition).* St. Louis: D. V. Mosby.

BADGER, E. (1981). Effects of parent education program on teenage mothers and their offspring. In K. G. Scott, T. Field, & E. G. Robertson (Eds.), *Teenage parents and their offspring.* New York: Grune & Stratton.

BAKWIN, H. (1973). The genetics of enuresis. In I. Kovin, R. C. MacKeither, & S. R. Meadow (Eds.), *Bladder control and enuresis* (pp. 73–78). Philadelphia: Lippincott.

BALSOM, P. J. (1973). Case study: Encopresis: A case with symptom substitution? *Behavior Therapy, 4,* 134–136.

BIBACE, R., & WALSH, M. E. (1980). Development of children's concepts of illness. *Pediatrics, 66,* 912–917.

BROWN, J. D., & SIEGEL, J. M. (1988). Exercise as a buffer of life stress: A prospective study of adolescent health. *Health Psychology, 7,* 341–354.

BRUNSWICK, A. F., & MERZEL, C. R. (1986). Biopsychosocial and epidemiologic perspectives on adolescent health. In N. A. Krasnegor, J. D. Arasteh, & M. F. Cataldo (Eds.), *Child health behavior: A behavioral pediatrics perspective.* New York: Wiley.

BURBACH, D. J., & PETERSON, L. (1986). Children's concepts of physical illness: A review and critique of the cognitive-developmental literature. *Health Psychology, 5*, 307–325.

BURTON, L. (1975). The family life of sick children. London: Routledge & Kegan Paul.

CALIFANO, J. A., JR. (1979). *Healthy people: The surgeon general's report on health promotion and disease prevention.* Washington, DC: U.S. Government Printing Office.

CAMPBELL, M. F. (1970). Neuromuscular uropathy. In M. F. Campbell & T. H. Harrison (Eds.), *Urology, Vol 2*. Philadelphia: Saunders.

CHASSIN, L., PRESSON, C. C., SHERMAN, S. J., & MCGREW, J. (1987). The changing smoking environment for middle and high school students: 1980–1983. *Journal of Behavioral Medicine, 10*, 581–594.

CHRISTOPHERSEN, E. R. (1989). Injury control. *American Psychologist, 44*, 237–241.

CHRISTOPHERSEN, E. R. (1986). Management of behavior problems in primary care settings. In N. A. Krasnegor, J. D. Arasteh, & M. F. Cataldo (Eds.), *Child health behavior: A behavioral pediatrics perspective*. New York: Wiley.

CHRISTOPHERSEN, E. R., & RAINEY, S. K. (1976). Management of encopresis through a pediatric outpatient clinic. *Journal of Pediatric Psychology, 4*, 38–41.

CHRISTOPHERSEN, E. R., & RAPOFF, M. A. (1979). Behavioral pediatrics. In O. F. Pomerleau & J. P. Brady (Eds.), *Behavioral medicine: Theory and practice* (pp. 99–123). Baltimore: Williams & Wilkins.

CLARREN, S. K., & SMITH, D. W. (1978). The fetal alcohol syndrome. *New England Journal of Medicine, 298*, 1063–1067.

CONGER, J. (1970). The treatment of encopresis by the management of social consequences. *Behavior Therapy, 1*, 386–390.

CZAJKOWSKI, D. R., & KOOCHER, G. P. (1986). Predicting medical compliance among adolescents with cystic fibrosis. *Health Psychology, 5*, 297–306.

DANAHER, B. G., SHISSLAK, C. M., THOMPSON, C. B., & FORD, J. D. (1978). A smoking cessation program for pregnant women: An exploratory study. *American Journal of Public Health, 68*, 896–898.

DOLEYS, D. M. (1977). Behavioral treatments for nocturnal enuresis in children: A review of the recent literature. *Psychological Bulletin, 84*, 30–54.

DOLEYS, D. M., CIMINERO, A. R., TOLLISON, J. W., WILLIAMS, C. L., & WELLS, K. D. (1977). Dry-bed training and retention control training: A comparison. *Behavior Therapy, 8*, 541–548.

DONOFRIO, J. C. (1979). A comparison of family verbal interaction patterns in families with an asthmatic, diabetic, and nondisabled child. Unpublished doctoral dissertation, State University of New York at Buffalo.

DROTAR, D. (1981). Psychological perspectives in chronic childhood illness. *Journal of Pediatric Psychology, 6*, 211–228.

DROTAR, D., OWENS, R., & GOTTHOLD, J. (1980). Personality adjustment of children and adolescents with hypopituitarism. *Child Psychiatry and Human Development, 11*, 59–66.

EDELMAN, R. I. (1971). Operant conditioning treatment of encopresis. *Journal of Behavior Therapy and Experimental Psychiatry, 2*, 71–73.

EVANS, R. I., HENDERSON, A. H., HILL, P. C., & RAINES, B. E. (1979). Current psychological, social, and educational programs in control and prevention of smoking: A critical methodological review. *Atherosclerosis Reviews, 6*, 203–245.

EVANS, R. I., & RAINES, B.E. (1982). Control and prevention of smoking in adolescents: A psychosocial perspective. In T. J. Coates, A. C. Peterson, & C. Perry (Eds.), *Promoting adolescent health: A dialogue on research and practice.* New York: Academic.

EVANS, R. I., ROZELLE, R. M., MITTLEMARK, M. B., HANSEN, W. B., BANE, A. L., & HAVIS, J. (1978). Deterring the onset of smoking in children: Knowledge of immediate physiological effects and coping with peer pressure, media pressure, and parent modeling. *Journal of Applied Social Psychology, 8,* 126–135.

FLAY, B. R. (1985). Psychosocial approaches to smoking prevention: A review of findings. *Health Psychology, 4,* 449–488.

FLAY, B. R., d'AVERNAS, J. R., BEST, J. A., KERSELL, M. W., & RYAN, K. B. (1983). Cigarette smoking: Why young people do it and ways of preventing it. In P. J. McGrath & P. Firestone (Eds.), *Pediatric and adolescent behavior medicine: Issues in treatment.* New York: Springer.

FOXX, R. M., & AZRIN, N. H. (1973). *Toilet training the retarded: A rapid program for day and nighttime independent toileting.* Champaign, IL: Research Press.

FREINDEN, W., & VAN HANDEL, D. (1970). Elimination of soiling in an elementary school child through application of aversive technique. *Journal of School Psychology, 8,* 267–269.

FRIAS, M. L. (1975). Prenatal diagnosis of genetic abnormalities. *Clinical Obstetrics and Gynecology, 18,* 221–236.

FRIMAN, P. C., & CHRISTOPHERSEN, E. R. (1986). Biobehavioral prevention in primary care. In N. A. Krasnegor, J. D. Arasteh, & M. F. Cataldo (Eds.), *Child health behavior: A behavioral pediatrics perspective.* New York: Wiley.

FURSTENBERG, F. F., Jr., BROOKS-GUNN, J., & CHASE-LANSDALE, L. (1989). Teen-aged pregnancy and childbearing. *American Psychologist, 44,* 313–320.

GEFFKEN, G., JOHNSON, S. B., & WALKER, D. (1986). Behavioral interventions for childhood nocturnal enuresis: The differential effect of bladder capacity on treatment progress and outcome. *Health Psychology, 5,* 261–272.

GOLDBERG, I. E., ROGHMANN, K. J., McINERNY, T. K., & BURKE, J. D. (1984). Mental health problems among children seen in pediatric practice: Prevalence and management. *Pediatrics, 73,* 278–293.

GORTMAKER, S. L. (1985). Demography of childhood chronic diseases. In N. Hobbs & J. M. Perrin (Eds.), *Issues in the care of children with chronic illness: A sourcebook on problems, services, and policies.* San Francisco: Jossey-Bass.

GROSS, R. T., & DORNBUSH, S. M. (1983). Enuresis. In M. D. Levine, W. B. Carey, A. C. Crocker, & R. T. Gross (Eds.), *Developmental-behavioral pediatrics* (pp. 573–586). Philadelphia: Saunders.

HALPERIN, S., BASS, J., MEHTA, K., & BETTS, K. (1983). Unintentional injuries among adolescents and young adults: A review and analysis. *Journal of Adolescent Health Care, 4,* 275–281.

HANSEN, W. B., GRAHAM, J. W., SOBEL, J. L., SHELTON, D. R., FLAY, B. R., & JOHNSON, C. A. (1987). The consistency of peer and parent influences on tobacco, alcohol, and marijuana use among young adolescents. *Journal of Behavioral Medicine, 10,* 559–580.

HANSON, C. L., CIGRANG, J. A., HARRIS, M. A., CARLE, D. L., RELYEA, G., & BURGHEN, G. A. (1989). Coping styles in youths with insulin-dependent diabetes mellitus. *Journal of Consulting and Clinical Psychology, 57,* 644–651.

HAUSER, S. T., JACOBSON, A. M., WERTLIEB, D., WEISS-PERRY, B., FOLLANSBEE, D., WOLSDORF, J. I., HERSKOWITZ, R. D., HOULIHAN, J., & RAJAPARK, D. C. (1986). Children with recently diagnosed diabetes: Interactions within their families. *Health Psychology, 5*, 273–296.

HOBBS, N., PERRIN, J. M., & IREYS, H. T. (1985). *Chronically ill children and their families.* San Francisco: Jossey-Bass.

HOFFERTH, S. L., & HAYES, C. D. (1987). *Risking the future: Adolescent sexuality, pregnancy, and childbearing: Vol 2. Working papers and statistical reports.* Washington DC: National Academy Press.

HOWARD, F. M., & HILL, J. M. (1979). Drugs in pregnancy. *Obstetrical and Gynecological Survey, 34*, 643–653.

JESSOR, R. (1984). Adolescent development and behavioral health. In J. D. Matarazzo, S. M. Weiss, J. A. Herd, N. E. Miller, & S. M. Weiss (Eds.), *Behavioral health: A handbook of health enhancement and disease prevention* (pp. 69–90). New York: Wiley.

KAROLY, P. (1982). Developmental pediatrics: A process-oriented approach to the analysis of health competence. In P. Karoly, J. J. Steffen, & D. J. O'Grady (Eds.), *Child health psychology: Concepts and issues* (pp. 29–57). New York: Pergamon.

KAZAK, A. E. (1989). Families of chronically ill children: A systems and social-ecological model of adaptation and change. *Journal of Consulting and Clinical Psychology, 57*, 25–30.

KIMMEL, H. D., & KIMMEL, E. (1970). An instrumental conditioning method for the treatment of enuresis. *Journal of Behavior Therapy and Experimental Psychiatry, 1*, 121–123.

KISTER, M., & PATTERSON, C. (1980). Children's conception of the cause of illness: Understanding of contagion and use of immanent justice. *Child Development, 51*, 839–846.

LaBARBA, R. C. (1984). Prenatal and neonatal influences on behavioral health development. In J. D. Matarazzo, S. M. Weiss, J. A. Herd, N. E. Miller, & S. M. Weiss (Eds.), *Behavioral health: A handbook of health enhancement and disease prevention* (pp. 41–55). New York: Wiley.

LANGMAN, J. (1975). *Medical embryology* (3rd ed.). Baltimore: Williams & Wilkins.

LANSKY, S. B., CAIRNS, N. U., HASSANEIN, R., WEHR, J., & LOWMAN, J. T. (1978). Childhood cancer: Parental discord and divorce. *Pediatrics, 62*, 184–188.

LAVIGNE, J. V., & RYAN, M. (1979). Psychological adjustment of siblings of children with chronic illness. *Pediatrics, 63*, 616–627.

LEVINE, M. D. (1975). Children with encopresis: A descriptive analysis. *Pediatrics, 56*, 412–416.

LOVIBOND, S. H. (1964). *Conditioning and enuresis.* Oxford, England: Pergamon.

MADDUX, J. E., ROBERTS, M. C., SLEDDEN, E. A., & WRIGHT, L. (1986). Developmental issues in child health psychology. *American Psychologist, 41*, 25–34.

MAGRAB, P. R. (1978). In P. R. Magrab, *Psychological management of pediatric problems, Vol. 1: Early life conditions and chronic disease* (pp. 3–14). Baltimore: University Park Press.

MATTSON, A. (1977). Long term physical illness in childhood: A challenge to psychosocial adaptation. In R. H. Moos (Ed.), *Coping with physical illness.* New York: Plenum.

MILLS, E. J., GRAUBARD, B. I., HARLEY, E. E., RHOADS, G. G., & BERENDES, H. W. (1984). Maternal alcohol consumption and birth weight: How much drinking is safe during pregnancy? *Journal of the American Medical Association, 252,* 1875–1879.

MINUCHIN, S., ROSMAN, B. L., & BAKER, L. (1978). *Psychosomatic families: Anorexia nervosa in context.* Cambridge, MA: Harvard University Press.

MOWRER, O. H., & MOWRER, W. (1938). Enuresis: A method for its study and treatment. *American Journal of Orthopsychiatry, 8,* 436–459.

MURRAY, D. M., PIRIE, P., LUEPKER, R. V., & PALLONEN, U. (1989). Five- and six-year follow-up results from four seventh-grade smoking prevention projects. *Journal of Behavioral Medicine, 12,* 207–218.

MURRAY, D. M., RICHARDS, P. S., LUEPKER, R. V., & JOHNSON, C. A. (1987). The prevention of cigarette smoking in children: Two- and three-year follow-up comparisons of four prevention strategies. *Journal of Behavioral Medicine, 10,* 595–612.

MUSICCO, N. (1977). Encopresis: A good result in a boy with UTP (Urinide-5-triphosphate). *American Journal of Proctology, 28,* 43–46.

NATIONAL ACADEMY OF SCIENCES. (1986). *Confronting AIDS: Directions for public health, health care and research.* Washington, D.C.: National Academy Press.

NATIONAL CENTER FOR HEALTH STATISTICS. (1989). *Health, United States, 1988.* (DHHS Publication No. PHS 89-1232). Washington, D.C.: U.S. Government Printing Office.

NATIONAL CENTER FOR HEALTH STATISTICS. (1988). *Vital statistics of the United States, 1986.* (Vol. 2, Mortality, Part A). (DHHS Publication No. PHS 88-1122). Washington, D.C.: U.S. Government Printing Office.

NATIONAL INSTITUTE ON ALCOHOL ABUSE AND ALCOHOLISM (NIAAA). (1986). *Media alert: FAS awareness campaign: My baby . . . strong and healthy.* Rockville, MD: National Clearinghouse for Alcohol Information.

NEALE, D. H . (1963). Behavior therapy and encopresis in children. *Behaviour Research and Therapy, 1,* 139–149.

NEWCOMB, M. B., & BENTLER, P. M. (1989). Substance use and abuse among children and teenagers. *American Psychologist, 44,* 242–248.

PARKER, L., & WHITEHEAD, W. (1982). Treatment of urinary and fecal incontinence in children. In D. C. Usso & J. W. Varni (Eds.), *Behavioral pediatrics: Research and practice* (pp. 143–174). New York: Plenum.

PEARSON, D. A., STRANOVA, T. J., & THOMPSON, J. D. (1976). Patient and program costs associated with chronic hemodialysis care. *Injury, 13,* 23–28.

PERLMUTTER, A. D. (1976). Enuresis. In T. P. Kelalis & L. R. King (Eds.), *Clinical pediatric urology.* Philadelphia: Saunders.

PERRIN, E. C., & GERRITY, P. S. (1981). There's a demon in your belly: Children's understanding of illness. *Pediatrics, 67,* 841–849.

PIAGET, J. (1930). *The child's conception of physical causality.* London: Kegan Paul.

PIERCE, C. M. (1985a). Encopresis. In H. I. Kaplan & B. J. Sadock (Eds.), *Comprehensive textbook of psychiatry/IV* (4th ed.) (pp. 1847–1849). Baltimore: Williams & Wilkins.

PIERCE, C. M. (1985b). Enuresis. In H. I. Kaplan & B. J. Sadock (Eds.), *Comprehensive textbook of psychiatry/IV* (4th ed.) (pp. 1842–1847). Baltimore: Williams & Wilkins.

PLESS, I. B., & PINKERTON, P. (1975). *Chronic childhood disorders: Promoting patterns of adjustment.* Chicago: Year Book Medical Publishers.

PLESS, I. B., & ROGHMANN, K. J. (1971). Chronic illness and its consequences: Observations based on three epidemiologic surveys. *Journal of Pediatrics, 79,* 351–359.

ROBERTS, M. C., & WRIGHT, L. (1982). Role of the pediatric psychologist as consultant to pediatricians. In J. M. Tuma (Ed.), *Handbook for the practice of pediatric psychology,* (pp. 251–289). New York: Wiley-Interscience.

RUSSO, D. C. (1986). Chronicity and normalcy as the psychological basis for research and treatment in chronic disease in children. In N. A. Krasnegor, J. D. Arasteh, & M. F. Cataldo (Eds.), *Child health behavior: A behavioral pediatrics perspective.* New York: Wiley.

SAUR, W. G. (1980). Social networks and family environments of mothers of multiply, severely handicapped children. Unpublished doctoral dissertation, Florida State University.

SCHAEFER, C. E. (1979). *Childhood encopresis and causes and therapy.* New York: Van Nostrand Reinhold.

SCHOENBORN, C. A., & BOYD, G. (1989). *Smoking and other tobacco use: United States, 1987.* (DHHS Publication No. PHS 89-1597). Washington DC: U.S. Government Printing Office.

SEVERSON, H. H., & LICHTENSTEIN, E. (1986). Smoking prevention programs for adolescents: Rationale and review. In N. A. Krasnegor, J. D. Arasteh, & M. F. Cataldo (Eds.), *Child health behavior: A behavioral pediatrics perspective.* New York: Wiley.

SIEGAL, M. (1988). Children's knowledge of contagion and contamination as causes of illness. *Child Development, 59,* 1353–1359.

STARFIELD, B., GROSS, E., WOOD, M., PANTELL, R., ALLEN, C., GORDON, I. B., MOFFATT, P., DRACHMAN, R., & KATZ, H. (1980). Psychosocial and psychosomatic diagnoses in primary care of children. *Pediatrics, 66,* 159–167.

STEINBAUER, P. D., MUSHIN, D. N., & RAE-GRANT, Q. (1974). Psychological aspects of chronic illness. *Pediatric Clinics of North America, 21,* 825–840.

STREISSGUTH, A. P., BARR, H. M., SAMPSON, P. D., DARBY, B. L., & MARTIN, D. C. (1989). IQ at age 4 in relation to maternal alcohol use and smoking during pregnancy. *Developmental Psychology, 25,* 3–11.

TALBOT, N. B., & HOWELL, M. C. (1971). Social and behavioral causes and consequences of disease among children. In N. B. Talbot, J. Kagan, and L. Eisenberg (Eds.), *Behavioral science in pediatric medicine* (pp. 1–89). Philadelphia: Saunders.

TASK FORCE ON PEDIATRIC AIDS. (1989). Pediatric AIDS and human immunodeficiency virus infection: Psychological issues. *American Psychologist, 44,* 258–264.

TRAVIS, G. (1976). *Chronic illness in children.* Stanford, CA: Stanford University Press.

TURNER, R. K., YOUNG, G. C., & RACHMAN, S. (1970). Treatment of nocturnal enuresis by conditioning techniques. *Behaviour Research and Therapy, 8,* 367–381.

WERNER, H. (1948). *Comparative psychology of mental development.* New York: Science Editions.

WILLIS, D. J., ELLIOT, C. H., & JAY, S. (1982). Psychological effects of physical illness and its concomitants. In J. M. Tuma (Ed.), *Handbook for the practice of pediatric psychology* (pp. 28–66). New York: Wiley-Interscience.

WRIGHT, L., SCHAEFER, A. B., & SOLOMONS, G. (1979). *Encyclopedia of pediatric psychology*. Baltimore: University Park Press.

YEATES, W. K. (1973). Bladder function: Increased frequency and nocturnal incontinence. In I. Kovin, R. C. MacKeither, & S. R. Meadow (Eds.), *Bladder control and enuresis* (pp. 151–155). Philadelphia: Lippincott.

YOUNG, G. C., & MORGAN, R. T. T. (1972). Overlearning in the conditioning treatment of enuresis. *Behaviour Research and Therapy*, *10*, 419–420.

ZALESKI, A., GERRARD, J. W., & SHOKIER, M. H. K. (1973). Nocturnal enuresis: The importance of a small bladder capacity. In I. Kolvin, R. C. MacKeither, & S. R. Meadow (Eds.), *Bladder control and enuresis* (pp. 95–102). Philadelphia: Lippincott.

ZELNICK, M., & KANTER, J. F. (1980). Sexual activity, contraceptive use and pregnancy among metropolitan area teenagers 1971–1979. *Family Planning Perspectives*, *12*, 230–237.

ZELNICK, M., & SHAH, F. K. (1983). First intercourse among young Americans. *Family Planning Perspectives*, *15*, 64–70.

ZIMMERMAN, J. L. (1980). The relationship between support systems and stress in families with a handicapped child. Unpublished doctoral dissertation, University of Virginia.

CHAPTER 16

# Geriatric Health Psychology

Most of us face aging with mixed emotions. We look forward to the future and the opportunities it provides, and we wish for a long life. We strive for independence and the ability to manage our own lives, and when we are young we look forward to the day when we may move out on our own. Yet we also know that aging is a continuing process, and we dread facing the limitations we fear may be associated with old age. Illness becomes more likely with advancing age, and some of the elderly are totally dependent on family, friends, or the health care system. However, some elderly people remain independent, dynamic individuals far longer than others. What are the common health problems associated with aging, and how inevitable is declining health and vitality? What psychological factors are important for the maintenance of good health in old age, and what strategies are available to reduce the impact of the biological changes related to aging? If health problems do exist, what psychological interventions are available to help the patient and his or her family cope with their effects? This chapter provides an overview of geriatric health psychology, the subfield of health psychology devoted to the study of aging.

# The Aging Process

Aging is usually thought of in predominantly biological terms, but it is important to recognize that there are also important psychological and social features involved in aging. *Biological aging* in an organism is "the process of change ... that ... over time lowers the probability of survival and reduces the physiological capacity for self-regulation, repair, and adaptation to environmental demands" (Birren & Zarit, 1985, p. 9). It thus refers to the natural changes occurring with age, as well as changes that occur as a result of illness or injury. *Primary aging* refers to the natural changes coincident with aging, whereas *secondary aging* refers to the changes that follow disease or other damage (Busse, 1977). *Psychological aging* refers specifically to changes in adaptational ability, such as changes in sensation, learning ability, and memory. Psychological aging therefore affects how well an individual may be able to deal with changes in the social or physical environment or cope with biological changes (Birren & Zarit, 1985). The study of psychological aging thus concentrates on age-related changes in how a person interacts with the environment and how she or he deals with age-related physiological alterations. *Social aging* refers to the changes in societal expectations and roles associated with aging, such as retirement and lowered activity levels, and the social problems related to aging, such as decreased financial resources and increasing use of the health care system (Birren & Zarit, 1985).

Biological, psychological, and social aging clearly interact. Lowered energy levels as a result of illness may clearly interfere with a person's ability to cope with daily life, so biological changes may impair psychological capacities. Financial difficulties may arise as a person on a fixed income has higher medical bills and becomes more dependent on care from others. On the other hand, if intellectual abilities remain unimpaired with age, a person may be much better able to cope with biological changes and develop replacement behaviors to counteract events such as declining eyesight or hearing. At the age of seventy-nine, the psychologist B. F. Skinner published a book describing how he has coped with aging (Skinner & Vaughan, 1983), and Skinner is still quite active and much in demand as a speaker at professional meetings. He advocates a variety of reminder strategies, such as using notebooks and hanging an umbrella on the doorknob immediately after hearing a weather forecast calling for rain so the umbrella will not be forgotten when he leaves the house. He also recommends maintaining a circle of friends with similar interests because discussions with these friends will reinforce intellectual activity and encourage continuing creativity. His adaptive psychological aging processes, especially his intellectual skills, have clearly allowed him to minimize or avoid many problems often associated with biological aging.

It will become increasingly important that more and more of the aged are able to emulate Skinner and remain active, productive members of society. Although people over 65 years of age accounted for only 4% of the U.S.

population in 1900, more than 11% of the current U.S. population is 65 and over. It is expected that 17% of the population will be elderly by the year 2010. It is also important to realize that the percentage of very old people is also increasing. Of those now over 65, 38% are over 75 and 9% are over 85; in 1900, the figures were 30% and 4%, respectively (U.S. Bureau of the Census, 1981; Zarit, 1986). The costs to society could be immense if such a high percentage of the population were heavy users of medical and social services, and the personal costs of an unhappy or unsatisfying old age to so many individuals would be incalculable.

Illness and disability rates increase with age, but it is by no means inevitable that illness and disability accompany aging. About 40% of the disabled in the U.S. are over 65, but only about 5% of those over 65 are in nursing homes or long-term care facilities. Only 17% of those over 65 require short-term hospitalization in a given year; this rate is not much higher than the 11% of those under 65 who require such care (Henriksen, 1978; Schaie & Willis, 1986). Indeed, it is becoming increasingly recognized that a steady deterioration in health is not unavoidable. Instead, good health may be maintained, followed by a brief, rapid decline at the end of life (Henry, 1985). If this pattern of health followed by rapid decline becomes the norm, and gradual deterioration the exception, then the increasing ratio of older to younger individuals may not lead to as serious a cost to society and individuals as could be imagined. The singular and collective experience the elderly possess could instead represent a major social asset.

# Health Problems Related to Aging

Aging is associated with an increase in the frequency of a variety of diseases. Heart disease has been reported to be present in 40% of people over 65 and in 50% of those over 75 (Kennedy, Andrews, & Caird, 1977), and the probability of suffering a stroke also increases with age. About 25% of the population over 65 reports the presence of arthritis, as compared to less than 1% of those under 17 years old (National Center for Health Statistics, 1976). Cancer is also more common among the elderly; people over 65 account for more than half of the cases of cancer in the United States and the incidence of cancer increases steadily with age (Crawford & Cohen, 1984). These diseases have been discussed in previous chapters, and will not be reviewed again here. Instead, this chapter will focus on diseases more specifically associated with aging and the biological changes related to the normal aging process.

## Sensory Changes and Arousal

There is a general decline in sensory abilities with age; the most noticeable declines occur in vision and hearing. The lens of the eye becomes less flexible and less transparent with age, leading to difficulties in focusing and to a need for more light in order to see well. Clouding of the lens also increases the risk for glare, as light rays are scattered as they enter the eye. Thus, the need for increased illumination levels may cause problems as higher-light levels often lead to more glare. The number of cones in the retina also decreases with age, leading to declining color vision and reduced visual acuity. (Kline & Scheiber, 1985). The aging person is thus at risk for feeling increasingly out of touch with the visual world, and this feeling may encourage withdrawal and restricted activity.

Hearing may deteriorate with age. *Presbycusis* refers to a constellation of age-related hearing changes, including an impairment in the ability to hear high-frequency sounds and to discriminate between sound frequencies, difficulties in speech discrimination, and increased problems in understanding distorted speech (Hinchcliffe, 1962). These losses are related to changes in the size, shape, and flexibility of the outer and middle ear, as well as to the loss of receptor cells and metabolic changes in the cochlea, the structure in the inner ear that transforms sound waves into neural impulses (Olsho, Harkins, & Lenhart, 1985). As with vision, changes in auditory sensitivity increase the risk that an older person may begin to feel increasingly more isolated from others and from previously enjoyed activites. Speech may become more difficult to hear and understand, and the ability to enjoy music may decrease as high-frequency sensitivity and frequency discrimination decline.

Changes in arousal may also occur with aging. Sleep patterns change with age; older persons spend less time in deep sleep and also dream less. Frequent awakenings during a night's sleep are also more common in older individuals. These awakenings may lead to daytime sleepiness, increased use of sleeping pills, and spending more time in bed in an attempt to get sufficient rest. Paradoxically, it appears that just the opposite is the best treatment for these sleep problems. Staying out of bed, perhaps even missing a night's sleep, and decreasing the use of sleeping medication is more likely to improve sleep (Woodruff, 1985).

Although some biological changes in sensation and arousal appear to be almost universally associated with aging, serious impairment is by no means inevitable. Declining vision and hearing may be corrected by glasses and hearing aids, and sleep problems may be counteracted. The most critical factor to consider is probably the degree of restriction that results from these biological changes. Remaining active and retaining a sense of control over one's life may go a long way toward increasing the probability of a rewarding and healthy old age, as will be discussed in more detail later in this chapter.

## Memory, Dementia, and Alzheimer's Disease

One of the best-known changes that occurs with aging is declining memory. The elderly often report that they feel less able to remember things as well as they did when they were younger and that they have greater difficulty retrieving already learned information from memory. Because of the frequency with which memory difficulties are reported, a great deal of research has been devoted to investigating the exact nature of the memory changes that are common in healthy and ill elderly people. This research has made it clear that memory changes are common, yet the nature of the changes is difficult to specify as a result of the complex nature of memory.

*Primary memory* refers to memory for immediate information, such as the ability to repeat a series of numbers just after it has been presented or the ability to remember the last few items in a list that has just been read. Primary memory appears to change relatively little with age, although a slight decline is common (Poon, 1985). People in their twenties are typically able to recall a list of six to seven letters immediately after presentation, whereas people in their seventies are able to recall an average of five and a half letters (Botwinck & Storandt, 1974). However, immediate memory for visual material appears to decline more with age than does immediate memory for verbal material. Haaland, Linn, Hunt, and Goodwin (1983) studied the performance of healthy adults over sixty-five years old on Russell's revision of the Wechsler Memory Scale (Russell, 1975). This memory test requires subjects to recall a story and to reproduce geometric designs from memory both immediately and thirty minutes after presentation. Immediate memory for the stories showed a slight decline with age, but immediate memory for designs showed a more dramatic decline. Memory after a delay of thirty minutes also declined with age, although the effect of age was more noticeable for visual than verbal material. Interestingly, no age-related differences were present for the percentage of information that was correctly recalled after thirty minutes. Although age affected the amount of information initially retained, it did not affect the amount of information that was forgotten over the thirty-minute span.

The thirty-minute recall portion of the Russell Memory Scale provides a test of *secondary memory*, or memory for information after it is no longer the focus of immediate attention. It has been regularly reported that secondary memory declines more with age than primary memory (Poon, 1985). However, the amount of decline with age can be counteracted with practice and by regulating the pace of learning, especially by allowing the learner to control the rate at which new information is presented. Secondary memory for such familiar material as names also declines less with age than secondary material for novel, or newly encountered, material (Poon, 1985). There may thus be ways to reduce the life interference that memory problems cause if older people adjust learning stategies by rehearsing what it is important to remember (e.g., repeating new phone numbers several times) and taking care to pace exposure to new material.

Although the data indicate that some degree of memory decline often accompanies aging, some older people experience a great deal of difficulty with memory and other intellectual abilities. *Dementia* is a disorder in which intellectual skills are severely impaired, and it is diagnosed when intellectual deterioration is severe enough that it interferes with normal social or occupational functioning. Symptoms of dementia include memory impairment, impaired judgment, language impairment such as aphasia, personality changes, and impaired abstract thinking, such as difficulties defining words and concepts. Dementia is diagnosed only when these symptoms are due to a physiological, or organic, cause rather than a psychological disorder (American Psychiatric Association, 1987). Dementia is much more common among the aged population than among younger people and has been estimated to affect up to 15% of the elderly if mild cases of dementia are included. The figure is probably closer to 5% if only moderate and severe cases are included. The majority of cases of dementia are due to two causes: multi-infarct dementia and primary degenerative dementia, also referred to as senile dementia (LaRue, Dessonville, & Jarvik, 1985). If the symptoms and neurological changes of senile dementia occur in a person younger than age sixty-five, the disorder is referred to as *Alzheimer's disease*, or presenile dementia. Alzheimer's is most common after the age of fifty and must have its onset before the age of sixty-five if it is to be correctly called Alzheimer's disease (Vogel, 1977). It has become clear that the underlying disease is the same, regardless of the patient's age (Richardson, Beal, & Martin, 1987). Due to the similarities between senile and presenile dementia, both are sometimes combined into a single category of dementias of the Alzheimer's type (DAT).

You may recall from Chapter 8 that an infarction occurs when tissue death results from a disruption in blood supply. In multi-infarct dementia the patient has experienced many small strokes, as an outcome of which many areas of the brain have been damaged. This may result in the symptoms of dementia if brain tissue damage has been severe enough to seriously impair intellectual functions. Which intellectual skills are impaired depends, of course, upon the areas of the brain that have been damaged, so patients with multi-infarct dementia may show a wide range of symptoms and degree of dysfunction. It may also be quite difficult to diagnose multi-infarct dementia because the areas of the brain damaged by the strokes may be quite small, and the damage thus quite difficult to detect (LaRue et al., 1985).

In contrast to the localized, "spotty" brain damage of multi-infarct dementia, primary degenerative dementia is characterized by a wide-ranging deterioration of the brain tissue. *Cortical atrophy* (a shrinking of the brain tissue itself) and *ventricular dilatation*, in which the normal spaces within the brain have become enlarged, are common. In addition, plaques, or small areas of dead-cell fragments, cover portions of the brain surface, and *neurofibrillary tangles* are present. Neurofibrillary tangles are nerve cells that have become filled with densely packed and twisted protein molecules (Dayan, 1978; LaRue et al., 1985).

The brains of dementia patients show more atrophy and a far greater number of plaques and tangles than do the brains of normal individuals (Dayan, 1978; LaRue et al., 1985). The plaques and tangles characteristic of DAT also appear to contain deposits of an abnormal substance, although the exact nature of this substance is still uncertain (Richardson et al., 1987). The reason why some people develop progressive degenerative dementia or Alzheimer's is currently unknown, although a variety of causes have been proposed. Genetic factors may be important, and it has also been reported that the brains of Alzheimer's patients have higher levels of aluminum accumulated in neurons than do the brains of nondemented individuals. A promising line of investigation concerns the finding that levels of the enzyme choline acetyltransferase are lower in the brains of DAT patients than in normals. This enzyme is necessary for the production of acetylcholine, a neurotransmitter important for learning and memory (LaRue et al., 1985).

## Psychological Disorders

As with all phases of life, old age is characterized by the presence of a variety of life crises. These crises carry with them opportunities for healthy adaptation and growth or the development of psychological difficulties. We have already discussed some biological changes and medical problems that may be associated with aging. It is important to remember that these changes not only involve physiological dysfunction but also require life-style and psychological adjustments on the part of the person experiencing the changes.

Butler and Lewis (1982) have noted that some specific life crises commonly occur in later life. The risk of widowhood is obviously increased in old age. Alterations in marital adjustment may also be required in view of the increased time a couple is likely to spend together after retirement and changes in activity patterns necessitated by aging. Sexual problems may also occur; although many older people remain sexually active, sexual activity may diminish as a result of illness or the normal aging process, and the loss of a spouse will clearly affect sexual behavior. Financial changes associated with a reduction in income and increased medical expenses are also common.

A sense of loss is a common theme cutting across all these crises. The loss may be interpersonal, as with the loss of a spouse; physical, as with illness or sensory loss; or financial. As might be expected, the risk for several psychological disorders increases with age. Depression and anxiety related to the anticipation or experience of loss are particularly common. Hale, Cochran, and Hedgepeth (1984) reported that the elderly produced consistently higher scores on the Brief Symptom Index, a self-report measure of psychological symptoms (Derogatis, 1977). The relationship of mental health in old age to physical health appears to be quite strong. Himmelfarb (1984) found no changes in psychological adjustment that could be attributed to aging alone but instead reported that physical health, social support, and a sense of control over one's health were particularly important predictors of mental health in individuals between the ages of fifty-five and eighty-nine. Parmelee, Lawton, and Katz (1989) found that depression in the elderly was significantly correlated with poor health and disability. It thus appears that aging itself is not a risk factor for increased psychological problems. Instead, psychological disorders may result from poor health and the loss of social support and control that sometimes accompany aging.

Depression in old age has received a great deal of research attention. This interest is due to two major factors: the frequency of depression and problems in differentiating between depression and dementia. Estimates of the frequency of depression in the elderly vary widely, dependent upon the nature of the depressive symptoms surveyed. When more serious symptoms are required for a diagnosis of depression, lower estimates of the frequency of depression result. About 10% to 15% of the geriatric population experience depression severe enough to warrant treatment (LaRue et al., 1985). Elderly people with medical problems are often depressed, yet their depression may go undetected by health care providers. Rapp, Parisi, Walsh, and Wallace (1988) found that only 8.7% of depressed geriatric medical patients were diagnosed as suffering from depression. In this study, 23 of 150 elderly medical patients were depressed, but nonpsychiatric physicians detected the presence of depression in only 2 of the 23 depressed patients. Psychological tests were significantly more sensitive to the presence of depression. Rapp and his colleagues therefore recommended that psychological testing be used to screen elderly medical patients for depression.

Depression may be very difficult to distinguish from dementia because of the overlap between the symptoms of the two disorders. Memory loss, concentration difficulties, a reduction of social and occupational activity, and complaints of physical problems are common in both. Between 5% and 15% of patients initially diagnosed as suffering from DAT have later been found to be suffering from depression (Feinberg & Goodman, 1984). It is very important that the correct diagnosis be made because depression and dementia vary greatly in their course and in the treatment options available. Dementia is an irreversible disease with a slow decline, whereas depression is quite treatable with medication and/or psychotherapy.

Memory testing may provide some clues for differentiating between depression and dementia. Although both demented and depressed persons may complain of memory problems, depressed patients may perform much better on memory tests than their complaints would suggest. Depression is commonly accompanied by a tendency to view oneself very negatively, and this negative self-evaluation may cause a depressed person to overestimate the magnitude of the problems he or she is experiencing. In fact, depressed persons may show little impairment on memory testing although they report many complaints of poor memory, such as a problem remembering jokes and reading material and tending to say the same thing twice (Williams, Little, Scates, & Blockman, 1987). Demented patients have also been found to forget things much more quickly than depressed patients. Although depressed patients may need a longer exposure time to acquire the same amount of information than do non-depressed persons, their rate of forgetting over a forty-eight-hour period has been found to be no different from normals. Demented patients forget much more material over this same interval (Hart, Kwentus, Taylor, & Harkins, 1987). Memory problems in depression may thus be related to attention and motivation difficulties that interfere with concentration, while DAT-related memory loss may be more closely related to an inability to store information in memory.

Of course, some elderly people may be suffering from dementia and may also be depressed. It has been estimated that about 30% of Alzheimer's patients are depressed (Teri & Uomoto, 1986). In these individuals, it is still worthwhile to consider the depression as a disorder worthy of treatment considering the improvement in the patient's emotional state that a reduction in depression might permit. However, memory ability is less likely to improve in these patients (Williams et al., 1987).

## Treatment Interventions

A review of the biological, social, and psychological events associated with aging discussed in the preceding pages reveals several common themes. Aging carries with it particular risks for (1) loss-related depression, social withdrawal, and inactivity; and (2) a sense of loss of control or competence when illness restricts activities or if memory changes are noticed. Treatment programs have thus been developed to alleviate or minimize these problems. Some treatment programs are relatively specific to the elderly population, whereas others are applications of interventions used with other age groups as well.

Biases against therapeutic work with the aged are sometimes present, and the health care system itself sometimes makes it difficult to provide services to elderly clients. Therapists are typically younger than their older potential clients, and some may mistakenly believe that intellectual decline is inevitable with old age and that older individuals would be poor candidates for treatment. In addition, reimbursement through Medicare is often limited for outpatient or psychological treatment, so care may be beyond the financial reach of many (Gatz, Popkin, Pino, & VandenBos, 1985). For example, consider that Medicare will reimburse for the costs of diagnosing Alzheimer's disease but not for treating the disease after diagnosis. The Medicare system justifies this practice by arguing that the disorder is incurable and Medicare is designed to pay for treatment rather than custodial care. However, that argument overlooks the benefits that accrue to the patient and the family when psychological treatment improves the patient's functioning and relieves the family's distress (Zarit & Zarit, 1982). As Gatz et al. (1985) have noted, there is substantial evidence that psychological intervention may be of benefit to the elderly, and biases against providing treatment are not supported by the evidence.

Social and behavioral factors clearly exert an influence on the health and survival rates of elderly individuals. Despite the biological changes associated with aging, biological forces do not exert such a profound effect that changes in behavior do not improve life expectancy. For example, Kaplan (1986) reported on a group of people over the age of 50 who were initially assessed in 1965 and then reevaluated in 1974 and 1983. Subjects who increased their activity level between 1965 and 1974 showed a 16% reduction in mortality risk between 1974 and 1983. A decrease in social contacts between 1965 and 1974 was associated with an increased mortality risk of about 20%. Psychosocial and behavioral changes may be of value regardless of age, and the biases and other obstacles complicating the elderly's access to psychological services are without foundation.

# Treatment of Depression

Although the basic principles of treatment for depression are the same in older and younger clients, some specific age-related issues may need to be addressed, and some techniques may need to be modified. It may be necessary to counter the belief that change is unlikely or impossible; this belief may be held by both the client and the therapist. Increasing the frequency of pleasant events is a common strategy in the treatment of depression, and it is important to consider the physical status of the patient when pleasant events are selected in order to minimize the risk of fatigue and discouragement. The rate of presentation of new information during therapy may need to be adapted to match the cognitive level of the client. This is particularly true if dementia is present. Therapy sessions may be tape-recorded for review after the session, or notebooks may be kept to encourage review of important information. In general, the therapist may need to be more patient, focused, and organized. However, if the therapist attends carefully to the individual needs and skills of the patient, he or she may remobilize the problem-solving skills that the patient has developed in the course of mastering earlier life challenges. In this sense, work with aging clients may be a very rewarding experience for both the client and the therapist (Zeiss & Lewinsohn, 1986).

Group therapy is often used with elderly patients. Group treatment may be more cost-effective, as more than one client may be treated during a session. Perhaps more important, the presence of other group members may help to reduce the sense of isolation some aged persons may experience, as they are able to see that others share similar problems and hear how others have attempted to solve these problems. Steur et al. (1984) compared two types of group psychotherapy with elderly clients. Half of the patients received group cognitive-behavioral therapy and half received group psychodynamic therapy. Cognitive-behavioral therapy focuses on thoughts and behaviors, working on the assumption that thoughts about behavior largely determine feelings. For example, if I noticed that I forgot a phone number, I might become very distressed if I interpreted that experience as meaning that I was beginning to suffer from dementia, but if I instead looked for other explanations, such as that I had not needed to remember that phone number for several months and I often forgot numbers under those circumstances even when when I was younger, my emotional distress would be minimal. The presence in the group of others with similar experiences should also act to reduce my distress about forgetting the phone number, and the other members could discuss how they interpreted their own occasional problems with memory. The patients in the cognitive-behavioral group therefore kept daily records of activities and pleasures, recorded and discussed daily thoughts that might be associated with depression, and generated new ways of viewing their experiences.

Psychodynamic therapy concentrates on gaining insight into the causes of behavior and emotions. For example, I may come to understand that the reason I am feeling depressed now is because I have been too passive and not asked others for what I wanted, and my passivity has been due to a fear that I would become a burden to others and they would reject me. Others in the group could help by discussing their own feelings about becoming dependent on others, and their support might help me to see that I am unlikely to be rejected and that I have a right to ask for what I want. Patients in the psychodynamic group worked with one another to gain insight into their behavioral and emotional patterns and used the support of the group to help encourage change. Steur et al. (1984) found no differences between the two types of treatment, although both groups were effective in reducing depression.

Therapies concentrating on behavior change to increase the frequency of pleasant events have been found to be useful. Patients suffering from a combination of dementia and depression have been helped by encouraging social contacts and distraction from thoughts of sad events. This type of approach works to reduce the *excess disability* that depression may lead to. Although some difficulties are inevitable when dementia is present, depression may intensify these problems and lead the patient to be more restricted than her or his medical condition demands (Teri & Uomoto, 1986).

Similar results have been reported by other investigators. Gallagher, Thompson, & Breckenridge (1986) found no significant differences between behavioral, cognitive, and psychodynamic treatment. In this study, treatment was administered individually rather than in groups; an average of 70% of the patients were either not depressed or substantially improved after 20 treatment sessions, and most patients maintained their gains over a 12-month period.

## Control and Competence Enhancement

A sense of control and the ability to deal competently with stressful events have been found to be associated with physical and psychological health (Husaini & Neff, 1980; McFarlane, Norman, Streiner, Roy, & Scott, 1980). Reports of agitation, loneliness, the number of sick days, and the number of medications taken have been found to be associated with how competent elderly people perceive themselves to be, with higher levels of competence perception related to better health (LiBethe & Levy, 1986). Although it is often difficult to know whether poor health leads to decreased feelings of competence and control or whether a lowered sense of competence results in poor health, treatment focused on increasing the sense of competence and control have been found to be useful for aging people.

Langer and Rodin (Langer & Rodin, 1976; Rodin & Langer, 1977) studied the effects on nursing home residents of an increased sense of control and responsibility. The hospital administrator spoke to one group of patients and emphasized the degree to which the patients' were responsible for themselves; these same patients were also given plants to care for. Another group of patients was addressed by the same administrator, but the administrator stressed the staff's responsibility for the patients' welfare; these patients also received plants, but the staff watered the plants for the patients. Excerpts from the patient-responsibility and the staff-responsibility messages are presented in Boxed Highlight 16.1. Both groups were patients in the same nursing home and received the same amount of attention from the staff. However, the group receiving the responsibility message chose and cared for their own plants, chose their movie night, and were able to give their opinions of how the staff handled complaints. Read the messages carefully, and notice how much more the personal-responsibility message encourages the patients to direct their own activites and care for themselves.

The patients receiving the message encouraging personal responsibility were found to be happier and more active than those receiving the message stressing staff responsibility (Langer & Rodin, 1976). A follow-up study conducted eighteen months later (Rodin & Langer, 1977) found significant differences in health status. The personal-responsibility patients showed an average gain in health, whereas the other patients showed a decline during the same time period. Most important, a difference in death rates was also found. The average death rate for the entire nursing home for the 18 months prior to the study was 25%. However, only 15% of the personal-responsibility patients died during the 18-month follow-up, whereas 30% of the other patients died.

Other studies have found similar benefits due to increased control. Relocation has been found to result in fewer health problems when individuals are able to have some degree of choice regarding the move, and the ability to control or predict when visitors would arrive and how long they could stay has been shown to have beneficial effects on health, activity, and psychological status (Schulz, 1976; Schulz & Brenner, 1977). Emphasizing the degree of control that elderly nursing home residents have over the length and timing of visitations can also favorably affect health status and enthusiasm for life (Haemmerlie & Montgomery, 1987). It seems that the knowledge that one has control, rather than the exercise of control, may be the active ingredient in these treatment programs. Rodin (1980) noted that the health and sociability of patients in a nursing home improved when the patients had a fifteen-minute period during which they knew a nurse would come when they called. Although patients called the nurse frequently during the early stages of the study, they exercised their control by calling the nurse less and less as the study progressed. You will remember that a similar effect was noted earlier in Chapter 14, regarding relaxation and EMG biofeedback. Prokop, Pratt, and Rhodes (1987) found that the degree of relaxation experienced was not

# Messages Stressing Personal Responsibility or Staff Responsibility for Nursing Home Residents

## PERSONAL RESPONSIBILITY MESSAGE

I brought you together today to give you some information about the Arden House. I was surprised to learn that many of you don't know about the things that are available to you and more important, that many of you don't realize the influence you have over our lives here. Take a minute to think of the decisions you can and should be making. For example, you have the responsibility of caring for yourselves, of deciding whether or not you want to make this a home you can be proud of and happy in. You should be deciding how you want your room arranged . . . whether you want to be visiting your friends who live on this floor or on other floors, whether you want to visit in your room or your friend's room . . . In other words, it's your life and you can make of it whatever you want . . .

Also, I wanted to take this opportunity to give you each a present from the Arden House. [A box of plants was passed around, and patients were given two decisions to make: first, whether they wanted a plant at all, and second, to choose which one they wanted. All residents did take a plant.] The plants are yours to keep and take care of as you'd like.

One last thing, I wanted to tell you that we're showing a movie two nights next week, Thursday and Friday. You should decide which night you'd like to go, if you choose to see it at all.

## STAFF RESPONSIBILITY MESSAGE

I brought you together today to give you some information about the Arden House. I was surprised to learn that many of you don't know about the things that are available to you; that many of you don't realize all you're allowed to do here. Take a minute to think of all the options that we've provided for you in order for your life to be fuller and more interesting. For example, you're permitted to visit people on the other floors and to use the lounge on this floor for visiting as well as the dining room or our own rooms. We want your rooms to be as nice as they can be, and we've tried to make them that way for you. We want you to be happy here. We feel that it's our responsibility to make this a home you can be proud of and happy in, and we want to do all we can to help you . . .

Also, I wanted to take this opportunity to give you each a present from the Arden House. [The nurse walked around with a box of plants and each patient was handed one.] The plants are yours to keep. The nurses will water and care for them for you.

One last thing, I wanted to tell you that we're showing a movie next week on Thursday and Friday. We'll let you know later which day you're scheduled to see it.

SOURCE: Adapted from E.J. Langer & J. Rodin. (1976). The effects of choice and enhanced personal responsibility for the aged: A field experiment in an institutional setting. *Journal of Personality and Social Psychology, 34,* 191–198. Copyright 1976 by The American Psychological Association. Adapted by permission.

related to how much a subject used the biofeedback signal but was instead related to how useful they found the signal to be. The knowledge that a useful relaxation tool was available was a more important determiner of relaxation than was the actual use of the tool, just as the knowledge that control over nursing visits was possible was more important to health than was actually calling the nurse.

It has been suggested that the elderly exercise control voluntarily in an effort to reduce distress about physical symptoms through the process of *vigilant coping*. Fewer older than younger people drop out of treatment for high blood pressure, and the elderly report more healthy habits than younger people. It apears that the elderly who are ill act to control the danger from physical problems and the emotional distress regarding illness by accepting treatment, and once treatment is accepted the elderly may ignore symptoms because treatment is presumably caring for the disorder responsible for the symptoms. This results in less emotional distress about the symptoms. The elderly who are well are less likely than younger people to delay seeking treatment when symptoms first appear. Whereas 62% of younger people have been reported to delay seeking treatment in the face of serious symptoms, only 13% of those who are older delay. Seeking treatment quickly resolves uncertainty about symptom interpretation and thus reduces the emotional distress. Exercising personal control through vigilant coping thus acts to maintain emotional equilibrium whether an elderly person is sick or well (Leventhal, Prohaska, & Leventhal, 1986).

Rodin (1986) has observed that three elements appear necessary if a control-enhancing intervention is to be successful. First, the options for control need to continue beyond the intervention period. For example, it would not be helpful if the only time a patient could control daily activities was during a time-limited treatment program and the staff began to control daily schedules after the program ended. It is therefore important that a permanent change in the environment be made if benefits to health are to be expected. Second, opportunities for practicing control and competent behavior must be provided. It is not enough just to tell someone that they can control their environment, they must also be allowed to experience that control, such as by being able to call a nurse or care for their own plants.

Third, individuals must know that their efforts will be reliably successful. It is important that all the staff members agree that patients in a nursing home should be able to control many aspects of their daily activities, or else the control will only be intermittently rewarded, and it will be clear that control is really dependent on the whims of the staff rather than the actions of the patients. For control to have a positive effect, it must be attributed to stable and internal sources within the patient, not to variable and external sources such as the attitudes of the staff.

Gatz et al. (1985) noted that all effective psychotherapy with the elderly employs similar mechanisms. Successful therapy fosters a sense of control, establishes constructive relationships between behavior and environmental changes, provides a sense of meaning, and establishes a relationship with the helper. In fact, these four mechanisms are not just a description of successful therapy but also a prescription for healthy aging: Maintain a sense of control and continue to be active so the effects of your actions may be seen in the environment. Stay in touch with others and maintain good interpersonal relationships. These actions should lead to an enhanced sense of meaning in life and may result in better physical and psychological health.

# Summary

Biological aging carries with it the risk of increased illness and physical decline. Senses may become less acute, and sleep and arousal patterns may change. Memory ability may decline, especially secondary memory and memory for visual material. Declining memory abilities and intellectual impairment are particularly severe in dementia. Dementia due to the occurrence of many small strokes is called multi-infarct dementia. Senile and presenile dementia, or dementias of the Alzheimer's type (DAT), are related to generalized deterioration of brain tissue. Cortical atrophy, ventricular dilatation, plaques, and neurofibrillary tangles are characteristics of DAT.

Life crises involving loss, such as widowhood, retirement, and financial changes, also become more likely with aging. Declining health, reduced social support, and a sense of loss of control may contribute to increased psychological distress and adaptive abilities. Depression and withdrawal in reaction to these losses is a particular risk.

Depression may be treated with behavioral, cognitive, and psychodynamic psychotherapy. All three approaches appear to be effective and equal in value. An enhanced sense of personal control and responsibility may also benefit the health of the aged. Many elderly people maintain control of their physical and psychological condition through vigilant coping, by seeking treatment for serious symptoms quickly, and by ignoring symptoms that are being treated.

However, aging need not result in serious psychological or physical problems; less than 5% of the elderly require care in a nursing home. Psychological and behavioral factors may exert a large influence on health, and physical changes in sensation and memory may be counteracted. Healthy aging may be promoted by retaining a sense of control, staying active, keeping a sense of meaning in life, and maintaining good interpersonal relationships.

# References

AMERICAN PSYCHIATRIC ASSOCIATION. (1987). *Diagnostic and statistical manual of mental disorders* (3rd ed., rev.). Washington, DC: Author.

BIRREN, J. E., & ZARIT, J. M. (1985). Concepts of health, behavior, and aging. In J. E. Birren & J. Livingston (Eds.), *Cognition, stress, and aging* (pp. 1–20). Englewood Cliffs, NJ: Prentice-Hall.

BOTWINCK, J., & STORANDT, M. (1974). *Memory, related functions, and age.* Springfield, IL: Charles Thomas.

BUSSE, E. W. (1977). Theories of aging. In E. W. Busse & E. Pfeiffer (Eds.), *Behavior and adaptation in late life* (2nd ed.) (pp. 8–30). Boston: Little, Brown.

BUTLER, R. N., & LEWIS, M. I. (1982). *Aging and mental health* (3rd ed.). St. Louis: Mosby.

CRAWFORD, J., & COHEN, H. J. (1984). Aging and neoplasia. *Annual Review of Gerontology and Geriatrics, 4,* 3–32.

DAYAN, A. D. (1978). The central nervous system: A. The neuropsychology of aging. In J. C. Brocklehurst (Ed.), *Textbook of geriatric medicine and gerontology* (pp. 158–185). New York: Churchill Livingstone.

DEROGATIS, L. R. (1977). *The SCL-90 Manual I: Scoring, administration, and procedures for the SCL-90.* Baltimore, MD: Johns Hopkins University School of Medicine, Clinical Psychometrics Unit.

FEINBERG, T., & GOODMAN, B. (1984). Affective illness, dementia, and pseudodementia. *Journal of Clinical Psychiatry, 45,* 100–103.

GATZ, M., POPKIN, S. J., PINO, C. D., & VANDENBOS, G. R. (1985). Psychological interventions with older adults. In J. E. Birren & K. W. Schaie (Eds.), *Handbook of the psychology of aging* (2nd ed.) (pp. 755–785). New York: Van Nostrand Reinhold.

GALLAGHER, D., THOMPSON, L. W., & BRECKENRIDGE, J. S. (1986, August). Maintenance of gains versus relapse following brief psychotherapy for depression. In M. A. Storandt (Chair), *Cognitive-behavioral therapies for older adults.* Symposium conducted at the meeting of the American Psychological Association, Washington, DC.

HAALAND, K. Y., LINN, R. T., HUNT, W. C., & GOODWIN, J. S. (1983). A normative study of Russell's variant of the Wechsler Memory Scale in a healthy elderly population. *Journal of Consulting and Clinical Psychology, 51,* 878–881.

HAEMMERLIE, F. M., & MONTGOMERY, R. L. (1987). Self-perception theory, salience of behavior, and a control-enhancing program for the elderly. *Journal of Social and Clinical Psychology, 5,* 313–329.

HALE, W. D., COCHRAN, C. D., & HEDGEPETH, B. E. (1984). Norms for the elderly on the Brief Symptom Index. *Journal of Consulting and Clinical Psychology, 52,* 321–322.

HART, R. P., KWENTUS, J. A., TAYLOR, J. R., & HARKINS, S. W. (1987). Rate of forgetting in dementia and depression. *Journal of Consulting and Clinical Psychology, 55,* 101–105.

HENRIKSEN, J. D. (1978). Problems in rehabilitation after age sixty-five. *Journal of the American Geriatrics Society, 26,* 510–512.

HENRY, J. P. (1985). Psychosocial factors, disease, and aging. In J. E. Birren & J. Livingston (Eds.), *Cognition, stress, and aging* (pp. 21–46). Englewood Cliffs, NJ: Prentice-Hall.

HIMMELFARB, S. (1984). Age and sex differences in the mental health of older persons. *Journal of Consulting and Clinical Psychology, 52,* 844–856.

HINCHCLIFFE, R. (1962). The anatomical locus of presbycusis. *Journal of Speech Disorders, 27,* 301–310.

HUSAINI, B. A., & NEFF, J. A. (1980). Characteristics of life events and psychiatric impairment in rural communities. *Journal of Nervous and Mental Disease, 168,* 159–166.

KAPLAN, G. A. (1986, August). Aging, health, and behavior: Evidence from the Alameda county study. In R. P. Abeles (Chair), *Health, behavior, and aging.* Symposium conducted at the meeting of the American Psychological Association, Washington, DC.

KENNEDY, R. D., ANDREWS, G. R., & CAIRD, F. I. (1977). Ischaemic heart disease in the elderly. *British Heart Journal, 39*, 1121–1127.

KLINE, D. W., & SCHEIBER, F. (1985). Vision and aging. In J. E. Birren & K. W. Schaie (Eds.), *Handbook of the psychology of aging* (2nd ed.) (pp. 296–331). New York: Van Nostrand Reinhold.

LANGER, E. J., & RODIN, J. (1976). The effects of choice and enhanced personal responsibility for the aged: A field experiment in an institutional setting. *Journal of Personality and Social Psychology, 34*, 191–198.

LARUE, A., DESSONVILLE, C., & JARVIK, L. F. (1985). Aging and mental disorders. In J. E. Birren & K. W. Schaie (Eds.), *Handbook of the psychology of aging* (2nd ed.) (pp. 664–702). New York: Van Nostrand Reinhold.

LEVENTHAL, H., PROHASKA, T. R., & LEVENTHAL, E. A. (1986, August). Health and illness behavior over the life span. In R. P. Abeles (Chair), *Health, behavior, and aging.* Symposium conducted at the meeting of the American Psychological Association, Washington, DC.

LIBETHE, J. A., & LEVY, L. H. (1986, August). *Stress, competence perception, and well-being in the elderly.* Poster presented at the meeting of the American Psychological Association, Washington, DC.

McFARLANE, A. H., NORMAN, G. R., STREINER, D. L., ROY, R., & SCOTT, D. J. (1980). A longitudinal study of the influence of the psychosocial environment of health status. *Journal of Health and Social Behavior, 21*, 124–133.

NATIONAL CENTER FOR HEALTH STATISTICS. (1976). *Vital statistics of the United States, Vol. 2, Part A.* Washington, D.C.: U.S. Government Printing Office.

OLSHO, L. W., HARKINS, S. W., & LENHART, M. L. (1985). Aging and the auditory system. In J. E. Birren & K. W. Schaie (Eds.), *Handbook of the psychology of aging* (2nd ed.) (pp. 332–377). New York: Van Nostrand Reinhold.

PARMELEE, P. A., LAWTON, M. P., & KATZ, I. R. (1989). Psychometric properties of the Geriatric Depression Scale among the institutionalized elderly. *Psychological Assessment, 1*, 331–338.

POON, L. W. (1985). Differences in human memory with aging: Nature, causes, and clinical implications. In J. E. Birren & K. W. Schaie (Eds.), *Handbook of the psychology of aging* (2nd ed.) (pp. 427–462). New York: Van Nostrand Reinhold.

PROKOP, C. K., PRATT, D. L., & RHODES, L. A. (1987, March). *Relaxation depth and perceived utility of biofeedback.* Paper presented at the meeting of the Southeastern Psychological Association, Atlanta, Georgia.

RAPP, S. R., PARISI, S. A., WALSH, D. A., & WALLACE, C. E. (1988). Detecting depression in elderly medical inpatients. *Journal of Consulting and Clinical Psychology, 56*, 509–513.

RICHARDSON, E. P., BEAL, M. F., & MARTIN, J. B. (1987). Degenerative diseases of the nervous system. In E. Braunwald, K. J. Isselbacher, R. G. Petersdorff, J. D. Wilson, J. B. Martin, & A. S. Fauci (Eds.), *Harrison's principles of internal medicine* (11th ed.) (pp. 2011–2027). New York: McGraw-Hill.

RODIN, J. (1986, August). Physiological mediators of health and behavior: Relationships in aging. In R. P. Abeles (Chair), *Health, behavior, and aging.* Symposium conducted at the meeting of the American Psychological Association, Washington, DC.

RODIN, J., & LANGER, E. J. (1977). Long-term effects of a control-relevant intervention with the institutionalized aged. *Journal of Personality and Social Psychology, 35*, 897–902.

RUSSELL, E. W. (1975). A multiple-scoring method for the assessment of complex memory functions. *Journal of Consulting and Clinical Psychology, 43*, 800–809.

SCHAIE, K. W., & WILLIS, S. J. (1986). *Adult development and aging* (2nd ed.). Boston: Little, Brown.

SCHULZ, R. (1976). Effects of control and predictability on the physical and psychological well-being of the institutionalized aged. *Journal of Personality and Social Psychology, 33*, 563–573.

SCHULZ, R., & BRENNER, G. (1977). Relocation of the aged: A review and theoretical analysis. *Journal of Gerontology, 32*, 323–333.

SKINNER, B. F., & VAUGHAN, M. E. (1983). *Enjoy old age*. New York: Norton.

STEUR, J. L., MINTZ, J., HAMMEN, C. L., HILL, M. A., JARVIK, L. F., MCCARLEY, T., MOTOIKE, P., & ROSEN, R. (1984). Cognitive-behavioral and psychodynamic group psychotherapy in the treatment of geriatric depression. *Journal of Consulting and Clinical Psychology, 52*, 180–189.

TERI, L., & UOMOTO, J. M. (1986, August). Depression and Alzheimer's disease. In M. A. Storandt (Chair), *Cognitive-behavioral therapies for older adults*. Symposium conducted at the meeting of the American Psychological Association, Washington, D.C.

U.S. BUREAU OF THE CENSUS. (1981). *Age, sex, race, and Spanish origin of the population by regions, divisions, and states: 1980*. (1980 census of the population supplementary reports, PC80-S1-1.) Washington, D.C.: U.S. Government Printing Office.

VOGEL, F. S. (1977). The brain and time. In E. W. Busse & E. Pfeiffer (Eds.), *Behavior and adaptation in late life* (2nd ed.) (pp. 228–239). Boston: Little, Brown.

WILLIAMS, J. M., LITTLE, M. M., SCATES, S., & BLOCKMAN, N. (1987). Memory complaints and abilities among depressed older adults. *Journal of Consulting and Clinical Psychology, 55*, 595–598.

WOODRUFF, D. S. (1985). Arousal, sleep, and aging. In J. E. Birren & K. W. Schaie (Eds.), *Handbook of the psychology of aging* (2nd ed.) (pp. 261–295). New York: Van Nostrand Reinhold.

ZARIT, S. H. (1986). Applications of clinical psychology to the problems of aging. *The Clinical Psychologist, 39*, 95–96.

ZARIT, S. H., & ZARIT, J. M. (1982). Families under stress: Interventions for caregivers of senile dementia patients. *Psychotherapy: Theory, Research, and Practice, 19*, 461–471.

ZEISS, A. M., & LEWINSOHN, P. M. (1986). Adapting behavioral treatment for depression to meet the needs of the elderly. *The Clinical Psychologist, 39*, 98–100.

# Training in Health Psychology

The preceding sixteen chapters have introduced the theoretical and applied aspects of health psychology. The major portion of this volume has described research regarding the treatment and prevention of various diseases as well as the promotion of health. Consistent with the current state of the art, we have focused our attention primarily on preventive and treatment interventions designed for individuals (e.g., biofeedback treatment for muscle contraction headaches) or small groups of people (e.g., cognitive-behavioral therapy for rheumatoid arthritis patients). Nevertheless, we have also included descriptions of preventive or health-promotion programs designed for large groups of individuals. It is clear, then, that there are currently many activities in which health psychologists engage.

Several psychologists have speculated about the professional activities of future health psychologists. For example, Coates and Demuth (1984) have suggested that the future *intervention targets* for health psychologists include health-policy-making organizations (e.g., Department of Health and Human Services, National Institutes of Health) in addition to the individuals, groups, organizations, and communities identified in this text. These authors have also indicated that, in addition to the direct service and teaching activities of today's health psychologists, future health psychologists will have to develop interventions that involve the media (e.g., cable television broadcasting systems that are devoted to health issues) as well as legal or economic systems (health insurance carriers). Finally, Coates and Demuth (1984) have noted that the future purposes of the health psychology community should include the development of technological advances (e.g., the development of improved methods for measuring colonic electrical activity or gastric acid secretions) and institutional changes (e.g., encouraging companies to provide financial rewards to employees who engage in health promotion efforts). These purposes will supplement the prevention, treatment, and scientific purposes of today's health psychologists. Figure 17.1 shows a model of the three dimensions of future health psychology activities.

Given the short history of health psychology and the many challenges that it faces in the future, it is necessary to raise the question of what are the most appropriate educational experiences for health psychology students. Fortunately, the Division of Health Psychology (Division 38) of the American Psychological Association (APA) has already begun to produce guidelines for the development of health psychology as a profession.

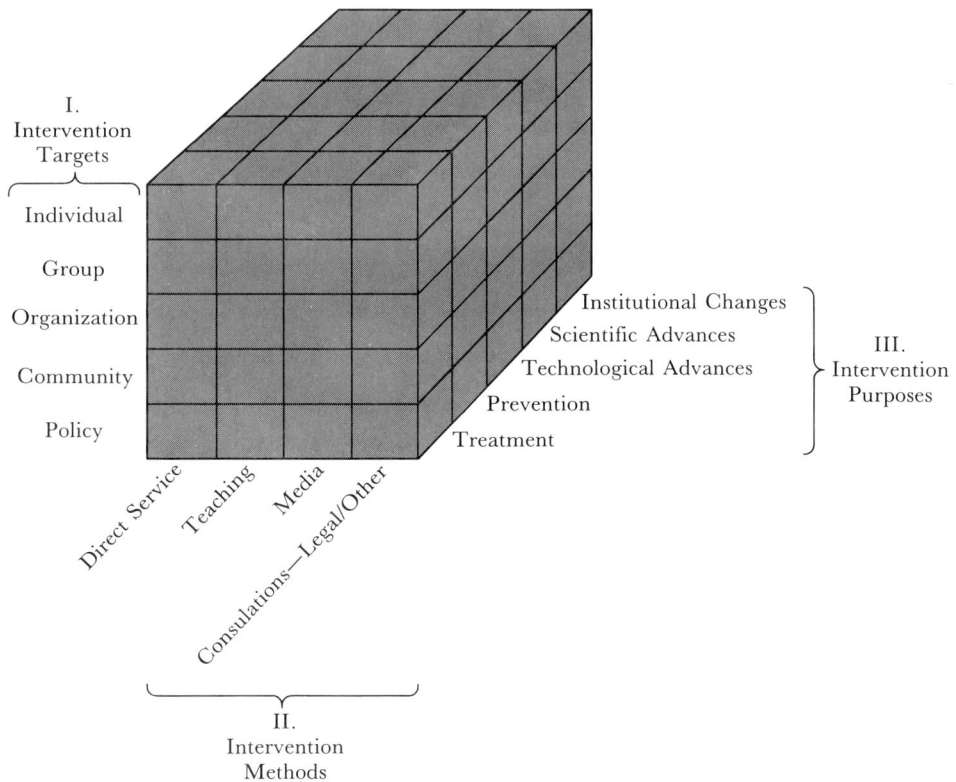

FIGURE 17.1  Three dimensions of health psychology activities. Adapted from "Dimensions of Counselor Functioning by W. H. Morill, E. R. Oetting, and J. C. Hurst, 1974, *Personnel and Guidance Journal, 52*, pp. 354–359.

# Training Standards in Health Psychology

## The Arden House Conference

In 1982, the Division of Health Psychology began to plan a national conference for the purpose of formulating standards for graduate and postgraduate education in health psychology (Weiss, 1983). The use of a national conference in planning the future course of a psychological specialty has a rich history in American psychology. Indeed, five major national conferences on training in clinical psychology were held between 1949 and 1973. The first of these conferences, held in Boulder, Colorado, in 1949, produced the guidelines for the training of clinical psychologists as both scientists and practitioners to which most clinical psychology training programs adhere today. (Matarazzo. 1983).

The Arden House conference (National Working Conference on Education and Training in Health Psychology) was held in Harriman, New York, in May 1983. The fifty-four delegates were chosen in an effort to provide representation to all areas of psychology that were relevant to health. The five-day conference produced several principles concerning training at the doctoral and postdoctoral level that are of great importance to undergraduate students who are interested in careers in health psychology.

The most important principle concerning those interested in a health psychology career is that the doctorate, or Ph.D., was identified as the entry-level degree for health psychology (Working Group on Predoctoral Education/Doctoral Training, 1983). Furthermore, consistent with the guidelines formulated at the 1949 Boulder conference in clinical psychology, the training of health psychologists as both scientists and practitioners was endorsed. In other words, it was recommended that students wishing to enter the field of health psychology must obtain a doctoral degree in psychology; the doctorate must be earned, in part, on the basis of the completion of a scientifically based doctoral dissertation as well as supervised apprenticeships involving both research and applied practical experiences.

The Arden House conference also produced guidelines for the required educational experiences in a health psychology training program. First, a health psychology training program must provide students with adequate training in *general psychology*. A program, therefore, must "require each student to demonstrate knowledge and use of: (a) scientific and professional ethics; (b) legal issues; (c) professional standards; (d) research design and methodology; (e) statistics; (f) psychological measurement; (g) history and systems of psychology" (Working Group on Predoctoral Education/Doctoral Training, 1983, p. 126). Moreover, a program must also provide training in *advanced research design, methodology*, and *statistics* that are relevant to health psychology (e.g., epidemiology, biostatistics) as well as the *biological* (e.g., physiological psychology, neuropsychology), *cognitive-affective* (e.g., learning, perception), *social* (e.g., social psychology, psychology of women), and *individ-*

*ual psychological* (e.g., personality theory, abnormal psychology) bases of behavior. These requirements may seem to be overly rigorous or excessive to undergraduate students, but they are consistent with the APA's accreditation guidelines for clinical psychology training programs.

The second set of required educational experiences for doctoral level students was composed of didactic and applied training specific to health psychology in the *biological* (e.g., genetics, stress and disease), *social* (e.g., communication skills, the health care system), and *psychological* (e.g., behavioral medicine, tests and measures) bases of health systems and behavior as well as in *health policy and organization* (e.g., health program evaluation, industrial and organizational systems).

The final set of required educational experiences consisted of didactic and applied training in professional health psychology activities. This training would include the assessment and treatment of health-related problems as well as consultation with health providers from other professional disciplines (e.g., physicians, nurses) and program evaluation. However, this set of experiences could be waived for those students who intend to engage only in research or policy-making activities following the completion of their training. Table 17.1 shows, in tabular form, the educational training requirements for health psychology students.

TABLE 17.1   Minimum knowledge and skill in three areas (generic, health, and professional) of psychology necessary for professional health psychologist. Students not seeking to provide direct service and/or professional credentialing need not receive professional training.[1]

| Area Training | Generic Psychology | Health Psychology | Professional |
|---|---|---|---|
| Knowledge and Skill | Statistics; research design; professional issues | Social bases of health and disease; biological bases of health and disease | Assessment |
| | | | Intervention |
| | History and systems | | |
| | | Psychological bases of health and disease; health policy and organization; health assessment and intervention | Consultation |
| | | | Evaluation |
| Three hour seminar course in each | Biological bases of behavior; Social bases of behavior; Cognitive/ Affective bases of behavior; Individual differences/psychological bases of behavior | | |

[1]Practica-professional (minimum 400 hours) and research internship (professional) — 1 year.

SOURCE:  Adapted from "Report" by Working Group on Predoctoral Education/Doctoral Training, 1983, *Health Psychology, 2* (Suppl. 1), pp. 123–130.

In order to ensure that training programs comply with the guidelines, the Arden House conference recommended the establishment of a Council of Directors of Health Psychology Training. This council has been established and includes representatives of doctoral-training programs in health psychology that can document their adherence to the guidelines. The council evaluates the credentials of new programs wishing to be admitted and those of member programs at specific time intervals (e.g., once every five years). The Council of Directors of Health Psychology Training is also responsible for enhancing the employment opportunities for health psychology graduates and communicating information regarding employment to the member programs.

In addition to establishing requirements for doctoral-training programs in health psychology, the Arden House conference also produced guidelines for required, one-year, predoctoral apprenticeships and recommended that health psychology graduates obtain two-year postdoctoral training fellowships before seeking employment. The national conference specified that the purpose of the apprenticeships was to allow health psychology students to integrate their basic knowledge in health psychology with the application or practice of health psychology skills (Working Group on Apprenticeship, 1983, p. 133). Those individuals who wish to pursue professional activities only in research or health policy-making would be required to obtain basic or applied research apprenticeships. The basic research apprenticeships should provide supervised experiences in

1. Posing questions and formulating hypotheses.
2. Using a variety of research methodologies.
3. Implementing research.
4. Analyzing data.
5. Publishing results in appropriate outlets.
6. Preparing grant proposals. (Working Group on Apprenticeship, 1983, p. 133)

The applied research apprenticeships in field settings should fulfill all of the criteria for the basic research apprenticeships and include supervised experiences in

1. Awareness and understanding of the roles, values, and vocabularies of others in the system.
2. Understanding the social, cultural, and environmental context.
3. Systems theory and analysis.
4. Ability to communicate effectively with other members of the system.
5. Consideration of the immediate and long-term impact of the health psychologist's activities on the setting.
6. Use of appropriate methodological and statistical techniques.
7. Assessment and intervention skills appropriate to the applied setting. (Working Group on Apprenticeship, 1983, p. 134)

Those who wish to engage in service delivery activities would be required to obtain applied apprenticeships in field settings. These apprenticeships should fulfill all of the criteria in the basic and applied research areas and provide supervised experiences in the delivery of health psychology services. These experiences would include assessment, intervention, and evaluation activities with patients or healthy individuals as well as consultation with other health-service providers. The apprenticeships must be located in interdisciplinary programs (e.g., medical centers, health maintenance organizations, schools of public health) that meet the current standards of the APA for accreditation of clinical and counseling psychology internship programs. Thus, the guidelines for health psychology apprenticeships are very similar to those that already exist for APA-approved clinical and counseling psychology internships.

The Arden House conference suggested that health psychology graduates also pursue two-year postdoctoral fellowships (similar to medical residencies) in order to acquire skills essential to the conduct of independent research and collaborative research with professionals in other health disciplines as well as the successful dissemination of information within the health psychology field and other disciplines (Working Group on Postdoctoral Research Training, 1983). Furthermore, those graduates who are interested in health-service delivery should pursue postdoctoral fellowships in order to obtain a broad general orientation to health service delivery and to become highly trained in specific competencies of the fellowship training program (e.g., rehabilitation of brain-injured individuals, health-promotion training for corporate employees, etc.) (Working Group on Postdoctoral Training for the Health Psychology Service Provider, 1983). The final training recommendation was that mechanisms be developed for evaluating and accrediting these fellowships by the APA's Education and Training Board as are clinical psychology internships and medical residencies by their respective accrediting agencies.

## Current Training Opportunities for Health Psychology Students

It must be remembered that the purpose of the Arden House conference was to develop *ideal* standards for education in health psychology. Thus, although great progress has been made in implementing these standards, it will still be several years before all of the conference's recommendations can be put into practice. It is essential, then, that today's undergraduate students become aware of the institutions that currently offer doctoral, apprenticeship, and postdoctoral training in health psychology. Moreover, undergraduates who wish to pursue careers in health psychology should use the following information and all other means possible (e.g., discussions with professors, reading of university bulletins) to determine the extent to which current training programs fulfill the educational requirements established at the national conference.

DOCTORAL TRAINING   The most recent survey of health psychology training in American and Canadian universities was conducted by Cynthia Belar and her associates (Belar, Wilson, & Hughes, 1982) in 1981. These psychologists sent questionnaires to 740 doctoral training programs and clinical internship sites in order to gather as much information as possible on health psychology training opportunities in North America. On the basis of the 310 questionnaires that were returned, it was found that 38 institutions offered doctoral training in health psychology. Students interested in doctoral level health psychology training should consult the survey results published by Belar, Wilson, and Hughes (1982) and write the thirty-eight identified institutions and others regarding their training opportunities. Students should be aware that many universities have modified or developed new health psychology curricula since the publication of the survey. They also should be aware that not all health psychology training programs are modeled on the Arden House guidelines. There are actually several different levels of these programs in North America.

The first level consists of a small number of programs that offer a PhD in Health or Medical Psychology. These programs are based on the Arden House guidelines and are designed for students who wish to pursue only research careers rather than provide clinical services to patients. The Albert Einstein College of Medicine and Uniformed Services University of the Health Sciences are two examples of institutions that offer this type of research training in health psychology.

The second level includes several training programs that most closely approximate the ideal standards established by the Arden House conference. These programs offer PhDs in psychology and APA-approved clinical training programs that emphasize health psychology. However, the research and clinical service training opportunities are enhanced by these programs' close relationships with university-affiliated, full-service medical centers. Examples of these programs include those found at the University of Alabama at Birmingham, University of Miami, University of Florida, and the University of Health Sciences of the Chicago Medical School. A similar program currently is being developed at the University of California-San Diego.

The third level is comprised of training programs that are organized in accord with Arden House training standards but are not associated with full-service, university-affiliated medical centers. The North Texas State University Behavioral Medicine program is an example of the third level of training.

The fourth level consists of training programs that offer PhDs in psychology with specialty tracks in areas such as clinical, social, or experimental-physiological psychology. Particular emphasis is given to various aspects of health psychology within the specialty tracks and many of the programs have relationships with full-service medical centers; the majority of health psychology training programs in North America are organized in this fashion. Examples of such programs include those found at Vanderbilt University, University of California-Los Angeles, Lousiana State University, State University of New York-Buffalo, Oregon Health Sciences University, University of California-Irvine, and the University of Georgia. Finally, a large number of doctoral programs in psychology offer several courses or clinical clerkships in health psychology. However, these courses and clerkships do not provide systematic and broad training in health psychology.

Detailed descriptions of several of the training programs just noted have been provided by Istvan and Hatton (1987). However, students might wonder if the differences among various health psychology training programs are of any practical significance. It should be noted that an American Board of Health Psychology has been established, and it will soon provide board certification to those psychologists who have acquired appropriate training and can document a high level of proficiency in their work. This board certification will be similar to that now required of medical doctors to practice in their speciality areas. We believe that board certification in health psychology eventually may become a requirement for the receipt of reimbursements from insurance companies for clinical service fees. Thus, we encourage health psychology students to seek out training programs that best provide educational experiences recommended by the Arden House conference.

APPRENTICESHIP TRAINING   There is currently no information regarding the availability of basic and applied predoctoral research apprenticeships in health psychology. However, W. Doyle Gentry and his colleagues (Gentry, Street, Masur, & Asken, 1981) have performed the most recent survey of health psychology training opportunities at predoctoral clinical internship (applied apprenticeship) sites. These investigators mailed questionnaires to the directors of all APA-approved internship programs in clinical and counseling psychology. The questionnaires were designed to assess the training opportunities for predoctoral interns in the diagnosis, treatment, and prevention of physical illness. Fifty-one percent of the internship programs responded to the questionnaires. Of the programs that did respond, 74% reported that formal training was available in the health psychology activities noted previously. In fact, 39% of the programs indicated that the health psychology training was required of all interns.

The questionnaire responses also indicated that the internship programs were generally staffed with appropriate faculty to provide health psychology training. Sixty-three percent of the programs reported having at least one faculty member with special interest or expertise in health psychology. Moreover, 42% of the programs indicated that new or more extensive health psychology training experiences were being planned for interns.

In summary, the questionnaire results suggested that, at the minimum, approximately 38% of all APA-approved, clinical internship programs offer formal health psychology training. Given that the questionnaires were distributed to the internship programs in 1978, it is certain that even greater opportunities exist for current doctoral students in health psychology to receive such training. Unfortunately, Gentry and his associates (1981) did not identify the specific internship programs that offered health psychology training. Current doctoral students in health psychology, therefore, must carefully investigate the training experiences that are available at the clinical internship programs before applying for admission.

POSTDOCTORAL TRAINING   There appears to be a wide variety of post-doctoral training opportunities available to new graduates with health psychology training. Belar and Siegel (1983) reported the results of a survey of 43 postdoctoral programs that provided advanced training in health psychology. These training programs provided a total of 105 postdoctoral positions; the majority of the trainee salaries ranged between $13,000 and $18,000 per year.

Belar and Siegel's (1983) results indicated there was a great deal of variability in the major emphases of the training programs. In addition, most of the programs reported multiple-training emphases. Clinical application and applied research emphases were reported in 70% and 90% of the programs, respectively. Basic science research was identified as a program emphasis by 44%, public or community-health emphasis was reported by 32%, and a public-policy emphasis was reported by 12% of the programs.

The postdoctoral training programs also reported opportunities for experience in multiple content areas within both the clinical and basic sciences. Eighty-three percent of the programs offered experience in the assessment and treatment of health problems, 75% offered experience in the etiology of disease, 66% gave training in rehabilitation activities, and 56% provided opportunities in the prevention of illness or in health promotion. Furthermore, the majority of the programs gave the trainees access to child, adolescent, adult, and geriatric populations.

# Career Opportunities for New Health Psychologists

It has been documented that, since the founding of the APA in 1892, the four primary career functions of psychologists have been teaching, research, professional-service delivery, and administration (Matarazzo, 1983). There is also evidence that recent health psychology graduates have devoted their professional energies nearly evenly among these four functions. Belar and her colleagues (1982) reported some information concerning the employment sites and activities of recent graduates of the health psychology training programs that they surveyed. It was found that 41% of the graduates were employed in university medical centers, 25% in universities or colleges, 17% in clinical treatment settings, 7% in private practice, 4% in the federal government, 2% in industrial settings, and the remainder were in some combination thereof. With respect to employment activities, the average graduate devoted 33% effort to clinical work, 26% to teaching, 24% to research, and 17% to administrative duties, consultation, or other work (Belar et al., 1982).

Additional information regarding the work activities of health psychologists was reported in a survey of the members of the APA's Division of Health Psychology (Morrow, Carpenter, & Clayman, 1983). The principal work settings for these individuals were universities or colleges (28%), medical centers (25%), and private practice (20%). Their professional activities, expressed in median percent time of involvement, included therapy (25%), research (15%), administration (10%), teaching (9%), and assessment (9%).

There is some evidence, however, that professional-service delivery may become a predominant activity of future health psychologists. Grzesiak (1984) examined the contents of 330 advertisements for new health psychology positions that were placed in the classified section of the *APA Monitor* (a monthly news magazine) between July 1982 and June 1983. It was found that nearly 50% of the positions emphasized professional-service-delivery skills. The remaining positions were academic positions requiring research, teaching, and perhaps service-delivery or administrative skills. Only 26% of the academic positions primarily required research skills. Thus, the most recent data suggest that there may be greater employment opportunities for some time for those health psychology graduates who can provide professional services in addition to research, teaching, administrative expertise, and other skills. Indeed, Matarazzo (1983) has suggested that a shift is likely to occur from the university as the main employment setting for health psychologists to business and industry as well as to private practice, group, and hospital settings that must serve the needs of persons with medical problems. This anticipated shift is in accord with the predictions of Coates and Demuth that were described at the beginning of this chapter.

# Summary

The 1982 Arden House conference has established ideal standards for graduate and postgraduate education in health psychology. The conference established the doctorate in psychology as the entry-level degree for students who wish to become health psychologists. Doctoral programs must offer training in both general and health psychology; they must also provide training in professional activities for those students who wish to deliver clinical services. In addition, one-year predoctoral apprenticeships are required of all students and two-year, postdoctoral training fellowships are recommended before graduates seek employment.

Health psychology training is currently provided by a large number of educational institutions. Most programs offer training in various aspects of health psychology within specialty tracks such as clinical or social psychology. Relatively few universities at present grant PhDs in Health or Medical Psychology or offer doctoral training that is organized in accord with the Arden House model. Nevertheless, Arden House training programs should increase in number, especially if board certification in health psychology becomes established as a requirement for insurance payments for clinical services.

Recent health psychology graduates have devoted their professional efforts nearly evenly among teaching, research, clinical services, and administration. However, there appears to be a trend developing for new health psychologists to devote greater time to clinical services as more employment opportunities are created in health care settings, business, and industry.

# References

BELAR, C. D., & SIEGEL, L. J. (1983). A survey of postdoctoral training programs in health psychology. *Health Psychology, 2,* 413–425.

BELAR, C. D., WILSON, E., & HUGHES, H. (1982). Health psychology training in doctoral psychology programs. *Health Psychology, 1,* 289–299.

COATES, T. J., & DEMUTH, N. M. (1984). An analysis of competencies and training needs for psychologists specializing in health enhancement. In J. D. Matarazzo, S. M. Weiss, J. A. Herd, N. E. Miller, & S. M. Weiss (Eds.), *Behavioral health: A handbook of health enhancement and disease prevention* (pp. 1196–1203). New York: Wiley.

GENTRY, W. D., STREET, W. J., MASUR, F. T., & ASKEN, M. J. (1981). Training in medical psychology: A survey of graduate and internship training programs. *Professional Psychology, 12,* 224–228.

GRZESIAK, R. C. (1982). *Employment opportunities in health psychology: Three and a half years of "monitor" advertisements, 1983.* Report to the Education and Training Committee, Division 38, American Psychological Association, Washington, D. C.

ISTVAN, J., & HATTON, D. C. (1987). Curricula of graduate training programs in health psychology. In G. C. Stone, S. M. Weiss, J. D. Matarazzo, N. E. Miller, J. Rodin, C. D. Belar, M. J. Follick, & J. E. Singer (Eds.), *Health psychology: A discipline and profession.* Chicago: University of Chicago Press.

MATARAZZO, J. D. (1983). Education and training in health psychology: Boulder or bolder. *Health Psychology, 2,* 73–113.

MORROW, G. R., CARPENTER, P. J., & CLAYMAN, D. A. (1983). A national survey of health psychologists: Characteristics, training, and priorities. *Health Psychologist Newsletter, 5,* 6–7.

WEISS, S. M. (1983). Planning the conference. *Health Psychology 2* (Supplement 1), 19–25.

WORKING GROUP ON APPRENTICESHIP. (1983). Report. *Health Psychology, 2* (Supplement 1), 131–134.

WORKING GROUP ON POSTDOCTORAL RESEARCH TRAINING. (1983). Report. *Health Psychology, 2* (Supplement 1), 135–140.

WORKING GROUP ON POSTDOCTORAL TRAINING FOR THE HEALTH PSYCHOLOGY SERVICE PROVIDER. (1983). Report. *Health Psychology, 2* (Supplement 1), 141–145.

WORKING GROUP ON PREDOCTORAL EDUCATION/DOCTORAL TRAINING. (1983). Report. *Health Psychology, 2* (Supplement 1), 123–130.

# Name Index

# Subject Index